Donald School Textbook

CURRENT STATUS OF CLINICAL USE
OF *3D/4D* ULTRASOUND
IN OBSTETRICS AND GYNECOLOGY

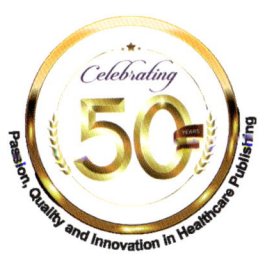

Donald School Textbook

CURRENT STATUS OF CLINICAL USE OF *3D/4D* ULTRASOUND IN OBSTETRICS AND GYNECOLOGY

Editors

Eberhard Merz MD PhD
Professor and Head
Center for Ultrasound and Prenatal Medicine
Frankfurt/Main, Germany
President, German Society for Ultrasound in Medicine (2006–2008)
President, Fetal Medicine Foundation (FMF) Germany
Vice President, International Academy of Perinatal Medicine
Director, Ian Donald Inter-University School of Medical Ultrasound
Frankfurt/Main, Germany

Asim Kurjak MD PhD
Professor
Department of Obstetrics and Gynecology
Medical School University of Zagreb and Sarajevo
Professor (Emeritus), University Sarajevo School of Science and Technology
President, International Academy of Perinatal Medicine
Founder and Director, Ian Donald Inter-University School of Medical Ultrasound
Zagreb, Croatia

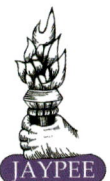

JAYPEE BROTHERS MEDICAL PUBLISHERS
The Health Sciences Publisher
New Delhi | London | Panama

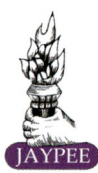 **Jaypee Brothers Medical Publishers (P) Ltd.**

Headquarters
Jaypee Brothers Medical Publishers (P) Ltd
4838/24, Ansari Road, Daryaganj
New Delhi 110 002, India
Phone: +91-11-43574357
Fax: +91-11-43574314
Email: jaypee@jaypeebrothers.com

Overseas Offices

J.P. Medical Ltd
83 Victoria Street, London
SW1H 0HW (UK)
Phone: +44 20 3170 8910
Fax: +44 (0)20 3008 6180
Email: info@jpmedpub.com

Jaypee-Highlights Medical Publishers Inc
City of Knowledge, Bld. 235, 2nd Floor
Clayton, Panama City, Panama
Phone: +1 507-301-0496
Fax: +1 507-301-0499
Email: cservice@jphmedical.com

Jaypee Brothers Medical Publishers (P) Ltd
Bhotahity, Kathmandu, Nepal
Phone: +977-9741283608
Email: kathmandu@jaypeebrothers.com

Website: www.jaypeebrothers.com
Website: www.jaypeedigital.com

© 2019, Jaypee Brothers Medical Publishers

Donald School Textbook: Current Status of Clinical Use of 3D/4D Ultrasound in Obstetrics and Gynecology

First Edition: **2019**

ISBN: 978-93-88958-82-0

Printed at: Samrat Offset Pvt. Ltd.

Dedicated to

Ian Donald and to our families.

Contributors

Juan Luis Alcázar MD PhD
Full Professor and Co-Chairman
Department of Obstetrics and
Gynecology
Clinica Universidad de Navarra
School of Medicine
Pamplona, Spain

Panagiotis (Panos) Antsaklis
MD PhD
Lecturer (Fetal and Maternal Medicine)
Alexandra Maternity Hospital
Medical School
University of Athens
Athens, Greece

Edward Araujo Júnior PhD
Associate Professor
Department of Obstetrics
Paulista School of Medicine
Federal University of São Paulo
(EPM-UNIFESP)
São Paulo-SP, Brazil

Guillermo Azumendi Pérez MD
Prenatal Ultrasound Unit
Centro Gutenberg
Málaga, Spain

Victoria Bitsadze MD
Professor
Department of Obstetrics and
Gynecology
The First IM Sechenov Moscow State
Medical University
Moscow, Russia

Francisco Jose Bonilla Bartret
MD PhD
Professor
Department of Obstetrics and
Gynecology
School of Medicine
Valencia, Spain

Fernando Bonilla-Musoles MD PhD
Professor
Department of Obstetrics and
Gynecology
School of Medicine
Valencia, Spain

Marisa Borenstein Guelman MD
Prenatal Ultrasound Unit
Centro Gutenberg
Málaga, Spain

Giuseppe Calì MD PhD
Head
Maternal Fetal Medicine Unit
Department of Obstetrics and
Gynecology
ARNAS Civico Di Cristina Benfratelli
Palermo, Italy

Sarah M Cohen MPH
Specialist
Department of Obstetrics and
Gynecology
Hadassah-Hebrew University Medical
Center
Mt Scopus
Jerusalem, Israel

Jing Deng MMed PhD
Medical Imaging Specialist
Barts Heart Centre and University
College London
London, UK

Hans Peter Dietz MD PhD
Professor (Obstetrics and Gynecology)
Department of Obstetrics, Gynecology
and Neonatology
Sydney Medical School Nepean
The University of Sydney
Kingswood, Australia

Sertaç Esin MD
Associate Professor
Baskent University
Perinatal Medicine Center
Ankara, Turkey

Francesco Forlani MD
Specialist
Department of Obstetrics and
Gynecology
ARNAS Civico Di Cristina Benfratelli
Palermo, Italy

Liat Gindes MD
Director of Ultrasound Unit
Department of Obstetrics and
Gynecology
Edith Wolfson Medical Center
Affiliated with the Sackler School of
Medicine
Tel Aviv University
Tel Aviv, Israel

Erich Hafner MD PhD
Professor
Donauspital am SMZ-Ost
Vienna, Austria

Uiko Hanaoka MD PhD
Lecturer
Department of Perinatology and
Gynecology
Kagawa University Graduate School
of Medicine
Kagawa, Japan

Toshiyuki Hata MD PhD
Professor and Chairman
Department of Perinatology and
Gynecology
Kagawa University Graduate School
of Medicine
Kagawa, Japan

Ulrich Honemeyer PhD MSc MBA
Associate Professor of Perinatology
Dubrovnik International University
Consultant Obstetrics and
Gynecology-Fetal Medicine
Alzahra Hospital NMC Sharjah
Sharjah, UAE

Katelyn T Horton BA
University of California
Berkeley, USA

Kenji Kanenishi MD PhD
Associate Professor
Department of Perinatology and
Gynecology
Kagawa University Graduate School
of Medicine
Kagawa, Japan

Ashok Khurana MD
Consultant in Reproductive
Ultrasound
The Ultrasound Lab
New Delhi, India

Sanja Kupesic Plavsic MD PhD
Professor
Department of Obstetrics and
Gynecology
Associate Dean
Office of Faculty Development
Paul L Foster School of Medicine
Texas Tech University Health Sciences
Center El Paso
El Paso, Texas, USA

Asim Kurjak MD PhD
Professor
Department of Obstetrics and
Gynecology
Medical School University of
Zagreb and Sarajevo
Professor (Emeritus)
University Sarajevo School of Science
and Technology
President
International Academy of Perinatal
Medicine
Founder and Director
Ian Donald Inter-University School of
Medical Ultrasound
Zagreb, Croatia

**Luciano Marcondes Machado
Nardozza** PhD
Associate Professor
Department of Obstetrics
Paulista School of Medicine
Federal University of São Paulo
(EPM-UNIFESP)
São Paulo-SP, Brazil

Alexander Makatsarya MD PhD
Professor of Obstetrics and
Gynecology
The First IM Sechenov Moscow State
Medical University
Department of Obstetrics and
Gynecology
Moscow, Russia

Eberhard Merz MD PhD
Professor and Head
Center for Ultrasound and Prenatal
Medicine, Frankfurt/Main, Germany
President, German Society for
Ultrasound in Medicine (2006–2008)
President, Fetal Medicine Foundation
(FMF) Germany
Vice President, International Academy
of Perinatal Medicine
Director, Ian Donald Inter-University
School of Medical Ultrasound
Frankfurt/Main, Germany

Baruch Messing MD
Head (Ultrasound Unit)
Department of Obstetrics and
Gynecology
Ma'ayane HaYeshua Medical Center
Bnei Brak, Israel
and
Department of Obstetrics and
Gynecology
Sheba Medical Center
Tel Hashomer, Israel

Gabriella Minneci MD
Specialist
Department of Obstetrics and
Gynecology
ARNAS Civico Di Cristina Benfratelli
Palermo, Italy

Danka Mlric Tesanic MD PhD
Specialist
Polyclinic GynaeArs
Private Practice of Obstetrics and
Gynecology, Zagreb, Croatia

Newton Osborne MD PhD
Professor
Department of Obstetrics and
Gynecology
Obadia Hospital
University of Panama
David, Panama

Sonal Panchal MD
Ultrasound Consultant
Dr Nagori's Institute for
Infertility and IVF
Ahmedabad, Gujarat, India

Sonila Pashaj MD PhD
Specialist
Center for Ultrasound and
Prenatal Medicine
Frankfurt/Main, Germany

Mishella I Perez BS RDMS RDCS
Specialist
Maternal Fetal Care and Genetics
Center
University of California
San Diego, USA
and
Department of Reproductive Medicine
University of California
San Diego, USA

Ritsuko Kimata Pooh MD PhD
President
Clinical Research Institute of Fetal
Medicine (CRIFM) PMC
Osaka, Japan

Dolores H Pretorius MD
Professor of Radiology
Maternal Fetal Care and Genetics
Center
University of California
San Diego, USA
and
Department of Radiology
University of California
San Diego, USA

Alessandro Quarto MD
Specialist
Università di Roma Tor Vergata
Division of Maternal Fetal Medicine
Ospedale Cristo Re
Roma, Italy

Francisco Raga MD PhD
Professor
Department of Obstetrics and
Gynecology
School of Medicine
Valencia, Spain

Giuseppe Rizzo MD
Professor of Obstetrics and
Gynecology
Università di Roma Tor Vergata
Division of Maternal Fetal Medicine
Ospedale Cristo Re
Roma, Italy
and
The First IM Sechenov Moscow State
Medical University
Department of Obstetrics and
Gynecology
Moscow, Russia

Liliam Cristine Rolo PhD
Adjunct Professor
Department of Obstetrics
Paulista School of Medicine
Federal University of São Paulo
(EPM-UNIFESP)
São Paulo-SP, Brazil

Leonid M Rovner
Medical Student
University of California
San Diego, USA

Aida Salihagić Kadić MD PhD
Professor
Department of Physiology
School of Medicine
University of Zagreb
Zagreb, Croatia

Cihat Şen MD
Professor
Memorial Hospital
Perinatal Medicine Center
Bahçelievler-Istanbul, Turkey

Israel Shapiro MD
Specialist
Department of Obstetrics and
Gynecology
Bnai-Zion Medical Center
Technion, Faculty of Medicine
Haifa, Israel

Lara Spalldi Barišić MD MA
PhD Candidate
Department of Obstetrics and
Gynecology
Private clinic Veritas
Zagreb, Croatia

Anja Šurina
Medical Student
Department of Physiology
School of Medicine
University of Zagreb
Zagreb, Croatia

Ebru Tarım MD
Professor in Perinatology
Ebru Tarim Clinic
Adana, Turkey

Sanja Tomasović MD PhD
Assistant Professor
Department of Neurology
University Hospital, Sveti Duh
Zagreb, Croatia
and
Medical Faculty
Josip Juraj Strossmayer University
of Osijek
Osijek, Croatia

Dan V Valsky MD
Specialist
Department of Obstetrics and
Gynecology
Hadassah-Hebrew University
Medical Center
Jerusalem, Israel

Oliver Vasilj MD PhD
Assistant
Department of Obstetrics and
Gynecology
University Hospital, Sveti Duh
Zagreb, Croatia

Eldar Volpert MD
Specialist
Department of Obstetrics and
Gynecology
Edith Wolfson Medical Center
Affiliated with the Sackler School
of Medicine, Tel Aviv University
Tel Aviv, Israel

Simcha Yagel MD
Professor and Head
Division of Obstetrics and Gynecology
Hadassah-Hebrew University Medical
Center
Jerusalem, Israel

Preface

Thirty years of 3D Ultrasound in Obstetrics and Gynecology represent an extraordinary success story in recent ultrasound history. However, as with many new technologies, the beginning was hampered by technical difficulties and doubts. Many ultrasound operators were initially skeptical regarding the clinical use of this new technique and viewed 3D ultrasound as a difficult, inconvenient, and even unnecessary method. A turnaround occurred with the First World Congress on 3D Ultrasound in Obstetrics and Gynecology in Mainz, Germany (September 5–6, 1997) and with the Second World Congress on 3D Ultrasound in Obstetrics and Gynecology in Las Vegas, USA (October 14–15, 1999). Since that time a tremendous progress could be observed in 3D/4D technology. 3D/4D ultrasound has profited greatly from the developments in computer technology and the construction of different 3D/4D transducers for automatic volume acquisition. The introduction of several display modes, a simplification of the operation process, faster rendering, continuous improvement of image quality, and the decrease in costs further contributed to the global spread of this technology.

In comparison with 2D ultrasound, 3D/4D sonography provides the operator with many advantages, such as the use of different visualization modes, precise control of a certain anatomical plane, digital long-term storage of the volumes without quality loss, and the possibility of performing virtual ultrasound examinations.

This book reflects the current state of 3D/4D Ultrasound in Obstetrics and Gynecology. The chapters in the book will provide you with an excellent overview of the possible applications of this technique.

Eberhard Merz
Asim Kurjak

Acknowledgments

The editors would like to thank all companies and engineers who contributed with their knowledge and skill to the developmental progress in 3D ultrasound during the past 30 years. The editors also want to thank all authors of this book for their excellent contributions. Recognition also applies to M/s Jaypee Brothers Medical Publishers (P) Ltd, New Delhi, India, for the perfect preparation work that allowed us to present this book at the Third World Congress for 3D Ultrasound in Dubrovnik, Croatia.

Contents

3D/4D Ultrasound for the Assessment of Ovarian Tumors

Juan Luis Alcázar

INTRODUCTION

Adnexal masses are a common clinical problem in gynecology. Most adnexal masses are benign, but few of them are malignant. An accurate diagnosis is essential for adequate management. Two-dimensional grayscale ultrasound (2D US) and color Doppler US have been proven as the best imaging technique for discriminating between benign and malignant adnexal masses.[1] However, there is still a group of masses difficult to classify.[2]

Three-dimensional US (3D US) has become a routine practice in many gynecologic US laboratories.[3] This technique overcomes some of the limitations of 2D US. This technique allows a surface rendering of the internal aspect of the cyst's wall. It can also present the masses in new different ways such as the so-called "inversion mode" or "silhouette mode" or it can represent the vascular tree of the tumor using a 3D reconstruction, or even allow a unique way for estimating the amount of vessels within the tumor or a part of the tumor.[4]

In this chapter, we shall review the role of 3D US in the evaluation of adnexal masses.

THREE-DIMENSIONAL GRAYSCALE ULTRASOUND

Grayscale 3D US aims to depict the macroscopic features of a given adnexal mass by using different ways of renderization.

Using surface rendering, Bonilla–Musoles et al. reported that 3D US was able to show papillary projections in the inner surface of the mass that were missed at 2D US in 7% of the cases. They found that sensitivity of 3D US was higher than that for 2D US (100% and 80%, respectively) and specificity was similar for both techniques (100% and 99%, respectively).[5] However, Hata el al. using a similar approach, found that 3D US showed higher specificity than 2D US (92.3% and 38.4%, respectively) with identical sensitivity (100%).[6]

Alcázar et al. reported findings in a series of 41 women with complex adnexal masses detected on 2D US who underwent 3D US for further assessment.[7] In this study, 3D US showed better sensitivity (100% versus 90%) and specificity (78% versus 61%) than 2D US for predicting ovarian malignancy but these differences were not statistically significant. However, 3D US reinforced examiner's diagnostic impression **(Figs. 1.1 to 1.4)**. Laban et al. also observed that 3D US was more sensitive (90% *versus* 81%) and specific (84% *versus* 79%) than 2D US.[8]

The main shortcomings of all these studies are that series are small and the prevalence of malignancy is high.

Several studies have assessed the reproducibility of 3D US when performed by different observers. All of them have found that this technique is reproducible among different observers.[9-11]

After reviewing these studies, it could be concluded that 3D US seems to have better diagnostic performance that 2D US for predicting malignancy in adnexal masses, but further better designed studies are needed to draw definitive conclusions.

There are some reports that have assessed the role of other rendering modes. Timor-Tirtsch et al. showed that the use of inverted mode could be useful for diagnosing hydrosalpinx[12] **(Figs. 1.5A and B)**. Alcázar et al. showed that the objective analysis of cyst content by calculating the so-called *mean gray value* could improve the performance of 2D US for the diagnosis of ovarian endometrioma.[13]

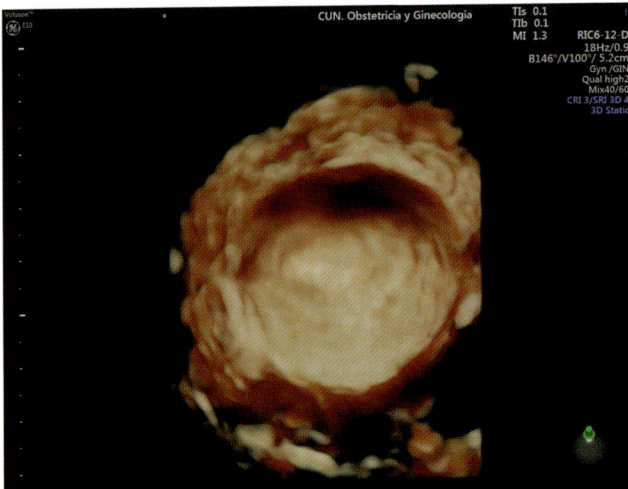

Fig. 1.1: Three-dimensional surface rendering of an ovarian simple cyst. A smooth internal wall is clearly observed. Histology revealed a serous cystadenoma.

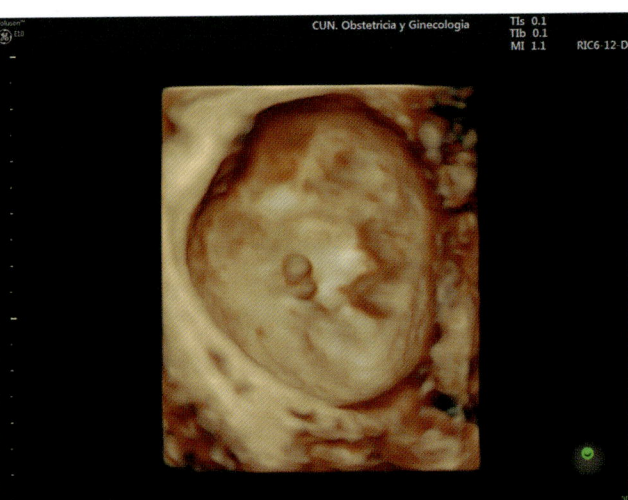

Fig. 1.2: Three-dimensional surface rendering of an ovarian cyst. In this case, a papillary projection arising from the internal wall is observed. Histology revealed a serous cystadenofibroma.

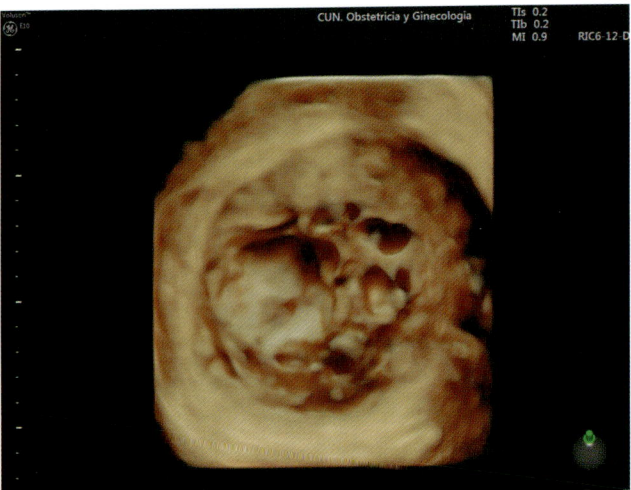

Fig. 1.3: Three-dimensional surface rendering of a multilocular ovarian cyst. Different locules are seen. Histology revealed a mucinous cystadenoma.

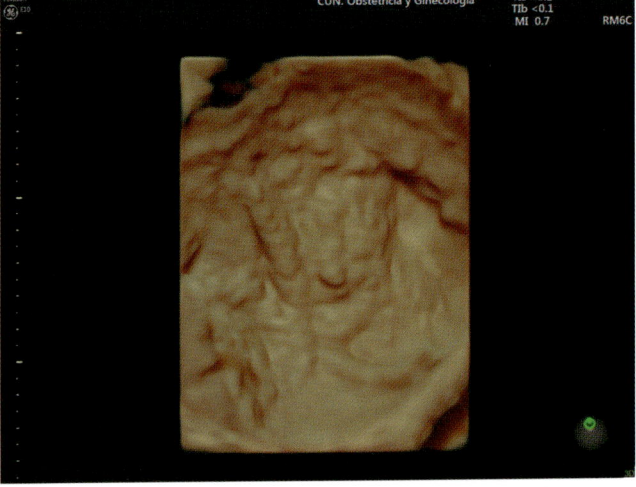

Fig. 1.4: Three dimensional surface rendering of a unilocular ovarian cyst showing an irregular internal surface. Histology revealed a serous borderline cystadenoma.

THREE-DIMENSIONAL POWER DOPPLER ULTRASOUND

Since the pioneering from Kurjak et al.[14] applying three-dimensional power Doppler ultrasound (3D PDU) for the differential diagnosis of ovarian tumors, there are many reports using this technique for this purpose.

By using 3D power Doppler angiography (3D PDA), it is possible to depict the vessels tree of ovarian tumors. The examiner can analyze the reconstructed vascular tree[14]

(**Figs. 1.6 and 1.7**). On the other hand, using dedicated software 3D PDU indexes can be calculated from the tissue or organ using the manual mode (**Figs. 1.8A and B**) or the spherical mode (**Figs. 1.9A and B**).

Cohen et al. evaluated 71 complex adnexal masses using this technique. They observed that the addition of 3D PDU improved the specificity of 2D US (75% versus 54%), with an identical sensitivity (100%) for both techniques.[15] However, 2D conventional color Doppler or 2D power Doppler was not used.

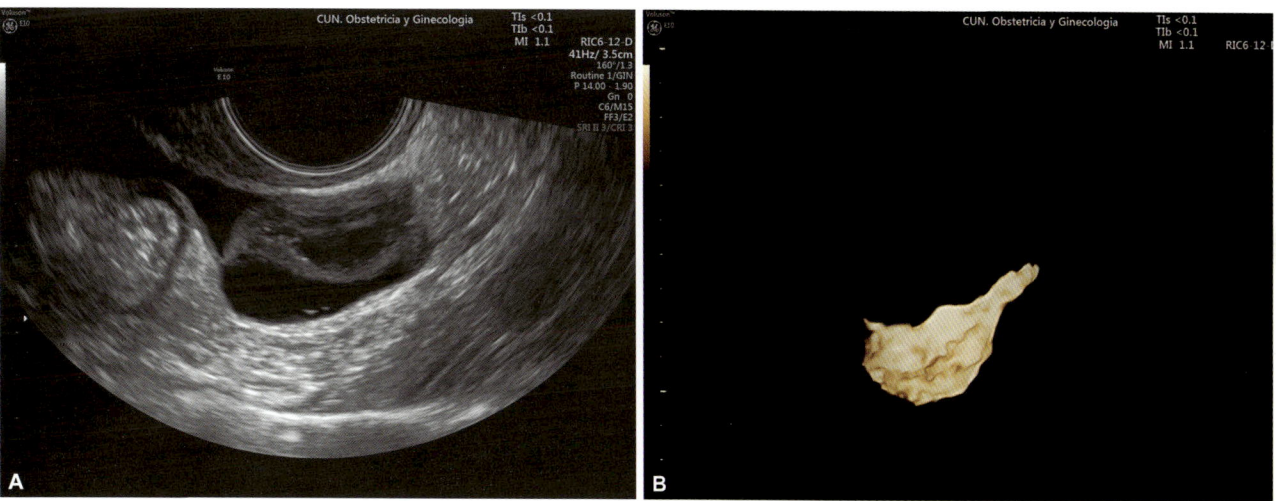

Figs. 1.5A and B: (A) Transvaginal ultrasound of a hydrosalpinx. (B) The same lesion as observed using the "inversion mode" on Three-dimensional ultrasound.

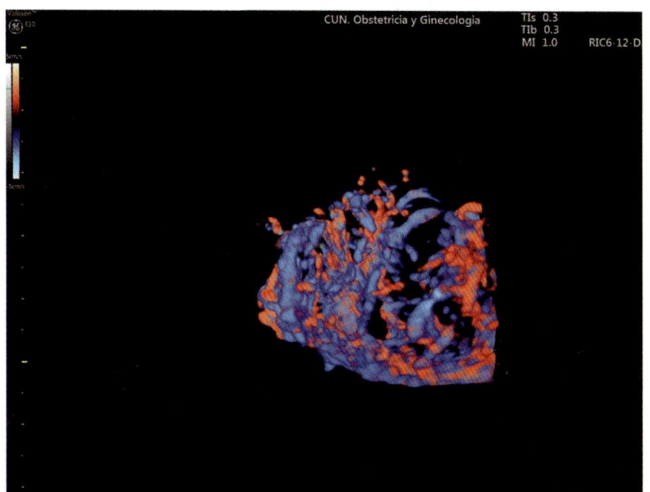

Fig. 1.6: Three-dimensional reconstruction of the vessel tree from an ovarian cancer. The chaotic distribution of vessels is shown.

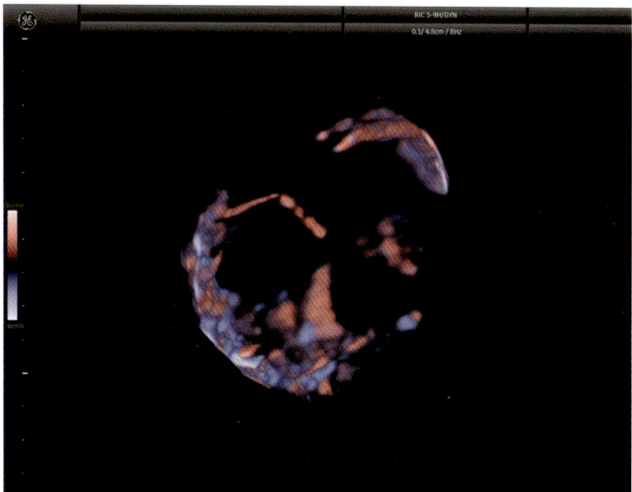

Fig. 1.7: Three-dimensional reconstruction of the vessel tree from an ovarian benign tumor. In this case, there is no chaotic distribution in the vessels network.

Alcazar et al. compared 2D power Doppler and 3D power Doppler and did not find differences between both techniques in terms of diagnostic performance.[16]

The first to use 3D PDA for distinguishing benign from malignant ovarian tumors using tumoral vascular tree architecture were Kurjak et al. They used a scoring system that included 3D US tumor vascular tree features and 2D US morphological features. The criteria for 3D PDA malignancy were the presence of chaotic vessel arrangement and complex branching pattern. In two different series, they found that this 3D PDU or 2D US-based scoring system showed better performance than 2D US alone.[14,17]

Chase et al. analyzed vascular architecture by 3D PDU in a series of 66 women diagnosed as having an adnexal mass. Their criterion for malignancy suspicion was the presence of chaotic vessel pattern. They also concluded that 3D US assessment of the vascular tree was useful for distinguishing benign and malignant ovarian masses.[18] Mansour et al. evaluated 400 patients with adnexal masses by 3D PDU. The pattern of vascularity of masses was interpreted as avascular, parallel, or chaotic, being

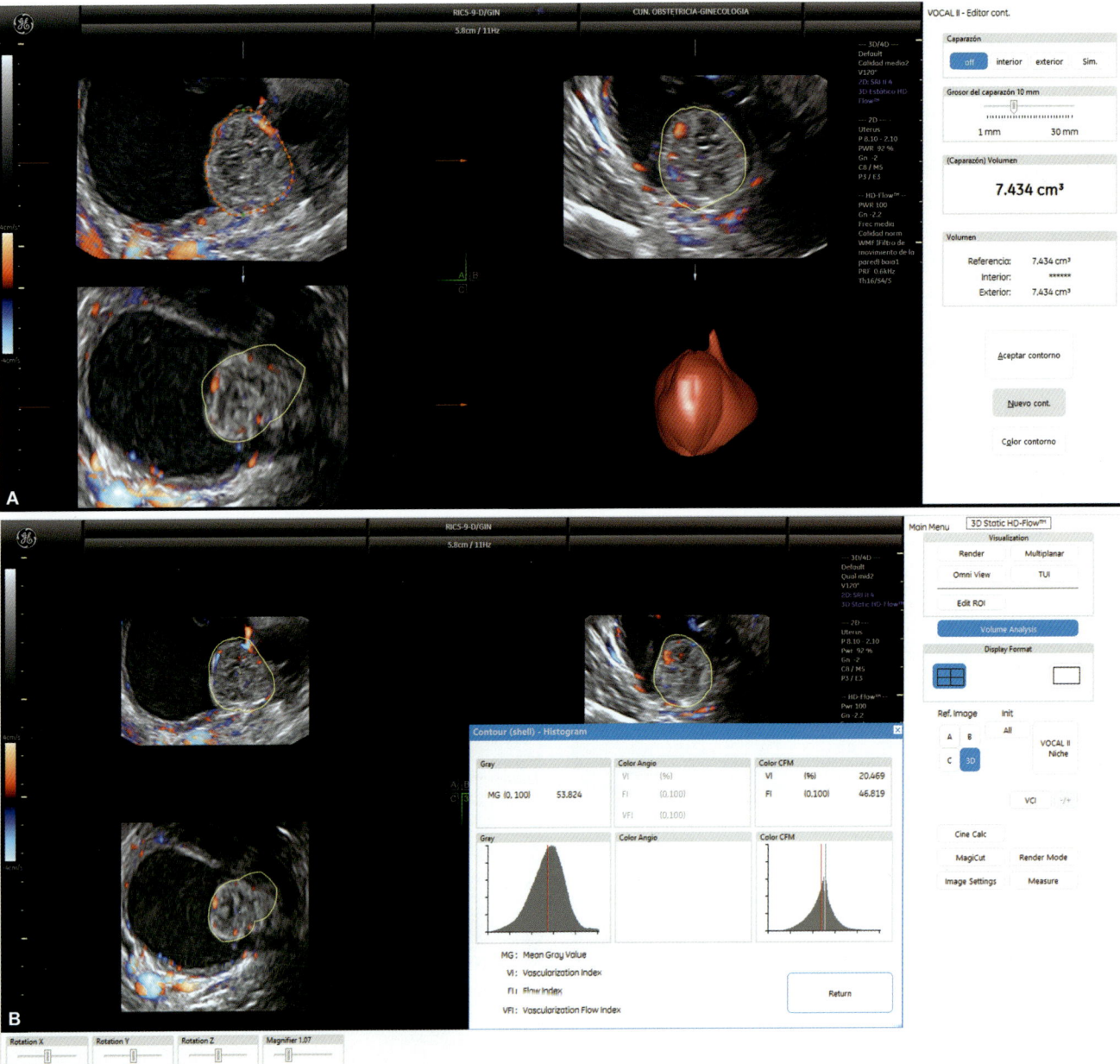

Figs. 1.8A and B: Three-dimensional vascular sampling from an ovarian tumor using the manual mode. (A) The solid is outlined and its volume calculated. (B) The three-dimensional vascular indices within this volume are calculated.

chaotic pattern suggestive of malignancy. They found that adding 3D PDU information to the risk of malignancy index (RMI) improved the diagnostic performance of this index.[19]

Kalmantis et al. found that sensitivity and specificity of 2D US increased when added 3D PDA.[20] However, Laban et al. used the criteria proposed by Kurjak in a series on 50 selected women with complex adnexal masses.[8] They reported that 3D PDU was not superior to 2D power Doppler. After this report, other studies from Sladkevicius

et al.[21] Alcázar et al.[22] and Dai et al.[23] reported similar findings.

More recently, there are some case reports showing that the 3D-PDU silhouette mode might be useful.[24] However, data are still too scanty to draw any conclusion.

It can be concluded that albeit potentially interesting, the assessment of the tumoral vascular network by 3D PDA has yielded conflicting results and its use is controversial.

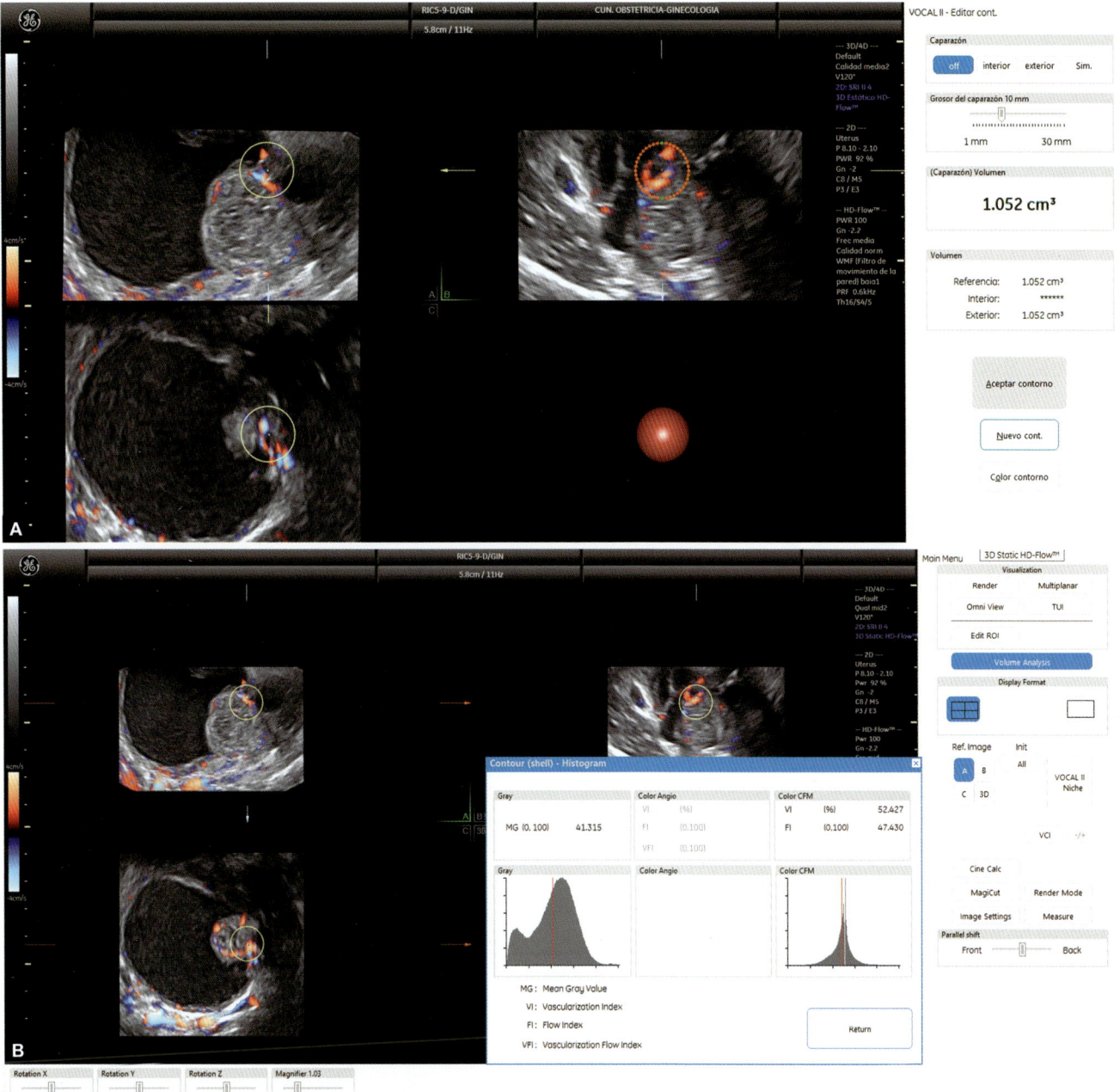

Figs. 1.9A and B: (A) Three-dimensional vascular sampling from the same ovarian tumor as in Figure 1.8, but using the spherical mode (volume—1.052 cc) from the most vascularized area. (B) The three-dimensional vascular indices within this sphere are calculated. Note that values are higher than those in Figure 1.8.

Alcázar et al. were the first to suggest the assessment of objective quantification of tumor vascularization by using the so-called 3D-PDU vascular indexes [namely vascularization index (VI), flow index (FI), and vascularization flow index (VFI)] within the most suspicious vascularized area from the tumor. In a selected series of 69 solid and cystic-solid masses with vascularization within the solid component, using manual sampling, they reported that all 3D-PDU vascular indexes were significantly higher in ovarian cancer as compared with benign tumors.[25] Geomini et al. evaluated 181 women with adnexal masses. This group included any kind of mass diagnosed at transvaginal US and performed the vascular assessment from the whole tumor. They found that FI, but not VI nor VFI, was significantly higher in ovarian cancer.[26]

Jokubkiene et al. proposed a different approach based on the use of a virtual 5-cc spherical sampling from the most vascularized area from the tumor.[27] They found that 3D PDU vascular indices from the spherical sample were higher in ovarian cancers as compared with benign tumors. However, they concluded that this information added no value to that obtained with grayscale assessment by an expert sonologist. Later on, Kudla et al. suggested the use of 1-cc spherical sampling instead of 5-cc.[28] They also reported that 3D PDU indices were significantly higher in ovarian cancer.

Abbas et al. compared the assessment of tumoral vascular network and 3D PDA-derived indices. Although 3D PDU-derived indices were higher in ovarian cancer, they concluded that vascular network assessment was better than 3D PDU-derived indices.[29]

Notwithstanding, three studies have been reported showing no differences in 3D PD indices between benign and malignant ovarian tumors.[30-32]

Regarding the reproducibility of this method, Alcazar et al. showed that both manual and spherical sampling assessment is reproducible between observers.[33-35]

From the clinical point of view, some studies have shown that the use of 3D PDU vascular indices could help for improving specificity of morphological grayscale and 2D power Doppler ultrasound (2D PDU) in selected ovarian tumors, which are difficult to classify using the latter technique. Alcázar and Rodriguez assessed 143 adnexal masses with vascularized solid components using manual sampling method. Using a cut-off VI more than or equal to 1.556% for classifying tumors as malignant, these authors reported that specificity improved a 33% retaining similar sensitivity.[36]

Kudla and Alcázar reported on a series of 138 women classified as malignant using 2D US and 2D power Doppler. They used 1-cc spherical sampling instead of manual sampling. Using a cut-off of VI more than or equal to 24.015%, 20 out of 26 benign tumors in this series were correctly classified as benign (specificity—77%), while 91% of malignant tumors were correctly classified as malignant.[37]

Vrachnis et al. also found that the use of 3D PDA could add valuable information to conventional 2D US.[38] However, as in other papers, the series is too small.

However, a prospective study reported by Utrilla–Layna et al. using the same method and cut-off for VI as proposed by Kudla and Alcazar, found that 3D PDU used as a third-step in the differential diagnosis of ovarian tumors did not improve the diagnostic accuracy of conventional 2D PDU. However, a suspicious VI (>24.015%) increases significantly the probability of malignancy.[39] Silvestre et al. also reported that 3D PDU indices have low accuracy for discriminating between benign and malignant tumors classified as inconclusive when using International Ovarian Tumor Analysis (IOTA) simple rules.[40]

Some studies have used contrast-enhanced 3D PDU. Huchon et al. reported that using contrast agent improved the visualization of vascular network and 3D PDA derived indexes were higher in malignant as compared with benign tumors. They concluded that 3D PDU could be useful in those cases where 2D US diagnosis is uncertain.[41] Zhang et al. also reported that contrast-enhanced 3D PDA could add valuable information in uncertain masses after 2D US.[42] Hu et al. reached similar conclusion in their study focused on small ovarian masses, reaching 100% accuracy.[43]

However, it should be borne in mind that the actual significance of these indices is not fully understood, there are some important technical limitations for this technique and standardization are lacking and its potential use in clinical practice is debated.[44-47]

FOUR-DIMENSIONAL POWER DOPPLER ULTRASOUND

Because of the problems mentioned above for 3D PDU, some authors have proposed the use of the spatiotemporal image correlation (STIC) technique, the so-called four-dimensional (4D) angiography.[48] This technique allows a detailed estimation of blood flow changes in the tissue under investigation within one cardiac cycle **(Figs. 1.10A and B)**. Using this technology, a new volumetric vascular index has been developed, the so-called volumetric pulsatility index (vPI).[49,50] This index should be low when blood flow increases in a given organ. In fact, Kudla and Alcazar demonstrated this in ovaries of women with polycystic ovarian syndrome.[51]

Alcázar et al. has reported a prospective study using a similar design than Utrilla–Layna et al. They found that vPI was significantly lower in malignant tumors as compared with benign ones. However, the addition of 4D

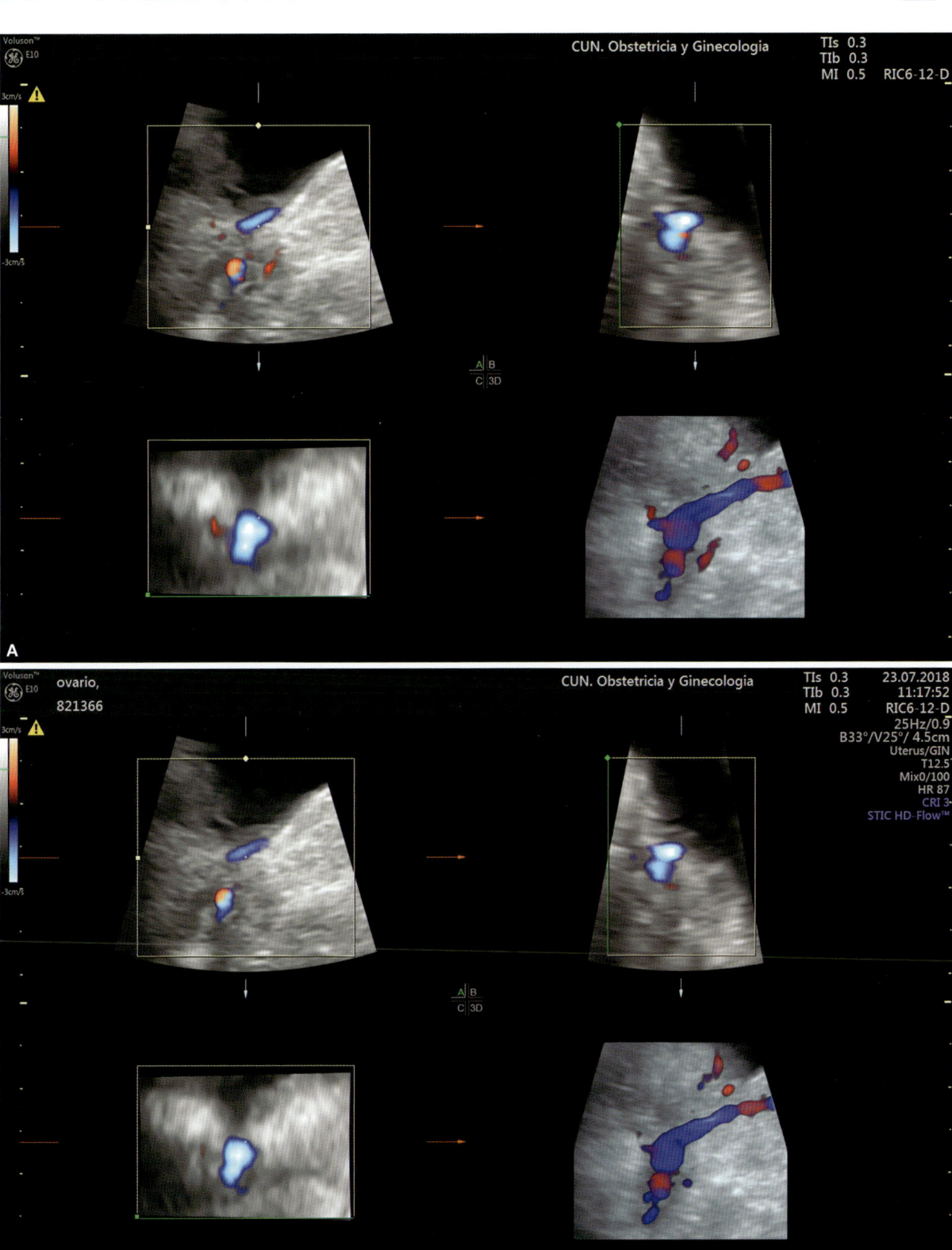

Figs. 1.10A and B: Four dimensional-spatiotemporal image correlation from the same area of an ovarian tumor. Vascular mapping changes from (A) systole to (B) diastole.

angiography did not improve the overall diagnostic performance.[52] This could be explained by the fact that the number of cases in which 4D angiography was used was small.

In conclusion, the use of 3D PDU and 4D angiography should be restricted to the research field and it should not be used in the clinical setting.

REFERENCES

1. American College of Obstetricians and Gynecologists' Committee on Practice Bulletins—Gynecology. Practice Bulletin No. 174: Evaluation and Management of Adnexal Masses. Obstet Gynecol. 2016;128:e210-26.
2. Valentin L, Ameye L, Jurkovic D, et al. Which extrauterine pelvic masses are difficult to correctly classify as benign or malignant on the basis of ultrasound findings and is there a way of making a correct diagnosis? Ultrasound Obstet Gynecol. 2006;27:438-44.
3. Alcázar JL. Three-dimensional ultrasound in Gynecology: Current status and future perspectives. Curr Women's Health Rev. 2005;1:1-14.
4. Alcázar JL. Three-dimensional ultrasound in gynecological practice. Report Med Imag. 2012;5:1-13.
5. Bonilla-Musoles F, Raga F, Osborne NG. Three-dimensional ultrasound evaluation of ovarian masses. Gynecol Oncol. 1995;59:129-35.
6. Hata T, Yanagihara T, Hayashi K, et al. Three-dimensional ultrasonographic evaluation of ovarian tumours: a preliminary study. Hum Reprod. 1999;14:858-61.
7. Alcázar JL, Galán MJ, García-Manero M, et al. Three-dimensional ultrasound morphologic assessment in complex adnexal masses a preliminary experience. J Ultrasound Med. 2003;22:249-54.
8. Laban M, Metawee H, Elyan A, et al. Three-dimensional ultrasound and three-dimensional power Doppler in the assessment of ovarian tumors. Int J Gynaecol Obstet. 2007;99:201-5.
9. Alcázar JL, García-Manero M, Galván R. Three-dimensional sonographic morphologic assessment of adnexal masses: a reproducibility study. J Ultrasound Med. 2007;26:1007-11.
10. Pascual MA, Graupera B, Hereter L, et al. Intra- and interobserver variability of 2D and 3D transvaginal sonography in the diagnosis of benign versus malignant adnexal masses. J Clin Ultrasound. 2011;39:316-21.
11. Sladkevicius P, Valentin L. Intra- and inter-observer agreement when describing adnexal masses using the International Ovarian Tumour Analysis terms and definitions: a study on three-dimensional ultrasound volumes. Ultrasound Obstet Gynecol. 2013;41:318-27.
12. Timor-Tritsch IE, Monteagudo A, Tsymbal T. Three-dimensional ultrasound inversion rendering technique facilitates the diagnosis of hydrosalpinx. J Clin Ultrasound. 2010;38:372-6.
13. Alcázar JL, León M, Galván R, et al. Assessment of cyst content using mean gray value for discriminating endometrioma from other unilocular cysts in premenopausal women. Ultrasound Obstet Gynecol. 2010;35:228-32.
14. Kurjak A, Kupesic S, Anic T, et al. Three-dimensional ultrasound and power Doppler improve the diagnosis of ovarian lesions. Gynecol Oncol. 2000;76:28-32.
15. Cohen LS, Escobar PF, Scharm C, et al. Three-dimensional ultrasound power Doppler improves the diagnostic accuracy for ovarian cancer prediction. Gynecol Oncol. 2001;82:40-8.
16. Alcázar JL, Castillo G. Comparison of 2-dimensional and 3- dimensional power-Doppler imaging in complex adnexal masses for the prediction of ovarian cancer. Am J Obstet Gynecol. 2005;192:807-12.
17. Kurjak A, Kupesic S, Sparac V, et al. Preoperative evaluation of pelvic tumors by Doppler and three-dimensional sonography. J Ultrasound Med. 2001;20:829-40.
18. Chase DM, Crade M, Basu T, et al. Preoperative diagnosis of ovarian malignancy: preliminary results of the use of 3-dimensional vascular ultrasound. Int J Gynecol Cancer. 2009;19:354-60.
19. Mansour GM, El-Lamie IK, El-Sayed HM, et al. Adnexal mass vascularity assessed by 3-dimensional power Doppler: does it add to the risk of malignancy index in prediction of ovarian malignancy? four-hundred case studies. Int J Gynecol Cancer. 2009;19:867-72.
20. Kalmantis K, Rodolakis A, Daskalakis G, et al. Characterization of ovarian tumors and staging ovarian cancer with 3-dimensional power Doppler angiography: correlation with pathologic findings. Int J Gynecol Cancer. 2013;23:469-74.
21. Sladkevicius P, Jokubkiene L, Valentin L. Contribution of morphological assessment of the vessel tree by three-dimensional ultrasound to a correct diagnosis of malignancy in ovarian masses. Ultrasound Obstet Gynecol. 2007;30:874-82.
22. Alcázar JL, Cabrera C, Galván R, et al. Three-dimensional power Doppler vascular network assessment of adnexal masses: intraobserver and interobserver agreement analysis. J Ultrasound Med. 2008;27:997-1001.
23. Dai SY, Hata K, Inubashiri E, et al. Does three-dimensional power Doppler ultrasound improve the diagnostic accuracy for the prediction of adnexal malignancy? J Obstet Gynaecol Res. 2008;34:364-70.
24. Sajapala S, AboEllail MA, Tanaka T, et al. Three-dimensional power Doppler with silhouette mode for diagnosis of malignant ovarian tumors. Ultrasound Obstet Gynecol. 2016;48:806-8.
25. Alcázar JL, Merce LT, Garcia Manero M. Three-dimensional power Doppler vascular sampling: a new method for predicting ovarian cancer in vascularized complex adnexal masses. J Ultrasound Med. 2005;24:689-96.
26. Geomini PM, Kluivers KB, Moret E, et al. Evaluation of adnexal masses with three-dimensional ultrasonography. Obstet Gynecol. 2006;108: 1167-75.

27. Jokubkiene L, Sladkevicius P, Valentin L. Does three-dimensional power Doppler ultrasound help in discrimination between benign and malignant ovarian masses? Ultrasound Obstet Gynecol. 2007;29:215-25.

28. Kudla MJ, Timor-Tritsch IE, Hope JM, et al. Spherical tissue sampling in 3-dimensional power Doppler angiography: a new approach for evaluation of ovarian tumors. J Ultrasound Med. 2008;27:425-33.

29. Abbas AM, Zahran KM, Nasr A, et al. Three-dimensional power doppler evaluation of adnexal masses. Which Parameter Performs Best? Thai J Obstet Gynecol. 2014;22:102-7.

30. Ohel I, Sheiner E, Aricha-Tamir B, et al. Three-dimensional power Doppler ultrasound in ovarian cancer and its correlation with histology. Arch Gynecol Obstet. 2010;281: 919-25.

31. Perez-Medina T, Orensanz I, Pereira A, et al. Three-dimensional angioultrasonography for the prediction of malignancy in ovarian masses. Gynecol Obstet Invest. 2013;75:120-5.

32. Niemi RJ, Saarelainen SK, Luukkaala TH, et al. Reliability of preoperative evaluation of postmenopausal ovarian tumors. J Ovarian Res. 2017;10:15.

33. Alcázar JL, Rodriguez D, Royo P, et al. Intraobserver and interobserver reproducibility of 3-dimensional power Doppler vascular indices in assessment of solid and cystic-solid adnexal masses. J Ultrasound Med. 2008;27:1-6.

34. Alcázar JL, Prka M. Evaluation of two different methods for vascular sampling by three-dimensional power Doppler angiography in solid and cystic-solid adnexal masses. Ultrasound Obstet Gynecol. 2009;33:349-54.

35. Kudla M, Alcázar JL. Does the size of three-dimensional power Doppler spherical sampling affect the interobserver reproducibility of measurements of vascular indices in adnexal masses? Ultrasound Obstet Gynecol. 2009;34: 732-4.

36. Alcázar JL, Rodriguez D. Three-dimensional power Doppler vascular sonographic sampling for predicting ovarian cancer in cystic-solid and solid vascularized masses. J Ultrasound Med. 2009;28:275-81.

37. Kudla MJ, Alcázar JL. Does sphere volume affect the performance of three-dimensional power Doppler virtual vascular sampling for predicting malignancy in vascularized solid or cystic-solid adnexal masses? Ultrasound Obstet Gynecol. 2010;35:602-8.

38. Vrachnis N, Sifakis S, Samoli E, et al. Three-dimensional ultrasound and three-dimensional power Doppler improve the preoperative evaluation of complex benign ovarian lesions. Clin Exp Obstet Gynecol. 2012;39:474-8.

39. Utrilla-Layna J, Alcázar JL, Aubá M, et al. Performance of three-dimensional power Doppler angiography as third-step assessment in differential diagnosis of adnexal masses. Ultrasound Obstet Gynecol. 2015;45:613-7.

40. Silvestre L, Martins WP, Candido-Dos-Reis FJ. Limitations of three-dimensional power Doppler angiography in preoperative evaluation of ovarian tumors. J Ovarian Res. 2015;8:47.

41. Huchon C, Metzger U, Bats AS, et al. Value of three-dimensional contrast-enhanced power Doppler ultrasound for characterizing adnexal masses. J Obstet Gynaecol Res. 2012;38:832-40.

42. Zhang X, Mao Y, Zheng R, et al. The contribution of qualitative CEUS to the determination of malignancy in adnexal masses, indeterminate on conventional US—a multicenter study. PLoS One. 2014;9:e93843.

43. Hu R, Xiang H, Mu Y, et al. Combination of 2- and 3-dimensional contrast-enhanced transvaginal sonography for diagnosis of small adnexal masses. J Ultrasound Med. 2014;33:1889-99.

44. Alcázar JL Three-dimensional power Doppler derived vascular indices: what are we measuring and how are we doing it? Ultrasound Obstet Gynecol. 2008;32:485-7.

45. Raine-Fenning NJ, Nordin NM, Ramnarine KV, et al. Evaluation of the effect of machine settings on quantitative three-dimensional power Doppler angiography: an in-vitro flow phantom experiment. Ultrasound Obstet Gynecol. 2008;32:551-9.

46. Raine-Fenning NJ, Nordin NM, Ramnarine KV, et al. Determining the relationship between three-dimensional power Doppler data and true blood flow characteristics: an in-vitro flow phantom experiment. Ultrasound Obstet Gynecol. 2008;32:540-50.

47. Martins WP. Three-dimensional power Doppler: validity and reliability. Ultrasound Obstet Gynecol. 2010;36: 530-3.

48. Kudla MJ, Alcázar JL. Spatiotemporal image correlation using high-definition flow: a new method for assessing ovarian vascularization. J Ultrasound Med. 2010;29: 1469-74.

49. Martins WP, Welsh AW, Lima JC, et al. The "volumetric" pulsatility index as evaluated by spatiotemporal imaging correlation (STIC): a preliminary description of a novel technique, its application to the endometrium and an evaluation of its reproducibility. Ultrasound Med Biol. 2011;37:2160-8.

50. Kudla MJ, Alcázar JL. Spatiotemporal image correlation with spherical sampling and high-definition flow: new 4-dimensional method for assessment of tissue vascularization changes during the cardiac cycle: reproducibility analysis. J Ultrasound Med. 2012;31:73-80.

51. Alcázar JL, Kudla MJ. Ovarian stromal vessels assessed by spatiotemporal image correlation-high definition flow in women with polycystic ovary syndrome: a case-control study. Ultrasound Obstet Gynecol. 2012;40:470-5.

52. Alcázar JL, Auba M, Ruiz-Zambrana A, et al. Evaluation of the 4D "Spatiotemporal Image Correlation" technology with high-definition color Doppler as third step for preoperative differential diagnosis of ovarian tumors. A prospective study. Donald School J Ultrasound Obstet Gynecol. 2018;12:1-8.

Fetal Organ Volume Measurements

Edward Araujo Júnior, Liliam Cristine Rolo, Luciano Marcondes Machado Nardozza

INTRODUCTION

The initial studies on the volumetric analysis of fetal organs dates back to the mid-1980s and involve the use of two-dimensional (2D) ultrasound, then in which fetal organs presented a regular ellipsoid geometric shape (length × width × height × 0.52).[1] In the early 1990s, with the advent of three-dimensional (3D) ultrasound, the volumetric analysis of fetal organs became more accurate because this technique allowed delineating the irregular external surface of organs, in contrast with 2D ultrasound, which rendered them as regular geometric structures.[2] The study by Riccabona et al.[3] was the first to compare 2D and 3D ultrasound volumes with actual volumes. These authors observed that for objects with irregular shapes, the percentage error was significantly lower in 3D ultrasound than in 2D ultrasound, whereas for regular objects, there was no significant difference between these two methods.

The first studies on the volumetric analysis of fetal organs date back to the beginning of the 1990s. Reference curves were constructed for different organs, including the cerebellum, lung, liver, and adrenal glands, using the multiplanar method or planimetry.[4-7]

In the early 2000s, a new volume calculation method designated virtual organ computer-aided analysis (VOCAL) was developed, and reference curves were created for the lungs, heart, cerebellum, kidneys, and spleen.[8-11] VOCAL was used in several clinical applications, including volumetric analysis of the lungs to predict pulmonary hypoplasia in fetuses with congenital diaphragmatic hernia (CDH),[12,13] fetal adrenal glands to predict preterm labor,[14] and fetal bladder in pregnant women with diabetes mellitus.[15] In addition, VOCAL combined with spatiotemporal image correlation (STIC)

allowed assessing fetal heart function.[16,17] VOCAL showed almost perfect intra- and interobserver agreement on the volume of fetal brain structures.[18]

Another volume calculation method developed in the mid-2000s was the eXtended Imaging VOCAL (XI VOCAL). This method was applied in the volumetric analysis of structures, including the embryo, yolk sac, and gestational sac, in the first trimester of pregnancy.[19-21] An in vitro study comparing the multiplanar method, VOCAL, and IX VOCAL with actual sizes indicated that IX VOCAL was superior to the others in assessing the size of structures with irregular shapes.[22] Reference curves were prepared for the fetal heart,[23] lateral ventricles of fetuses with malformations of the central nervous system,[24] cranial structures in fetal growth restriction (FGR),[25] and healthy and hydronephrotic kidneys.[26]

Another commercially available volume calculation method is sonography-based automated volume count (SonoAVC). The main applications include identifying and counting the number of follicles in controlled ovarian stimulation for human reproduction techniques,[27,28] but this method has also been used to evaluate the volume of fetal organs, including cardiac cavities[29] and renal pelvis.[30,31]

Another important application of the volumetric analysis of fetal organs is predicting birth weight and intrauterine nutritional status. Studies have shown that 3D ultrasound is more accurate than 2D ultrasound in predicting birth weight[32,33] and monitoring the nutritional status of fetuses at risk of growth disorders.[34,35]

The objective of this chapter is to describe the main techniques of volumetric analysis of fetal organs using 3D ultrasound and its potential clinical applications.

METHODS USED FOR VOLUMETRIC ANALYSIS OF FETAL ORGANS USING 3D ULTRASOUND

Multiplanar Method

This method consists of measuring the size of fetal organs in three orthogonal planes (axial, transverse, and coronal). It includes defining a plane on which the outer surface of the organ is delineated to determine an area; at the same time in another plane, a cursor moves along an axis to define new planes to be marked. The distance of the displacement of the cursor is measured by the operator and usually ranges from 0.5 mm to 3.0 mm; depending on the size of the fetal organ. At the end of the cursor movement on the analyzed structure, the device sums the delimited areas automatically and provides its size **(Figs. 2.1A and B)**.

Virtual Organ Computer-aided Analysis

This method allows the fetal organ to be analyzed to be rotated on an axis, and the consecutive planes that determine organ measurement are gradually shown on the screen of the equipment. The organ ends are demarcated using measurement calibrators, and the external surface of the structure is delimited either manually or in

sphere mode. The angle of rotation can be 6°, 9°, 15°, or 30° with the delimitation of 30 planes at 6° and of six adjacent and sequential planes at 30°. The device calculates an area in each delimited plane and at the end of the rotation, the software automatically calculates the volume and makes a 3D reconstruction of the organ **(Figs. 2.2A and B)**.

eXtended Imaging Virtual Organ Computer-aided Analysis

This technique consists of delimiting areas in adjacent sequential planes arranged on the apparatus screen. The examiner defines the first and last planes and the number of intermediate planes between these limits (5, 10, 15, or 20). Each plane boundary determines an area; after scanning all planes, the equipment automatically provides the organ volume, the reconstructed 3D image, the distance between the intermediate planes, and the distance between the first and last planes **(Figs. 2.3A and B)**.

Sonography-based Automated Volume Count

This volumetric analysis method can be used in the following two modes—(1) SonoAVC follicle and (2) SonoAVC general. The former is used to determine follicular volume

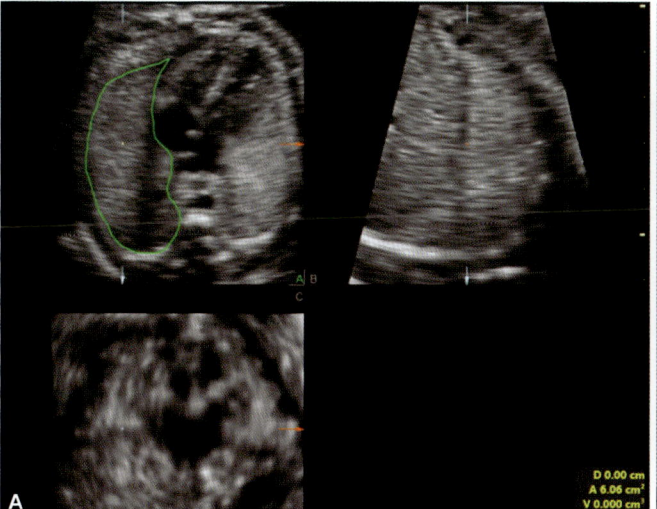
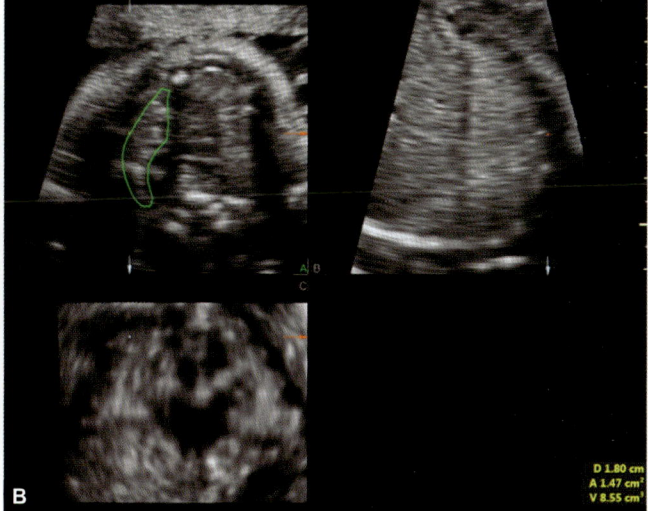

Figs. 2.1A and B: Calculation of fetal right lung volume measurement by multiplanar method. (A) Plane A (axial) is selected with reference, which is rotated about the z-axis so that the lung is positioned at 12 h. The B plane (sagittal) is selected and the cursor is arranged at the level of the mid-point of fetal diaphragm. The first area of the lung in the A plane is delimited manually, while in the B plane the cursor moves from the base to the lung apex at intervals of 3.0 mm; (B) When the cursor reaches the lung apex in plane B, the last area in plane A is delimited, with the apparatus automatically providing the organ volume.

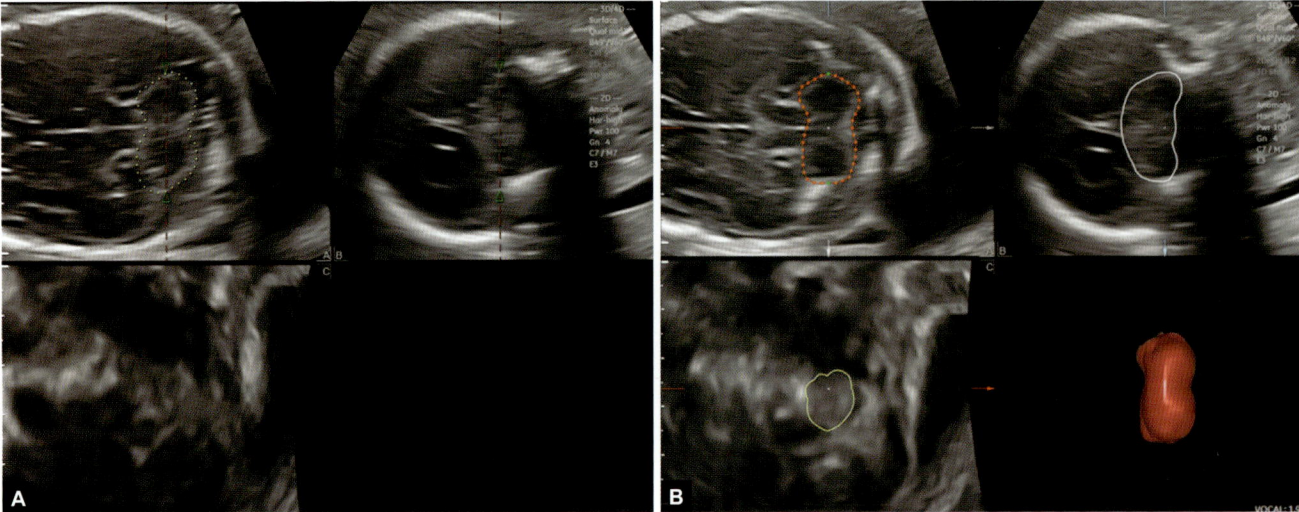

Figs. 2.2A and B: Fetal cerebellum volume measurement by the virtual organ computer-aided analysis (VOCAL) method. (A) Plane A is selected with reference, which is rotated about the z-axis so that the cerebellum is set in 12 h at the level of transverse cerebellum diameter measurement. Calipers are positioned at the extremities of the organ. The outer surface of the organ is delimited in a manual manner, and with each rotation (30°) a new area is delimited; (B) At the end of the rotational process (6 planes), the apparatus provides the rebuilt image of the structure with its volume.

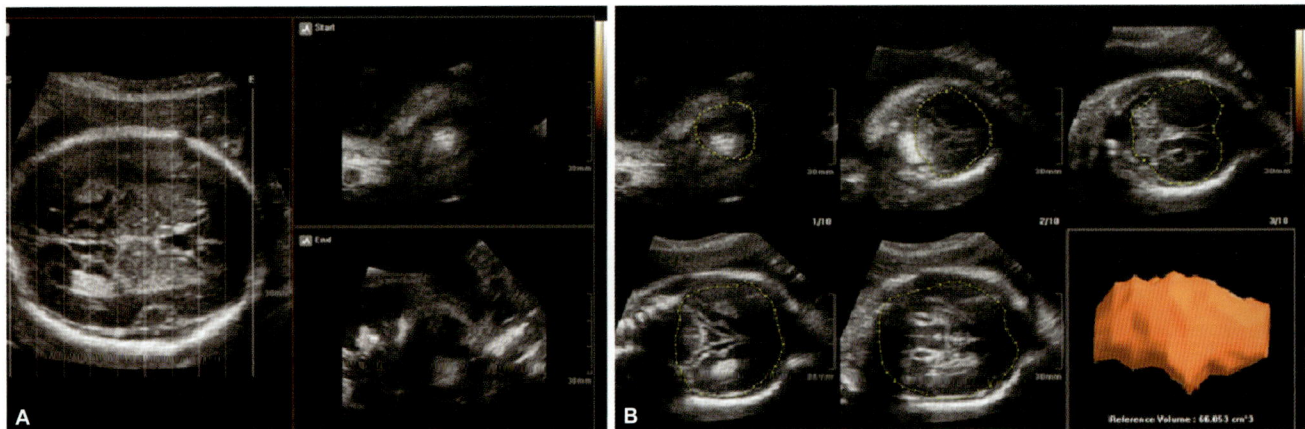

Figs. 2.3A and B: Fetal brain volume measurements by eXtended imaging virtual organ computer-aided analysis (XI VOCAL) method. (A) The initial and the last sectional planes are positioned at the proximal and distal cortex. Afterward, 10 sequential areas are delimited in the axial view; (B) Finishing the last area delimitation, the equipment automatically provides the 3D reconstructed image of the fetal brain with its volume.

and diameter and the latter is used to measure the overall volume, in this case, the fetal organs. The operator initially defines the region of interest, i.e. what part of the obtained volume will be analyzed. In SonoAVC follicle, the program determines the volume (V), three orthogonal diameters (dx, dy, and dz), the mean of these three diameters (md), and the volume-based diameter (vD) of all the anechoic structures in the region of interest.

After determining the volume, the operator should assess whether all follicles were identified, the presence of nonfollicular structures identified as follicles, and the presence of gross errors when estimating follicular volume. In SonoAVC general, the size is not measured automatically, and the operator needs to click on the option corresponding to the desired volume, e.g. fetal heart chamber volume **(Fig. 2.4)**.

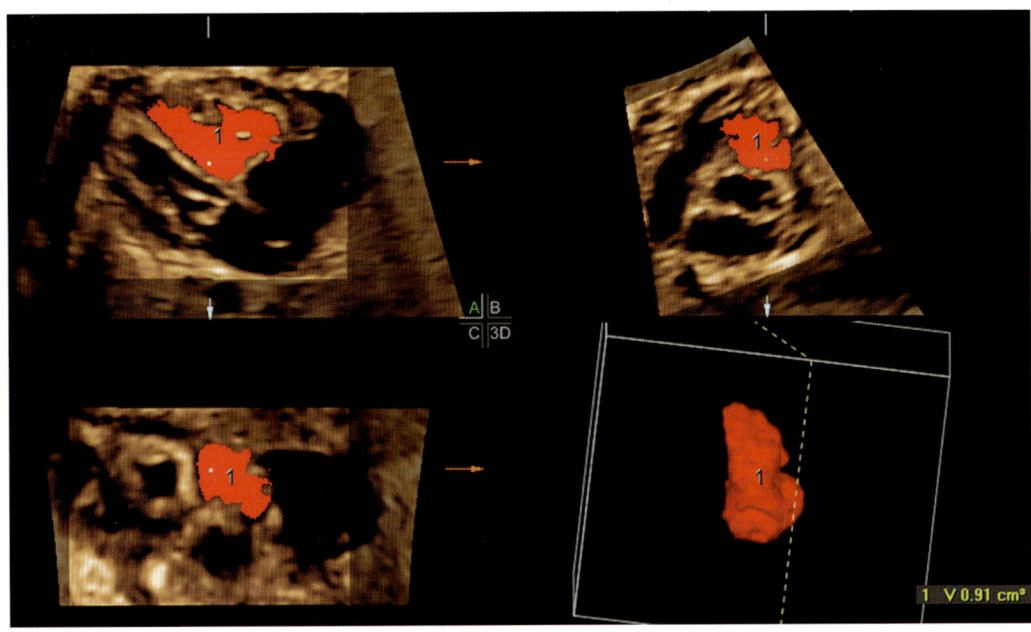

Fig. 2.4: Fetal heart right ventricle volume measurement during systole by sonography-based automated volume count (SonoAVC) method.

EVALUATION OF FETAL CARDIAC VOLUME

The study by Chang et al.[36] was the first to evaluate fetal cardiac volume using 3D ultrasound. The heart volume of 50 healthy fetuses was assessed at 20–30 weeks of gestation, and 2D ultrasound (length × width × height × 0.5233) and 3D ultrasound were compared with the multiplanar method. This method used a slice sequence of the four-chamber plane with a 1.0-mm interval. These authors observed that 3D ultrasound was more reproducible than 2D ultrasound, and the 2D ultrasound volumes were larger than those obtained using 3D ultrasound. The volumes obtained by 2D ultrasound were made equivalent to those obtained using 3D ultrasound by performing polynomial regression and obtaining a new 2D constant (0.4563). The 2D volumes calculated with this new constant did not differ from those obtained using 3D ultrasound.

Peralta et al.[8] found reference values for fetal cardiac volume using VOCAL. A total of 650 normal pregnancies were evaluated at 12–32 weeks of pregnancy using VOCAL with a rotation angle of 30°. The mean cardiac volume was increased significantly with gestational age from 0.6 mL at 12 weeks of gestation to 4.3 mL at 20 weeks and 26.6 mL at 32 weeks.

Barreto et al.[22] obtained reference values for fetal heart volume at 20–34 weeks of pregnancy using XI VOCAL with 10 sequential planes. Cardiac volume was increased with gestational age with mean values of 3.09 mL at 20 weeks of gestation, 9.18 mL at 26 weeks, and 24.89 mL at 34 weeks.

EVALUATION OF FETAL CEREBELLAR VOLUME

The study by Chang et al.[4] was the first to measure fetal cerebellar volume. Reference values were determined in 231 singleton pregnancies by the multiplanar method. Cerebellar volume was strongly correlated with gestational age and fetal biometric parameters.

Araujo Júnior et al.[37] performed a prospective longitudinal study with 52 healthy pregnant women at 20–32 weeks of pregnancy, and fetal cerebellar volume was calculated using VOCAL with a rotation angle of 30°. There was a correlation between cerebellar volume with gestational age and biometric parameters. Furthermore, the equation for fetal cerebellar volume formulated by Chang et al.[4] in the Chinese population of Taiwan may not apply to the Brazilian population because of the marked ethnic differences between these groups.

The VOCAL was used to measure the volume of intracranial structures, including the thalamus, frontal lobe, and cerebellum. Overall, 39 FGR fetuses and 39 appropriate-for-gestational-age (AGA) fetuses were evaluated. Cerebellar volume was significantly smaller in FGR fetuses than in AGA fetuses (6.0 ± 2.1 vs 5.0 ± 1.7; p = 0.001).[38]

EVALUATION OF FETAL LUNG VOLUME

The lungs have been the most investigated fetal organ using volumetric analysis because of the clinical applicability of predicting pulmonary hypoplasia in fetuses with CDH and other conditions, including skeletal dysplasias and preterm premature rupture of membranes.

Britto et al.[39] conducted a longitudinal study with 61 pregnant women at 24–32 weeks of gestation and obtained reference values for fetal lung volume using 3D ultrasound. The volume of each lung was calculated using VOCAL with a rotation angle of 30°. The mean right lung volume ranged from 12.5 ± 0.7 cm³ at gestational week 24 to 31.8 ± 1.8 cm³ at week 32. The mean left lung volume ranged from 9.2 ± 0.9 cm³ at 24 weeks of pregnancy to 22.0 ± 1.6 cm³ at 32 weeks. There was a strong correlation between lung volume and gestational age and estimated fetal weight.

In fetuses with CDH, fetal lung volumes (observed or expected total lung volume) were more accurate in predicting mortality than lung area measurements using 2D ultrasound. The accuracy of measuring fetal lung volume and area is approximately 80% and 70%, respectively.[40,41] Fetuses with isolated CDH with observed or expected total lung volumes smaller than 0.35 have a higher risk of death than those with larger volumes. This result is relevant because fetal endoscopic tracheal occlusion can be performed in these fetuses, and this procedure is associated with increased postnatal survival.[42,43]

Volumetric analysis of the lungs may also predict hypoplasia in risk conditions other than CHD, including preterm premature rupture of membranes, skeletal malformations, hydrothorax, and bilateral renal dysplasia. Gerards et al.[44] evaluated 33 pregnancies with different degrees of risk, and lung volume was measured by the multiplanar method. Of the 33 pregnancies, 16 presented pulmonary hypoplasia on clinical or radiological examination or necropsy. Volumetric analysis of the lungs using 3D ultrasound was more accurate than 2D ultrasound and had sensitivity and specificity of 94% and 82%, respectively. Barros et al.[45] analyzed the prediction of pulmonary hypoplasia in fetuses with skeletal dysplasias at 20–32 weeks of pregnancy. Skeletal dysplasia was lethal

in 18 fetuses (75%). Lung volume was obtained using VOCAL at a rotation angle of 30°, and 3D ultrasound showed a sensitivity of 83.3%, specificity of 100%, positive predictive value of 100%, and negative predictive value of 66.7%.

ASSESSMENT OF FETAL ADRENAL GLAND VOLUME

The study by Chang et al.[7] was the first to evaluate the volume of fetal adrenal glands using 3D ultrasound. The volume was measured in 119 healthy fetuses at 21–40 weeks of gestation using the multiplanar method. Fetal adrenal gland volume was highly correlated with estimated fetal weight and gestational age, and reference values were obtained at each analyzed gestational age.

Helfer et al.[46] obtained reference values for fetal adrenal gland size in 204 normal singleton pregnancies at 24–37 weeks of pregnancy using VOCAL at a rotation angle of 30°. The mean size ranged from 0.179 cm³ at gestational week 24 to 0.592 cm³ at week 37. Size was strongly correlated with gestational age and fetal biometric parameters and presented good inter- and intraobserver reproducibility.

Turan et al.[47] measured fetal adrenal gland volume using VOCAL, fetal zone volume using 2D ultrasound, and cervical volume using transvaginal ultrasound for predicting delivery within 7 days in 74 pregnant women at 21–34 weeks of gestation. Adrenal gland size measured using 3D ultrasound and fetal zone size measured using 2D ultrasound were superior to uterine cervix size in predicting preterm delivery. In a similar study, Ibrahim et al.[48] compared fetal adrenal gland size measured using VOCAL, fetal zone size using 3D ultrasound, cervical size using transvaginal ultrasound, and cervicovaginal fetal fibronectin for predicting delivery within 7 days in 75 women at 28–36 weeks of pregnancy. Adrenal gland size and fetal zone size had the highest accuracy with sensitivity and specificity of 92.6% and 95.8%, and 92.6% and 89.6%, respectively.

EVALUATION OF FETAL THYMUS VOLUME

The size of the fetal thymus by 3D ultrasound was obtained in 28/37 cases (77.7%) using VOCAL at gestational weeks 12–35. There was a good correlation between fetal thymic size and gestational age. In 12 cases, the size was measured using STIC to assess the variability of adrenal gland volume during systole and diastole, which was minimal.[49] Tonni et al.[50] measured thymus volume in 100 fetuses from 18 weeks to 23 weeks and 6 days. The thymus was identified in the three vessels and trachea view, and color Doppler was performed to identify the internal mammary arteries. The thymic volume was obtained by VOCAL at a rotation angle of 30°; the mean volume ranged from 1.25 cm³ at gestational week 18 to 2.62 cm³ at week 23. Olearo et al.[51] determined the thymic size by VOCAL in small for gestational age (SGA) fetuses, FGR fetuses, and controls from 20 weeks to 37 weeks and 6 days. The thymic volume or abdominal circumference ratio was significantly lower in SGA fetuses than in controls and was significantly lower in FGR fetuses with umbilical artery Doppler changes than in SGA and FGR fetuses with normal umbilical artery Doppler.

ASSESSMENT OF FETAL LIMB VOLUME

The first studies that measured fetal limb volume using 3D ultrasound were performed in the early 2000s using the multiplanar method.[52,53] Chang et al.[52] conducted a cross-sectional study with 202 pregnant women at 20–40 weeks of gestation to determine reference values for fetal arm volume by the multiplanar method. The mean arm volume ranged from 6.31 mL at gestational week 20 to 74.63 mL at week 40, and there was a good correlation between the arm volume and gestational age. In 2003, the same research group performed a cross-sectional study with 204 pregnant women at 20–40 weeks of pregnancy to identify reference values for fetal thigh volume by the multiplanar method. The mean thigh volume ranged

from 8.99 mL at 20 weeks of gestation to 128.89 mL at 40 weeks with a good correlation between thigh volume and gestational age and fetal biometric parameters.[53]

Lee et al.[54] proposed the term "fractional limb volume," which corresponded to the 50% portion of the limb diaphysis that contains the largest amount of soft tissues and is therefore the most relevant for the evaluation of nutritional disorders, besides being more feasible than the multiplanar method because it excludes the epiphyses of fetal limbs **(Figs. 2.5A and B)**.

Fetal limb volume was also assessed using XI VOCAL. Cavalcante et al.[55] conducted a cross-sectional study with 425 normal pregnancies at 20–40 weeks of pregnancy and evaluated fetal arm volume using XI VOCAL with 10 plane sequences. The mean arm volume ranged from 4.45 cm³ at 20 weeks of gestation to 59.95 cm³ at 40 weeks and was strongly correlated with gestational age. Araujo Júnior et al.[56] performed a cross-sectional study involving 425 normal pregnancies at 20–40 weeks of pregnancy and measured fetal thigh volume using XI VOCAL with 10 plane sequences; the mean thigh volume ranged from 7.34 cm³ at 20 weeks of gestation to 115.68 cm³ at 40 weeks and was strongly correlated with gestational age.

Studies from the mid-1990s reported that fetal limb volume measurements obtained using the multiplanar method were more accurate than those obtained using 2D ultrasound in predicting birth weight.[32,33] Chang et al.[32] examined 100 pregnant women between 32 and 42 weeks of pregnancy and measured fetal limb volume 48 h before delivery; 2D ultrasound formulae were compared with

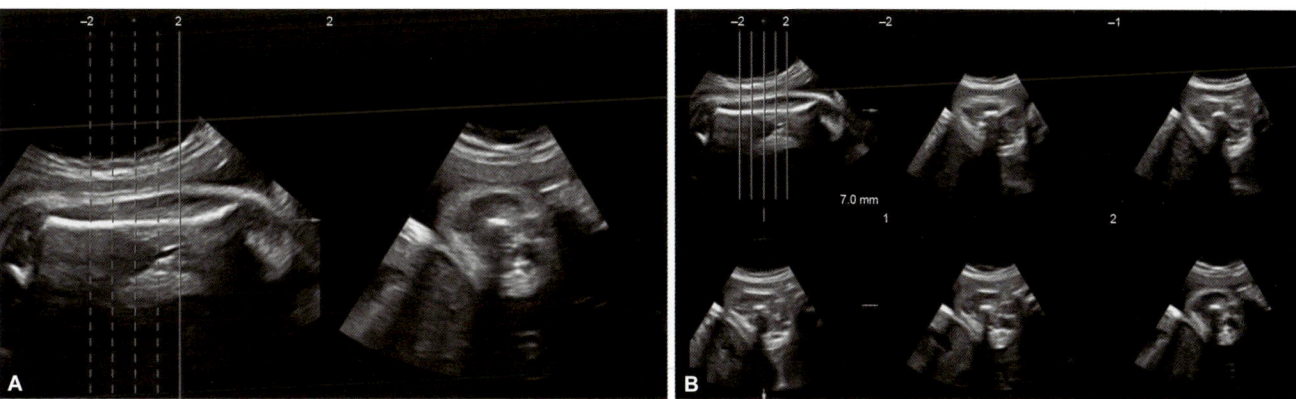

Figs. 2.5A and B: Fetal fractional thigh volume measurement. (A) The reference plane is placed in the mid-point of femur length and two equidistant right and left planes are formed; (B) After the delimitation of external surface of the fetal limb in the axial plane, the software provides the final volume.

actual birth weights. The authors proposed a new equation [birth weight (g) = 1080.87350 + 22.44701 × thigh volume (mL)], and its error, percentage error, absolute error, and absolute percentage error were significantly lower than those of 2D ultrasound formulae. Liang et al.[33] analyzed 105 pregnant women at 32–43 weeks of gestation and measured fetal arm volume within 48 h before delivery. The 2D ultrasound results were compared with actual birth weights. The error, percentage error, and absolute error of the new equation [birth weight (g) = 1088.6 + 36.024 × arm volume (mL)] were significantly lower than those of 2D ultrasound equations.

Suboptimal fetal growth and nutrition may increase the risk of chronic diseases during adulthood. Catalano et al.[57] reported that measurements of body composition, lean body mass, and fat mass, may be an anthropometric refinement in fetal growth assessment. In addition, the fat mass of the newborn represents 14% of the total weight postpartum, and fetal subcutaneous fat and changes in lean body mass during pregnancy can be monitored by measuring the mean circumference of the arm and thigh. Fetal fat may be a more sensitive and specific marker of abnormal intrauterine growth compared with lean body mass index because of the increased rate of growth with advancing gestational age.

The diagnosis of fetal growth disorders cannot be based on cross-sectional studies because the fetuses present biological variations and distinct genetic growth potentials. For this reason, Lee et al.[34] proposed an individualized assessment of growth using fractional arm volume, arm circumference, and humeral diaphysis length as parameters. There was a linear increase in the three parameters up to 28 weeks of gestation, and accelerated deposition of subcutaneous tissue and muscle in fetuses with normal growth after this period. Therefore, fractional arm volume may detect early changes in soft tissues and serve as a good parameter for the early detection of fetal growth disorders.

CONCLUSION

Fetal organ volume measurements by 3D ultrasound is more reliable than 2D ultrasound, because of the irregular surface of fetal organs. Multiplanar, VOCAL, and XI VOCAL techniques are consistent and reproducible; however, multiplanar is more time-consuming. Fetal lung volume measurements show the main clinical applications, mainly in the prediction of pulmonary hypoplasia

in cases of CDH. Fetal limb volume measurement shows applications in the prediction of birth weight and intrauterine status nutrition.

REFERENCES

1. Jeanty P, Romero R, Hobbins JC. Fetal limb volume: a new parameter to assess fetal growth and nutrition. J Ultrasound Med. 1985;4:273-82.
2. Riccabona M, Nelson TR, Pretorius DH, et al. Distance and volume measurement using three-dimensional ultrasonography. J Ultrasound Med. 1995;14:881-6.
3. Riccabona M, Nelson TR, Pretorius DH. Three-dimensional ultrasound: accuracy of distance and volume measurements. Ultrasound Obstet Gynecol. 1996;7:429-34.
4. Chang CH, Chang FM, Yu CH, et al. Assessment of fetal cerebellar volume using three-dimensional ultrasound. Ultrasound Med Biol. 2000;26:981-8.
5. Chang CH, Yu CH, Chang FM, et al. Volumetric assessment of normal fetal lungs using three-dimensional ultrasound. Ultrasound Med Biol. 2003;29:935-42.
6. Chang CH, Yu CH, Chang FM, et al. The assessment of fetal liver volume by three-dimensional. Ultrasound Med Biol. 2003;29:1123-9.
7. Chang CH, Yu CH, Chang FM, et al. Assessment of fetal adrenal gland volume using three-dimensional ultrasound. Ultrasound Med Biol. 2002;28:1383-7.
8. Peralta CF, Cavoretto P, Csapo B, et al. Lung and heart volumes by three-dimensional ultrasound in normal fetuses at 12-32 weeks' gestation. Ultrasound Obstet Gynecol. 2006;27:128-33.
9. Araujo Júnior E, Pires CR, Nardozza LM, et al. Correlation of fetal cerebellar volume with other fetal growth indices by three-dimensional ultrasound. J Matern fetal Neonatal Med. 2007;20:581-7.
10. Tedesco GD, Bussamra LC, Araujo Júnior E, et al. Reference range of fetal renal volume by three-dimensional ultrasonography using the VOCAL method. Fetal Diagn Ther. 2009;25:385-91.
11. You JH, Lv GR, Liu XL, et al. Reference ranges of fetal spleen biometric parameters and volume assessed by three-dimensional ultrasound and their applicability in spleen malformations. Prenat Diagn. 2014;34:1189-97.
12. Ruano R, Benachi A, Joubin L, et al. Three-dimensional ultrasonographic assessment of fetal lung volume as prognostic factor in isolated congenital diaphragmatic hernia. BJOG. 2004;111:423-9.
13. Ruano R, Aubry MC, Barthe B, et al. Three-dimensional ultrasonographic measurements of the fetal lungs for prediction of perinatal outcome in isolated congenital diaphragmatic hernia. J Obstet Gynaecol Res. 2009;35:1031-41.
14. Turan OM, Turan S, Buhimschi IA, et al. Comparative analysis of 2-D versus 3-D ultrasound estimation of the fetal adrenal gland volume and prediction of preterm birth. Am J Perinatol. 2012;29:673-80.

15. Maged AM, Abdelmoneim A, Said W, et al. Measuring the rate of fetal urine production using three-dimensional ultrasound during normal pregnancy and pregnancy-associated diabetes. J Matern Fetal Neonatal Med. 2014;27:1790-4.

16. Molina FS, Faro C, Sotiriadis A, et al. Heart stroke volume and cardiac output by four-dimensional ultrasound in normal fetuses. Ultrasound Obstet Gynecol. 2008;32:181-7.

17. Simioni C, Nardozza LM, Araujo Júnior E, et al. Heart stroke volume, cardiac output, and ejection fraction in 265 normal fetuses in the second half of gestation assessed by 4D ultrasound using spatio-temporal image correlation. J Matern Fetal Neonatal Med. 2011;24:1159-67.

18. Albers MEWA, Buisman ETIA, Kahn RS, et al. Intra- and interobserver agreement for fetal cerebral measurements in 3D-ultrasonography. Hum Brain Mapp. 2018;39: 3277-84.

19. Araujo Júnior E, Nardozza LM, Rolo LC, et al. Reference range of embryo volume by 3-D sonography using the XI VOCAL method at 7 to 10 + 6 weeks of pregnancy. Am J Perinatol. 2010;27:501-5.

20. Araujo Júnior E, Nardozza LM, Rolo LC, et al. Assessment of yolk sac volume by 3D-sonography using the XI VOCAL method from 7 to 10 + 6 weeks of pregnancy. Arch Gynecol Obstet. 2011;283:1-4.

21. Nardozza LM, Rolo LC, Araujo Júnior E, et al. Comparison of gestational sac volume by 3D-sonography using planimetric, virtual organ computer-aided analysis and extended imaging virtual organ computer-aided analysis methods between 7 and 11 weeks of pregnancy. Acta Obstet Gynecol Scand. 2010;89:328-34.

22. Barreto EQ, Milani HJ, Araujo Júnior E, et al. Reliability and validity in vitro volume calculations by 3-dimensional ultrasonography using the multiplanar, virtual organ computer-aided analysis (VOCAL) and extended imaging VOCAL methods. J Ultrasound Med. 2010;29:767-74.

23. Barreto EQ, Milani HJ, Haratz KK, et al. Reference intervals for fetal heart volume from 3-dimensional sonography using the extended imaging virtual organ computer-aided analysis method at gestational ages of 20 to 34 weeks. J Ultrasound Med. 2012;31:673-8.

24. Haratz KK, Oliveira PS, Rolo LC, et al. Fetal cerebral ventricle volumetry: comparison between 3D ultrasound and magnetic resonance imaging in fetuses with ventri-culomegaly. J Matern Fetal Neonatal Med. 2011;24: 1384-91.

25. Caetano AC, Zamarian AC, Araujo Júnior E, et al. Assessment of intracranial structure volumes in fetuses with growth restriction by 3-dimensional sonography using the extended imaging virtual organ computer-aided analysis method. J Ultrasound Med. 2015;34: 1397-405.

26. Nam KH, Cho A, Kwon JY, et al. Feasibility of measuring 3-dimensional renal parenchymal volume to predict post-natal renal function in near-term fetuses with congenital hydronephrosis: a preliminary study. J Ultrasound Med. 2012;31:955-62.

27. Raine-Fenning N, Jayaprakasan K, Clewes J, et al. SonoAVC: a novel method of automatic volume calculation. Ultrasound Obstet Gynecol. 2008;31:691-6.

28. Salama S, Arbo E, Lamazou F, et al. Reproducibility and reliability of automated volumetric measurement of single preovulatory follicles using SonoAVC. Fertil Steril. 2010; 93:2069-73.

29. Rizzo G, Capponi A, Pietrolucci ME, et al. Role of sonographic automatic volume calculation in measuring fetal cardiac ventricular volumes using 4-dimensional sonography: comparison with virtual organ computer-aided analysis. J Ultrasound Med. 2010;29:261-70.

30. Duin LK, Nijhuis JG, Scherjon SA, et al. Comparison of conventional versus three-dimensional ultrasound in fetal renal pelvis measurement and their potential prediction of neonatal uropathies. J Matern Fetal Neonatal Med. 2016;29:2494-9.

31. Duin LK, Willekes C, Vossen M, et al. Reproducibility of fetal renal pelvis volume assessed by three-dimensional ultrasonography with two different measurement techniques. J Clin Ultrasound. 2013;41:230-4.

32. Chang FM, Liang RI, Ko HC, et al. Three-dimensional ultrasound-assessed fetal thigh volumetry in predicting birth weight. Obstet Gynecol. 1997;90:331-9.

33. Liang RI, Chang FM, Yao BL, et al. Predicting birth weight by fetal upper arm volume with use of three-dimensional ultrasonography. Am J Obstet Gynecol. 1997;177:632-8.

34. Lee W, Deter RL, McNie B, et al. The fetal arm: individualized growth assessment in normal pregnancies. J Ultrasound Med. 2005;24:817-28.

35. Lee W, Balasubramaniam M, Deter RL, et al. Fractional limb volume—a soft tissue parameter of fetal body composition: validation, technical considerations and normal ranges during pregnancy. Ultrasound Obstet Gynecol. 2009;33: 427-40.

36. Chang FM, Hsu KF, Ko HC, et al. Fetal heart volume assessment by three-dimensional ultrasound. Ultrasound Obstet Gynecol. 1997;9:42-8.

37. Araujo Júnior E, Guimarães Filho HA, Pires CR, et al. Validation of fetal cerebellar volume by three-dimensional ultrasonography in Brazilian population. Arch Gynecol Obstet. 2007;275:5-11.

38. Benavides-Serralde A, Hernández-Andrade E, Fernández-Delgado J, et al. Three-dimensional sonographic calcula-tion of the volume of intracranial structures in growth-restricted and appropriate-for-gestational age fetuses. Ultrasound Obstet Gynecol. 2009;33:530-7.

39. Werneck Britto IS, de Silva Bussamra LC, Araujo Júnior E, et al. Reference range of fetal lung volume by 3D-ultrasonography using the rotational method (VOCAL). J Perinatal Med. 2009;37:161-7.

40. Ruano R, Takashi E, da Silva MM, et al. Prediction and probability of neonatal outcome in isolated congenital diaphragmatic hernia using multiple ultrasound parameters. Ultrasound Obstet Gynecol. 2012;39:42-9.

41. Ruano R, Lazar DA, Cass DL, et al. Fetal lung volume and quantification of liver herniation by magnetic resonance

imaging in isolated congenital diaphragmatic hernia. Ultrasound Obstet Gynecol. 2014;43:662-9.

42. Deprest J, Gratacos E, Nicolaides KH. Fetoscopic tracheal occlusion (FETO) for severe congenital diaphragmatic hernia: evolution of a technique and preliminary results. Ultrasound Obstet Gynecol. 2004;24:121-6.

43. Ruano R, Yoshisaki CT, da Silva MM, et al. A randomized controlled trial of fetal endoscopic tracheal occlusion versus postnatal management of severe isolated congenital diaphragmatic hernia. Ultrasound Obstet Gynecol. 2012; 39:20-7.

44. Gerards FA, Twisk JW, Bakker M, et al. Fetal lung volume: three-dimensional ultrasonography compared with magnetic resonance imaging. Ultrasound Obstet Gynecol. 2007;29:533-6.

45. Barros CA, Rezende Gde C, Araujo Júnior E, et al. Prediction of lethal pulmonary hypoplasia by means of fetal lung volume in skeletal dysplasias: a three-dimensional ultrasound assessment. J Matern Fetal Neonatal Med. 2016;29:1725-30.

46. Helfer TM, Rolo LC, Okasaki NA, et al. Reference ranges of fetal adrenal gland and fetal zone volumes between 24 and 37+6 weeks of gestation by three-dimensional ultrasound. J Matern Fetal Neonatal Med. 2017;30: 568-73.

47. Turan OM, Turan S, Funai EF, et al. Ultrasound measurement of fetal adrenal gland enlargement: an accurate predictor of preterm birth. Am J Obstet Gynecol. 2011;204:311.

48. Ibrahim MI, Sherif A, El-Kady M, et al. Can three-dimensional ultrasound measurement of fetal adrenal gland enlargement predict preterm birth? Arch Gynecol Obstet. 2015;292:569-78.

49. Re C, Bertucci E, Weissmann-Brenner A, et al. Fetal thymus volume estimation by virtual organ computer-aided analysis in normal pregnancies. J Ultrasound Med. 2015;34:847-52.

50. Tonni G, Rosignoli L, Cariati E, et al. Fetal thymus: visualization rate and volume by integrating 2D- and 3D-ultrasound during 2nd trimester echocardiography. J Matern Fetal Neonatal Med. 2016;29:2223-8.

51. Olearo E, Oberto M, Oggè G, et al. Thymic volume in healthy, small for gestational age and growth restricted fetuses. Prenat Diagn. 2012;32:662-7.

52. Chang CH, Yu CH, Chang FM, et al. Assessment of normal fetal upper arm volume by three-dimensional ultrasound. Ultrasound Med Biol. 2002;28:859-63.

53. Chang CH, Yu CH, Chang FM, et al. Three-dimensional ultrasound in the assessment of normal fetal thigh volume. Ultrasound Med Biol. 2003;29:361-6.

54. Lee W, Deter RL, Ebersole JD, et al. Birth weight prediction by three-dimensional ultrasonography: fractional limb volume. J Ultrasound Med. 2001;20:1283-92.

55. Cavalcante RO, Araujo Júnior E, Nardozza LM, et al. Nomogram of fetal upper arm volume by three-dimensional ultrasound using extended imaging virtual organ computer-aided analysis (XI VOCAL). J Perinat Med. 2011;39:717-24.

56. Araujo Júnior E, Cavalcante RO, Nardozza LM, et al. Fetal thigh volume by 3D sonography using XI VOCAL: reproducibility and reference range for Brazilian healthy fetuses between 20 and 40 weeks. Prenat Diagn. 2011;31:1234-40.

57. Catalano PM, Tyzbir ED, Allen SR, et al. Evaluation of fetal growth by estimation of neonatal body composition. Obstet Gynecol. 1992;79:46-50.

Ultrasound and Folliculogenesis

Fernando Bonilla-Musoles, Newton Osborne, Francisco Raga
Francisco Jose Bonilla Bartret

INTRODUCTION

No one disagrees that ultrasounds along with gyneco-logic endocrinology have been two major advances in our specialty and that they have been the fundamental enablers of the revolution that has occurred in assisted reproduction technology (ART).[1,2] Without ultrasound, ART as we now know it would be inconceivable. The main steps in this "revolution" were:

- Introduction of vaginal probes by Kratochwil in Vienna.
- Description of endometrial changes, folliculogenesis, and the diverse types of endometrium by Hackelöer in Hamburg.
- Disappearance of laparoscopic follicular aspiration because of the introduction of ultrasound-guided transvaginal aspiration, developed by Feichtinger, also in Vienna.
- Three-dimensional (3D) and four-dimensional (4D) ultrasound have improved and eased folliculogenesis control.

The 4D enables us to capture new planes of vision, improves image quality, and introduces new ultrasound modes [high definition (HD) live and silhouette, auto-matic volume calculation (AVC), virtual organ computer-aided analysis (VOCAL), inverse mode, etc.] that allows great resolution and evaluation of pelvic organs.

In recent years, the spectacular advances with 4D ultrasonography have generated a new revolution in ART.

In spite of these advances, a review of the literature leads us to raise more questions:

- How can an evaluation of folliculogenesis be improved?

- How can we better evaluate existing antral follicles (AF)?
- How can we know the best moment to administer human chorionic gonadotropin (hCG) for the induction of ovulation?
- What is the effect of the dominant follicle luteinization on growing follicles that remain?
- When should a luteal body be considered active, regressive, or luteinized and not broken?

Lastly, discussions related to ultrasound characteris-tics of the endometrium (thickness, morphology, vas-cularization, delimitation, and volume) are so ample that it is no simple matter to develop a protocol that guides to an adequate evaluation of the concept of endometrial receptivity.

Commentary about the value of color Doppler and Doppler energy along with the recent advances in the varied modes of 3D or 4D visualization **(Figs. 3.1 to 3.3)** will merit a separate chapter.

ULTRASONOGRAPHIC NOTIONS FOR FOLLICULOGENESIS CONTROL

Among the available means for adequate control of folliculogenesis, only ultrasound is capable of showing the evolution of follicular growth over short-time spans. Folliculogenesis starts 70–74 days prior to ovulation. That is, two and a half cycles prior to its own ovulatory cycle.

About 400–500 primordial and primary follicles initiate growth in a different ovarian area each time, with the mechanisms that control each area are still unknown.

- Why in this area?
- Why in this specific ovary?

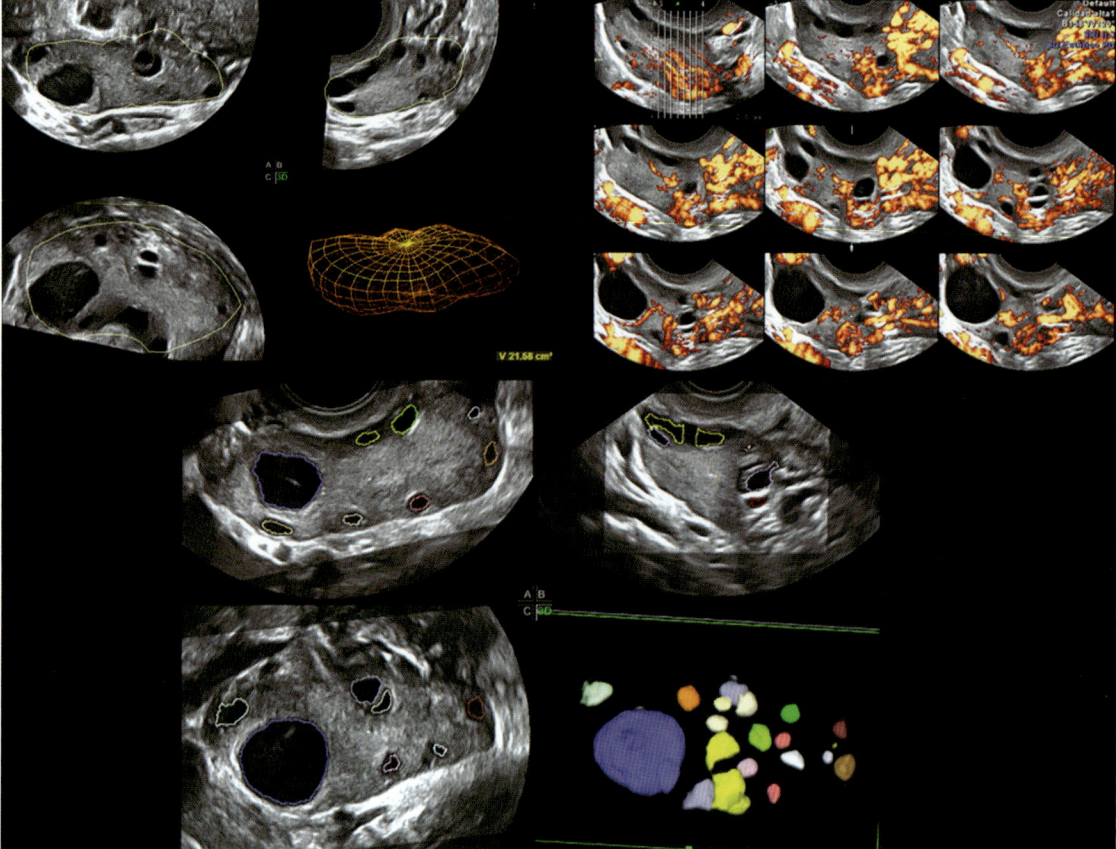

Fig. 3.1: Nowadays used ultrasound modes for folliculogenesis monitoring are used which are more definitive than the 2D vaginal ultrasound used in the past. Above and left, the three-orthogonal planes and histogram showing the total ovarian volume calculation which is of interest when looking to the ovarian reserve. To the right Doppler energy and tomography ovarian cuts are shown. This mode increases the findings by using only color Doppler. Below, 2D in orthogonal planes and automatic volume calculation from the existing antral follicles. Each follicle is showed in a different color. It is easy to count and measure each follicle. The dominant follicle is clearly depicted in blue color.

These events take place independently of the action of hormones from the hypophysis **(Figs. 3.1 to 3.3)**.

Although the mechanism by which these cells start their growth is not known, it is known that there is an increase of local growth factors and an increase in follicular microvasculature. Furthermore, it is known that the layer of granulosa cells is functional and remains intact. The larger number of cells in the granulosa layer will result in a greater number of gonadotropin [follicle-stimulating hormone (FSH) and luteinizing hormone (LH)] receptors, and as a consequence, with a greater probability of follicular.

Ovarian folliculogenesis has three well-established phases **(Fig. 3.4)**:
- Recruitment of the follicular cohort
- Selection of 20–25 AF during the peak of intercyclical FSH during the previous cycle

- Dominance and maturation of one, and exceptionally, more than one follicle.

The end of the vast majority of antral and pre-AF will be their atresia by apoptosis **(Fig. 3.4)**.

Antral Follicles

There are two basic exploratory ultrasound applications during these events—(1) visualization and (2) AF count in the basal state.

The number of existing AF in basic ultrasound and, although in lesser magnitude, the ovarian volume, is of great importance for knowledge about ovarian reserve. In order to develop an evaluation protocol, it is agreed that the count of AF must be done during the first days of the menstrual cycle. Nevertheless, AF count can be carried out at any phase of the menstrual cycle. Small follicles (2–3 mm) can be seen and measured with vaginal probes.

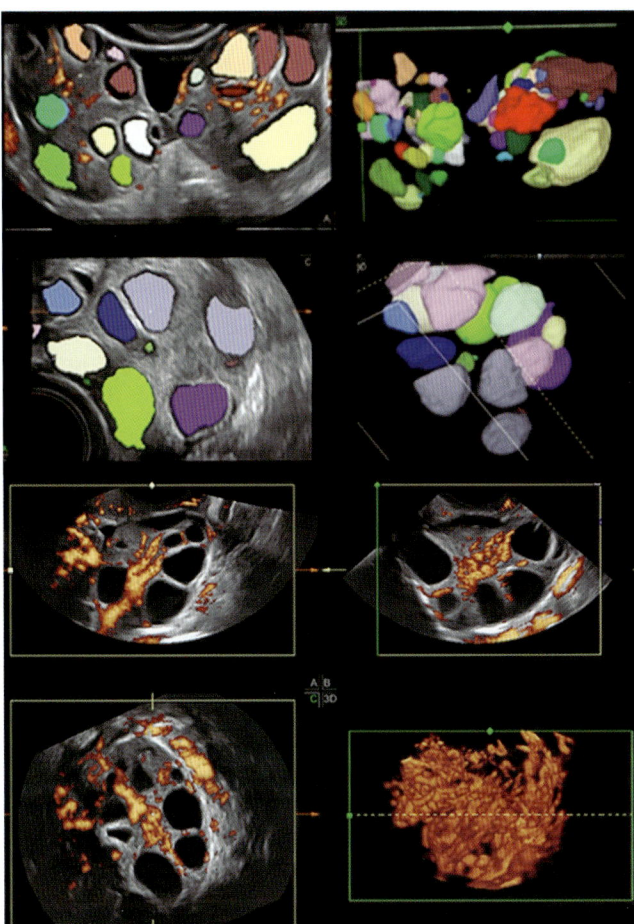

Fig. 3.2: Folliculogenesis. Vascular image around each follicle obtained with 3D angiography and color power Doppler. It is clearly depicted that only preovulatory follicles dispose of a great vascularity located around the whole follicle, which will allow fluid transvasation to the follicular fluid without increasing its internal fluid pressure. It can be observed that only antral preovulatory follicles dispose of this enormous perifollicular vascularization. In the above picture, the same follicles observed with automatic volume calculation mode.

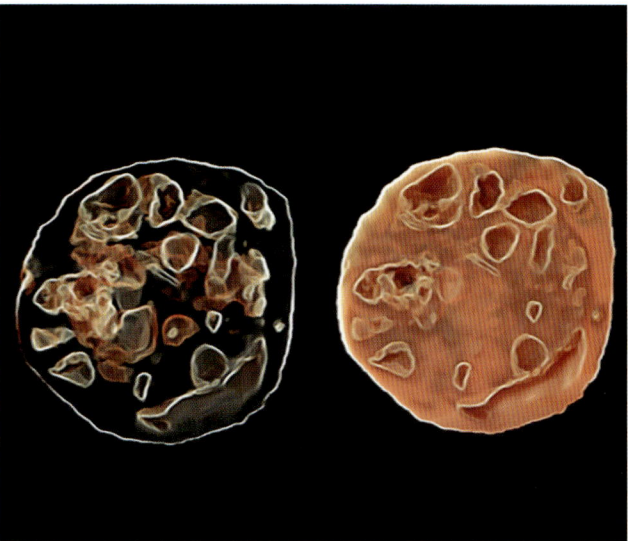

Fig. 3.3: Spontaneous folliculogenesis. The new ultrasound mode "silhouette" shows a better delimitation of the structure profile and allows a clear delimitation of each antral follicle.

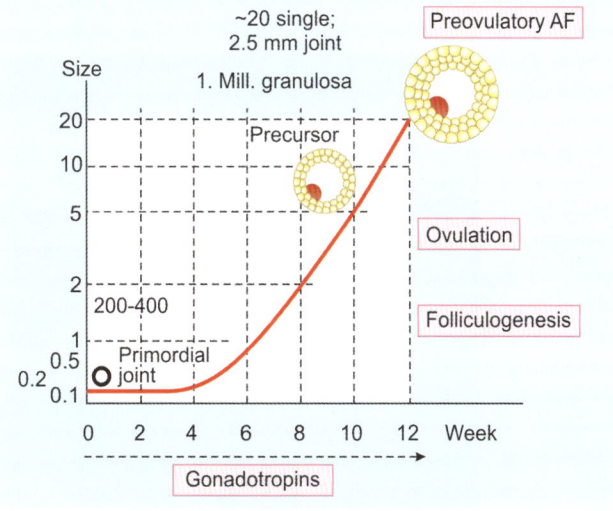

Fig. 3.4: Human folliculogenesis schema. Estimate follicular development (in weeks) from primordial to preovulatory follicle.

Visualization is much simpler using the different 3D modes—inverse, AVC, VOCAL, and silhouette (**Figs. 3.5 and 3.6**).

Folliculogenesis Control

Vaginal 2D or 3D ultrasound allows optimal evaluation (daily or at short intervals) of follicular growth. When farmers want to determine the best time to pick their oranges, they do not need to check on them daily. They must wait several days to notice size and color changes that indicate when picking must be done. It is the same with follicles. It is advisable to have the first ultrasound evaluation on the second or third day of the cycle. Subsequent evaluations in induced cycles will be done 6 days after the administration of gonadotropins or 4–5 days after administration of clomiphene.

We are of the opinion that ultrasound evaluation is sufficient for adequate folliculogenesis control in natural cycles as well as in ART cycles. Additional evaluation of estradiol concentrations has not proven to add additional

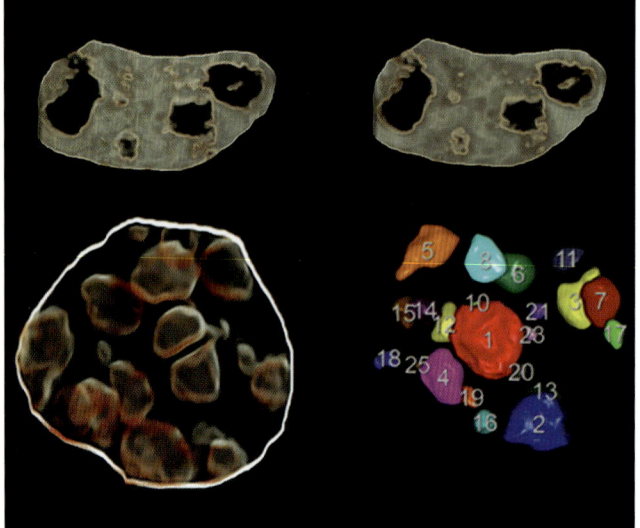

Fig. 3.5: Above—silhouette mode of a normal ovarian section showing three growing and various atretic follicles. Below—antral follicles count with automatic volume calculation, in colors and silhouette modes. Thanks to these new modes, our knowledge's and the calculation form of the antral follicles for the ovarian reserve have dramatically changed in the last years.

information that is crucial for adequate control of ovarian stimulation cycles for in vitro fertilization or intracytoplasmic sperm injection (IVF or ICSI). In the vast majority of cases, ultrasound is enough. In this way, laboratory overwork and unnecessary additional charges are avoided.

FOLLICULOGENESIS IN NATURAL CYCLE

Folliculogenesis varies depending on whether it is spontaneous or induced. As mentioned above, the first (or basal) ultrasound should be performed on the second or third day of the cycle. This would provide approximate knowledge of ovarian reserve.

Follicles between 2 mm and 9 mm are part of the cohort of small AF that are starting the process of maturation. Shortly after, a dominant follicle, distinguished by greater size and faster growth, will appear. The remaining AF will cease to grow or become atretic. It is from this moment that if so desired, hormonal determinations and ultrasound controls every 48 h can be done.

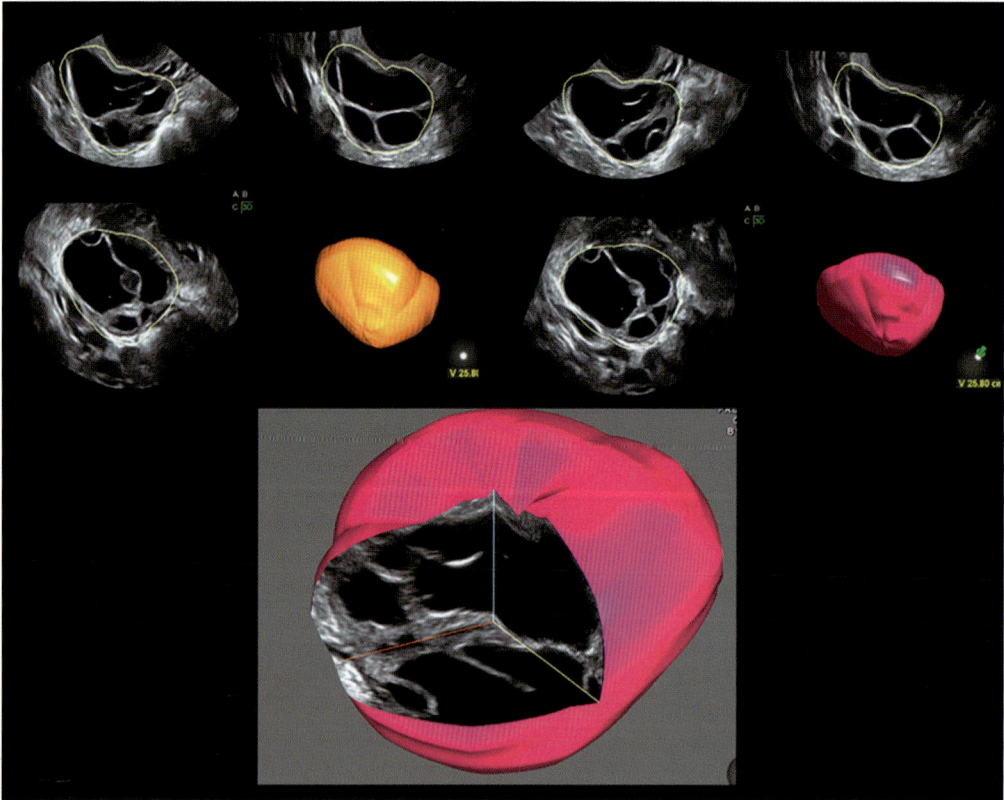

Fig. 3.6: Automatic volume calculation using virtual organ computer-aided analysis mode. We observe the whole ovarian surface and indoor, the follicles. This calculation, recommended by the Rotterdam classification in cases of polycystic ovaries is, in our opinion, less valuable than the simple antral follicle count.

Follicle growth and 17β-estradiol production occur in parallel. The follicle is considered to be mature when it produces ~ 250 pg/mL of 17β-estradiol.

Since in natural cycles, the relation of follicular growth to estradiol production occurs in a linear manner up to the 10th day of the cycle, these determinations can be avoided. Follicle growth after the 10th day is not linear, but exponential. The closest follicle gets to ovulation, the fastest is its growth. The follicle grows between 1 mm/day and 1.2 mm/day up to the 10th day and a mean growth of 1.8 mm/day at the end of the proliferative phase.

Prior to ovulation, the dominant follicle measures 22–25 mm (occasionally, between 18 mm and 36 mm), and this growth is the only marker that will predict with certainty ovulation **(Figs. 3.7 to 3.10)**.

An approximated summary would be discussed in **Box 3.1**.

There are other ultrasound images that predict an approaching ovulation, but they are not always visible.

Visualization of the Cumulus Oophorus

The cumulus oophorus can be seen 20% of the times with transvaginal ultrasound. However, with 3D/4D/HD live it can be seen 50% of the times as well as follicles larger than 18 mm always **(Figs. 3.11 to 3.13)**.

The cumulus oophorus appears less than 24 h prior to ovulation. What we are really observing are the more mature follicles, which are likely to contain metaphase II oocytes, and therefore, ideal for fertilization (or for aspiration in cases of cycles induced for IVF/ICSI).

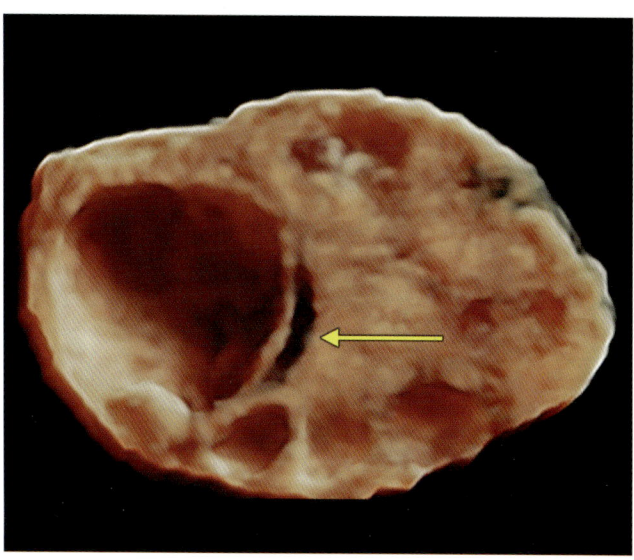

Fig. 3.7: Dominant also called De Graaf follicle. Next to the follicle various small antral follicles. The arrow shows a part of the granulosa sheet uncoupling, an ultrasound sign of imminent ovulation.

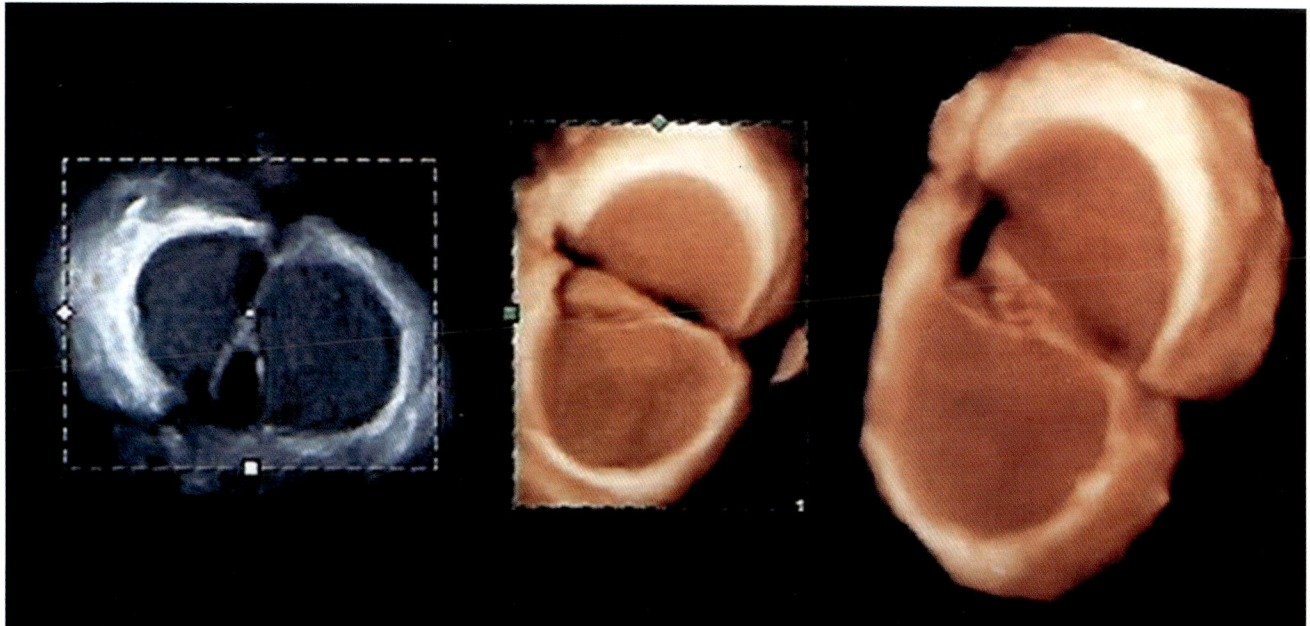

Fig. 3.8: Ripe preovulatory follicle. We are visualizing the whole follicle cavity. 2D or 3D ultrasound is visualized in a case of spontaneous ovulation. The size arrives 21–25 mm.

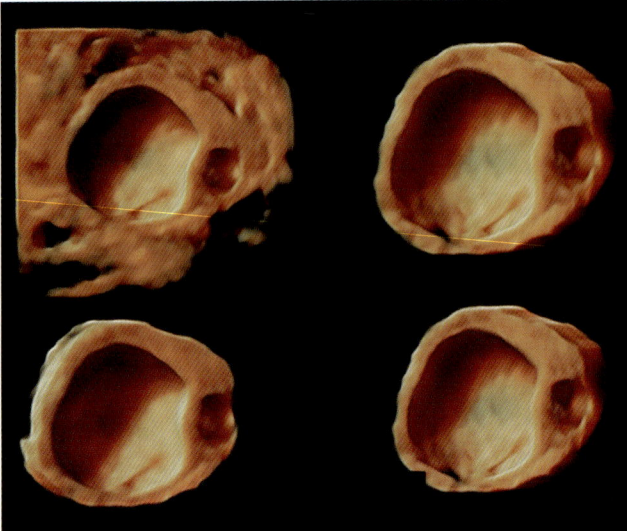

Fig. 3.9: Mature follicle in a proliferation phase high definition live ultrasound with various light focus orientations.

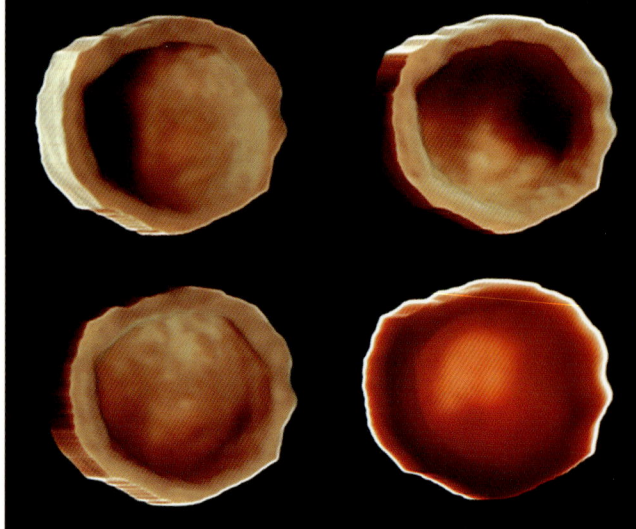

Fig. 3.10: Mature follicle. High definition live. This mode allows to see the whole inner part of the follicle observed from different light angles appearing lights and shadows which increase the vision quality, also maximal luminescence can be employed (below right).

Box 3.1: Ultrasound characteristics mature preovulatory or de Graaf follicle.

Size ≥21–25 mm, in spontaneous cycle

Size ≥18 mm, in stimulation with clomiphene and/or human menopausal gonadotropin

Size ≥15 mm, in stimulation with gonadotropins

Production above 250 pg/mL of 17β-estradiol

Visualization of the cumulus oophorus

Visualization of the rosebush thorns sign or irregular contour

Visualization of the uncoupling of the granulosa

Uncoupling of the Granulosa

- It occurs in 5–12 h prior to ovulation (**Fig. 3.14**).
- It occurs when the theca becomes edematous under the effect of hyaluronidase.
- It appears as an irregular, dark halo.
- As is the case with the previous sign, it is difficult to observe with transvaginal sonography. But with 3D/4D/HD live, it can be seen 50% of the times in ovulatory follicles. As is the case with visualization of the cumulus, it is a sign that indicates a potential for follicular maturation.

Appearance of the "Rosebush Thorns"

In these cases, the granulosa layer is already irregular, it is undulating, breaking apart, and indentations appear

toward the interior of the follicle (**Fig. 3.14**). These last two images coincide with the onset of luteinization. As was the case with the two last images, it is difficult to observe with transvaginal ultrasound (18%), and should be looked for with 3D and HD live (60%).

Ovulation

Upon rupture of the wall of the follicle follicular fluid escapes, a phenomenon that is not explosive, but that may take from a few seconds to 30–45 minutes.

Many ultrasound signs have been described, both with transabdominal and transvaginal ultrasound, but we will list the ones we consider to be of clinical interest.

- Sudden follicle disappearance (a not very useful indirect sign. It is more important, if it is accompanied by a simultaneous appearance of fluid in Douglas's sac).
- Appearance of the typical corpus luteum images:
  - After a few minutes, the follicular antrum fills partially or totally with blood with simultaneous appearance of the typical image of "hemorrhagic" corpus luteum, of irregular shape, internal echoes, and frequently thickened wall. This is the first really pathognomonic image and it is found in practically 100% of cases (**Fig. 3.15**).
  - After the appearance of this, the corpus luteum takes one of the three US presentation forms, all absolutely pathognomonic of ovulation

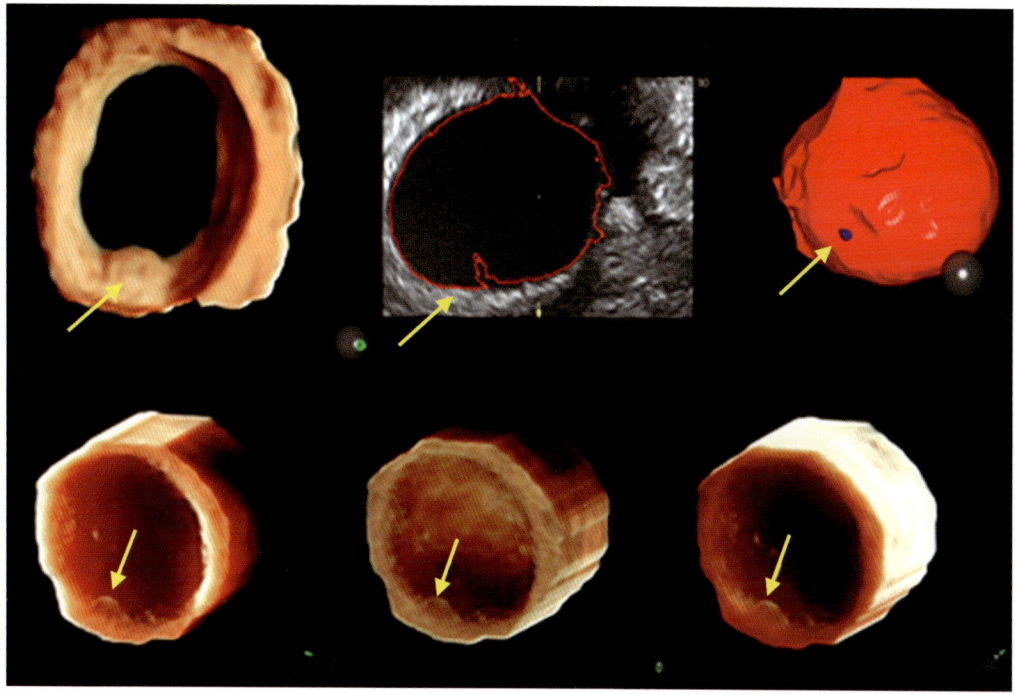

Fig. 3.11: Cumulus oophorus marked with yellow arrows and observed with 4D, high definition live, and virtual organ computer-aided analysis (above). Below three cuts of the same cumulus oophorus using high definition live.

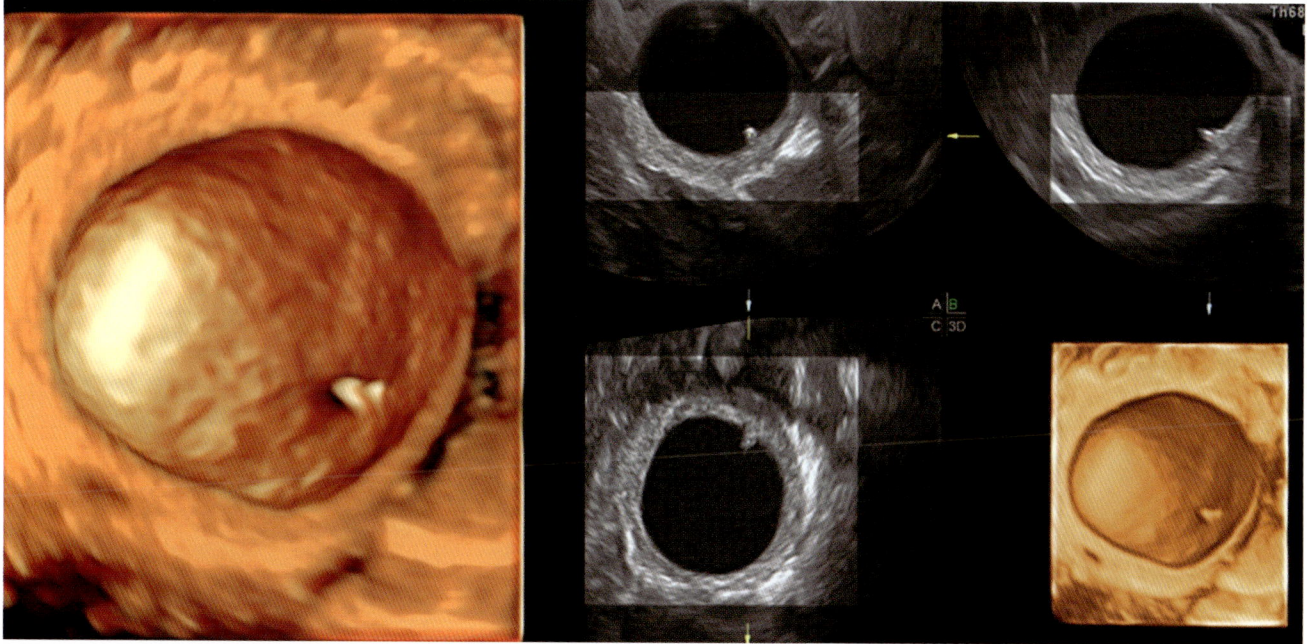

Fig. 3.12: Cumulus oophorus.

– It is important to emphasize that two of the ultrasound images, the reticular, and especially the eco-gray, may be unnoticed with 2D transvaginal ultrasound, especially if Doppler is not used **(Fig. 3.16)**.

Corpus Luteum

The 3D ultrasound images of the corpus luteum are:
- *Three-layered corpus luteum:* The corpus luteum reveals an external hyper-refringent layer with

transvaginal 2D, due to thickening of the theca wall, an intermediate gray layer, due to the refringence of the luteinized theca granulose, and an internal and central dark layer that is due to blood accumulation. This is the most common image. It is present in 90% of cases **(Figs. 3.16 and 3.17)**.

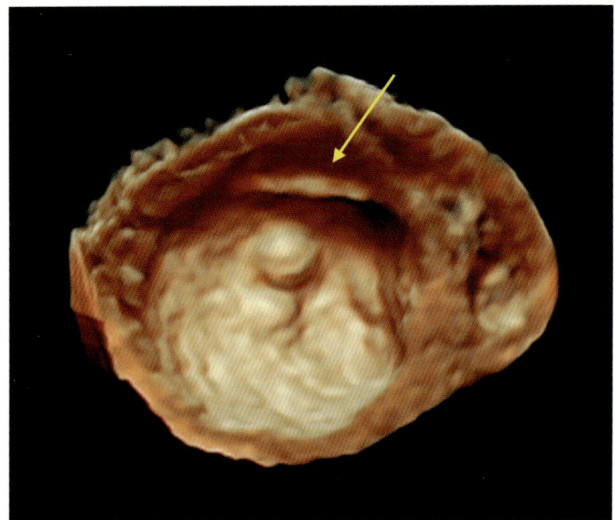

Fig. 3.13: Cumulus oophorus, in his upper part we see the uncoupling of a part of the granulosa (arrow).

- *Corpus luteum with a reticular pattern:* This image usually appears 48–72 h after ovulation. It is produced by a clot, reticulin fibers, collagen, and disseminated luteinized cells that they confer a reticular aspect to the corpus luteum **(Fig. 3.18)**.
- *Eco-gray corpus luteum:* This image is difficult to differentiate from ovarian stromal, but very simple to observe with Doppler, since the characteristic intense peripheral vascularization of very low resistance that is known as "ring of fire," appears **(Fig. 3.19)**. Without Doppler, it may remain unnoticed and be confused with ovarian stromal. With 3D Doppler, diagnosis is very easy **(Fig. 3.19)**.
- This image is produced by the luteinized granulosa-theca that is occupying the entire follicular cavity without the presence of blood or clots. It is typical after day 21 of the cycle **(Figs. 3.19 and 3.20)**.
- Given the enormous vascularization that is produced by the invasion of vessels from the luteinized theca-granulosa, Doppler study is of extraordinary help.
- The corpus luteum attains a 2–3 cm size, but it can easily grow to 5 cm, and may be confused with pathologic cysts or other tumors.
- This image disappears with menstruation.

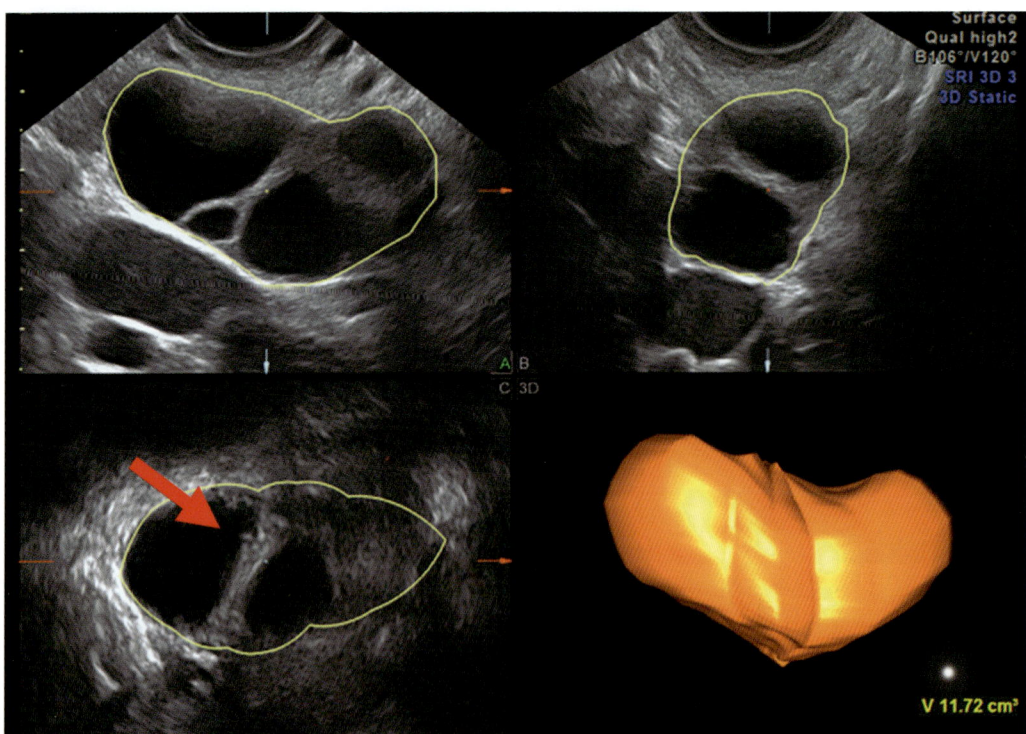

Fig. 3.14: Rosebush thorns (red arrow).

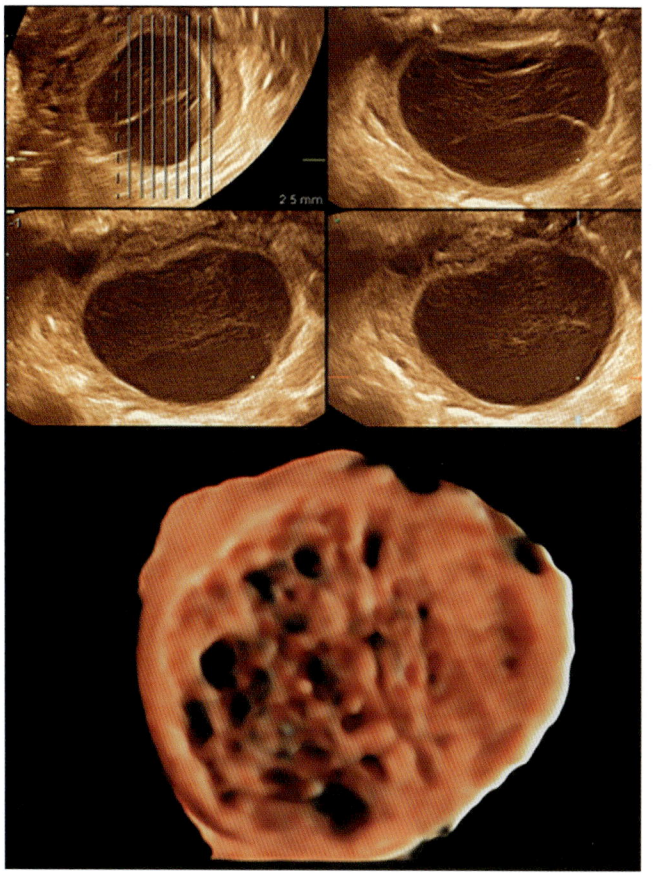

- All of these ovarian changes will be accompanied by corresponding endometrial changes that we will address further ahead.
- Follicles that persist after day 14 without presenting corpus luteum imaging, and naturally, without Doppler effect, changes are unruptured luteinized follicles (ULF).
- These are not unusual (they are observed in 6% of induced cycles).

DOPPLER IN A NATURAL CYCLE

- Except for 24 h prior to ovulation when perifollicular vascularization can be detected, Doppler has no application in spontaneous folliculogenesis.
- Neither does it predict hyperstimulation in induced cycles.
- During the 24 h prior to ovulation, the dominant follicle is surrounded by, a low resistance, thin vascular layer that occupies 50–75% of the follicular periphery **(Fig. 3.21)**.

Corpus Luteum Functionality

- Doppler study evaluates corpus luteum function, which becomes an exceptional application of ultrasound.

Fig. 3.15: Hemorrhagic corpus luteum depicted with 3D tomographic and high definition live views.

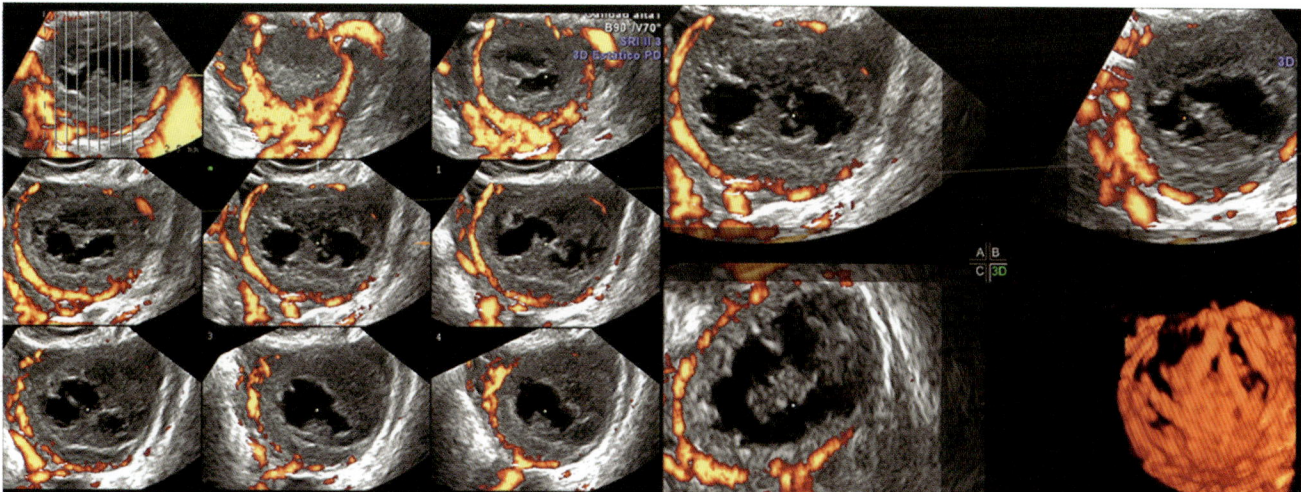

Fig. 3.16: Three-layered corpus luteum visualized with three-orthogonal planes and power Doppler. The central part is clearly depicted as eco negative image (blood). At is around, an eco-gray sheet, the luteinized granulosa-theca sheet, and in the outer part and with numerous vessels showing the typical image of "the ring of fire" a more white sheet.

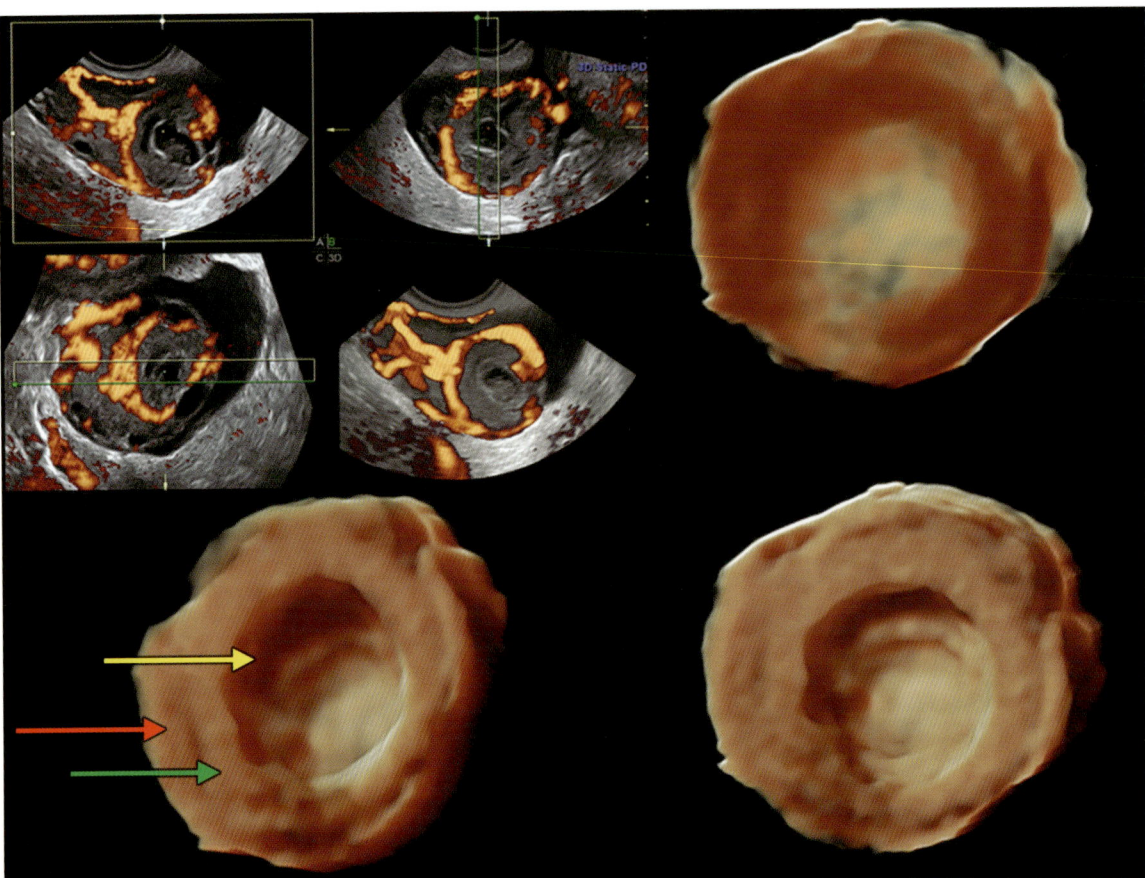

Fig. 3.17: Three-sheet high definition live corpus luteum. The yellow arrow shows the cavity, the green the granulose, and the red one the theca layer. The above left part of the figure shows the "fire ring" power Doppler, typical image, as well as the corpus luteum in maximum luminescence (above right).

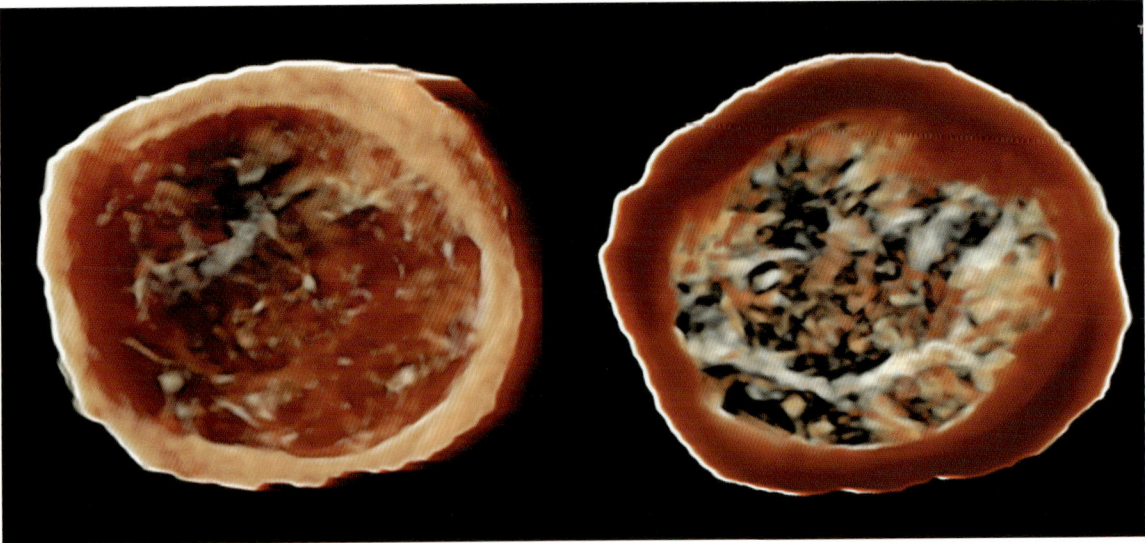

Fig. 3.18: Corpus luteum reticularis. Observe how well the reticulum is visualized using high definition live and maximum luminescence.

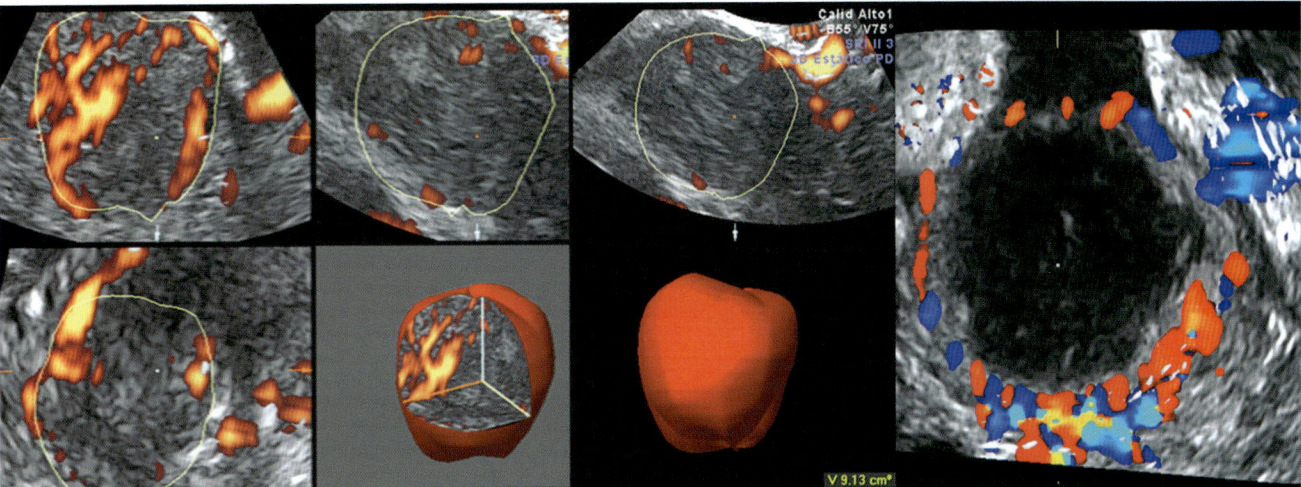

Fig. 3.19: An eco-gray corpus luteum with the characteristic "ring of fire" produced by the enormous quantity of vessels, which are surrounding the preovulatory follicle as well as the corpus luteum. We are showing the "ring" with color and Doppler energy. In the center image, and in red color, the volume of the corpus luteum is calculated with virtual organ computer-aided analysis.

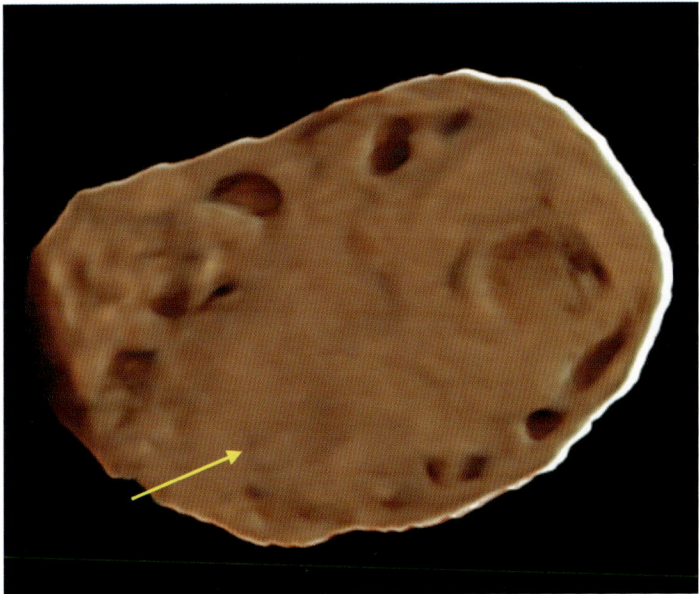

Fig. 3.20: Gray corpus depicted with high definition live (arrow). This image is difficult to differentiate from ovarian stromal, but very simple to observe with Doppler, since the characteristic intense peripheral vascularization of very low resistance that is known as "ring of fire".

- The luteinized granulosa-theca is rich in thick and very low resistance blood vessels.
- Because of this, the "ring of fire" above mentioned that is formed by all the vessels that surround the corpus luteum periphery are pathognomonic of a mature follicle and subsequently, of the corpus luteum. It is present in all cases, independently of the type of corpus luteum that appears **(Figs. 3.16, 3.19, and 3.21).**
- Measurement of resistive and pulsatility indexes provide us with knowledge of its functional activity. We can also evaluate whether there is corpus luteum insufficiency, if impedance remains high or if there is an increase in impedance during the secretory phase.

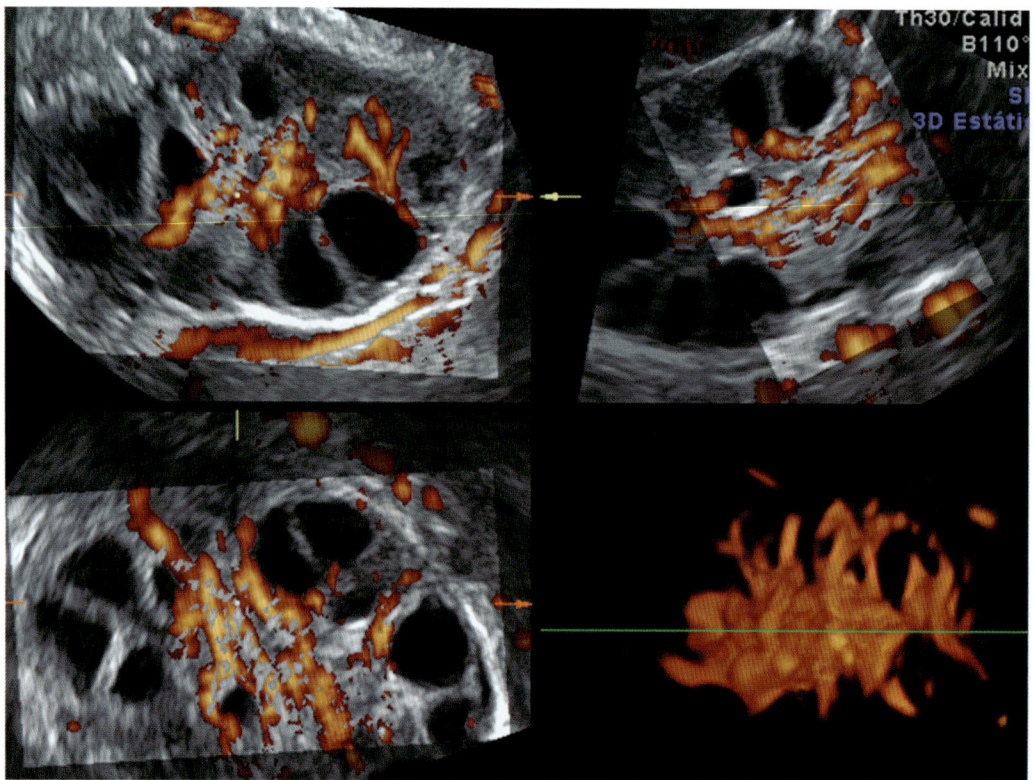

Fig. 3.21: Hyperstimulation showed with Doppler energy. Many ovulatory follicles all showing "ring of fire" are depicted. We also show the 3D angio-Doppler vascularity (below right).

FOLLICULOGENESIS IN AN INDUCED CYCLE

- Any protocol of medical ovulation induction is "antiphysiological".
- All of these protocols (clomiphene and letrozole included) produce hyperstimulation as a consequence, by selecting a greater number of follicles that develop faster and in a shorter time.
- Although this effect seems to be theoretically counter-productive, it really is not, because humans have millions of primordial and primary follicles to be used from the 7th month of intrauterine life on.
- At puberty, between 11 years and 13 years of age, the ovary has 350,000 follicles that will produce 400–450 ovulations during reproductive life.
- In other words, ovarian reserve is high.
- Medical induction of multiple follicles with subsequent ovulation will not end their supply prematurely.
- This knowledge is fundamental for ultrasound control and evaluation of the differences between spontaneous and induced folliculogenesis.

- In induced folliculogenesis, a base ultrasound should be done to evaluate ovarian reserve.
- The following ultrasound should be done 5 or 6 days after stimulation with gonadotropins or 3–4 days of finishing clomiphene or letrozole induction.
- It does not make sense to evaluate earlier with ultrasound.
- Neither should estradiol levels be done in those days.
- Follicular growth is not synchronic. Existing AFs initiate their growth, but they initiate it at different times and at different speeds.
- This lack of synchrony is one of the basic problems of ovulation induction.
- The growth rate is faster than with spontaneous ovulation.
- Follicles grow exponentially and much faster.
- Once hCG is administered to liberate ovulation with a follicular diameter of 17–18 mm, follicles continue growing for about 40 h.
- Follicle growth does not occur in parallel with 17β-estradiol production.

- The global level represents the total production of all follicles.
- But since growth is not synchronic, i.e. production by follicles of different sizes and growing at different speeds, they will produce different quantities of estradiol.
- The global level must be divided by the total number of follicles observed to estimate the approximate production of each one.
- The number obtained is therefore only an approximation.
- There are some follicles that produce much estradiol and others a scant amount.
- The value obtained from this division presupposes that all follicles produce identical amounts of hormone, which is not true.
- The largest follicle does not always contain the most mature oocyte, neither is it always the one with the highest hormonal production.
- For this reason, it is advisable to aspirate all follicles that exceed 14 mm and all those that show an oocyte-cumulus complex.
- As it may be noticed, ultrasound is a basic need for adequate control of a cycle by ovarian stimulation.
- The cycle will be canceled when more than 10 AFs are observed and/or estradiol is above 2,500 pg/mL.
- An exception, of course, will be when ovulation induction is done with a subcutaneous agonist, the so called "agonist bolus."

DOPPLER IN AN INDUCED CYCLE

- Although there was an expectation that with ultrasonography it would be possible to avoid the potentially grave complication of ovarian hyperstimulation syndrome, we believe that neither 2D nor 3D angiography can effectively prevent it **(Fig. 3.21)**.
- This complication can occur independent of the size or number of ovarian perifollicular or medullar vessels existent.
- Basically, the follicular growth and number must be monitored while stimulation is under way.

NEW ULTRASOUND MODES

Ultrasound should guide the moment of hCG administration for:

- The collection of the greatest number of best quality oocytes

- Obtaining in this way good embryos, and,
- Increasing the rate of gestations.

The new ultrasound modes, applied to ovulation induction, are contributing relevant data in relation to the actual modes used in reproduction—AVC, inverse mode, VOCAL, HD Live, and Silhouette.

Automatic Volume Calculation and Virtual Organ Computer-aided Analysis

Advantages provided:

- Semiautomatic evaluation of AF number, their diameters and the volume of their follicular fluid in a much more precise way than was up to now done **(Figs. 3.22 to 3.25)**.
- This is of utmost importance for prediction of ovarian response and selection of stimulation protocol.
  - Volumetric appraisal of each AF.
    - This has allowed us to find out that:
      - A 1 mL volume corresponds with a diameter more than 12 mm.
      - A 4 mL volume corresponds with a diameter more than 18–20 mm.
      - A 7 mL volume corresponds with a diameter more than 24 mm.
    - The value obtained with this technology correlates better with the degree of oocyte maturation observed after aspiration.
  - From all this we have deduced something very important for clinical care:
    - The dominant follicle will not affect the fertilization of smaller AF that is also aspirated for IVF procedures.
    - Aspiration of follicles larger than 12–14 mm allows recovery of phase II oocytes.
    - Following hCG administration, the greatest number of mature oocytes is obtained from follicles between 18 mm and 20 mm. It is not necessary to wait for larger follicles. Because of this, more than only larger AF can be aspirated with a likelihood of obtaining oocytes.
    - The VOCAL mode is especially interesting in the volumetric evaluation either of the wall ovary as well as for each AF **(Figs. 3.6, 3.19, and 3.26)**. Ovarian volume is nowadays considered diagnostic criteria in polycystic ovarian syndrome (PCOS).

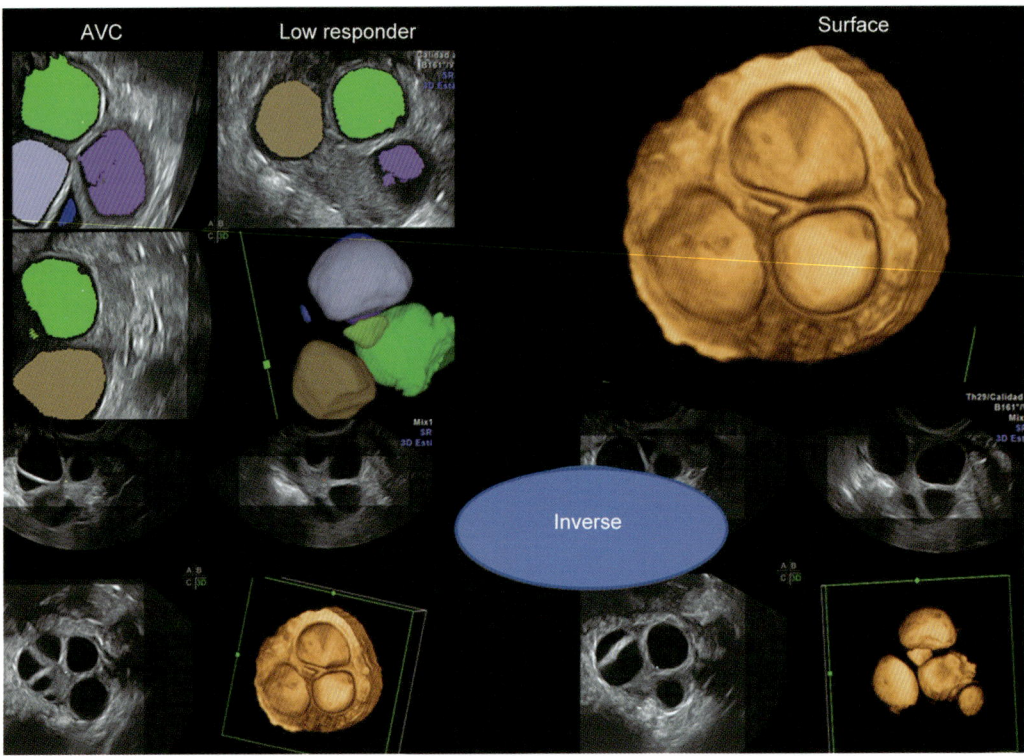

Fig. 3.22: Image of a low ovarian reserve. Automatic volume calculation and surface mode are showing very few follicles in the cortical part of the ovary (automatic volume calculation, above left, surface 3D mode above right and below left, and inverse mode below right).

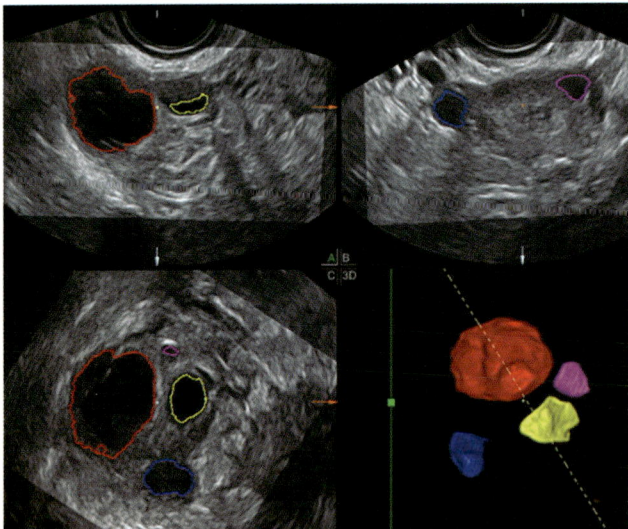

Fig. 3.23: Low ovarian reserve image. Only four antral follicles are shown with 2D but also, and very specially, when using automatic volume calculation (below right).

Inverse Mode

- This is a very interesting mode for evaluation of the number and volume of AF **(Figs. 3.26 and 3.27)**. It is useful for calculating ovarian reserve.
- By applying this mode, the ovarian parenchyma is not seen. The echo-negative follicles become echo-positive.
- Recently, use of this mode has come into question because it seems that small AFs are not seen **(Fig. 3.28)**.

HD Live and Silhouette Modes

As we have insisted repeatedly, HD live has been the first ultrasound mode, following the introduction of high frequency vaginal probes that have improved image quality **(Fig. 3.29)**.

Silhouette mode has been introduced recently. It helps define more neatly the images **(Fig. 3.30)**. We allude to this mode in several figures.

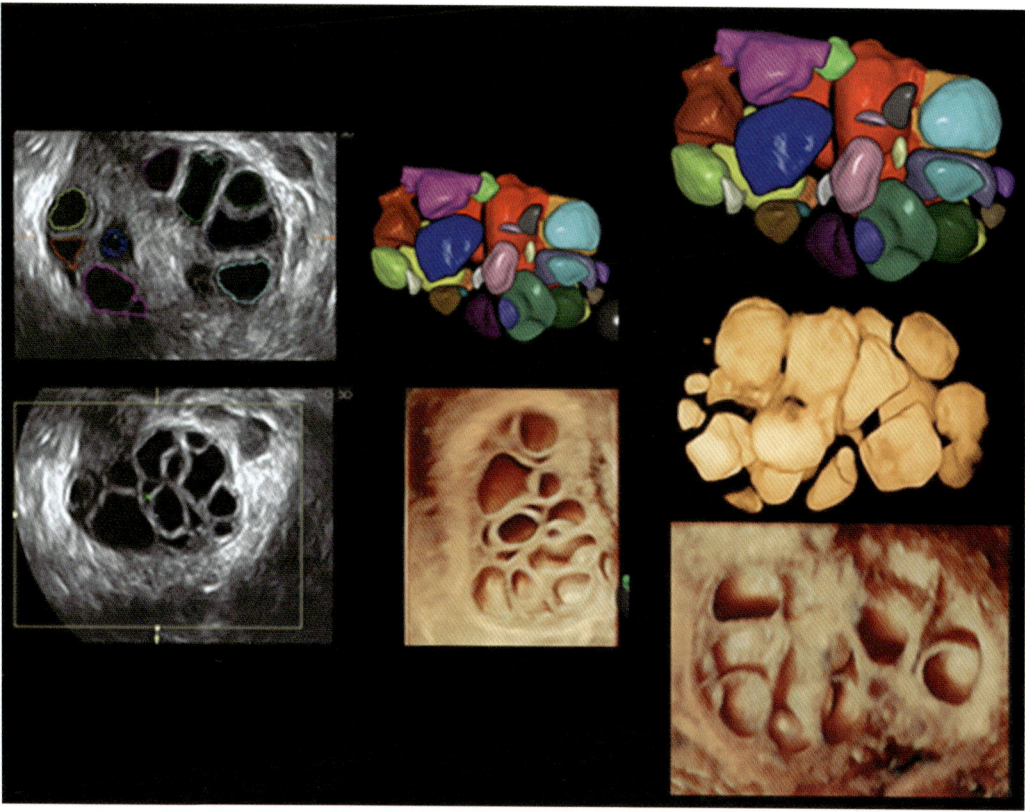

Fig. 3.24: Excellent answer to gonadotropins due to existing a very good ovarian reserve. 2D/3D, high definition live, inverse mode, and automatic volume calculation, of a hyperstimulated ovary. The existing antral follicle, better observed than in 2D, appears indifferent colors. The computer calculates automatically the number, their measurements and volume.

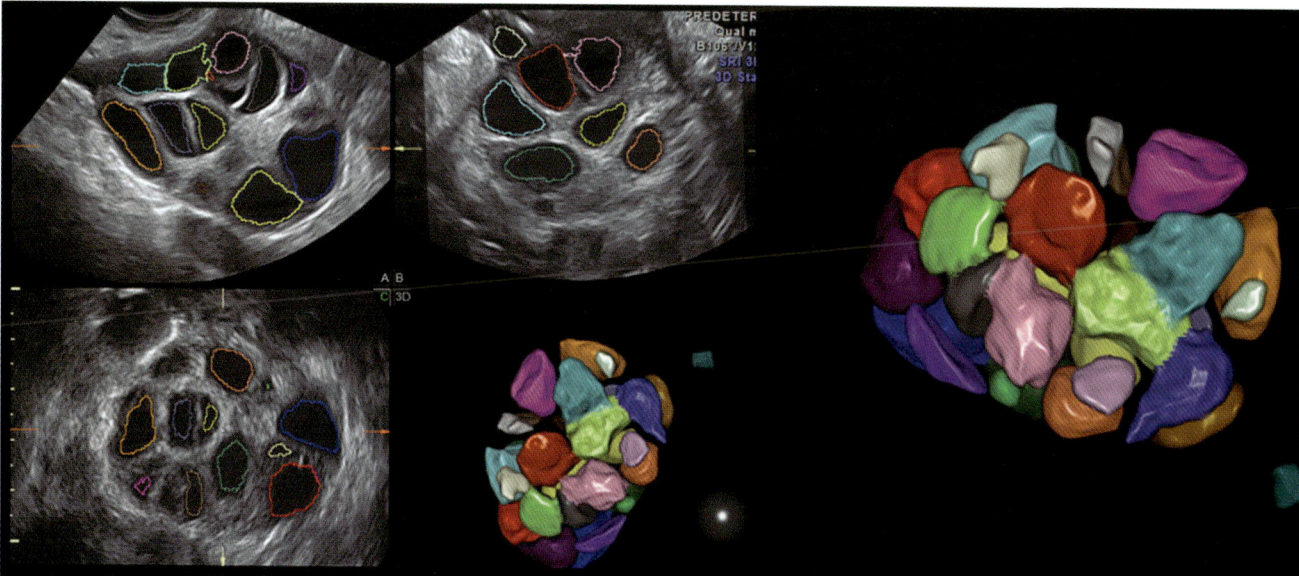

Fig. 3.25: Automatic volume calculation mode. High response to ovulation induction, risk of hyperstimulation. Newly each antral follicles appear with a different color and the software will calculate its volume. In this way, the follicles to be punctured can be selected.

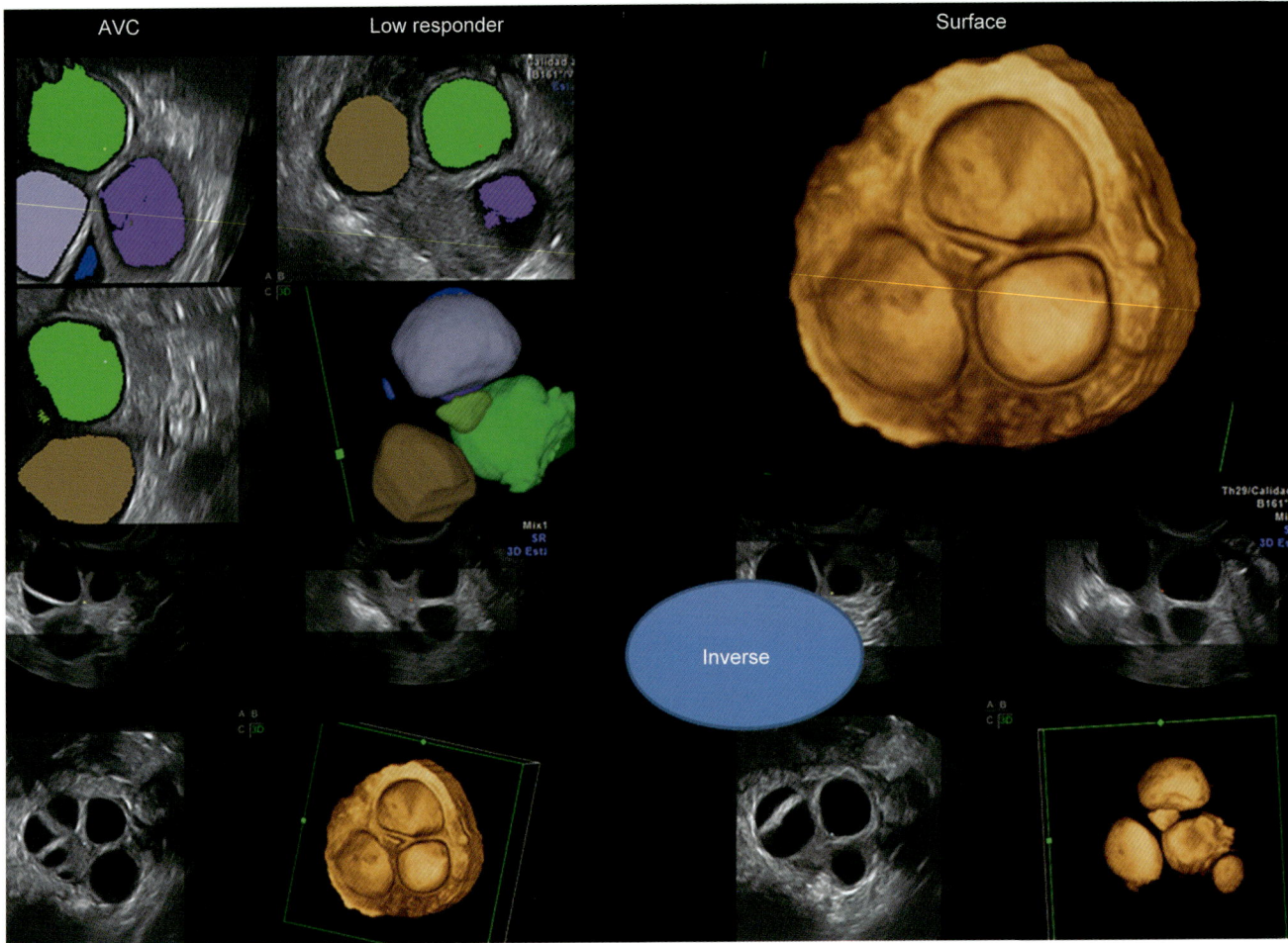

Fig. 3.26: Inverse mode of an ovary with an excellent reserve.

STUDY OF THE ENDOMETRIUM

In folliculogenesis, almost as important as the impact on oocytes is the effect on the endometrium, also known as endometrial receptivity.

Ultrasound parameters associated with reproductive results in IVF or ICSI cycles:

- Endometrial thickness
- Endometrial pattern (echogenicity and homogeneity)
- Volume, and
- Vascularization findings with 3D or 4D.

Endometrial Thickness

Although still a controversial subject, we considered more than 8 mm an adequate endometrial thickness. However, we recognize that gestations are possible with lesser thicknesses, even less than 4–5 mm.

Echogenicity and Homogeneity

The best reproductive results are obtained in IVF or ICSI cycles, when the trilaminar line is observed during the periovulatory period.

Endometrial Volume

Not one woman became pregnant when endometrial volume was less than 2 mL. Gestation occurred only in 5% of women with a 2–3 mL volume, and in all cases where gestation was achieved the volume was more than 6 mL (**Figs. 3.31 and 3.32**).

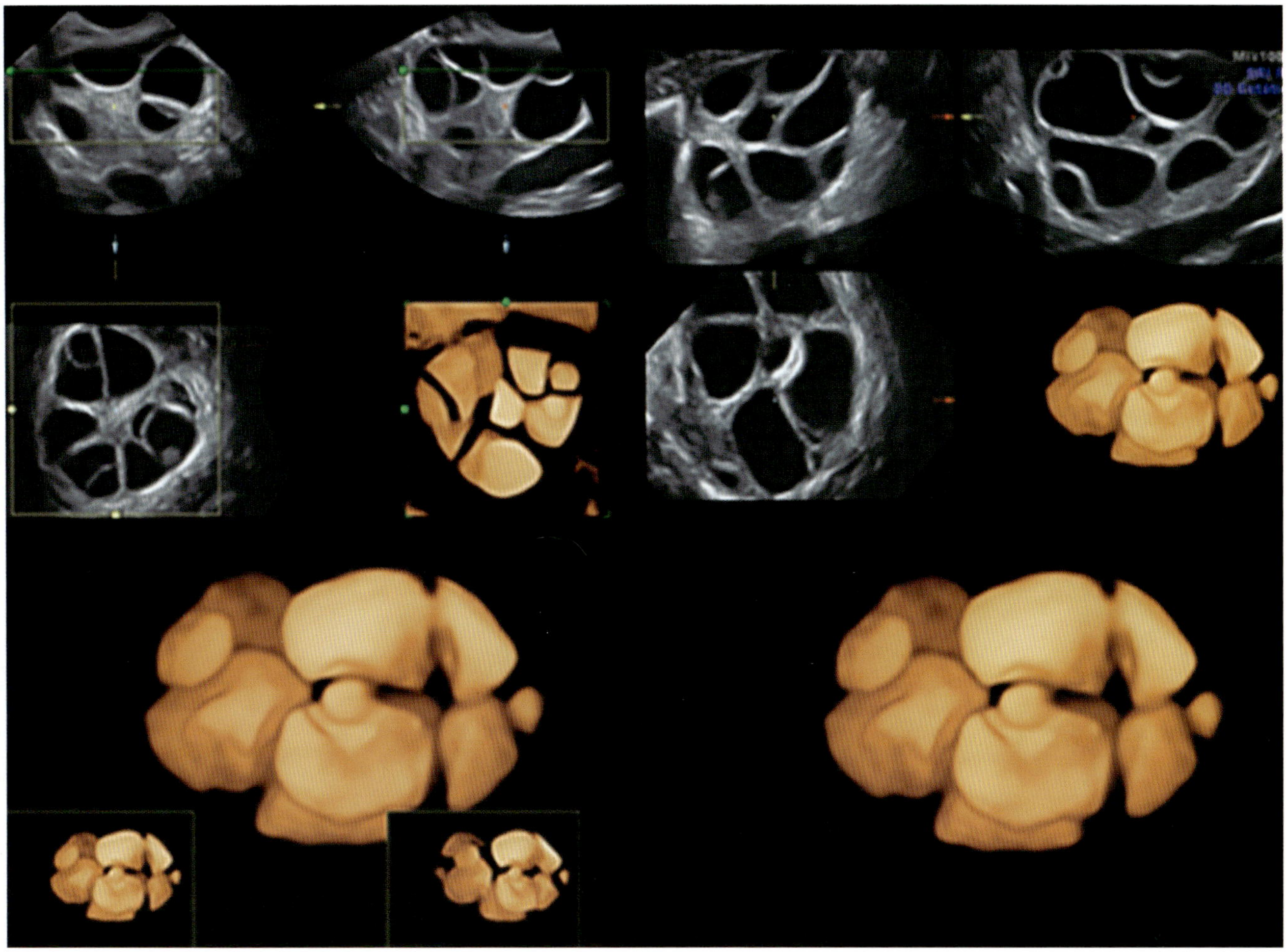

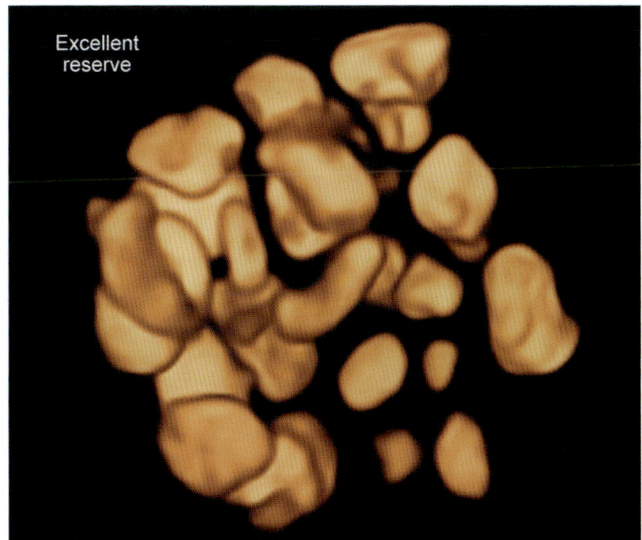

Fig. 3.27: Antral follicle calculation using inverse mode in a case of hyperstimulation.

Fig. 3.28: Inverse mode of an ovary with excellent reserve. Each follicle appears in yellow color.

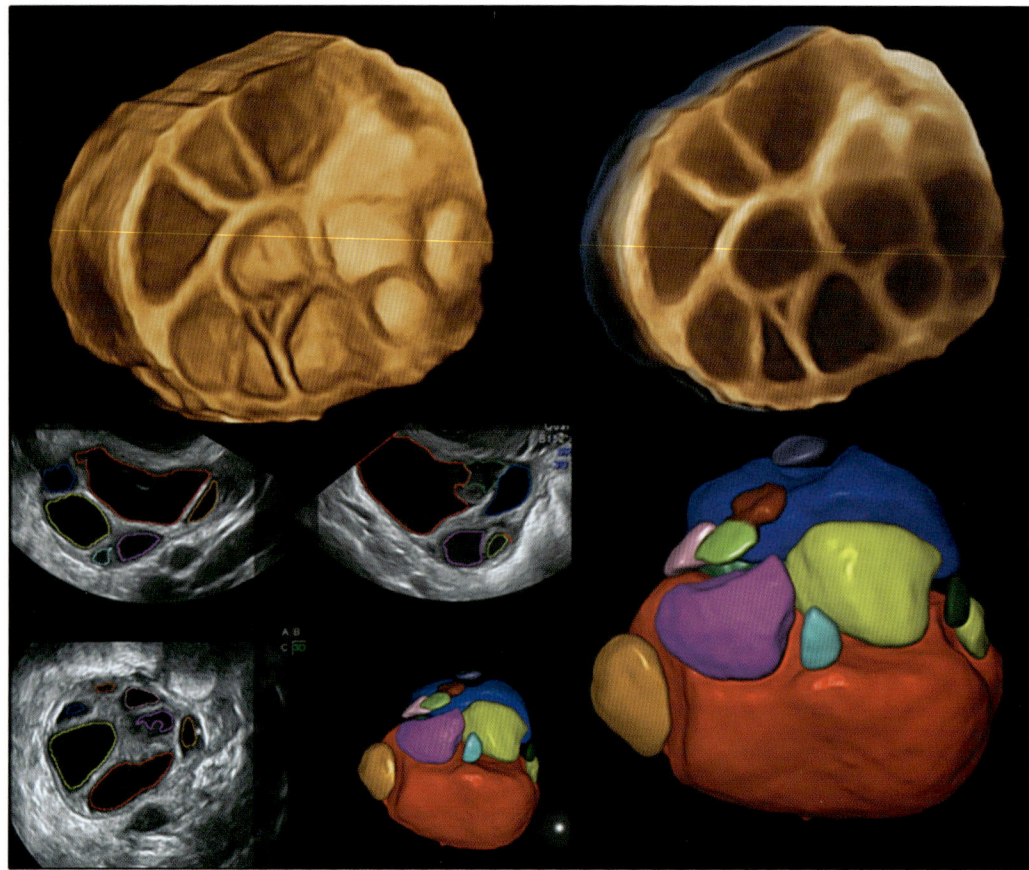

Fig. 3.29: 3D high definition live and automatic volume calculation in a hyperstimulated ovary. Look at the quality of the obtained images. Compare with the 2D vaginal images (below left) in orthogonal planes.

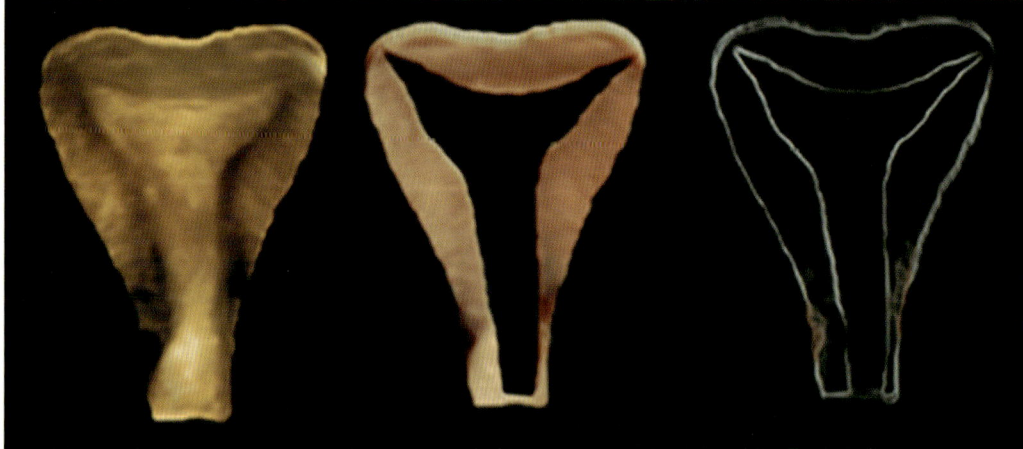

Fig. 3.30: Mode 3D high definition live, and using magic cut, of the cavity. Silhouette of a normal endometrium.

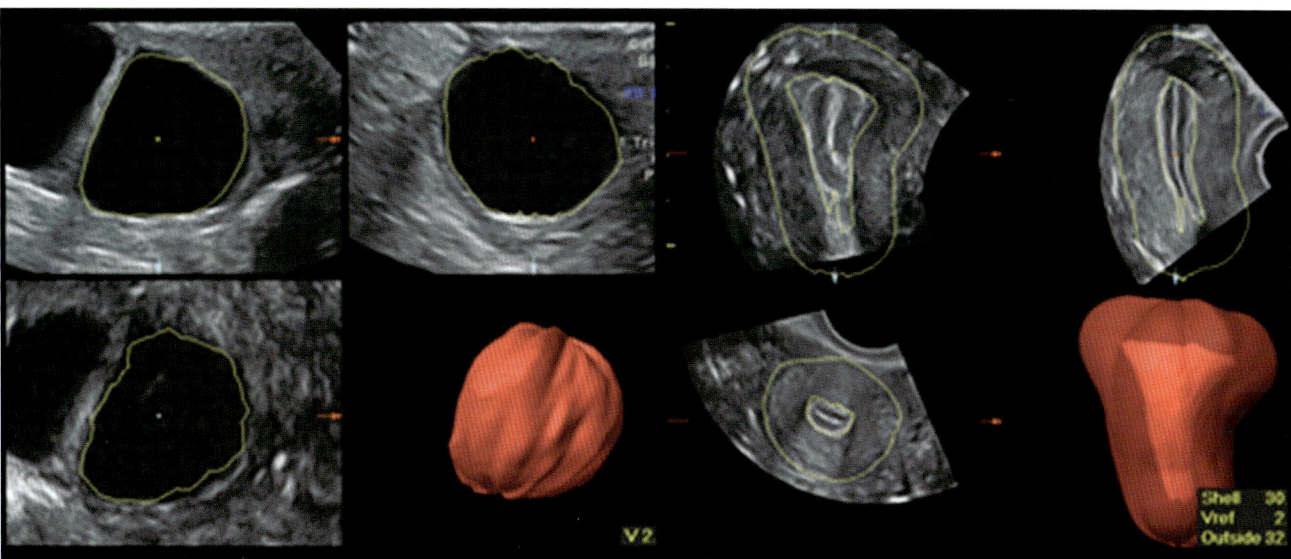

Fig. 3.31: Virtual organ computer-aided analysis mode. This is the ideal technique to evaluate the ovarian response as well as the uterine receptivity. To the left the picture shows how we are measuring the follicular volume. To the right the endometrial volume, which appears very well defined from the myometrium.

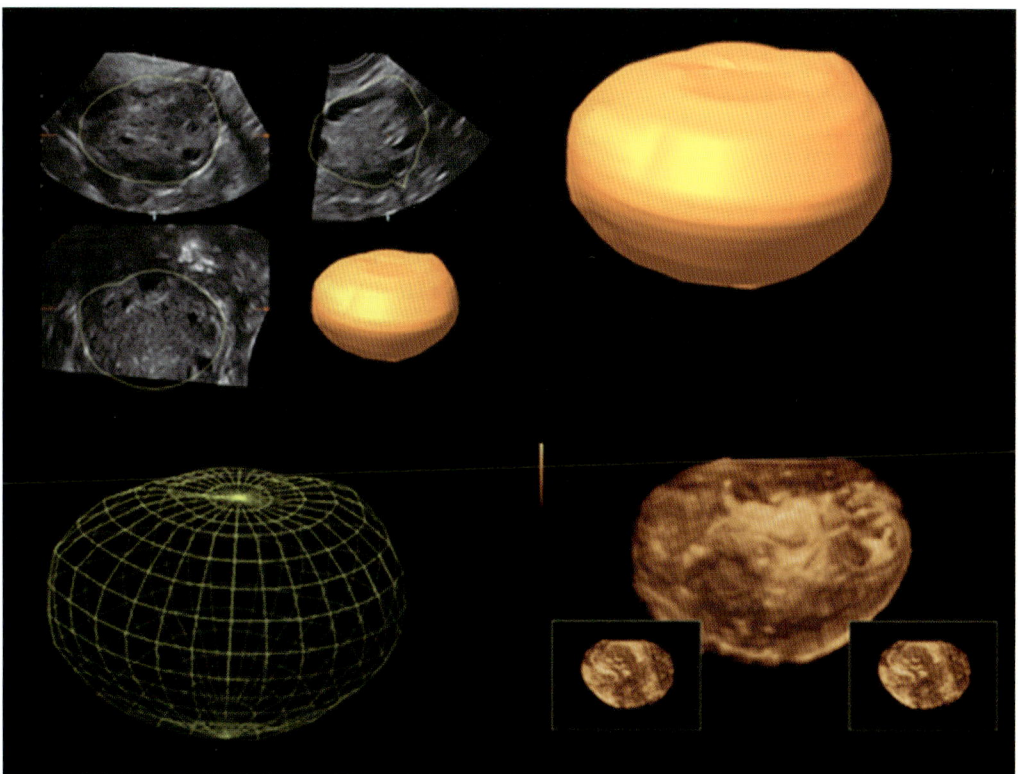

Fig. 3.32: 3D, virtual organ computer-aided analysis, and reconstruction form modes (below left). We see an ovary with scarce reserve and its corresponding volume automatically calculated with the virtual organ computer-aided analysis mode. The ovary is very small and the ultrasound machine brings electronically volume values (above and right, yellow color).

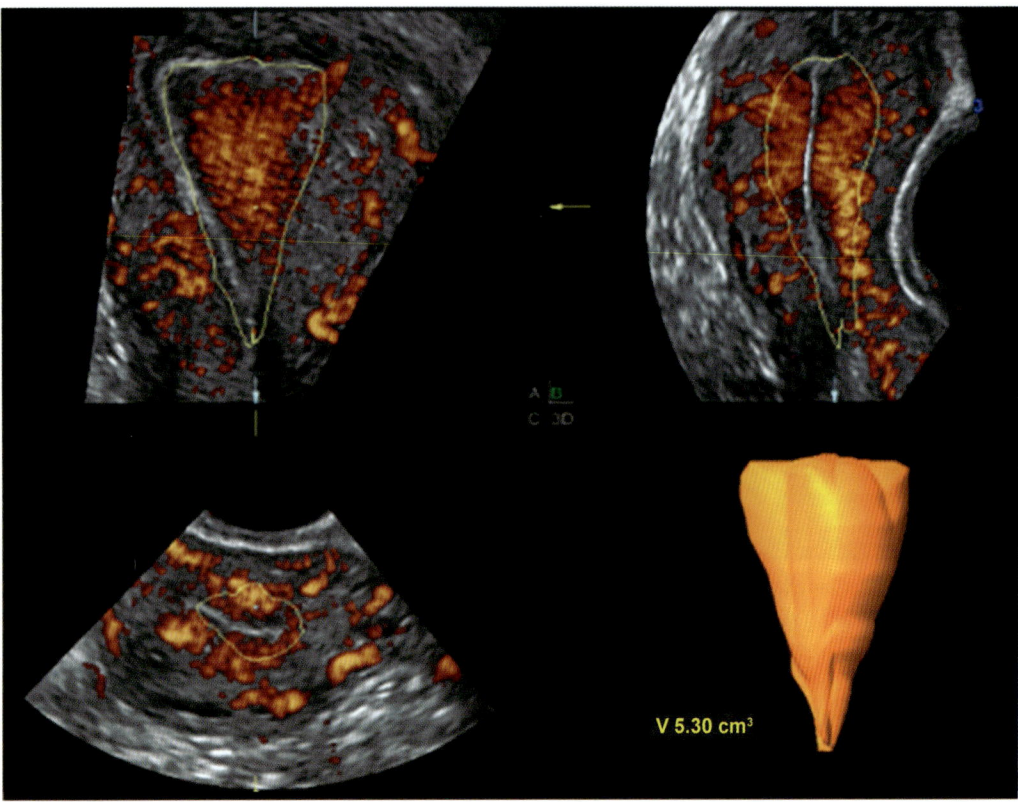

V 5.30 cm³

Fig. 3.33: Virtual organ computer-aided analysis of a normal uterus also with 3D Doppler angiography. A clear endometrial, subendometrial, and myometrium vascularization is depicted.

Endometrial Vascularization

Angio-power 3D Doppler must be used for this evaluation. There is a significant correlation between vascular indexes and reproductive success **(Fig. 3.33)**.

OVARIAN ENDOCRINOLOGIC PATHOLOGIES

Polycystic ovarian syndrome is the most common endocrinopathy in the reproductive age, affects the 12–21%, and after the advanced age, the second cause of infertility in women.

It is a complex endocrine situation due to its heterogeneity and the existing doubts about its etiology.

Various groups of investigators suggest that the origin of PCOS is genetic (polygenic) and/or one androgenic medium ambientalis effect during the fetal live, which involves the programming of the metabolic or endocrine axis, more specifically metabolism of carbohydrates and the adrenal secretion

Due to that, its diagnosis is based in clinical, biologic, and morphologic criteria its definition has suffered various revisions:

- In the consensus conference of the National Institute of Health (NIH) in 1990, the PCOS was defined as:
  - Chronic anovulation with
  - Clinic and/or biochemical hyperandrogenism, excluding other etiologies, which are clinically similar, such as thyroid or adrenal dysfunctions.
- En the year 2003, the Rotterdam consensus of the European Society for Human Reproduction or American Society of Reproductive Medicine (ESHRE or ASRM) proposed that the diagnosis must include two of the following criteria:
  - Oligo and/or anovulation,
  - Clinic and/or biochemical hyperandrogenism, and
  - Polycystic ovaries using ultrasound
    - Also excluding other etiologies as above mentioned.
- This syndrome is ultrasound characterized by:
  - Numerous small same sized peripheric AF
  - With an increased medullary tissue

– And monotonous and persistent ovarian central vascularization without cyclic changes.

– Ultrasound is nowadays an essential part of the diagnostic criteria and 3D, HD live **(Fig. 3.34)** VOCAL, inverse mode **(Fig. 3.35)**, and silhouette **(Fig. 3.36)** show more definitive images than transvaginal 2D.

■ The size of the ovarian medullaris is not considered in the Rotterdam criteria—we considered this part important for the diagnosis due to bigger size. Only using this new technology **(Fig. 3.37)** the real medullaris size can be estimated.

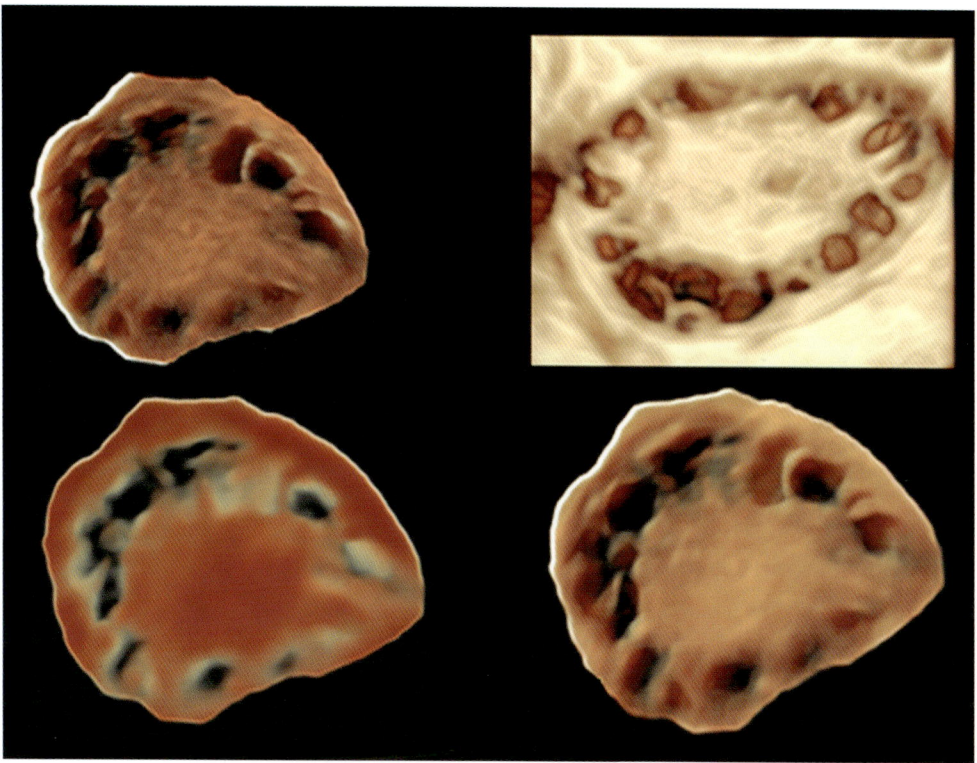

Fig. 3.34: 3D, 4D, and high definition live of typical polycystic ovarian syndrome.

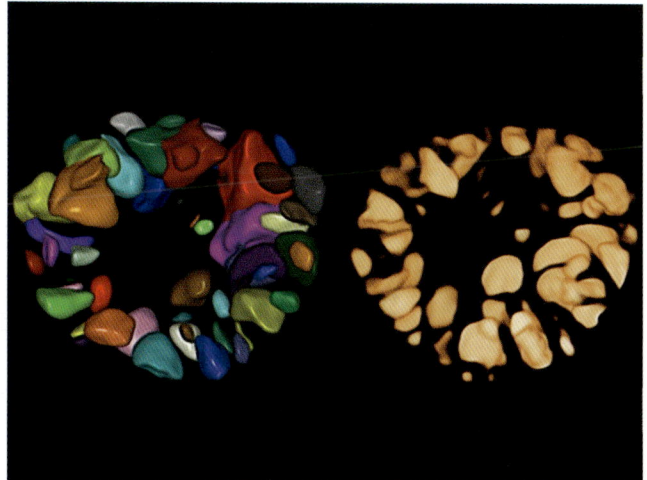

Fig. 3.35: Virtual organ computer-aided analysis, left, and inverse mode, right, of a polycystic ovarian syndrome.

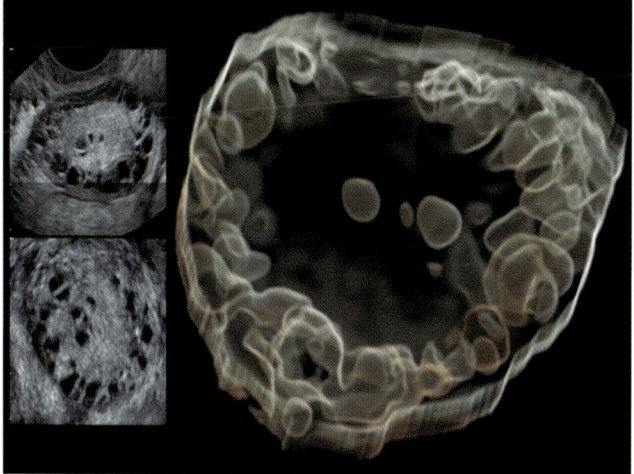

Fig. 3.36: Transvaginal 2D ultrasound, left, and the new silhouette mode, right, in typical polycystic ovarian syndrome.

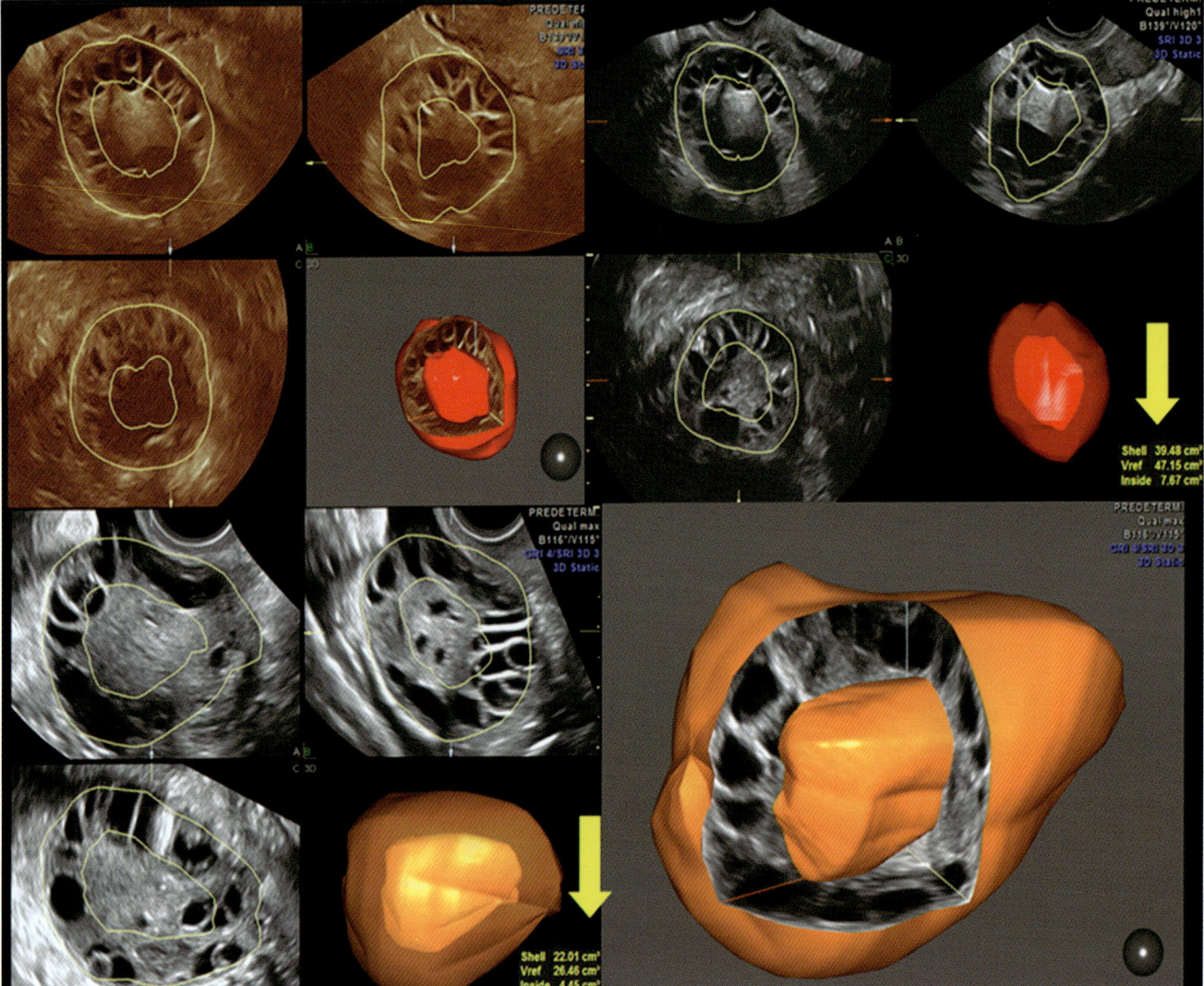

Fig. 3.37: Double niche section of the ovarian medullaris shows in red and yellow color. The computer calculates its real size (yellow arrows).

REFERENCES

1. Bonilla-Musoles F, Castillo JC, Caballero O, Raga F, Bonilla Jr. F: Ultrasonidos y Foliculogénesis. In: Ultrasonidos en Obstetricia, Reproducción y Ginecología. Madrid. Editorial Médica Panamericana; 2018. pp. 509-527.

2. Bonilla-Musoles F, Dolz M, Raga F, Moreno J. Reproducción Asistida: Abordaje en la práctica clínica. Madrid: Editorial Médica Panamericana; 2010.

Application of 3D in First Trimester

Marisa Borenstein Guelman, Guillermo Azumendi Pérez

INTRODUCTION

The first trimester of pregnancy is the most critical moment for the embryo and fetal development in terms of rapid changes and modification of its internal and external appearance. It is a very complex process that we were not able to see or understand completely. The modern ultrasound (US) equipment and all the available tools enable us to identify some of these changes as early as 5–7 weeks after last menstrual period (LMP).

The relevance of three-dimensional US (3D) in the detection and demonstration of fetal abnormalities has already been proven. Some of the 3D or four-dimensional (4D) tools have shown some benefit compared with the two-dimensional (2D) US when a malformation is present in particular to visualize the problem from different perspectives, to obtain other doctors, opinion, to share volumes with colleagues and as academic or teaching material. In addition, 3D images are usually clearer for parents to understand the problem or the normality of the small fetus. The surface mode and the multiplanar mode of display are the most used in these situations. In summary, we could say there are five main aspects of the 3D or 4D US to mention that are relevant during the first trimester of pregnancy—(1) the multiplanar approach of the embryo and fetus; (2) the ability to obtain planes that are not accessible with 2D US; (3) the possibility to do an off-line analysis of acquired 3D or 4D volumes and telemedicine; (4) the images are usually easier to interpret for parents when displayed with surface mode; and (5) the increasing amount of tools available to process fetal images and perform different measurements.

The objective of this chapter is to briefly explain which are the potential applications of 3D US during the first trimester of pregnancy in the embryonic and fetal periods. The main tools that will be discussed are listed in **Table 4.1**. Not all the available tools are useful in the first trimester and therefore we will focus on those applications that are of interest although some of them are not widely available.

SURFACE MODE

The study of the embryo from week 5 to 9–10 after last menstrual period (LMP) is called sonoembryology and it is based on the observation performed by Carnegie in 1914, when he described 23 different developmental stages of the embryo. In the past, all the studies were carried out with microscopic magnetic resonance, which has low resolution and it was time-consuming. As the US machines got better resolution and with the introduction of high-resolution transvaginal (TV) probes, it is now possible to perform the so-called 3D US sonoembryology. The images obtained during this period are of great resolution but a learning curve is needed to improve the interpretations of such images. Several studies reported the feasibility of this assessment and its benefits including the use of a novel 3D tool for surface rendering called high definition (HD) live.[1-8] This approach of the embryo allows the operator to identify with great detail the developmental changes that the embryo experiences day-to-day during this period. Some may believe this is only science fiction, but thanks to the advance of the technology, it is a reality.

The combination of high frequency TV probes, sono-embryology, and HD live silhouette is being referred as the "see-through fashion".[9]

All the structures in the uterus are seen with this approach including decidua and chorion, yolk sac, embryo, and umbilical cord. There is still difficulty in the

Table 4.1: 3D or 4D ultrasound tools used in the first trimester of pregnancy.

3D or 4D ultrasound tool	Application in first trimester
Surface mode: Renderization (different settings to display—HD live, dynamic render, silhouette, and studio)	• Sonoembryology (5th–10th week development of the embryo, decidua, and yolk sac) • Visualization of external defects • Provide nice pictures for parents
Multiplanar mode (standard volume manipulation with reference dots, TUI, and OmniView)	• Identification of adequate planes to perform measurements • Volume manipulation • Interpretation of fetal defects
Volume calculation (VOCAL and SONOAVC)	Calculate volume of any fetal structure, placenta and amniotic sac
STIC (spatiotemporal image correlation)	From 11 weeks onwards, better if TV approach of the fetal heart

(3D HD: Three-dimensional high definition; 4D: four-dimensional; SONOAVC: sonography-based automated volume count; TUI: tomographic ultrasonographic imaging; TV: transvaginal; VOCAL: virtual organ computer-aided analysis)

visualization of the amniotic membrane since it is too thin to be clearly identified with 3D US **(Figs. 4.1A to E)**.

Detection or suspicion of embryo abnormalities should be taken with care, since expert opinion is required before counseling the parents regarding abnormal findings in this early stage of pregnancy. The 3D sonoembryology is extremely useful as a research and investigation field, which is rapidly increasing our knowledge about such a complex biological process as it is the embryonic period. The reader could refer to specific texts for more detailed information about embryo development and sonoembryology.[1-9]

At the end of the 10th week, the fetal period begins and there is a rapid growth of fetal structures with a great differentiation in several internal organs. The surface of the fetus is also modified due to an increase in fetal movements and its position in the uterus. At 10–12 weeks, the fetus lies horizontal, which facilitates its visualization and by the end of the 13th week, they lie more vertical, probably due to the vertical growth of the uterus. At 11–13[+6] weeks of gestation, the scan is performed for the assessment of markers of chromosomal abnormalities, fetal anatomy evaluation, and screening for preeclampsia.[10-12] In the past, this scan was performed with abdominal approach in many centers but with the introduction of high-frequency TV prove the combination of both abdominal and vaginal approach provides a remarkable improvement in the visualization of the fetal anatomy. In this respect, images obtained by high-frequency TV probes are of much better resolution compared with the ones obtained abdominally and this is critically important

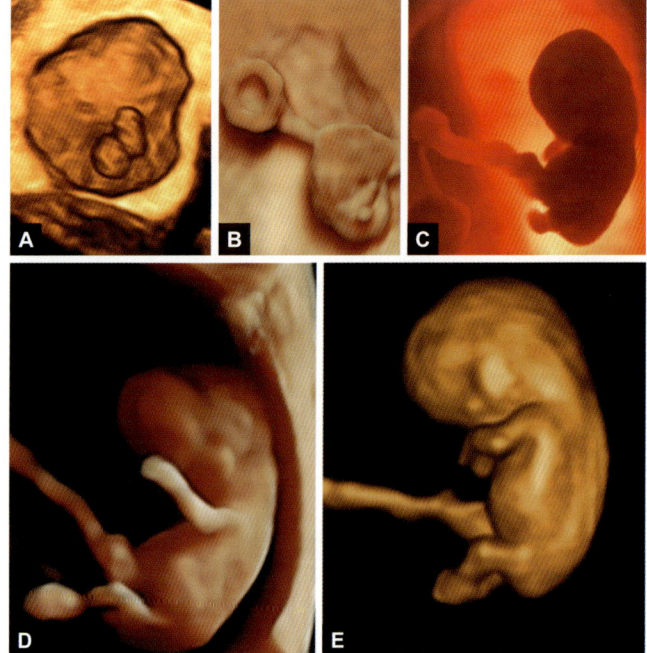

Figs. 4.1A to E: Three-dimensional images of embryos in the first trimester displayed with different surface mode renderization—(A) embryo at 6 weeks and yolk sac very close to it with surface mode; (B) Embryo at 7 weeks and yolk sac separated from the embryo displayed with HD live; (C) Embryo at 8 weeks with HD live; (D) Embryo at 9 weeks with HD live, note the physiologic umbilical hernia; and (E) 10 weeks embryo with standard surface mode.

in the acquisition of volume, since the quality of the volume is in direct relation to the quality of the 2D image. Surface mode of 3D or 4D US is useful during this scan to show nice pictures and fetal movement to the parents with a spectacular bonding effect. There are a number of different modes of display the 3D renderization—in from the classical surface mode to the *dynamic rendering or fetoscopic view* that creates a sensation of more depth in the volume; *HD live* that allows a great modification in term of illumination of the image increasing the facial features and gestures; *HD live silhouette* that improves the definition of borders and *studio HD* which is a recent introduction in some US brands that combines different algorithms to produce a much more realistic image of the fetal surface with the chance to modify three different parameters of light, background, and focus **(Figs. 4.2 to 4.4)**.

The skeletal mode of display is the one used to show the fetal bones and it is useful in facial or spine abnormalities. It was possible to describe the development of facial and skull bones in the first trimester in normal and syndromic fetuses **(Figs. 4.5A and B)**.[13,14]

There are a large number of fetal defects that can be detected at this stage of pregnancy with conventional 2D US by transabdominal and TV approach.[15]

The 3D US is also useful to demonstrate these fetal abnormalities using the surface mode as in abdominal wall and facial defects, abnormal extremities, and umbilical cord cysts **(Figs. 4.6 and 4.7)**. In addition, the multiplanar volume navigation becomes essential for a correct

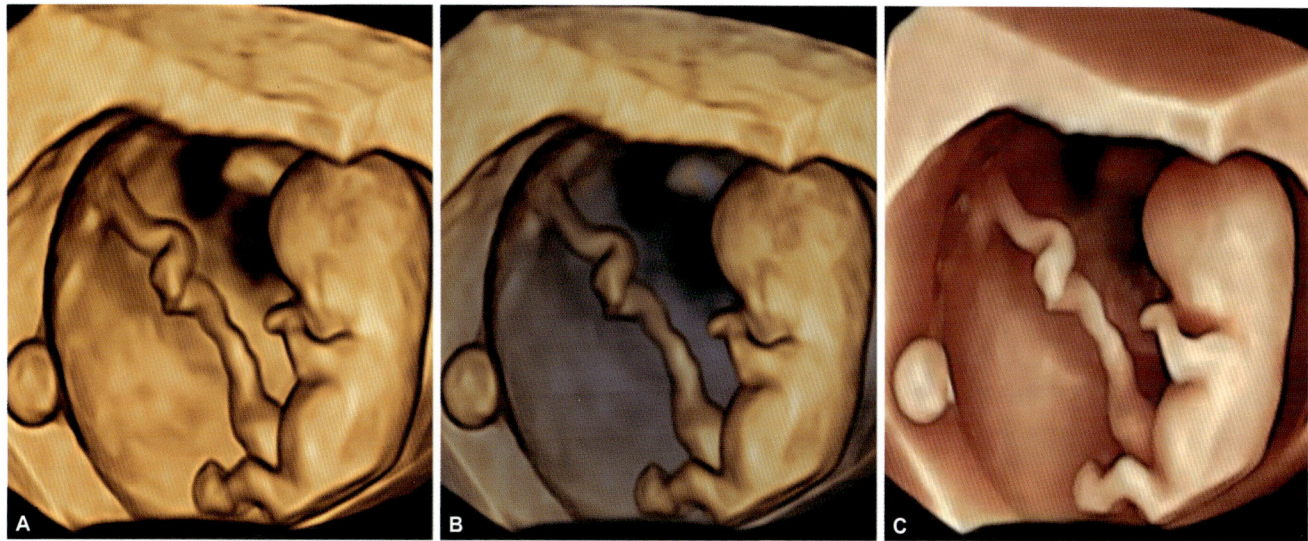

Figs. 4.2A to C: Three-dimensional image of a normal fetus at 12 weeks of gestation displayed with three different renderization surface modes: (A) Standard surface mode; (B) Dynamic rendering (note that structures far from the transducer appear darker, in blue in this case); and (C) HD live that provides a more realistic image with increase in the sensation of volume in the fetus.

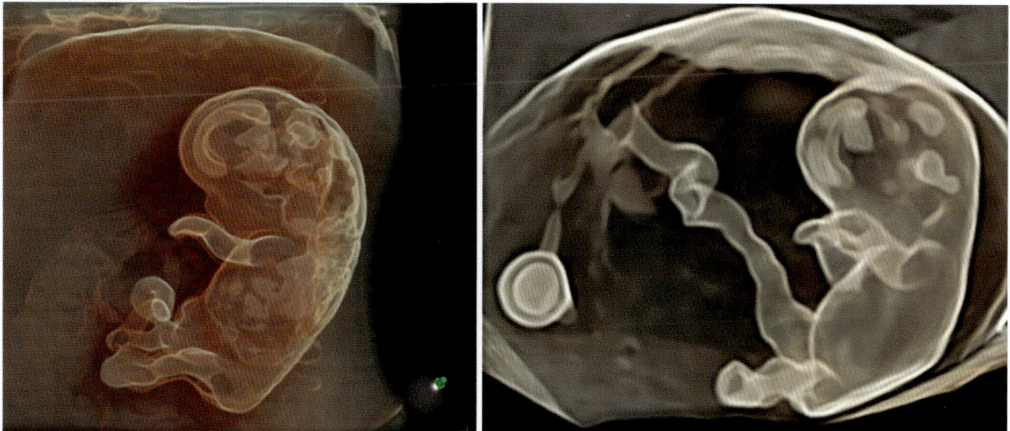

Fig. 4.3: Three-dimensional images of a normal fetus at 11 weeks of gestation displayed with HD live silhouette.

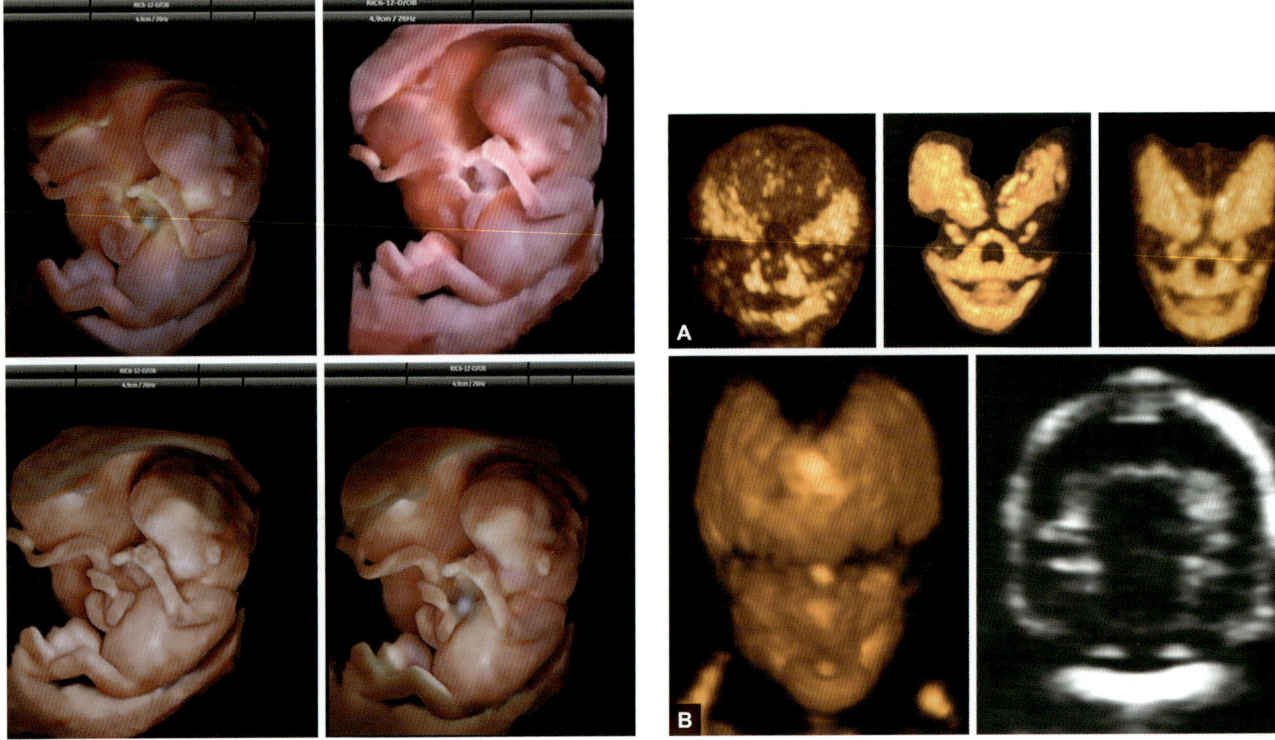

Fig. 4.4: Three-dimensional images of a normal fetus at 12+4 weeks displayed with HD studio. There are many different options for modification that can be applied to this mode.

Figs. 4.5A and B: (A) Development of the metopic suture in normal fetuses at 11, 12, and 13 weeks of gestation demonstrated with skeletal mode of renderization; (B) Abnormal metopic suture in a fetus at 12+5 weeks of gestation with holoprosencephaly and trisomy 13.

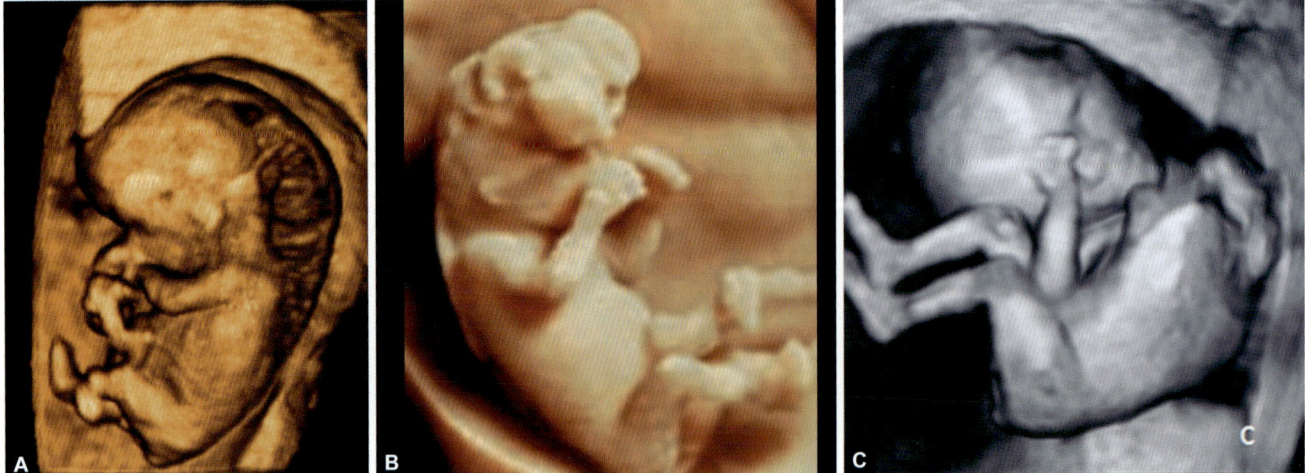

Figs. 4.6A To C: Three-dimensional images demonstrating different fetal abnormalities at 11–13+6 weeks that had been diagnosed with 2D ultrasound and were displayed in surface mode after the acquisition of 3D volumes, in order to store them and to show to the parents more clearly the abnormality present in the fetus; (A) Cystic hygroma at 11+0 weeks; (B) Anencephaly at 11+2 weeks; (C) Body stalk anomaly at 12 weeks (note the abnormal position in which the fetus lies in the uterus; with 4D ultrasound abnormal movements could also be observed).

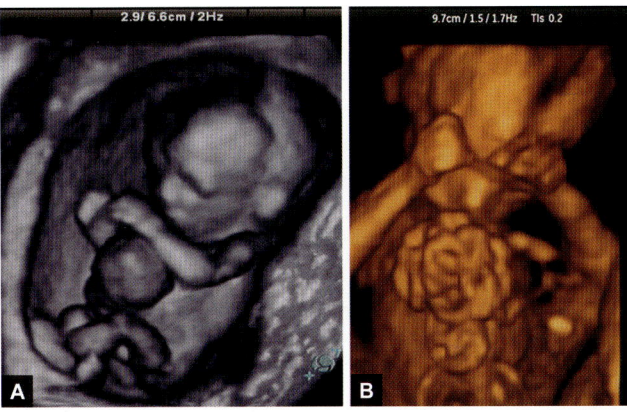

Figs. 4.7A and B: Three-dimensional images showing abdominal wall defects at 11–13+6 weeks; (A) Large omphalocele containing liver in a chromosomally normal fetus at 12+6 weeks; (B) Gastroschisis in a fetus at 13+4 weeks.

diagnosis in many situations during the first trimester US in combination with the surface mode of display, in particular abnormalities of the facial bones have been described.[16-19] Analysis of such volumes is fairly simple and quick and could be done during the live scan on the US machine or as an off-line analysis with the appropriate software in the computer. Multiplanar approach will be discussed later in this chapter.

The use of 4D US during the first trimester has not been reported as useful for diagnostic purposes; however, it is of great importance for parents to be able to see the fetus moving. Fetuses at 11–14 weeks show plenty of movements in normal situations, with great jumping and waving hands and due to the size of the fetus, it can be imaged completely on the screen (this is not always possible in the 2nd trimester of pregnancy). There are still not so many facial expressions as seen later in pregnancy and images are of slim funny fetuses. The use of 4D US is mainly dedicated to the cardiac assessment with spatiotemporal image correlation (STIC), a tool that is not used routinely and is mainly reserved to the expert in fetal heart evaluation and in cases of cardiac abnormalities.

MULTIPLANAR MODE

The multiplanar mode of display the volume is one of the first tools to be developed in 3D US. This mode facilitates the visualization of any fetal structure in the three planes of the space in any desired position. It is useful in its standard or basic mode in which one reference dot can be moved along the volume in the x, y, and z axes; the reference dot represents the single intersection point of the three axes in space. The volume is usually displayed in three panels named A, B, and C in order to visualize all the possible planes simultaneously.

The multiplanar mode of display is widely available in all 3D US machines; it is as useful in live scanning as in off-line analysis. It is fairly easy to manipulate provided the operator is aware of the normal anatomy of the fetus. To remark is the importance of the multiplanar mode in the description of adequate planes in the fetus to perform measurements or anatomical survey, for example the perfect mid-sagittal plane **(Fig. 4.8)** to ensure the correct plane of the fetal head to measure nuchal translucency (NT), facial angle, nasal bones assessment and intracranial translucency (IT) evaluation.[20,21] The same applies to the adequate coronal view to identify the nasal bones in the retronasal triangle **(Figs. 4.9 and 4.10)**.[22]

There are two main advantages of the multiplanar mode—the possibility to explore the anatomy of the fetus easily and the chance to store the volumes for further analysis or consultation with the expert. The interpretation of images and the understanding of the anatomic relationship between structures is another advantage of this. For example, the assessment of the presence or absence of the nasal bone can be performed in vivo during the scan with a simple acquisition of the fetal profile (well-contrasted 2D image, nasal bone parallel to the probe, and small acquisition angle between 30°–40°). Following this acquisition, the multiplanar mode is displayed in three planes or with tomographic ultrasound imaging (TUI) and adequate visualization of the nasal bones can be obtained in sagittal or coronal view to ensure that both nasal bones are present, or one or both are absent **(Figs. 4.9 to 4.11)**.

The combination of 2D US with some 3D tools such as multiplanar, TUI, and renderization in skeletal or surface mode provides a good idea of the normality or the defect in the fetus in the first trimester **(Figs. 4.12A and B)**. The multiplanar mode is the most used 3D tool in the assessment of fetal defects in the 2nd and 3rd trimester of pregnancy. It is of great importance in the study of central nervous system (CNS) and cardiac malformations.

Other tools such as TUI (GE Medical Systems, Zipf, Austria) or the equivalent in other companies, i.e. Multi Slice View (Medison, Seoul, Korea) and OmniView simplify the navigation and have been used to calculate algorithms for automatization mainly in the cardiac assessment in combination with STIC (see below).

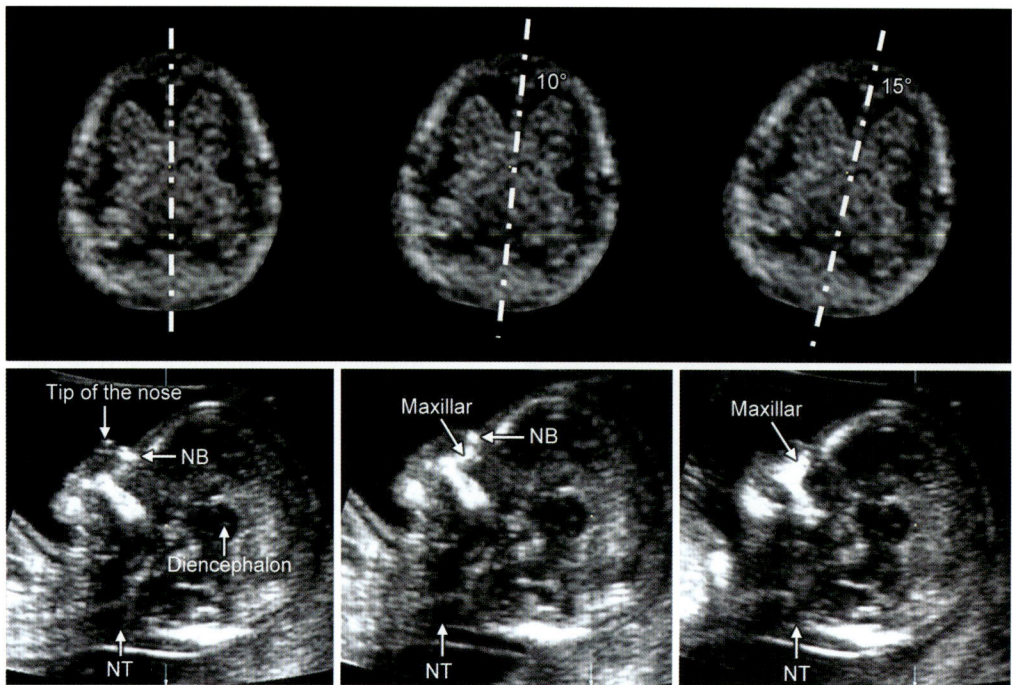

Fig. 4.8: Effect of the modification of the position of the head in the appearance of the fetal profile; rotation of 10° or 15° modifies the aspect of the profile: the visualization of the zygomatic process of the maxilla between the nose and the upper palate and the tip of the nose that is not seen after the rotations.

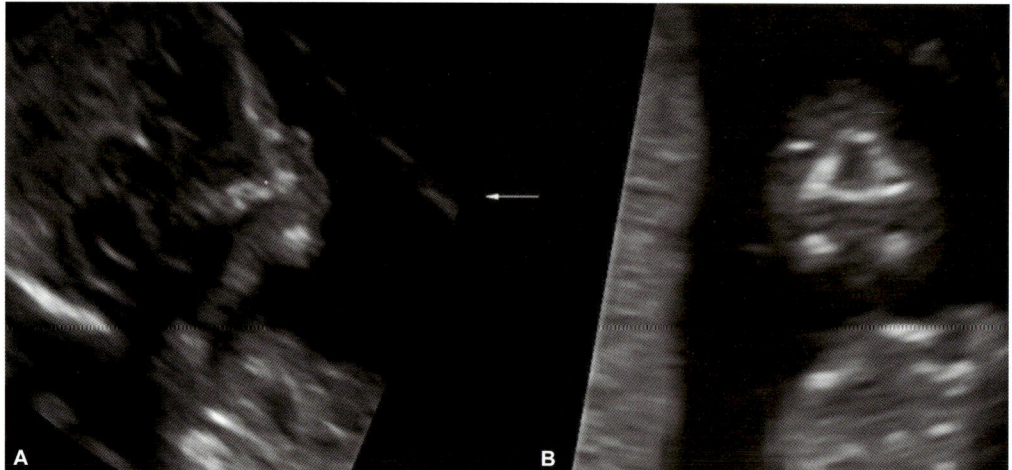

Figs. 4.9A and B: Image of the fetal profile at 12 weeks displayed with multiplanar mode showing only A and B plane (sagittal and coronal views respectively). The acquisition plane is the one recommended for the midsagittal assessment with the transducer parallel to the nose. After rotation of the plane A (fetal profile) in the z-axis, a coronal view is obtained in B. In this view, it is possible to assess the retronasal triangle, both nasal bones simultaneously and the mandibular gap. All these structures appear normal in this fetus.

These automatic tools are not yet available for first trimester volumes.

The TUI provides a series of parallel images contained in the volume and in the selected plane and displayed as in tomography imaging. Many images can be analyzed at the same time with no need of further manipulation. It is particularly useful in the first and second trimester for nasal bone assessment, if the fetus is in the correct position to obtain a volume **(Fig. 4.11)**. In contrast, OmniView allows the operator to trace a

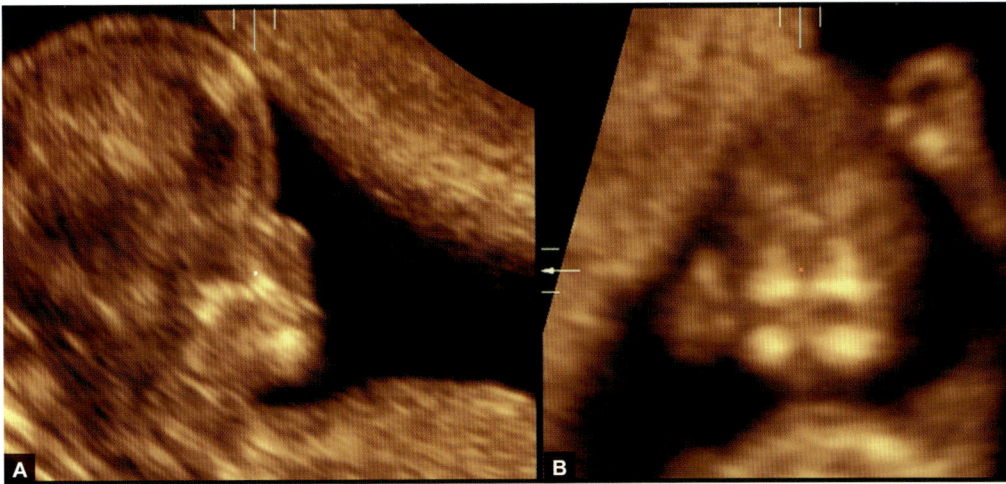

Figs. 4.10A and B: Image of the fetal profile in a fetus with trisomy 21 at 13 weeks displayed with multiplanar mode showing A and B planes in a fetus with absent nasal bones. Note in the sagittal view that the line is not thicker or brighter compared with the skin above; in the coronal view the retronasal triangle is incomplete due to the absence of the nasal bones.

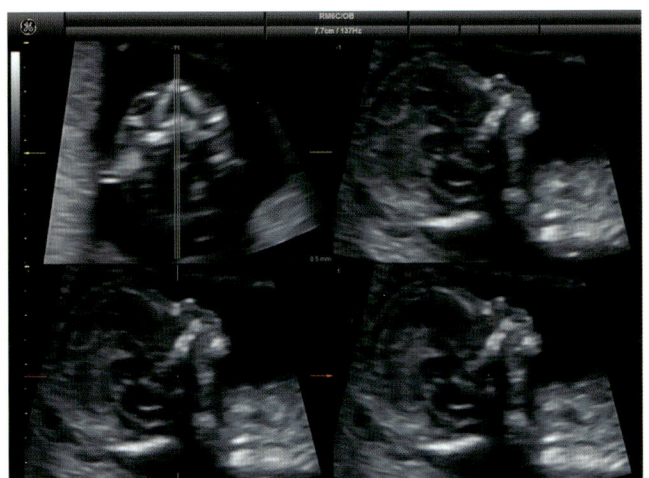

Fig. 4.11: TUI (tomographic ultrasound imaging) in a normal fetus at 12+3 weeks demonstrating the presence of both nasal bones at each side of the perfect mid-sagittal plane of the fetal face. The reference image corresponds to the transverse view of the face so that the parallel sequence of images is displayed in the sagittal view to assess the nasal bones simultaneously. The distance between the lines is 0.5 mm and both pictures on the right side named 1 and −1 correspond the parallel images from the midline. Note that the appearance of the brain is slightly different when moving away from the midline.

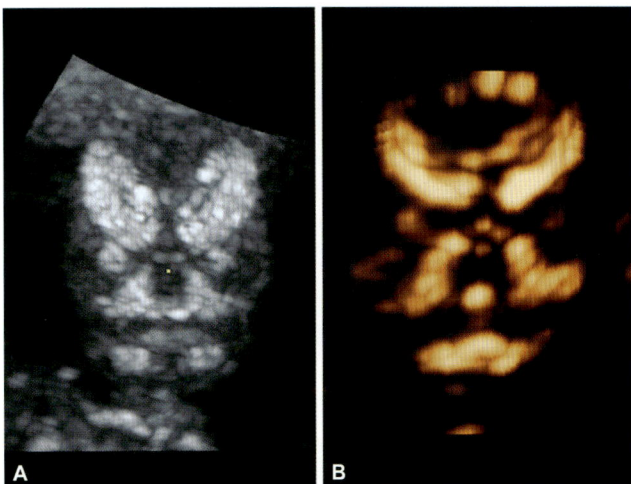

Figs. 4.12A and B: The multiplanar mode of display set the concept for the renderization of the coronal view of the face, simulating the retronasal triangle but with renderization mode. A normal fetus at 12 weeks in A and a bilateral cleft in a fetus with trisomy 13 at 12 weeks in B.

Sonography-based NT (SonoNT) software derives from multiplanar algorithm but in the routine use of automated NT measurement, 3D US is not needed.[23]

These are indirect benefits of the multiplanar mode, because the 3D volumes were used as a research tool to describe many important structures in the fetus and this knowledge has helped many doctors to perform better US examinations in the first trimester.

series of three different types of lines, straight, curved, or of free traced and displays the correspondent region of the volume **(Fig. 4.13)**. This mode of navigation is much more intuitive than the one with reference dots.

We want to emphasize how useful the multiplanar mode of the 3D US was to understand and describe anatomic aspects of the fetus. In the present, at least some of the detectable abnormalities in the fetus can be suspected or diagnosed with a high-resolution 2D evaluation. In particular, the incorporation of the coronal view in a routine 2D US at 11–14 weeks of gestation is extremely useful and we recommend performing this approach with volume navigation and in real-time 2D US.

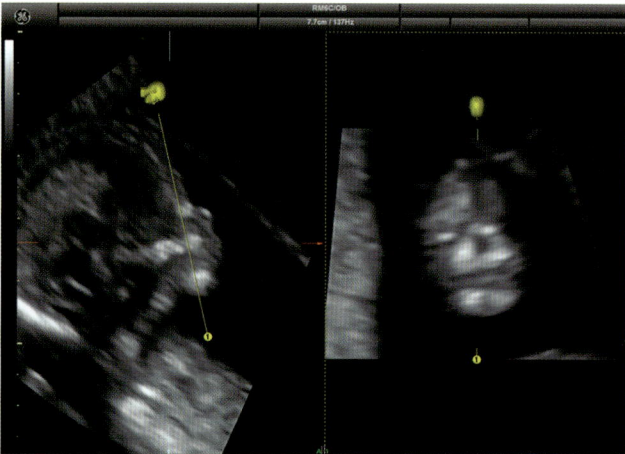

Fig. 4.13: Retronasal triangle demonstrated with OmniView in a normal fetus at 13 weeks of gestation. The reference image on the right corresponds to the fetal profile in which the OmniView line is drawn as a straight line and the coronal view is displayed on the left showing all the structures that appear on the line; in this case the retronasal triangle is observed.

VOLUME CALCULATION

Volume calculation is possible during the first trimester of pregnancy but its utility is not as relevant in prenatal US. There are many different ways to perform the volume calculation after the acquisition but not all of them are widely available. Inversion mode and VOCAL (virtual organ computed-aided analysis) were the first to be introduced. VOCAL is based on the calculation done on a volume after a series of rotations and tracing of the contour of the selected structure. This technique is fairly precise but is time-consuming and requires well-defined borders to ensure that the tracing is correct. At the end of the process, the volume calculation is given and a nice colorful reconstruction can be displayed. It gives the chance to edit the tracing in case of mistakes. To apply VOCAL, the operator has to establish the number of rotations that will be done, when more steps are selected, more reliable the measurement will be, increasing the time spent to achieve such result. If the shape of the desired structure is irregular, the tracing is more difficult and less precise. Volume calculation of several fetal structures and the placenta has been reported. But unfortunately, after a decade or more, none of these publications made a great difference in terms of diagnosis of abnormalities or preeclampsia detection in the first trimester **(Figs. 4.14 and 4.15)**.[24-30] One study reported low intraobserver agreement in the assessment of placenta volume.[31] Studies performed later concluded that the reproducibility of

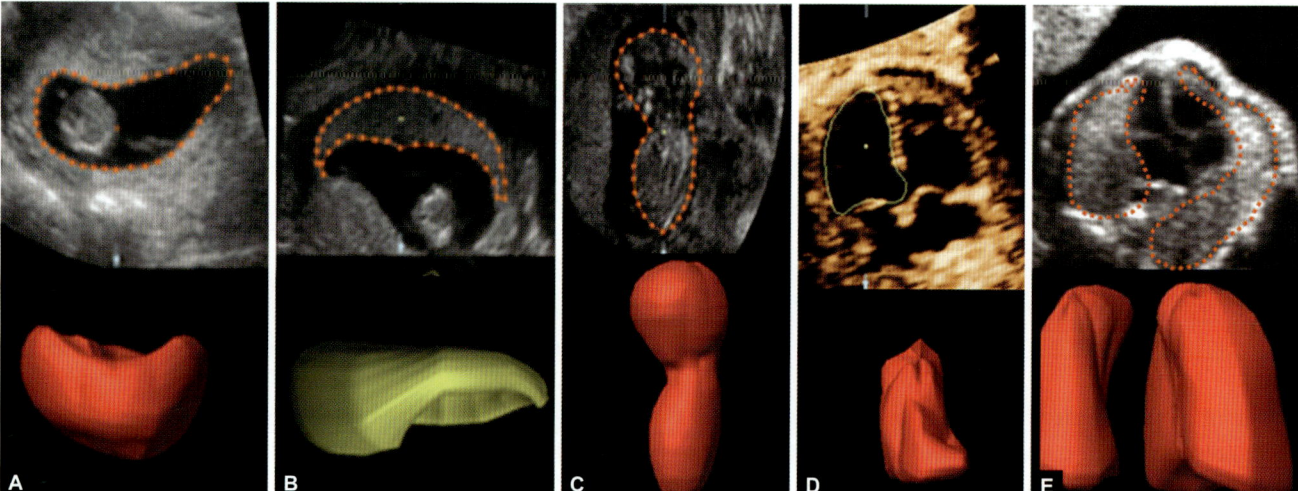

Figs. 4.14A to E: Virtual organ computer-aided analysis in the assessment of gestational sac (A), amniotic sac (B) and fetus (C) volumes in the first trimester of pregnancy and cardiac structures (D) and lungs (E) volumes in second trimester.

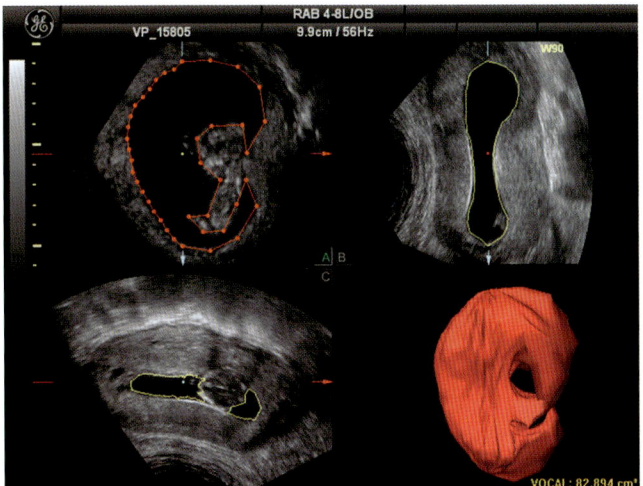

Fig. 4.15: Gestational sac volume calculated with virtual organ computer-aided analysis. Note that the irregular shape of the fetus makes the tracing more difficult and need more rotation steps (15° angle) to ensure the accuracy of the measurement.

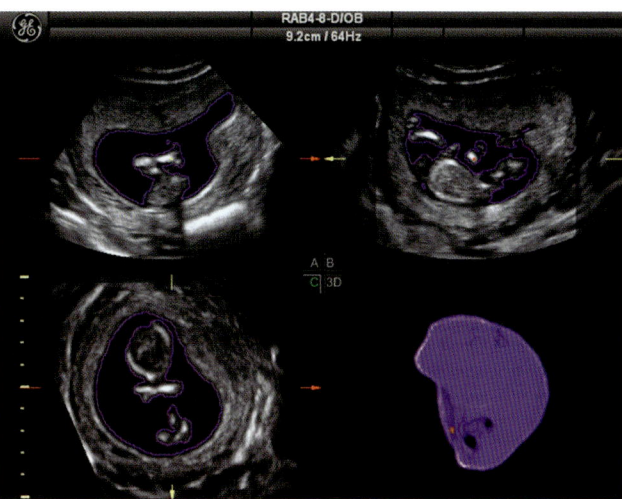

Fig. 4.16: Gestational sac volume calculated with sonography-based automated volume count follicle. The semiautomatic calculation recognizes very well the borders of the fetus due to the contrast between the anechoic amniotic fluid and the hypoechoic fetus. No further adjustments or editing is needed.

VOCAL is not as good as the reproducibility obtained with a new tool called *SonoAVC* (sonography-based automated volume count) general or follicle **(Fig. 4.16)**. Several studies analyzed the relationship between the volume of the placenta in the first trimester measured with VOCAL and the risk of preeclampsia and fetal growth restriction in second and third trimester. They concluded that the volume calculation is feasible but they could not prove association for clinical use.[29-30]

Sonography-based automated volume count was designed to count the number of follicles present in the ovaries after stimulation in assisted reproduction treatment. In addition, the size of each follicle could be independently estimated.[32] SonoAVC works by identification of anechoic or hypoechoic fluid-filled structures with a well-defined limits and it is a semiautomatic process that requires that the operator obtains a volume and selects the region of interest for the software to make the calculations. It takes only a few seconds to get the results on the screen. Each follicle gets a color in order to simplify its localization in the ovary and they are counted and listed by the size. This tool has been used in prenatal US as well but later the application for general use became available to distinguish from the follicle count that initially was developed **(Figs. 4.17A to D)**. The new software improved the assessment when hypoechoic structures are involved and limits are not always as clear as in

the ovaries. Therefore, the SonoAVC general is the one that should be used in obstetric 3D US. Several studies reported on the volume calculation of fetal structures and gestational sac measurements with this technique **(Figs. 4.17A to D)**.[33-38] These studies remark that the volume calculation of such fetal structures and gestational sac is feasible with SonoAVC and that the tool is easy to use. Most of these studies concluded that SonoAVC provides a calculation in less time compared with VOCAL when calculating the volume of the fetal stomach, renal pelvis, fetal volume, and gestational sac volume. Moreover, those studies that compared the whole calculation process between VOCAL and SonoAVC concluded that the ability to perform the calculations was similar, but the reproducibility was much better when performed the semiautomated SonoAVC calculation. In one study, SonoAVC was used to assess bladder size and urine production in twin-to-twin transfusion syndrome. Only a few studies report that SonoAVC requires more editing of the volume compared with VOCAL, but SonoAVC appears to be faster overall.

SPATIOTEMPORAL IMAGE CORRELATION

The STIC is a 4D tool exclusively designed to assess the fetal heart providing moving or still images. The way it works is with the acquisition of the heart beating followed

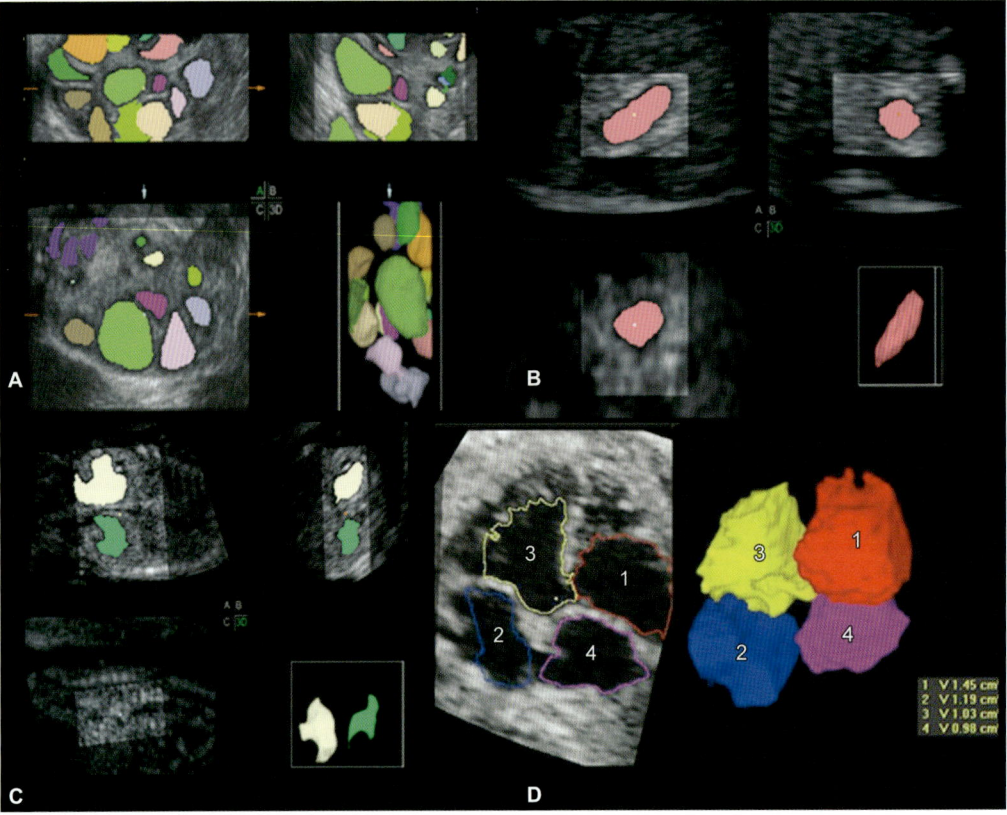

Figs. 4.17A to D: Volume calculation with sonography-based automated volume count: (A) Ovary with stimulation in IVF, (B) Fetal stomach at 16 weeks, and (C) renal pelvis in a fetus at 15 weeks with hydronephrosis and (D) Cardiac chambers at 18 weeks.

by the reconstruction of a complete cardiac cycle based on the fetal heart rate. The software asks to the operator to agree with the fetal heart rate estimated before giving the volume images. The series of images that will be available for analysis are reconstructed images from the 2D mode or color Doppler mode or both. The probe performs a slow sweep over the area of interest selected depending on the gestational age and the fetal cardiac size; it varies from 7.5 seconds to 15 seconds and the sweep angle from 15° to 40°. It is recommend working with a 2D cardiac setting in order to obtain high-contrasted images. Once the STIC is obtained, the volume can be manipulated in the three planes when displayed with the multiplanar mode (standard, TUI, and OmniView). Renderization and inversion mode can be useful to demonstrate flow in the cardiac chambers and vessels; volume of the chambers can be analyzed with VOCAL and SonoAVC.[32,37,39]

Its use in first trimester is recommended always with high frequency TV probes. Publications report that it is not so easy to obtain volumes of high quality and in certain cases the assessment with 2D US in real time is still of better resolution. However, the experts consider the STIC[40,41] as a useful 4D tool (**Figs. 4.18A to C**) in the evaluation of cardiac defects in the first trimester of pregnancy.[42-46] The value of the STIC at any gestational age is the possibility to send volumes for second opinion through Internet with no need to send the patient far away for reassurance. Many different algorithms have been published to facilitate cardiac assessment during the second and third trimester including the automatization of the steps to obtain basic cardiac planes.[47] Other reports combined OmniView with STIC to produce different algorithms to simplify cardiac assessment in the acquired volume.[48,49] Unfortunately, they are not yet available for first trimester. As in all other 3D or 4D tools, a learning curve is needed to acquire correct STIC volume in the first trimester and extra time to learn how to manipulate these particular volumes of the fetal heart. In fact, the manipulation of such volumes also requires at least a minimum knowledge about the fetal heart anatomy.

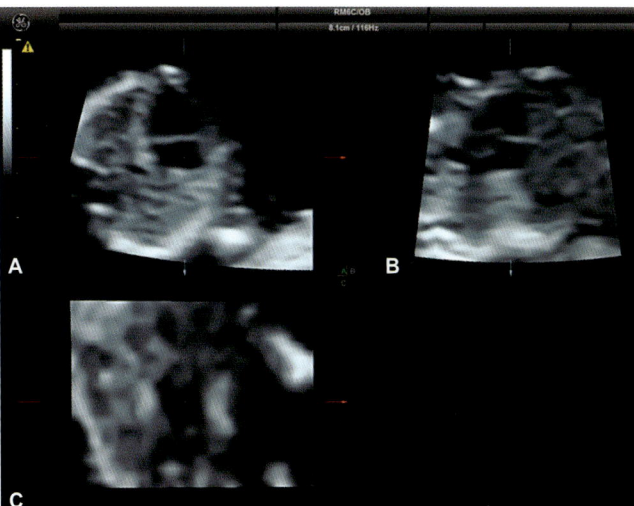

Figs. 4.18A to C: Multiplanar display of a 4D volume obtained with spatiotemporal image correlation (STIC) in a fetus at 13+5 weeks of gestation. The acquisition plane (plane A) that in this case corresponds to the apical four chambers view of the heart is the plane with better resolution. In first trimester STIC volumes, this is critically important since the other planes B and C may not be as useful for analysis. Therefore, in abnormal cases, more than one volume is needed to demonstrate the defect.

TELEMEDICINE

The 3D or 4D US in the first, second, and third trimesters has given the opportunity for doctors to exchange images, volumes, and videos easily. This is called telemedicine and in our opinion it is one of the most useful applications of the 3D. It is true that there are lovers and detractors of 3D or 4D US, but the combination of this technology and the Internet is a great advantage compared with the 2D US in the assessment of fetal abnormalities in a distant location without the need of seeing the patient in real-time scanning. However, it is not true that any volume is useful for analysis and care must be taken to acquire adequate volumes in each anatomical area and, in particular, when a fetal defect is suspected. For this reason, we suggest to obtain more than one volume of the area of interest in more than one orientations to ensure that the whole defect is contained in the information stored. Many studies reported on the benefits of the telemedicine.[50,51] It is clear that in the routine clinical practice, for those with less experience or who do not have the opportunity to work in a medical team, the possibility of sending volumes away to a colleague, asking for a second opinion is critically important and for teaching purposes as well. Along this line, we believe that learning how to obtain a 3D volume is at least as important as how to interpret the acquired information. We, therefore, encourage the readers to get adequate training in 3D to improve the results achieved.

SUMMARY

Is it really essential to have a 3D or 4D US machine in our practice to carry out a first trimester scan? The answer is no. However, as most of the practitioners do have one nowadays, it is important to point out its benefits and limitations.

It is clear that 3D images obtained with TV high-resolution probes to visualize the embryo with all the new renderization modes are spectacular but with little use in medical diagnosis yet. However, as the fetus gets bigger, 3D US can show the fetus very nicely and demonstrate some of the abnormalities that affect the fetal surface and that had been previously seen on 2D. Moreover, 4D US in this phase of pregnancy, by visualizing the fetus with constant movements, creates early bonding with the family.

The use of the multiplanar mode of display is extremely useful in its standard mode or with TUI and OmniView in the demonstration of facial abnormalities, which are very common in association with chromosomal abnormalities. This 3D mode is essential for teaching in an offline process that can be carried out in a computer with no patient or US machine, allowing plenty of time for navigation in the stored volume.

The limitations include the less resolution of the 2D US in the first trimester compared with a second trimester fetus as for example in internal organs and the heart. Therefore, images of good quality and volumes are more difficult to obtain for multiplanar navigation of cardiac assessment with STIC. In some situation, not even with TV approach is possible to store good volumes increasing the scanning time or the need to reschedule the patient for another visit. It is not possible to avoid a learning curve in acquisition and manipulation of volumes, in particular with the surface mode, since new tools become available every year, and update of information on how to use them is always recommended.

REFERENCES

1. Pooh RK, Kurjak A. Novel application of three-dimensional HD live imaging in prenatal diagnosis from the first trimester. J Perinat Med. 2015;43(2):147-58.

2. Pooh RK, Shiota K, Kurjak A. Imaging of the human embryo with magnetic resonance imaging microscopy and high resolution transvaginal 3-dimensional sonography: human embryology in the 21st century. Am J Obstet Gynecol. 2011;204:77.e1-16.

3. Pooh RK, Kurjak A. 3D/4D sonography moved prenatal diagnosis of fetal anomalies from the second to the first trimester of pregnancy. J Matern Fetal Neonatal Med. 2012;25:433-55.

4. Martinez Ten P, Gomez Ruiz ML, Santacruz B. Sono-embriologia. Aportación de la ecografía 3D. In: Gallo M, Martinez–Ten P, Espinosa A (Eds). Ecografía Tridimensional (3D/4D) en el embarazo. España: Amolca, Actualidades médicas CA; 2013. pp. 63-77.

5. Kurjak A, Pooh RK, Merce LT, et al. Structural and functional early human development assessed by three-dimensional and four-dimensional sonography. Fertil Steril. 2005;84:1285-99.

6. Benoit B, Hafner T, Kurjak A, et al. Three-dimensional sonoembryology. J Perinat Med. 2002;30:63-73.

7. Zanforlin Filho DM, Araujo Junior E, Guiaräes Filho HA, et al. Sonoembryology by three-dimensional ultrasono-graphy: pictorial essay. Arch Gynecol Obstet. 2007;276: 197-200.

8. Blaas HG, Eik-Nes SH. Sonoembryology and early prenatal diagnosis of neural anomalies. Prenat Diagn. 2009;29: 312-15.

9. Pooh RK. Sonoembryology by 3D HD live silhouette ultrasound—what is added by the "see-through fashion"? J Perinat Med. 2016;44:139-48.

10. Quezada MS, Gil MM, Francisco C, et al. Screening for trisomies 21, 18 and 13 by cell-free DNA analysis of mater-nal blood at 10-11 weeks' gestation and the combined test at 11–13 weeks. Ultrasound Obstet Gynecol. 2015;45: 36-41.

11. Kagan KO, Wright D, Spencer K, et al. First-trimester screening for trisomy 21 by free beta human chorionic gonadotropin and pregnancy-associated plasma protein-A: impact of maternal and pregnancy characteristics. Ultrasound Obstet Gynecol. 2008;31:493-502.

12. Rolnik DL, Wright D, Poon LCY, et al. ASPRE trial: performance of screening for preterm pre-eclampsia. Ultrasound Obstet Gynecol. 2017;50:492-5.

13. Faro C, Benoit B, Wergrzyn P, et al. Three-dimensional sonographic description of the fetal frontal bones and metopic suture. Ultrasound Obstet Gynecol. 2005;26: 618-21.

14. Faro C, Wegrzyn P, Benoit B, et al. Metopic suture in fetuses with holoprosencephaly at 11-13+6 weeks of gestation. Ultrasound Obstet Gynecol. 2006;27:162-6.

15. Syngelaki A, Cheleman T, Dagklis T, et al. Challenges in the diagnosis of fetal non-chromosomal abnormalities at 11-13 weeks. Prenat Diagn. 2011;31:90-102.

16. Sepulveda W, Wong AE, Martinez-Ten P, et al. Retronasal triangle: a sonographic landmark for the screening of cleft palate in the first trimester. Ultrasound Obstet Gyencol. 2010;35:7-13.

17. Martinez-Ten P, Adiego B, Illescas T, et al. First trimester diagnosis of cleft lip and palate using three-dimensional ultrasound. Ultrasound Obstet Gynecol. 2012;40:40-6.

18. Sepulveda W, Wong AE, Viñals F, et al. Absent mandibular gap in the retronasal triangle view: a clue to the diagnosis of micrognathia in the first trimester. Ultrasound Obstet Gynecol. 2012;39:152-6.

19. Rembouskos G, Cicero S, Londo D, et al. Assessment of the fetal nasal bone at 11-14 weeks of gestation by three-dimensional ultrasound. Ultrasound Obstet Gynecol. 2004;23:232-6.

20. Plasencia W, Dagklis T, Pachoumi C, et al. Frontomaxillary facial angle at 11 + 0 to 13 + 6 weeks: effect of plane of acquisition. Ultrasound Obstet Gynecol. 2007;29:660-5.

21. Borenstein M, Persico N, Kaihura C, et al. Frontomaxillary facial angle in chromosomally normal fetuses at 11 + 0 to 13 + 6 weeks. Ultrasound Obstet Gynecol. 2007;30: 737-41.

22. Adiego B, Martinez-Ten P, Illescas T, et al. First-trimester assessment of nasal bone using retronasal triangle view: a prospective study. Ultrasound Obstet Gynecol. 2014;43: 272-6.

23. Moratalla J, Pintoffl K, Minekawa R, et al. Semi-automated system for measurement of nuchal translucency thickness. Ultrasound Obstet Gynecol. 2010;36:412-6.

24. Falcon O, Cavoretto P, Peralta CF, et al. Fetal head-to-trunk volume ratio in chromosomally abnormal fetuses at 11+0 to 13+6 weeks of gestation. Ultrasound Obstet Gynecol. 2005;26:755-60.

25. Peralta CF, Cavoretto P, Csapo B, et al. Lung and heart volumes by three-dimensional ultrasound in normal fetuses at 12-32 weeks' gestation. Ultrasound Obstet Gynecol. 2006;27:128-33.

26. Falcon O, Wegrzyn P, Faro C, et al. Gestational sac volume measured by three-dimensional ultrasound at 11 to 13 + 6 weeks of gestation: relation to chromosomal defects. Ultrasound Obstet Gynecol. 2005;25:546-50.

27. Wegrzyn P, Faro C, Falcon O, et al. Placental volume measured by three-dimensional ultrasound at 11 to 13 + 6 weeks of gestation: relation to chromosomal defects. Ultrasound Obstet Gynecol. 2005;26:28-32.

28. Wegrzyn P, Fabio C, Peralta A, et al. Placental volume in twin and triplet pregnancies measured by three-dimensional ultrasound at 11 + 0 to 13 + 6 weeks of gestation. Ultrasound Obstet Gynecol. 2006;27:647-51.

29. Farina A. Systematic review on first trimester three-dimensional placental volumetry predicting small for gestational age infants. Prenat Diagn. 2016;36:135-41.

30. Arakaki T, Hasegawa J, Nakamura M, et al. Prediction of early and late-onset pregnancy induced hypertension using placental volume on three-dimensional ultrasound and uterine artery Doppler. Ultrasound Obstet Gynecol. 2015;45:539-43.

31. Larsen ML, Naver KV, Kjaer MM, et al. Reproducibility of 3-dimensional ultrasound measurements of placental volume at gestational ages 11-14 weeks. Facts Views Vis Obgyn. 2015;28:203-9.

32. Raine-Fenning N, Jayaprakasan K, Clewes J, et al. SonoAVC: a novel method of automatic volume calculation. Ultrasound Obstet Gynecol. 2008;31:691-6.

33. Borenstein M, Azumendi Perez G, Molina Garcia F, et al. Gestational sac volume: comparison between SonoAVC and VOCAL measurements at 11 + 0 to 13 + 6 weeks of gestation. Ultrasound Obstet Gynecol. 2009;34: 510-4.

34. Sur SD, Jayaprakasan K, Jones NW, et al. A novel technique for the semiautomated measurement of embryo volume: an intraobserver reliability study. Ultrasound Med Biol. 2010;36:719-25.

35. Duin LK, Willekes C, Vossen M, et al. Reproducibility of fetal renal pelvis volume assessed by three-dimensional ultrasonography with two different measurement techniques. J Clin Ultrasound. 2013;41:230-4.

36. Kist WJ, Slaghekke F, Papanna R, et al. Sonography-based automated volume count to estimate fetal urine production in twin-to-twin transfusion syndrome: comparison with virtual organ computer-aided analysis. Am J Obstet Gynecol. 2011;205:574.e1-5.

37. Rizzo G, Capponi A, Pietrolucci ME, et al. Role of sonographic automatic volume calculation in measuring fetal cardiac ventricular volumes using 4-dimensional sonography: comparison with virtual organ computer-aided analysis. J Ultrasound Med. 2010;29:261-70.

38. Rizzo G, Capponi A, Pietrolucci ME, et al. Sonographic automated volume count (SonoAVC) in volume measurement of fetal fluid-filled structures: comparison with virtual organ computer-aided analysis (VOCAL). Ultrasound Obstet Gynecol. 2008;32:111-2.

39. DeVore GR, Falkensammer P, Sklansky MS, et al. Spatiotemporal image correlation (STIC): new technology for evaluation of the fetal heart. Ultrasound Obstet Gynecol. 2003;22:380-7.

40. Viñals F, Poblete P, Giuliano A. Spatiotemporal image correlation (STIC): a new tool for the prenatal screening of congenital heart defects. Ultrasound Obstet Gynecol. 2003;22:388-94.

41. Comas C, Azumendi G, Alonso I, et al. Spatiotemporal image correlation (STIC) as a new screening tool for prenatal detection of congenital heart defects. The first Spanish experience. Ultrasound Rev Obstet Gynecol. 2006; 6:45-57.

42. Turan S, Turan OM, Ty-Torredes K, et al. Standardization of the first-trimester fetal cardiac examination using spatiotemporal image correlation with tomographic ultrasound and color Doppler imaging. Ultrasound Obstet Gynecol. 2009;33:652-6.

43. Bennasar M, Martínez JM, Olivella A, et al. Feasibility and accuracy of fetal echocardiography using four-dimensional spatiotemporal image correlation technology before 16 weeks' gestation. Ultrasound Obstet Gynecol. 2009;33: 645-51.

44. Wiechec MT, Nocun AA. Early fetal heart assessment using 4D ultrasound–STIC technique in 11th-13 + 6 scans. Ultrasound Obstet Gynecol. 2008;32:333.

45. Espinoza J, Lee W, Viñals F, et al. Collaborative study of 4-dimensional fetal echocardiography in the first trimester of pregnancy. J Ultrasound Med. 2014;33:1079-84.

46. Votino C, Cos T, Abu-Rustum R, et al. Use of spatiotemporal image correlation at 11-14 weeks' gestation. Ultrasound Obstet Gynecol. 2013;42:669-78.

47. Abuhamad A, Falkensammer P, Reichartseder F, et al. Automated retrieval of standard diagnostic fetal cardiac ultrasound planes in the second trimester of pregnancy: a prospective evaluation of software. Ultrasound Obstet Gynecol. 2008;31:30-6.

48. Yeo L, Romero R, Jodicke C, et al. Simple targeted arterial rendering (STAR) technique: a novel and simple method to visualize the fetal cardiac outflow tracts. Ultrasound Obstet Gynecol. 2011;37:549-56.

49. Yeo L, Romero R, Jodicke C, et al. Four-chamber view and 'swing technique' (FAST) echo: a novel and simple algorithm to visualize standard fetal echocardiographic planes. Ultrasound Obstet Gynecol. 2011;37:423-31.

50. Viñals F, Mandujano L, Vargas G, et al. Prenatal diagnosis of congenital heart disease using four-dimensional spatiotemporal image correlation (STIC) telemedicine via an Internet link: a pilot study. Ultrasound Obstet Gynecol. 2005;25:25-31.

51. Tajada M, Rueda S, Bolillos MJ, Herráiz N, Gonzalez de Agüero R. Tele-Ecogtrafía en el diagnóstico Prenatal de Cardiopatias Congénitas.(Telemedicine in the diagnosis of prenatal cardiac defects) Oral comunication in II International Course in Fetal Medicine organized by Ultrasound and Prenatal Diagnosis Unit, Gutenberg Clinic, Málaga, Spain 24-26th Sept 2009.

5

3D Ultrasonography and 3D Power Doppler in the Evaluation of Placenta Accreta Spectrum

Giuseppe Calì, Francesco Forlani, Gabriella Minneci

INTRODUCTION

Following the constant rise in cesarean deliveries occurred in the last decades, the anomalies of placental implantation and invasion have become an emerging pathology. Severe forms of invasive placentation unexpectedly encountered at the time of delivery can lead to dramatic consequences such as uterine rupture in labor, peripartum hemorrhage, necessity of hysterectomy, massive blood transfusions. In this scenario, prenatal diagnosis plays a key role in the individuation of patients at risk, who should be referred to tertiary centers. If the diagnosis of abnormal placentation is confirmed, the next step should be to state the degree of placental invasion. 2D ultrasonography (US) is the technique mainly employed in the diagnosis of placenta accreta spectrum (PAS) disorders, but its accuracy is enforced by the complementary use of 3D US and 3D power Doppler.

PLACENTA ACCRETA SPECTRUM AND ULTRASOUND DIAGNOSIS

Placenta accreta spectrum disorders include three forms of abnormal placentation:[1]

1. Placenta accreta (or adherent), when the villi adhere to the myometrium without invasion
2. Placenta increta, when the villi invade the myometrium
3. Placenta percreta, when villi invade the full thickness of the myometrium including the uterine serosa and sometimes adjacent pelvic organs.

According to the lateral extension of the myometrial invasion and the number of cotyledons involved, PAS disorders can also be divided in focal, partial or total. There is not a specific clinical symptomatology of PAS and in many forms of acretism, there is not bleeding during the gestation. So clinicians have to suspect its presence if the patient has recognized risk factors. These include placenta previa, previous curettage, multiparity, maternal age over 35 years, medically assisted reproduction techniques, adenomyosis, hysterotomic scars and, above all, previous cesarean deliveries (CD), in particular if associated with placenta previa. The increasing rate of these events has caused the rising incidence of PAS in the Western countries in the last decades.[2] In the last 40 years, cesarean section rates around the world have risen from less than 10% to over 30%. One of the consequences has been a 10-fold increase in the incidence of PAS.[1] In 2013, a systematic review[3] reported 19% of incidence in women at risk, with a previous cesarean section and with anterior placenta previa diagnosed in the third trimester of pregnancy.

At delivery, PAS disorders expose to a high risk of intra- and postoperative complications, including severe hemorrhage with possible necessity of hysterectomy and massive blood transfusions. So, an accurate prenatal diagnosis is essential to reduce maternal mortality and morbidity. It allows to plan the timing of the delivery, to organize a multidisciplinary team with adequate experience, to predispose the availability of compatible blood, to evaluate the therapeutic options considering the surgical difficulties and the eventual patient's wish of preserving her fertility.

Nowadays ultrasound is the main technique used in the prenatal diagnosis of PAS.

Recently an International AIP Expert Group has proposed some standardized ultrasound criteria in order to reduce the diagnostic errors linked to the subjective interpretation of the examination:[4]

- *Loss of the clear zone*: Loss or irregularity of hypoechoic area between placenta and myometrium.
- *Placental vascular lacunae*: Presence of numerous lacunae (more than three), some of which wide and irregular, in the placental parenchyma. They often are characterized by turbulent flow visible on grayscale and color Doppler imaging.
- *Interruption of the bladder wall*: Loss or interruption of the hyperechoic line between uterine serosa and bladder lumen (bladder line).
- *Myometrial thinning*: The thickness of the myometrium overlying the placenta is less than 1 mm or undetectable.
- *Placental bulge*: Deformation of the uterine serosa caused by the abnormal protrusion of placental tissue into neighboring organs, typically bladder. Uterine serosa appear distorted.
- *Focal exophytic mass*: Placental tissue breaks through uterine serosa and extends beyond it. It is visible if the bladder is filled and it is related to the most severe PAS disorders.
- *Uterovesical hypervascularity*: Striking amount of color Doppler signal between myometrium and posterior wall of the bladder, showing closely packed tortuous vessels with multidirectional flow and aliasing artifact.
- *Subplacental hypervascularity*: Striking amount of color Doppler signal in the placental bed, showing closely packed tortuous vessels with multidirectional flow and aliasing artifact.
- *Bridging vessels*: Vessels appearing to extend from placenta, across myometrium and beyond serosa into bladder or other organs, often running perpendicular to myometrium.
- *Intraplacental hypervascularity*: Complex vascularization with tortuous and irregular vessel, visible with 3D color Doppler.

In D'Antonio's meta-analysis,[3] the loss of the clear zone showed sensibility of 66.2% and specificity of 95.7%; placental lacunae showed sensibility of 77.4% and specificity of 95%; bladder line anomalies presented sensibility of 49.6% and specificity of 99.7%. Grayscale and color Doppler imaging showed overall sensibility of 90.7%, specificity of 96.9%, and odd ratio of 98.5%.

A recent prospective longitudinal study of 2018[5] highlighted that if ultrasound is employed in a population at risk, its diagnostic accuracy is excellent, with sensibility and specificity of 100%. In particular, the specificity of the examination increases if more diagnostic criteria are used. Probably the increased awareness of the pathophysiology of PAS disorders, the greater attention to the selection of patients at risk, the improvements of ultrasound devices and the bigger experience of operators, have allowed to achieve these results in the last years.

ROLE OF 3D ULTRASONOGRAPHY AND 3D POWER DOPPLER

Two-dimensional ultrasonography is the gold standard in the diagnosis of PAS disorders. Nevertheless, the importance of an accurate evaluation of the severity of the condition suggests the opportunity to employ all the available imaging techniques in an attempt to improve prenatal diagnostic accuracy.

In fact, surgical complications and hemorrhagic risk associated with PAS vary significantly according to the extent of placental invasion, the severity of uteroplacental hypervascularization and the involvement of bladder and parametrium.

Three-dimensional ultrasonography seems to afford advantages over 2D in the imaging of PAS. It provides images that are not obtainable with 2D US, thanks to its multiplanar capability which allows the visualization of structures from multiple viewpoints. 3D power Doppler permits the dynamic assessment of uteroplacental vascularity, leading to a more accurate and clearer configuration of the abnormal placentation. So, tridimensional ultrasonography and 3D power Doppler have become frequent in the study of placental development and vascularization, leading to an evaluation not just qualitative but also quantitative.

Three-dimensional power Doppler allows to acquire multiplanar images on coronal, axial and sagittal planes and with rotational technique permits to visualize the placenta–bladder interface more accurately, giving a much more coherent view of the extent of placental invasion. It allows a better study of the degree of bladder invasion, an information with great impact on the subsequent counseling, and management.

Until a few years ago, there were not consistent studies in literature about the evaluation of the myometrial invasion degree and the possibility to differentiate between placenta accreta, increta, and percreta before the delivery. In 2000, Chou et al. stated that 3D power Doppler permits a quantitative analysis of the level of placental neovascularization, so representing an important examination complementary to 2D ultrasound.[6] In 2009, Chou et al.[7] proposed some 3D US diagnostic criteria in case of suspect abnormal placental invasion and bladder involvement:

- Loss of the echolucent space between the bladder and the placenta in coronal and axial scans
- Invasion of the bladder by the infiltrating placenta with irregularity and disruption of the normal bladder wall architecture and/or a focal exophytic placental mass projecting into the bladder in coronal and axial scans.
- Aberrant blood vessels extending into the bladder in rotational technique.

In 2009, Shih et al. published a prospective study about the role of 3D power Doppler in the diagnosis of PAS versus 2D ultrasound and color Doppler.[8] In 39 cases of PAS histologically confirmed, the best diagnostic sign was the presence of chaotic vascularization with confluent and tortuous vessels, with sensitivity of 97% and specificity of 92%. The employment of 3D ultrasound with power Doppler increased the diagnostic information obtainable with tridimensional technique. The same study also discussed the method limitations, particularly those resulting from SIGNAL post-processing, such as the threshold and transparency settings, as well as those related to the relative weighting of the power Doppler

signals in the elaboration of data with "glass-body" technique.

In 2013, these results were confirmed in a prospective study we conducted on 187 patients with placenta previa and previous cesarean delivery, among which 41 with placenta accreta histologically confirmed.[9] We used a 3D ultrasound system with transabdominal and transvaginal transducers. Transabdominal 3D power Doppler was employed to map the vascularization of the placental parenchyma and of the uterine serosa–bladder interface. 3D volumes were obtained and processed, either on the ultrasound monitor or using the 4D view software application. With a 180° rotation process, we visualized the sagittal and coronal sections. 3D power Doppler showed that the hypervascularization observed in the uterus–bladder interface extended from side-to-side in all cases of placenta percreta, with sensibility of 90% and specificity of 100% **(Figs. 5.1A and B)**. We used bladder filling of 300 mL for evaluating the uterine serosa-bladder interface. In this condition, the irregular and tortuous vascularization of the whole placental thickness and the vascularization of the whole uterine serosa-bladder interface strongly suggested the most severe forms of PAS.

This result should be interpreted with caution, because the prospective studies in literature are few. Moreover, 3D power Doppler is usually employed after 2D color Doppler and this could be a bias in the comparison between the techniques. So further studies are

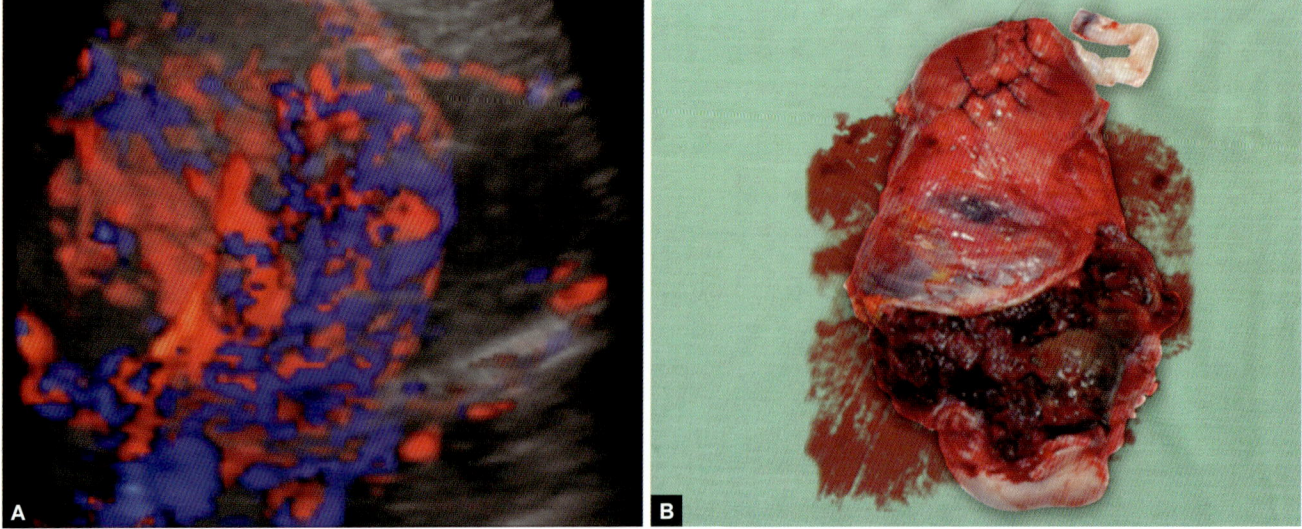

Figs. 5.1A and B: (A) 3D power Doppler image showing a remarkable vascularization involving the total bladder–uterine interface from side to side; (B) Surgical specimen showing the loss of myometrial tissue in the anterior uterine wall in a case of placenta percreta.

required to evaluate the diagnostic performance of 3D ultrasonography used as main instrument in the examination of PAS.

Few years ago, Collins et al.[10] proposed a new quantitative 3D ultrasound technique permitting reliable prenatal identification of PAS, in an attempt to obtain adequate preparation and management. The technique puts in evidence the largest area of confluent power Doppler signal, called "Area of Confluence" (Acon). It can differentiate between the presence and absence of PAS, and is associated with the histopathologic and clinical severity of the condition, thus predicting the clinical risk. The parameter shows 100% sensitivity and 8% false-positive rate, suggesting that this technique could be useful for an accurate prenatal diagnosis or screening. Acon could help in removing subjectivity in the evaluation of the increased vascularity associated with PAS. However, further validation is necessary before it could be clinically available.

Virtual Cystoscopy

A careful study of the degree of bladder involvement is an information with great impact on the subsequent surgical management of PAS disorders. Preoperative knowledge about the degree of bladder invasion can be useful in order to predict the risk of bladder injury, to estimate the entity of bleeding during surgery, to predict technical surgical difficulties and to evaluate the possible insertion of ureteral stents before surgery.

Conventional cystoscopy can identify lesions occupying the full thickness of the bladder wall but does not provide details on vascularization of the placental basal layer adjacent to the urothelium, whose extent is directly related to the degree of PAS disorders.

In the diagnostic workup of our patients with diagnosis of PAS disorders, we introduced in 2014[11] the 3D high-definition flow "sonographic virtual cystoscopy", employed for the analysis of the vascular topography of the uterine–bladder interface. We filled the bladder with 300 mL of liquid for an optimal evaluation of the uterine–bladder interface and, after volume acquisition, we analyzed the image with glass-body rendering, observing the contiguity of posterior bladder wall with the abnormal site of placental insertion in case of placenta percreta. So the hypervascularization of the serosa–bladder interface under the urothelial tissue was documented allowing the preoperative detection of the degree of myometrial

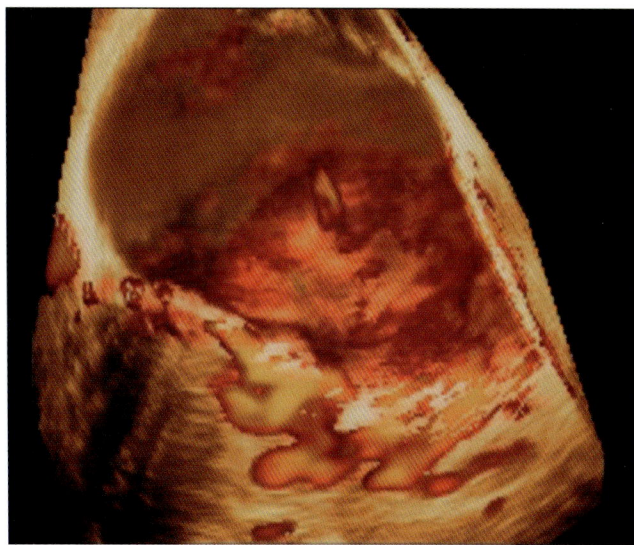

Fig. 5.2: Virtual cystoscopy: This technique allows to state the extent of vascularization below the bladder mucosa, before bladder wall perforation.

infiltration and involvement of the bladder mucosa **(Fig. 5.2)**. Very clear details of the same district can be observed employing a 3D volume-rendering technology called "Crystal Vue". This emerging technique is based on image-contrast enhancement and can be used for processing and rendering of acquired 3D volumes. In our experience, we used Crystal Vue in the study of the hypervascularization of the bladder wall, creating a highly detailed virtual cystoscopy. As shown in **Figures 5.3A and B**, Crystal Vue puts in evidence the irregularity and disruption of the normal bladder wall architecture in a case of percretism.[12]

The accurate preoperative knowledge of the degree of bladder wall invasion is important for planning the timing of delivery and the surgical approach and to anticipate potential technical difficulties. 3D ultrasonography has a key role for this purpose.

2D and 3D Ultrasound Detection of Bladder–Uterovaginal Anastomoses

High degrees of PAS are often characterized by the presence of a rich vascular anastomotic system between bladder, uterus, and vagina. Normally, the connection between uterine arteries and bladder arteries is microscopic; while in case of PAS, these vessels enlarge and present an important neovascularization. The result is a complex vascular network involving the superior,

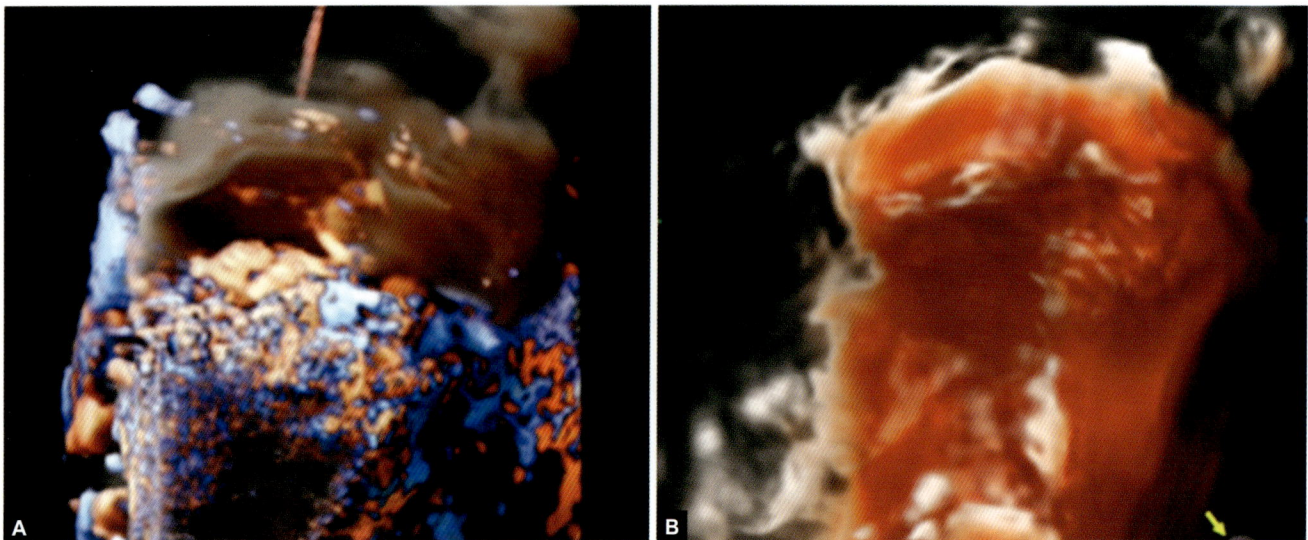

Figs. 5.3A and B: Virtual cystoscopy realized with Crystal Vue technology. The images show with great detail and efficacy of the extensive and chaotic hypervascularization (A) and the disruption (B) of the uterine serosa–bladder interface, strongly suggesting percretism.

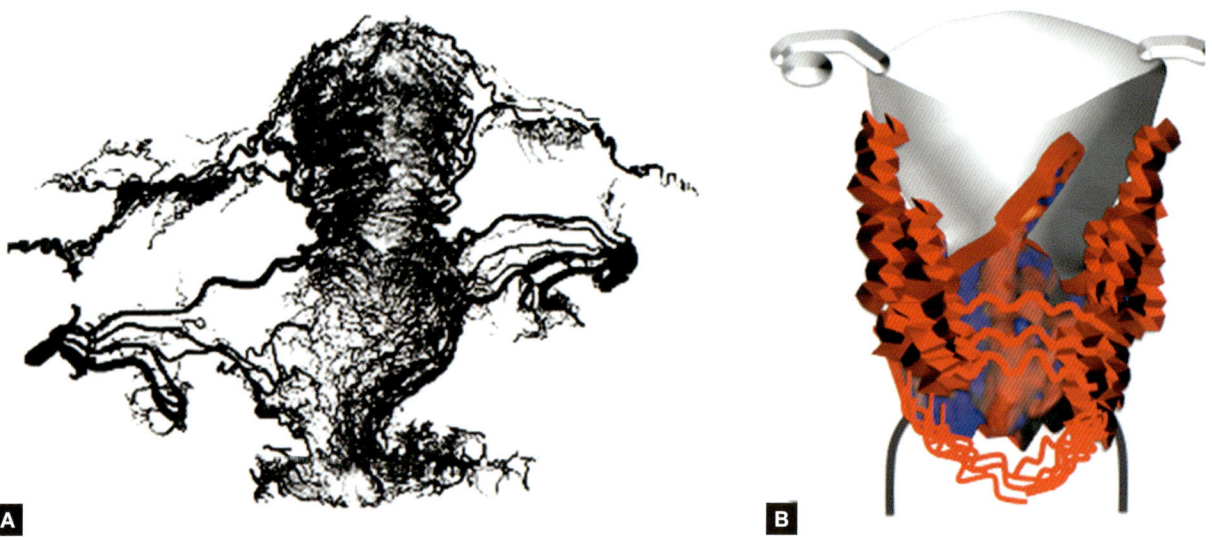

Figs. 5.4A and B: (A) Complex vascular anastomotic system between bladder, uterus and vagina. In normal circumstances, the connection between bladder arteries and uterine arteries is microscopic, while (B) in presence of abnormal placentation these vessels enlarge and present important neovascularization
Courtesy: Prof Palacios Jaraquemada (A).

medial, and inferior vaginal and the lower vesical arteries **(Figs. 5.4A and B)**.

The role of the interventional radiologist is fundamental in the multidisciplinary team required for an optimal management of PAS disorders. Thanks to the employment of embolization techniques, we can reach

vascular control, an important step to reach satisfactory results in the surgical treatment of PAS. Since the vessels involved arise from the internal pudendal artery, endovascular hemostasis is not possible through ligation or other methods of closure of the uterine arteries or the anterior divisions of the iliac internal artery. To obtain a targeted embolization, it is necessary to identify the presence of the abnormal vascular connections of the genital tract. A study of 2016 reported the feasibility of ultrasound evaluation of bladder–uterovaginal anastomoses (the "BUV system") in patients with suspect of PAS disorder, using 2D grayscale, color Doppler and 3D power Doppler US. The ultrasound equipment used was a Samsung WS80A with Elite with a 3D transabdominal transducer of 3.8 MHz and a transvaginal transducer of 6.5 MHz. The power Doppler setting was pulse repetition frequency of 0.9 kHz, with the wall filter set to "low". Ultrasound images were evaluated using the 3D multiplanar and the 3D color and power Doppler angiographic application software performed off-line. On conventional 2D ultrasound, patients showed the classic signs of PAS (placental lacunae, loss of the hypoechoic space between the bladder and the myometrium, Doppler abnormalities involving the uterus–bladder interface). The vascular inflow to the lower uterine segment was evaluated with transvaginal scans. 3D power Doppler was applied on sagittal images showing the lower uterine segment and the vagina, with a partially full bladder. On color Doppler, large anastomotic connections between lower uterine segment, vagina, and bladder were visualized, presenting a low-resistance blood flow **(Fig. 5.5)** via axial views through the vaginal fornix, the abnormal anastomotic connections appeared as diffuse pericervical

vascularization with multiple anastomotic connections extending superiorly to the bladder and inferiorly through the vagina **(Fig. 5.6)**. To detect the BUV, anastomoses in a patient with PAS disorder is an important information which can improve the prenatal diagnosis, potentially anticipating technical difficulties during surgery and post-surgical outcomes.[13]

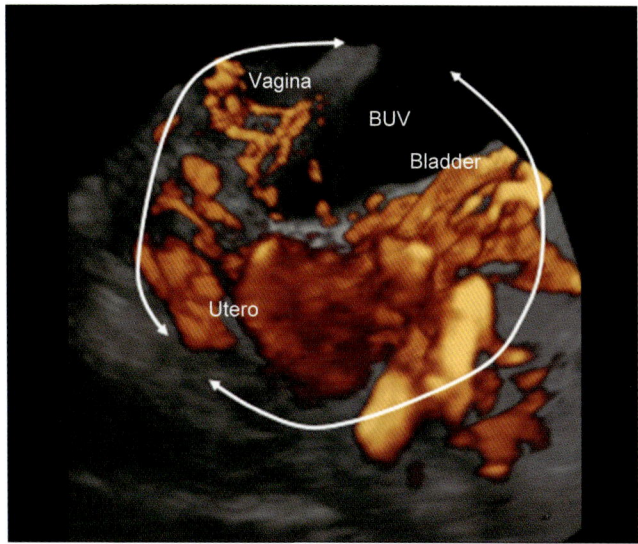

Fig. 5.5: Transvaginal sagittal lateral scan: the picture shows the large anastomoses characterizing the bladder–uterus–vagina (BUV) system.

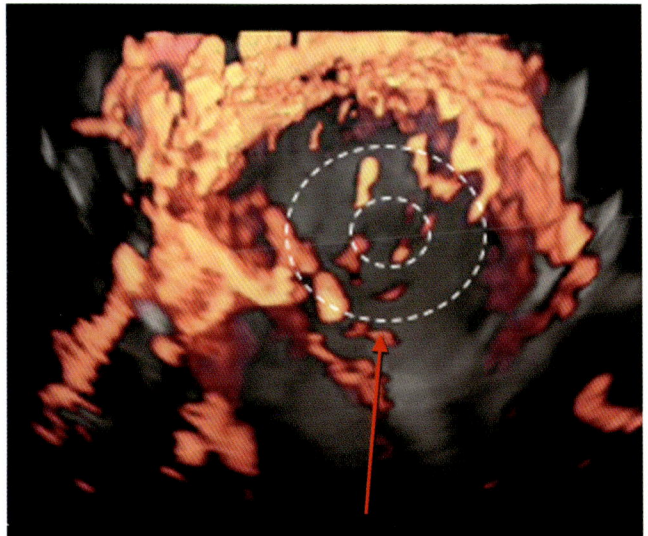

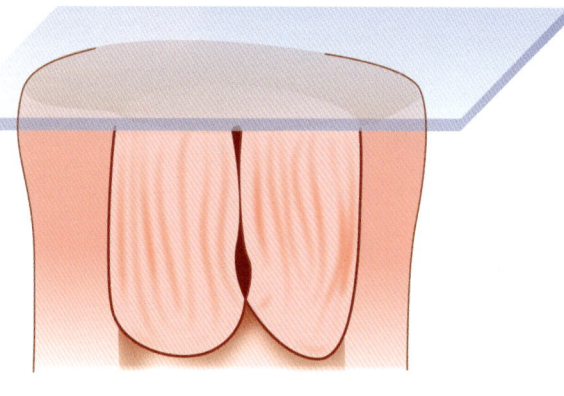

Fig. 5.6: Transvaginal axial scan: vascularity of vagina and vaginal fornix in an axial section.

CONCLUSION

Nowadays no single diagnostic technique affords complete assurance for the diagnosis of PAS. From literature data, diagnostic accuracy seems to increase using more ultrasound criteria. 2D ultrasonography is the gold standard in the diagnosis of abnormal placentation, but 3D US represents an important complementary examination for making or excluding PAS disorders and for stating the degree of placental invasion of the myometrium and the neighboring organs. Literature presents just few prospective studies about the role of 3D in this pathologic condition and objective diagnostic criteria have not been defined yet. Moreover, diagnosis is subjective with accuracy depending on the experience of the operator.[10] 3D power Doppler technique seems to have got good intraoperator but low interoperator reproducibility, because it needs a rigorous standardization of predetermined machine settings. We need new confirmatory, multicenter studies to identify common and objective 3D ultrasound criteria, to reduce interoperator variability.[9]

REFERENCES

1. Jauniaux E, Bhide A, Kennedy A, et al. FIGO consensus guidelines on placenta accreta spectrum disorders: Prenatal diagnosis and screening. Int J Gynecol Obstet. 2018;140:274-80.
2. Calì G. Le anomalie dell'invasione placentare. EDITEAM; 2015.
3. D'Antonio F, Iacovella C, Bhide A. Prenatal identification of invasive placentation using ultrasound: systematic review and meta-analysis. Ultrasound Obstet Gynecol. 2013;42:509-17.
4. Alfirevic Z, Tang AW, Collins SL, et al. Proforma for ultrasound reporting in suspected abnormally invasive placenta (AIP): an international consensus. Ultrasound Obstet Gynecol. 2016;47:276-8.
5. Cali G, Forlani F, Timor-Trisch I, et al. Diagnostic accuracy of ultrasound in detecting the depth of invasion in women at risk of abnormally invasive placenta: A prospective longitudinal study. Acta Obstet Gynecol Scand. 2018;97:1219-27.
6. Chou MM, Ho ES, Lee YH. Prenatal diagnosis of placenta previa accreta by transabdominal color Doppler ultrasound. Ultrasound Obstet Gynecol. 2000;15(1): 28-35.
7. Chou MM, Chen WC, Tseng J, et al. Prenatal detection of bladder wall involvement in invasive placentation with sequential two-dimensional and adjunctive three-dimensional ultrasonography. Taiwan J Obstet Gynecol. 2009;48:38-45.
8. Shih JC, Palacios Jaraquemada JM, Su YN, et al. Role of three-dimensional power Doppler in the antenatal diagnosis of placenta accreta: comparison with gray-scale and color Doppler techniques. Ultrasound Obstet Gynecol. 2009;33(2):193-203.
9. Calì G, Giambanco L, Puccio G, et al. Morbidly adherent placenta: evaluation of ultrasound diagnostic criteria and differentiation of placenta accreta from percreta. Ultrasound Obstet Gynecol. 2013;41:406-12.
10. Collins SL, Stevenson GN, Al-Khan A, et al. Three-dimensional power doppler ultrasonography for diagnosing abnormally invasive placenta and quantifying the Risk. Obstet Gynecol. 2015;126(3):645-53.
11. Calì G, Forlani F. Picture of the month. Three-dimensional sonographic virtual cystoscopy in a case of placenta percreta. Ultrasound Obstet Gynecol. 2014;43:481-2.
12. Minneci G, Foti F, Cali G. Crystal Vue technology in the study of the uterine-bladder interface in a case of abnormally invasive placenta. Donald School J Ultrasound Obstet Gynecol. 2017;11(3):177-8.
13. Calì G, D'Antonio F, Forlani F, et al. Ultrasound detection of bladder-uterovaginal anastomoses in morbidly adherent placenta. Fetal Diagn Ther. 2017;41:239-40.

6

Nomenclature of Three-dimensional and Four-dimensional Ultrasound in Obstetrics, Gynecology, and Fetal Echocardiography

Jing Deng

INTRODUCTION

Since three-dimensional (3D)[1-3] and four-dimensional (4D)[4-6] ultrasound were developed for women's and fetal cardiac imaging in 1980s and 1990s, they have become increasingly matured for clinical applications.[7-14]

A recent review by the 3D Special Interest Group (3D SIG) of the International Society of Ultrasound in Obstetrics and Gynecology (ISUOG) has found that, of a total of 287 formal articles (excluding its World Congress Abstracts) published during 2012 in the journal—Ultrasound in Obstetrics and Gynecology (UOG), 99 (34%) had included 3D, 4D or terms closely related to 3D/4D ultrasound imaging (VOCAL, STIC, etc.) **(Table 6.1)**.[15]

Table 6.1: Prevalence of 3D/4D articles published in Ultrasound in Obstetrics and Gynecology in 2012.

Publication types	No. of 3D/4D articles	No. of total articles	%
Picture of the month	6	9	67
Review	7	15	47
Original paper	66	161	41
Opinion	4	11	36
Miscellaneous	2	6	33
Letter to editor	7	32	22
Referee commentary	2	12	17
Case report	2	15	13
Correspondence	3	23	13
Randomized trial	0	3	00
Grand total	99	287	34

However, multidimensional imaging terms used in those publications were inconsistent in articles not just by different author groups, but also by same author groups or even within a single article.

Therefore, the prevalence of 3D/4D imaging techniques used for women's medical research and clinical care and the inconsistency in using relevant 3D/4D terms have demonstrated an ever increased need for implementation of standardized terminology since the first article in this regard was published in UOG over 15 years ago.[16]

The 15 years have also witnessed the advent of greatly improved or newly available technologies. For example, fetal cardiac gating has become online with (mechanical) spatiotemporal image correlation (STIC)[17] progressing to electronic STIC (eSTIC).[9] Dense matrix-array transducers have replaced sparse ones,[18] enabling real-time 3D visualization of the in utero heart and greatly improving prenatal diagnosis of cardiovascular malformations even without the need for fetal cardiac gating[16,19] or even without holding the probe still.[20] 3D display modes and volumetric quantification tools have become more sophisticated and automated than ever before.[21,22]

All these have made it necessary to refine old terms or define new terms (including "new" trademark names), and to address subsequent issues that may often confuse or mislead users (sometimes even experienced users). For example, what is *"real-time" 3D imaging*? Does *4D ultrasound* necessarily mean *real-time 3D ultrasound*? Will *real-time 3D* imaging signal the end of *slice-reconstructed 3D* imaging and *cardiac gating* (including STIC)? Is an *eSTIC 3D* scan a real-time 3D scan? If no is the answer to the latter three questions, should other concepts such as *direct volume scan* and *indirect volume scan*[16,23] be used in regard to a 3D ultrasound system's capability of imaging slow or fast moving obstetric, genital parts and beyond?[10,24-34]

Based on the author's own 3D/4D experiences, with invaluable suggestions from the ISUOG 3D SIG (see Acknowledgments) and with a review of related literature, this chapter attempts to define various 3D or 4D terms (*in bold italics*) with rationales behind these definitions and with a focus on most frequently but often inconsistently or misused terms.

It needs to be pointed out that nomenclature proposed here is preferred by the author personally, with most but not all of the terms being agreed by all members of the 3D SIG then. Therefore, it is hoped that this chapter can also provoke further discussions to help the 3D community reach a better consensus on preferred 3D/4D terms.

Although theoretical, the discussion is of practical help for objective selection of competent 3D/4D systems for specific scientific and clinical applications.

DIMENSIONALITY IN MEDICAL IMAGING: 3D AND 4D

Potential Confusions

When time is treated as a dimension, a two-dimensional (2D) display can mean either a display with one temporal dimension and one spatial dimension (such as in early M-mode only fetal echocardiography[35,36]) or a display with only two spatial dimensions (as seen in early, static cross-sectional ultrasound).[37] Similarly, a 3D display can mean either a display with one temporal dimension and two spatial dimensions (as seen in real-time cross-sectional ultrasound)[38,39] or a display with three-spatial dimensions (as seen in static 3D ultrasound).[2,40]

Recommended Use of 3D and 4D

To avoid these confusions, it is advisable to restrict the use of "dimension(s)" or "dimensional" only to indicate spatial dimension(s) while using "time" or "temporal", "motion" or "moving", or "dynamics" or "dynamic" to indicate the temporal dimension. In other words, avoid terming M-mode as a 2D mode, or real-time cross-sectional (or 2D) ultrasound as a 3D modality. One exception is for 4D (four-dimensional or four dimensions) which can be unmistakably used to indicate the three-spatial dimensions plus the temporal dimension. Though,

this is not absolutely definite as "more and subordinate dimensions" do exist. Please refer to a namesake section in this refereed article.[16]

Key Points

- The term *4D (ultrasound) imaging* equals to the term *dynamic 3D (ultrasound) imaging*. However, *4D* imaging is not necessarily equal to *real-time 3D* imaging because *4D* imaging can be achieved by *slice-reconstructed* or *subvolume-reconstructed 4D* approach (with motion gating necessary for a dynamic target, or by *real-time 3D* approach (using a dense 2D-array transducer with gating being usually unnecessary). For more about gating necessity see Chapter 7 on Four Relativity Issues in Four-dimensional Ultrasonography.

- Non-strictly speaking, *real-time 3D* means *real-time 4D*. However, there is an unnecessary duplication in the latter phrase, as both *real-time* and *4D* (the temporal dimension + three spatial dimensions) contain the meaning of "temporal". Hence, the use of *real-time 4D* should be avoided. Otherwise, we could call real-time 2D as real-time 3D (two spatial dimensions + the temporal dimension in real-time), which is not entirely unreasonable but could mislead readers into thinking of imaging a 3D space while it actually concerns only cross-sectional (2D) imaging.

REAL-TIMENESS

Current Usage

Several terms have been used to describe high volume-rate scanning for 3D/4D imaging (see terms frame rate and volume rate below). The most commonly used (and probably the most attractive) one is *real time*, such as *real-time 3D*, *real-time 4D*, and *real-time volumetric* imaging. These catchphrases are usually introduced by manufacturers for commercial promotion, but the actual volume rates to which they refer vary greatly (*c.* 8 ~ 60 Hz).

Proposed Definition

According to the Oxford Dictionary, *real time* means the actual time during which a process or event occurs, especially one analyzed by a computer, in contrast to time subsequent to it when computer processing may be done, a recording replayed, or the like.

In terms of ultrasonography or other imaging modalities, it should be used to indicate a system's ability of visualizing dynamic morphology or morphological dynamics while the anatomical data are being acquired over the time, or with a negligible delay no longer than the *persistence of vision* between the acquisition and the visualization. It is generally stated that the human eye and brain retain a visual impression for about 1/25th of a second (so comes the standard cinematic rate of approximately 25 frames per second).[41]

Hence, real-time 2D or 3D imaging should only be used to indicate a system capable of displaying 2D or 3D images (1) virtually as they are acquired, and (2) at about or above the cinematic rate—25 Hz (Hz = frames per second, i.e. *fps*, in 2D imaging, or = volumes per second, i.e. *vps*, in 3D/4D imaging).

Key Points

The exact visual persistence time depends on the brightness of the image and perhaps individual variations, but most people would probably agree that a rate less than 20 Hz will likely produce "jerky" movies. Strictly speaking, therefore, a 3D ultrasonography incapable of a volume rate at or above 20 Hz should not be qualified as a real-time 3D system. Our clinical research has shown that, for the 18 ~ 28 gestational weeks scanned with latest, state-of-art matrix-array 4D systems, a volume rate range between 20 Hz and 30 Hz can achieve satisfactory recognition of both gross and fine cardiac structures **(Figs. 6.1, 6.2 and Table 6.2)**.[20,42]

The term "real-time" should not be used to describe systems only capable of displaying images with certain delay after data acquisition (such as 4D fetal echocardiography using STIC or eSTIC gating) even if they can online reconstruct 4D images of the fetal heart at a rate of 20 Hz or higher.

When talking about real-time imaging, we are actually talking about whether an imaging system is capable to "fool" our visual persistence. Therefore, it should not be used to imply whether a system's frame rate or volume rate is necessarily adequate for visualizing the dynamics of an object for specific scientific or clinical purposes. For example, a 25 Hz "real-time" ultrasound scanner is unable to distinguish isovolumetric contraction (IVC) or isovolumetric relaxation (IVR) phases of the fetal heart. This is because the time to form an image at such a frame

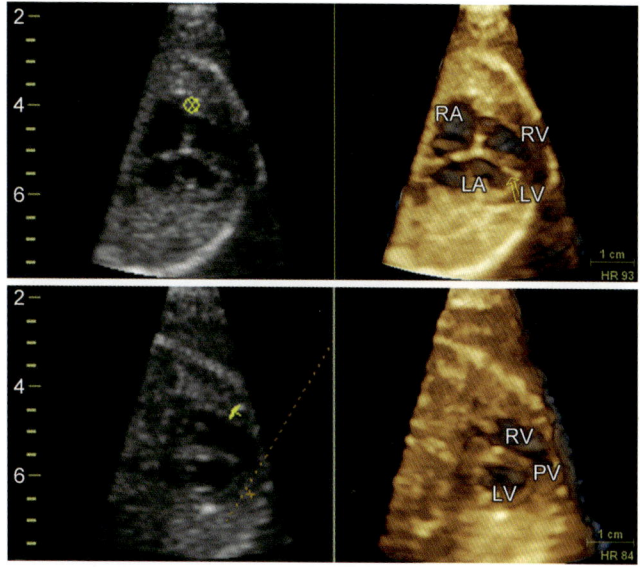

Fig. 6.1: Real-time 3D imaging of a 25-week fetal heart using a latest dense matrix-array ultrasound transducer (4Vc, GE E95). The scan corresponds to Quick One Scan (in Figure 7.2, Chapter 7) if the clinical interest is only in assessing most gross and some fine structures of the heart during long cardiac phases (Figure 7.3). Hence, not only gating is unnecessary but the probe can even be manually moved during the 4D scan without causing obvious motion artifact. HR 84, 93 were the maternal heart rates. (RA and RV: right atrium and ventricle; LA and LV: left atrium and ventricle; PV: pulmonary valve) [visible in video clips on our website: *www.medphys.ucl.ac.uk/mgi/jdeng* under Fetal Heart > album 7 entry].

rate or volume rate is 40 ms, much longer than the IVC (*c.* 25 ms) and IVR (*c.* 20 ms) (Figure 7.3, Chapter 7). In this regard, the terms *direct* or *indirect volume scans* can be used (see "Direct and Indirect Volume Scanning" below).

ONLINE AND OFFLINE

Current Usage

Before acquired data can be visualized in 3D (using multiplanar reformatted 2D, and/or surface or volume rendered 3D displays), some post-processing has to be carried out, taking time on the ultrasound system or on another reviewing computer. Computing terms *online* and *offline* are often used to indicate, respectively, the post-processing and visualization performed on the same acquisition system that also acquires the data, and those performed on a separate system using 3D/4D data transferred from an ultrasound acquisition system.

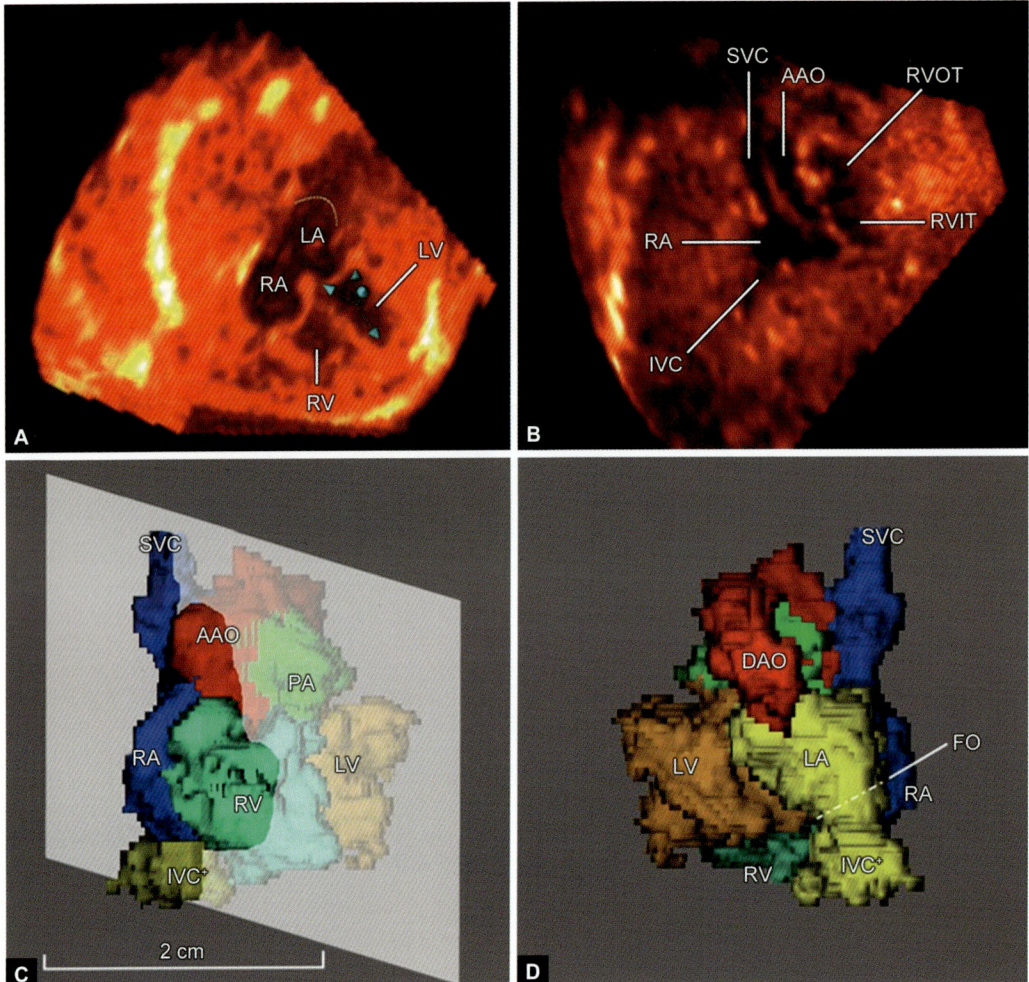

Figs. 6.2A to D: Real-time 3D imaging of a 21-week fetal heart using another dense matrix-array ultrasound transducer (X7-2, Philips IEE33). (A) In this usual 3D surface view, the upper half of the chest is "removed" to reveal the four cardiac chambers in the lower half. Note that the spatial relationships and sequential connections of cardiovascular structures between the two halves cannot be straightforwardly displayed. Also note that, because of inhomogeneous echogenicity between the left posterior atrial wall and the remaining cardiac walls, the left atrium (LA) appears larger than it is. During semi-automated virtual casting, a 3D barrier (dotted curve) can be placed by an operator to stop a "seed" from growing beyond the border. The arrows in the left ventricle (LV) illustratively show how a "seed" placed inside a cardiac chamber grows in all direction to detect endocardium; (D) Cross-sectional view of the right heart system reformatted from the (light gray) cutting plane in (C), showing anatomical detail. The cast view can guide multiplanar reformatting in a way much easier to understand than a usual 3D surface view can do; (C and D) Negative 3D surface view after virtual casting. The front (C) and back (D) 3D cast views show straightforwardly the spatial relationships and connections of all major structures. Note that the inferior vena cava and its tributaries from the liver (IVC+) and the LA are cast together due to normal physiological shunting through foramen ovale (FO). Also note that the LA is not over-segmented due to the barrier set in (A). (AAO and DAO: ascending and descending aorta; PA: pulmonary artery; RA and RV: right atrium and ventricle; RVIT and RVOT: right ventricular inflow and outflow tracts; SVC: superior vena cava. Corresponding 3D/4D movies are available on our website at *www.medphys.ucl.ac.uk/mgi/jdeng* under Fetal Heart > album 6 entry.
Source: Reprinted with permission from Deng J, Rodeck CH. Current applications of fetal cardiac imaging technology (invited review). Curr Opin Obstet Gynecol. 2006;18(2):177.

Proposed Definitions

Online means that necessary procedure(s), e.g. motion gating, can be carried out rapidly (but not necessarily in real-time) so that resultant 3D images can be displayed in real-time (e.g. using a real-time matrix-array system performing a *direct volume scan*) (see "Direct and Indirect Volume Scanning" below), or immediately after

Table 6.2: Approximate dimensions of various cardiac structures between 16 weeks and 40 weeks of gestation.

Anatomy			Approximate dimension/thickness (systole ~ diastole if applicable) mm	
			16 weeks	*40 weeks*
Gross structures	The whole heart	Long-axis	15	75
		Short-axis	10	50
	Four chambers		1~3	10~16
	Ventricular walls and muscular septum		1~2	4~6
	Lumen of the great vessels		2	10
	Some papillary muscles		1	4
Fine structures	Membranous septa, valves, trabeculations, most papillary muscles, moderator bands		From 0.5 to 2	

an acquisition (e.g. using STIC or eSTIC gated, slice-reconstructed or subvolume-reconstructed 4D scans), usually by/on the same system.

Offline denotes that necessary procedure(s) are carried out, or resulting 3D images are displayed with a considerable delay after the acquisition, e.g. several minutes or even hours after an acquisition, no matter whether or not they are displayed on the acquisition system or on another system.

Key Points

- As networked, multisystem data acquisition, processing and visualization are now commonplace, the physical boundary between online and offline has become hazy, and the corresponding definitions should no longer over-emphasize this boundary. The new definitions here emphasize on how fast a system (or a set of networked systems) is capable of producing clinical information in relationship to a particular patient scan. *Online* connotes such a short (processing) time (usually not more than a few seconds or maximally a few minutes) that the patient can still be kept on the scanning couch. Thereafter, if further acquisitions are indicated by the online results, these can be performed without recalling the patient. Hence, although STIC or eSTIC is not a real-time 4D technique, it is an online one.
- *Offline* implies such a long (processing) time (usually several minutes or even hours) that the patient may have to be sent off after a scan. If further acquisitions are necessary, the patient has to be called into the scanning room again or to be examined in a new session.

FRAME RATE AND VOLUME RATE

Current Usage

Many articles have used frame rate regardless whether 2D or 3D imaging is concerned. The need for distinguishing frame rate from volume rate is best illustrated in STIC imaging where the real-time 2D imaging frame rate can be as high as 150 Hz (fps), but reconstructed 4D imaging volume rate is usually 10–40 Hz (vps) for a reasonably large volume size. With matrix-array transducer technology, volume rate during real-time 3D scanning can be as high as 20~30 Hz with a reasonable imaging volume size and spatial resolution, and even up to over 60 Hz at the cost of spatial resolution and/or volume size.[42,43]

Proposed Usage

- *Frame rate* (unit: frames per second, fps or Hz) should be only referred to the number of 2D images (frames) achieved by cross-sectional imaging per unit time, usually per second.
- *Volume rate* (unit:volumes per second, vps or Hz) should be used to indicate the number of the volumes achieved by a 3D/4D system.

Key Points

- When talking about a cross-sectional imaging rate per unit time, *frame rate* should be used no matter if an imaging system/mode performs a routine 2D scan or a volume scan for 3D or 4D reconstruction.
- *Volume rate* can either refer to a real-time volume rate, such as that during matrix-array real-time 3D scanning, or to a reconstructed volume rate obtained by motion-gated 4D reconstruction such as using STIC.

REGION OF INTEREST VERSUS IMAGING PLANE SIZE AND VOLUME OF INTEREST VERSUS IMAGING VOLUME SIZE

Current Usage

Many publications have used *region of interest (ROI)*, even when talking about 3D/4D scanning, where, strictly, the concern should be a *volume of interest (VOI)* in relationship to *imaging volume size* during a 3D/4D scan.

Proposed Usage

We would suggest constraining the use of *ROI* only during 2D scanning of a study while using *VOI* during 3D/4D scanning of the study. Use *imaging volume size* to indicate whether or not a 3D or 4D mode can provide sufficiently large imaging volume to embrace the entirety of, or just part of a VOI.

Key Points

The differentiating use of *ROI* with imaging plane size from *VOI* with imaging volume size can remind an operator to ensure that the inseparable entirety of the VOI should be fully embraced by the imaging volume during direct volume scanning (see "Direct and Indirect Volume Scanning" below). Take for example the 3D measurement of the left ventricle stroke volume, which is: LVSV = the end-diastolic LV volume—the end-systolic LV volume. Now the interest is the LV volumetric change (rather than the entire heart). The operator should make sure that the imaging volume is sufficiently large to embrace the largest LV boundary at all times through the cardiac cycle before recording a direct volume scan.

What about if the imaging volume is not full enough, resulting in part of the LV boundary not captured in the 4D dataset? Or, if the operator is now interested in the volumetric change of the entire heart and connecting great vessels and their branches? If to increase the imaging volume would degrade temporal and/or spatial resolution, subvolume-reconstruction 4D mode must be employed. The scan has become an *indirect volume scan* (see "Direct and Indirect Volume Scanning" below), and gating must be used to avoid motion (stitching) artifacts **(Figs. 6.3A and B)**.

MULTIPLANAR VERSUS MULTISLICE REFORMATTING/DISPLAY, THREE-ORTHOGONAL PLANES VERSUS TRIPLANAR DISPLAYS, TOMOGRAPHIC DISPLAY VERSUS PARALLEL-PLANE, AND OMNI-VIEW VERSUS CURVED PLANE

Multiplanar versus Multislice Reformatting/Display

Among the four term pairs in the heading of this section, this pair is the most inclusive one concerning all sorts of 2D views obtained (reformatted) from a 3D/4D dataset **(Fig. 6.4)**. Because of its 3D/4D property, multiple planes can simultaneously be displayed with known spatial relationship in the volume and between each other 2D views, allowing better comprehension of spatially complex structures than using conventional multiple slices (with unknown or inaccurate spatial relationship between each other, which we have to use our mental power to figure out).

The inclusiveness of the term is also reflected in that reformatted views are not required to be necessarily orthogonal or in parallel to each other, and that even curved plane or OmniView (as termed by some manufacturers) can be used for obtaining 2D views of special interest.[44,45]

As "*curved plane*" rather than "curved slice" has been an existing scientific/imaging phrase, we would therefore recommend to use *multiplanar reformatting (MPR)*, instead of multislicing, when concerning reformatting 2D views (or 2D views reformatted) from a volume dataset.

Biplanes, Triplanes, and Orthogonal Planes

In theory, an unlimited number of 2D views can be reformatted from a volume from any viewing angles or points. In practice, only a limited number of 2D views is needed at one time.

Biplane plane: It was the first to be developed for endoscopic imaging (such as transvaginal ultrasound or transesophageal echocardiography). At its infancy, it was two perpendicularly-intersecting ultrasound beam planes simultaneously cross-sectioning an organ of interest. There was no imaging data in between the two planes **(Fig. 6.5)**.

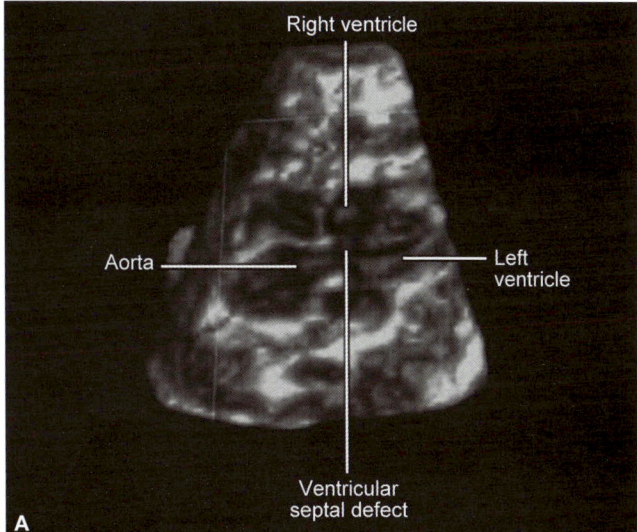

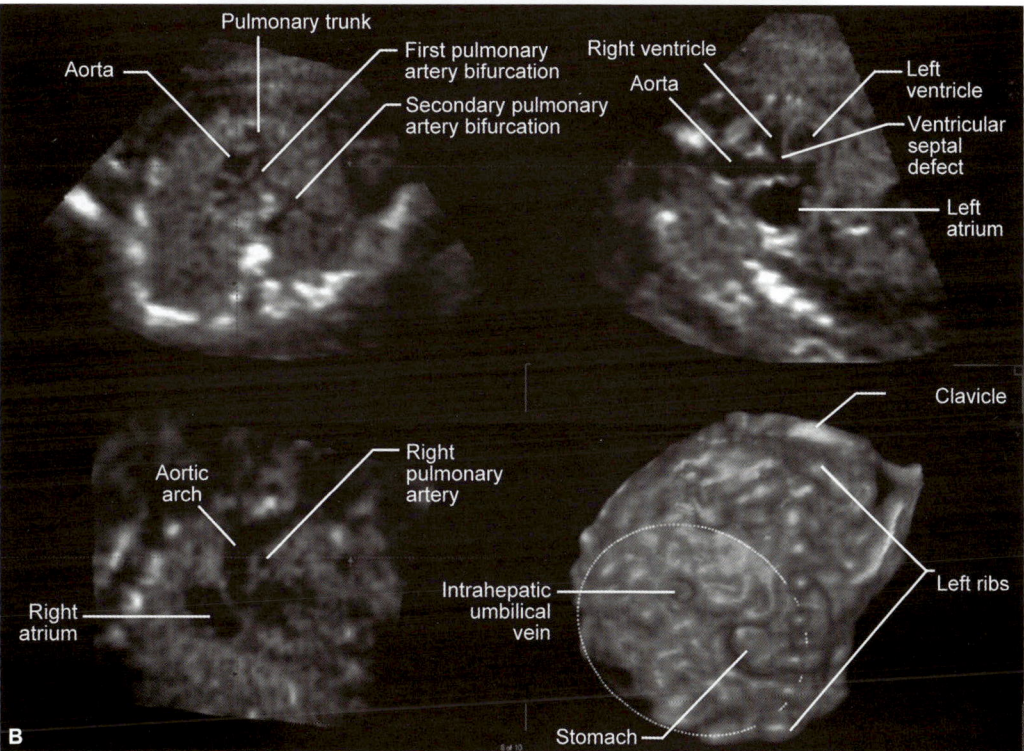

Figs. 6.3A and B: Four-dimensional (4D) ultrasound imaging of a 21-week-old fetal heart in part and in totality. (A) Real-time 3D surface display of the open heart revealed a ventricular septal defect during a "live 3D" scan; (B) The whole chest and upper abdomen were also acquired by a full volume combined from four gated subvolumes. Three imaging planes, reformatted offline, demonstrated simultaneously all three features required for confirmative diagnosis of fetal tetralogy of Fallot: the ventricular septal defect, the overriding aorta and the narrowed pulmonary trunk. The detailed visualization of the entire course of the pulmonary artery and branches (including the secondary branches) is very important for helping parental counseling and surgical planning. (Video clips on our website: *www.medphys.ucl.ac.uk/mgi/jdeng* under Fetal Heart > Album 5 entry).
Source: Reprinted with permission from John Wiley & Sons, Ltd.

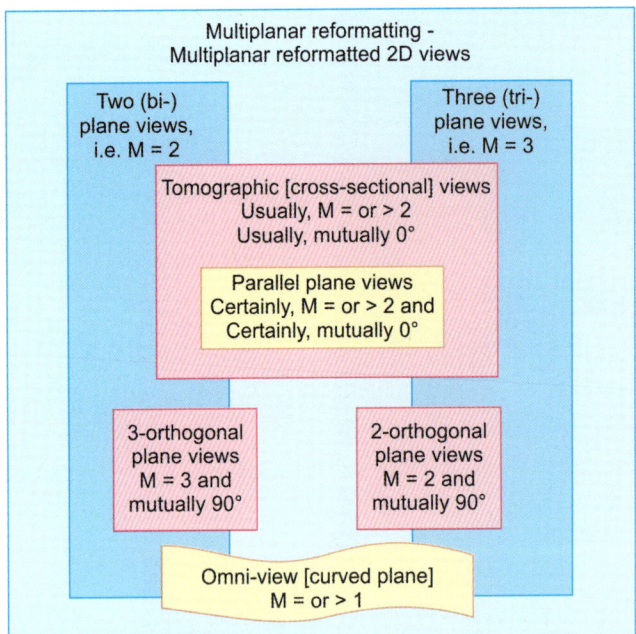

Fig. 6.4: Multiplanar reformatting. Illustration of the relationship among (and overlapping over) terms describing different reformatted 2D views from a 3D dataset, depending on their multiple number (M) and angle (°) to each other plane/view and whether they are flat or curved planes/views.

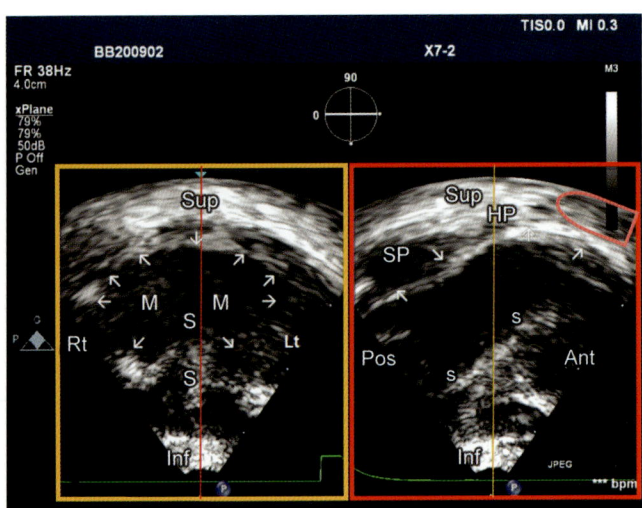

Fig. 6.5: Biplane (Philips' tradename: X-Plane) imaging of the infant tongue. The two-framed images are perpendicularly across each other along the red-yellow line. The submental position of a matrix-array ultrasound transducer (Fig. 7.5) is indicated by a small blue circles with a letter P in each image. The yellow-framed coronal view shows the connective tissue (bright) separation (S) between the two lateral muscular (dark) areas (M) of the tongue. In the human body, the separation should normally be on the midsagittal plane. With the red line cutting through or very close to the separation, a true midsagittal view is obtained in the red frame, showing a wavy (peristaltic) upper surface (arrows) of the tongue together with the nipple (open pink arrow) during breastfeeding. The peristalsis from the reader's right to left is dynamically displayed in the video clips on our website: *www.medphys.ucl.ac.uk/mgi/jdeng* under Baby Breast/Bottle Feeding. (Ant: anterior; HP: hard palate; Inf: inferior; Lt: left; Pos: posterior; Rt: right; SP: soft palate; Sup: superior). *Source*: Reprinted with permission from Burton P, Deng J, McDonald D, et al. Real-time 3D ultrasound imaging of infant tongue movements during breast-feeding. Early Hum Dev. 2013;89(9):635-41.

Triplane or multiplane: With the advent of dense matrix-array transducer technology enabling real-time volumetric imaging, biplane, and triplane views can be obtained from an imaging volume in any angles, but usually from two or three axial planes to form biplane or triplane views, and with or without additional plane(s) parallel to the transducer footprint to form *triplane or multiplane* views (**Fig. 6.6**).

Three-orthogonal display: It is a type of multiplanar display that shows three mutually perpendicular 2D planes/views (**Fig. 6.7**).[6] Therefore, the term should only be used in such a context (i.e. three planes intersecting each other at 90°). When not confined to this context, a display with two, three, or more planes should only be called "bi-, tri-, or multiplane display".

Tomographic Slices versus Parallel-plane Views

In terms of reformatting a series of 2D views parallel to each other, the author prefers to term them as *parallel planes* (or slices, views, displays, etc.). This is because the phrase directly indicates that the serial planes have an angle of 180° to each other (**Fig. 6.8**). In this context, the phrase "tomographic planes" is less indicative as it only refers to serial cross-sectional images from an ultrasound beam, X-ray or magnetic field imaged volume. By CT or MR scanning of the human body, you can obtain a series of sagittal tomograms (which are in parallel to each other) or a set of transverse tomograms (also in parallel to each other), but any of the sagittal tomograms and any of the transverse tomogram are not in parallel to each other.

Curved Plane versus Omni-view

Strictly speaking, curve means a line that bends continuously and has no straight parts or sharp angles. As MPR is used for a simplified display of an area (usually a path) of interest which in real anatomy does not always lie on a flat plane or may have flat segments or sharp angles

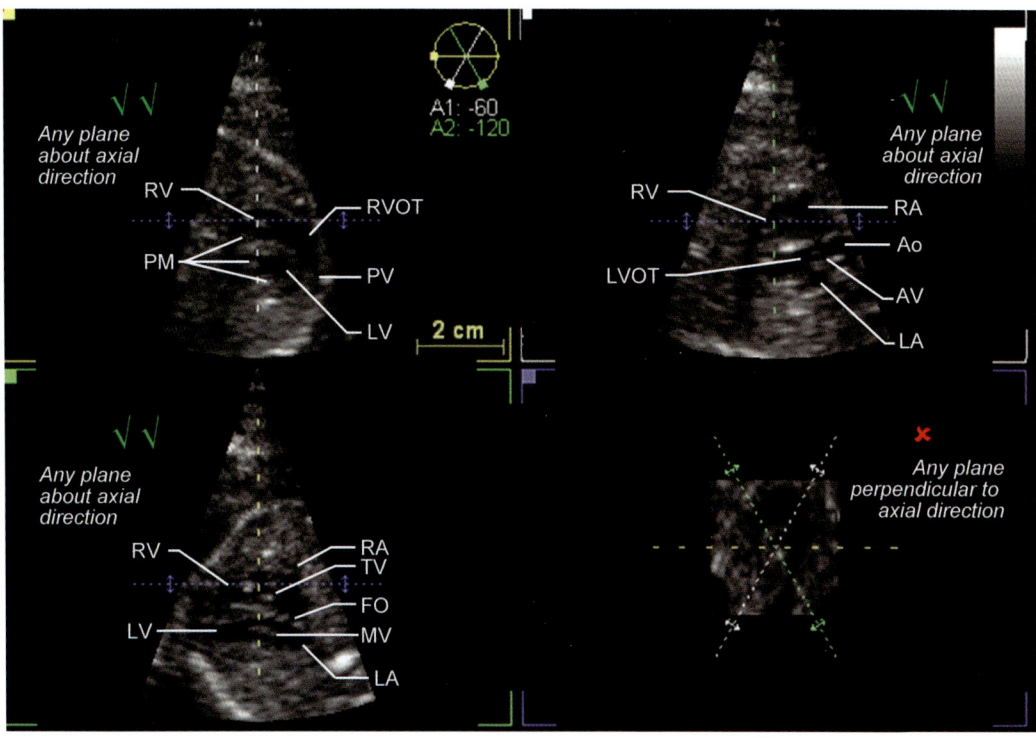

Fig. 6.6: Matrix-array transducer provides virtually identical, good-quality resolution for images reformatted from any planes about the ultrasound propagation (axial) direction while poor-quality resolution for images from planes perpendicular to the axial direction (dotted white and green lines). Upper left: LV short axis views, also showing one papillary muscle (PM) in the right ventricle (RV), two PMs in the left ventricle (LV), and RV outflow tract (RVOT) and the pulmonary valve (PV). Lower left: Four-chamber view, also showing the tricuspid and mitral valve (TV, MV), and the foramen ovale (FO) between the right and left atria (RA, LA). Upper right: Five-chamber view, also showing the aortic valve (AV) between LV outflow tract (LVOT) and the aortic root (Ao). Lower right: cardiac structures in the so-called plane C reformatted at the dotted blue line level are hardly recognizable (also see the section on Types of Spatial Resolution: Slice-reconstruction 3D versus Real-time 3D Scans and Fig. 7.7, both in Chapter 7).

along the path, the phrase *omni-view* should be preferred **(Fig. 6.9).**[45]

Key Points

- Note that, without simultaneousness, multiplanar views do not necessarily mean real MPR views. You can obtain multiple (including three individual orthogonal) planar views even using a conventional cross-sectional transducer if it is manually moved around a mother's abdomen without a time constraint. Obviously, three views obtained in this way are not what MPR really means because they are not within the same 3D/4D coordinate system.
- Bi-, tri- or multiplanes are several types of multi-planar reformatted planes with a specified number of resulting two, three or more planes, but with the angle between any of the two planes not necessarily specified.

- Orthogonal or parallel planes are two types of multi-planar reformatted planes with a specified angle between resulting planes (90° or 180°).
- A series of parallel planes/views often has an equal interval between each two consecutive slices and identical slice thickness, but the phrase itself does not necessarily indicate these.

INVERSION MODE/NEGATIVE SURFACE DISPLAY VERSUS VIRTUAL CASTING/DIGITAL CASTING

Current Usage

Although usual 3D surface display is a natural way of visualizing internal morphologies of the heart and vessels, it usually requires part of the dataset to be cut away to disclose them. This can impair 3D sequential assessment as the structures in the removed part and their

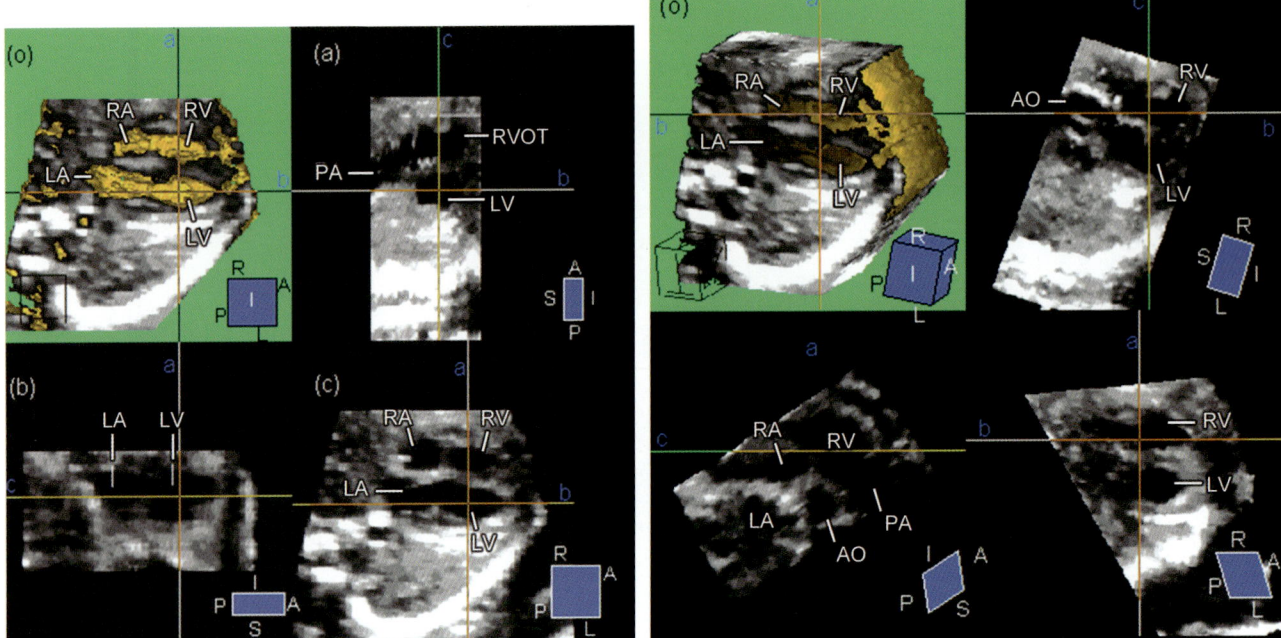

Fig. 6.7: Three orthogonal planes/ views. Interactive multiplanar reformatting of the 3D object (a 17-week fetal heart) with different orientations providing unlimited sets of three orthogonal views using only one scan 3D dataset (o). Only shown here are (Left panel): (a) left ventricular short axis view; (b) left heart two-chamber view; (c) four-chamber view; (Right panel): (a) long axis view of left heart, (b) cardiac base short axis view, and (c) bi-ventricular view. The positions of the planes (a), (b), and (c) were indicated by the intersection lines a, b, and c. RA and RV: right atrium and ventricle. LA and LV: left atrium and ventricle. AO: aorta; PA: pulmonary artery; RVOT: right ventricular outflow tract. A, I, L, P, R and S are anatomical orientations.
Source: Reprinted with permission from Deng J, Gardener JE, Rodeck CH, et al. Fetal echocardiography in three and four dimensions. Ultrasound Med Biol. 1996;22(8):979-86.

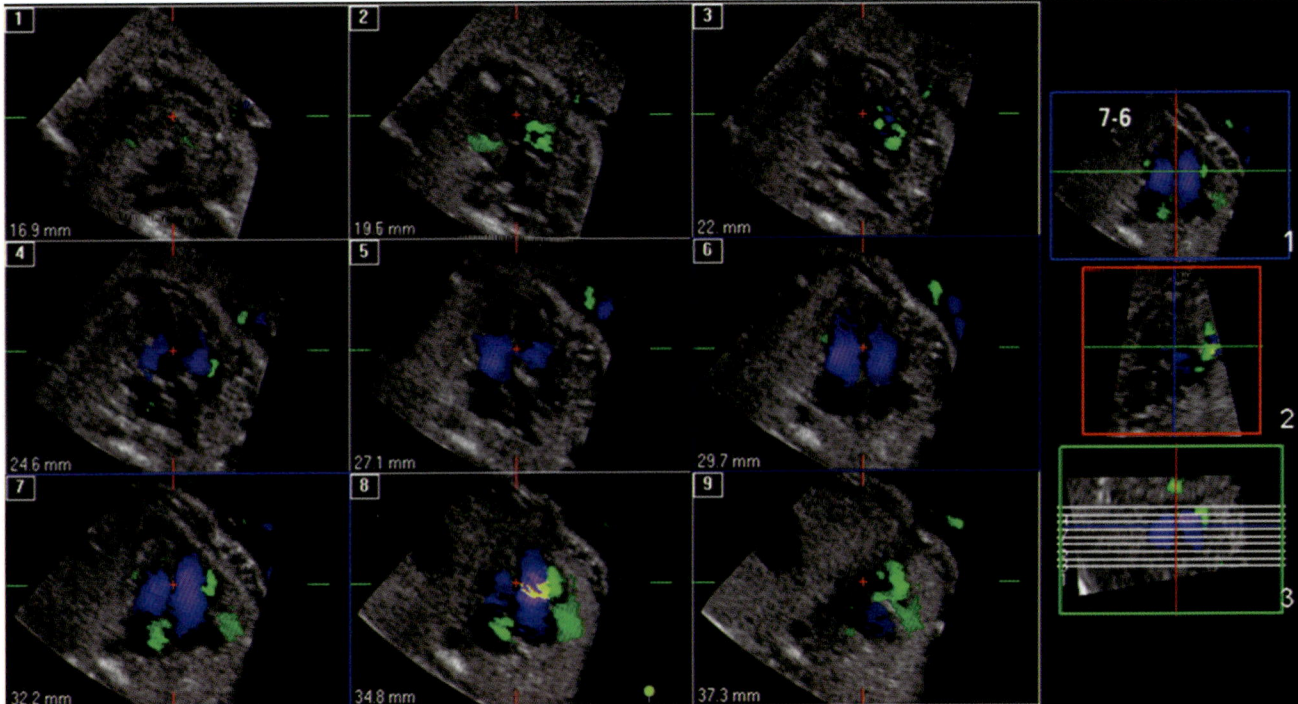

Fig. 6.8: Parallel reformatted fetal chest transverse views showing various cardiac structures and color Doppler flow.
Courtesy: Philip Ultrasound.

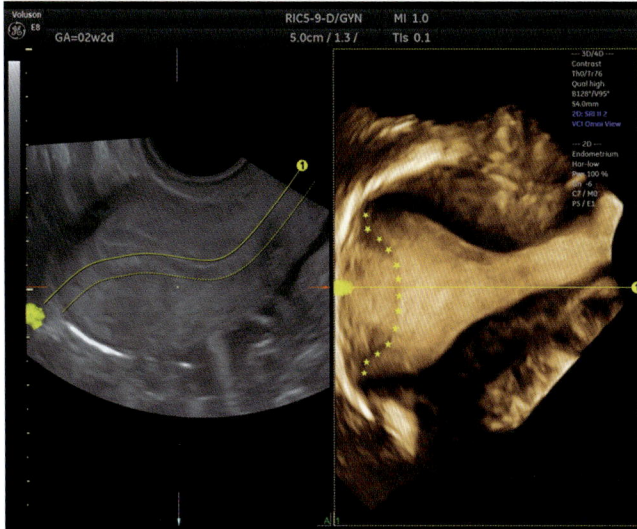

Fig. 6.9: The use of Omni-view polyline reformatting to demonstrate the internal configuration of the uterus. This technology allows the operator to follow the endometrial path. The coronal plane, naturally curved in many cases, can be fully visualized in a single view.
Courtesy: Dr Stefania Tudorache.
Source: Reprinted with permission from Tudorache S, Florea M, Dragusin R, et al. 3D Ultrasound Assessment of the Uterus: Why an Accuracy Study for Mullerian Congenital Anomalies is not Feasible, while Screening Already is, and should be done. J Clin Diagn Res. 2017;5:134.

relationships to those in the displayed part cannot be imaged in their entirety **(Fig. 6.10C)**.

A commonly used solution is to invert echogenicity (brightness, or black and white) of a 3D dataset (so comes the name *inversion mode*) **(Figs. 6.10A and B)**, and then apply a simple threshold so that hollow cardiac chambers are shown in solid (hence, also termed as *negative surface display*) **(Figs. 6.10C and D)**[46] as if they were obtained by postmortem casting, thus being also called *virtual casting* and *digital casting* **(Figs. 6.2C and D)**.[47] This makes easier not only spatial relationship comprehension (in particular, complicated vessel malformations),[48] but also volumetric quantification.[49]

Proposed Usage

It is recommended to constrain the *inversion mode* to the method of simply inversing gray-scale echogenicity, while using *virtual casting* to refer to display methods that are more intellectually analogs to the process of postmortem casting. The analogy is beyond the scope of this chapter, but can be found by comparing these two studies.[50,51]

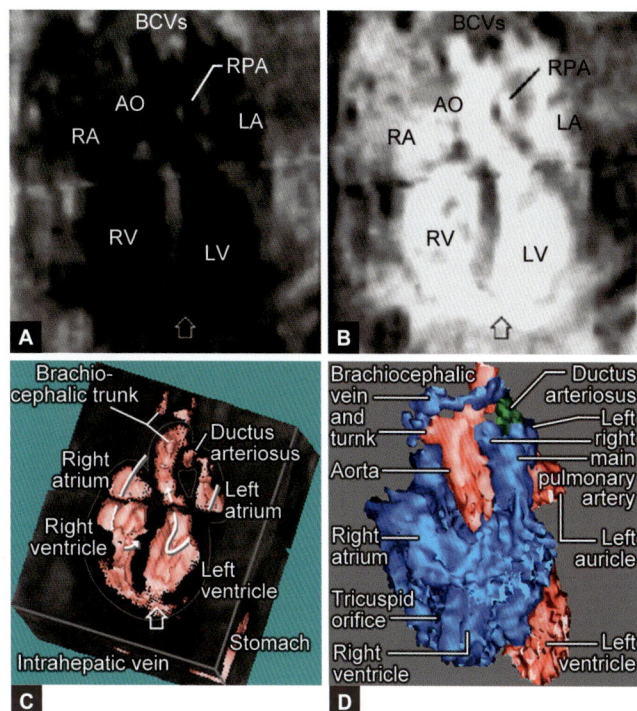

Figs. 6.10A to D: A 22-week-old fetal cardiac images from a single 3D ultrasound data, using (A) (original) gray-scale 2D display where the cardiovascular cavities are mostly shown as an echogenic or very hypoechogenic areas, (B) gray-scale inverted 2D display where the same cavities are mostly shown as very hyperechogenic areas, (C) usual 3D surface display and (D) gray-scale inverted (inversion mode) 3D surface display of the same 3D dataset. In (C), it is necessary to cut open by "image surgery" the 3D volume and remove part of it (here the top half) in order to reveal the four chambers and great vessels (with their internal surfaces displayed in pink and thin grey lines indicate the external borders of the heart and vessels). Open arrows: drop-out artifacts, see text. Although the image quality is virtually textbook-like, the structures in the cutoff (top) half cannot be displayed in the same view. In inversion mode 3D surface display (D) the cardiovascular cavities shown are shown in solid and in their entirety, helping comprehend the spatial relationships of the structures, which is almost of the same quality as a postmortem luminal cast. BCVs: brachiocephalic vessels. RPA: right pulmonary artery. For a better perception of 3D effect, please refer to our website at *www.medphys. ucl.ac.uk/mgi/jdeng/* under *Fetal Heart* entry).
Source: Reprinted with permission from Deng J, Ruff CF, Linney AD, et al. Simultaneous use of two ultrasound scanners for motion-gated three-dimensional fetal echocardiography. Ultrasound Med Biol. 2000;26(6):1021-32.

Key Points

The *inversion mode* only works well with largely homogeneous data; thus, the inhomogeneous datasets commonly encountered blunt its usefulness.[47] For example, different parts of the myocardium may present very different echogenicity whereas a part of myocardium may have the same echogenicity as that of a part of the blood pool, resulting in drop-out artifacts in both non-inversion and inversion modes **(Figs. 6.10B and C)**.

Although *visual casting* involves more intelligent detection of the internal surfaces with inhomogeneous ultrasound data processing, it is sometimes semi-automated. For instance, a 3D barrier has to be placed by an operator to stop a "seed" from growing beyond the border **(Fig. 6.2A)**.

The *inversion mode* should not be confused with 3D images using various Doppler modes such as power,[52,53] color[54] or B-mode,[55,56] where Doppler signals are independent of gray-scale signals and need no inversion to form 3D images.

However, inversion mode can be mixed with one of Doppler modes shown in **Figures 6.11A to D** where gray-scale inversion mode is mixed with color Doppler mode.[54]

DIRECT AND INDIRECT VOLUME SCANNING

Current Need

In terms of real-time 3D imaging (see "Real-Time"ness above), it concerns only whether or not a 3D ultrasound system is capable of providing an imaging volume at a cinematic rate, i.e. c. 25 Hz (vps). If yes, this creates persistence of vision in the human brain,[41,43] thus, it is an observer's subjective concept.

In medical imaging, however, what matters is the ability to distinguish and analyze an anatomy's dynamic events, rather than to see it moving continuously in our mind. The unreliability (and potential risk if in a clinical situation) of the latter is analogs to the "wagon-wheel effect" illusion: the wheels of a car running forward too quickly is perceived by us as rotating in reverse due to temporal aliasing artifact.[57] Hence, there is a need for introducing objective terms to describe whether a scanning system is capable of achieving what really matters.

Proposed Two New Terms/Concepts

Direct volume scan refers to any volume scan in which a VOI is scanned (1) in an instant (i.e., with sufficient temporal resolution), (2) in detail (i.e., with sufficient spatial resolution), (3) in totality (i.e., with sufficient VOI coverage), and (4) in a fitting environment (i.e., with

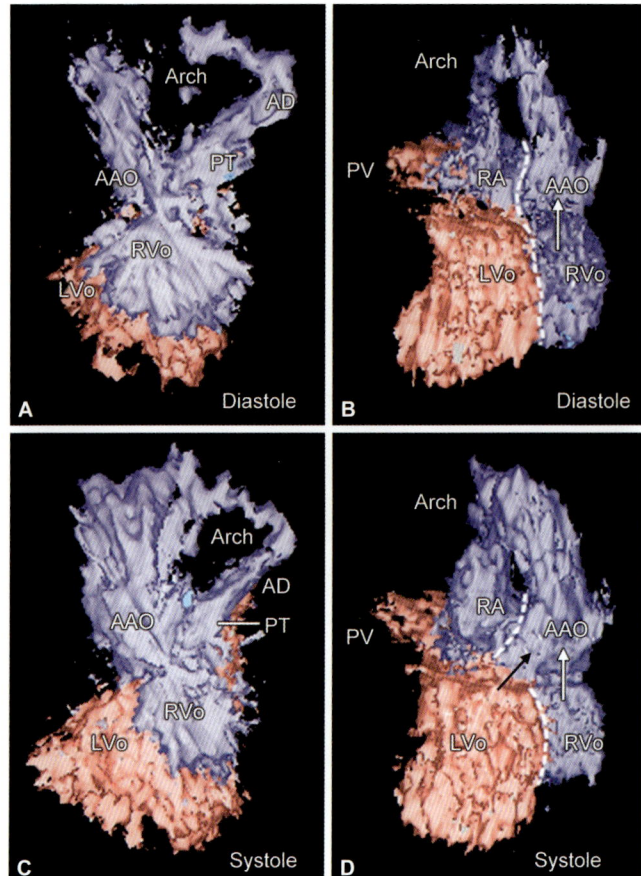

Figs. 6.11A to D: Images reconstructed from a 4D dataset created using both color Doppler and inverted gray-scale information from a 22-week-old fetus. The flows and structures are colored according to anatomical orientation (not flow direction). (A) and (C) are viewed right superioanteriorly; (B) and (D) are obtained by rotating the object in (A) and (C) about 90° to the reader's right. The dotted lines separate the ascending aorta (AAO) from the right atrium (RA) and the right from the left ventricular outlet (RVo from the LVo). (A) and (B) shows that the AAO arises exclusively from the RVo (white arrow) as does the pulmonary trunk, suggesting a double-outlet right ventricle. Because they are diastolic views when blood flow in the AAO and PT is slow, narrow flow paths are imaged. (C) and (D) are systolic views when blood flow is fast (thus wider paths are imaged). Note that the shunting flow from the LVo through the ventricular septal defect (black arrow) reveals the overriding of the aorta only seen in systole with the narrowed PT. The overall diagnosis is tetralogy of Fallot, but there is associated double-outlet right ventricle, the aorta being supported by the right ventricle for most of the cardiac cycle. AD, arterial duct; PV, pulmonary vein; Arch, aortic arch.
Source: Reprinted with permission from Deng J, Yates R, Sullivan ID, et al. Dynamic three-dimensional colour Doppler ultrasound of human fetal intracardiac flow. Ultrasound Obstet Gynecol. 2002;20(2):131-6.

sufficient functional freedom) **(Figs. 6.1 and 6.2, and Fig. 6.3A)**. If any of the above four conditions is not met, it is defined as an indirect volume scan **(Fig. 6.3B)**.

Key Points

The two new concepts consider the relativity between volumetric imaging speed (volume rate) and VOI moving speed. They also deal with at least three other relativity issues of clinical significance. Due to their complexity and importance in 4D imaging, they are dealt with in Chapter 7.

ACKNOWLEDGMENTS

The author is very grateful to the following 3D/4D experts in the ISUOG 3D SIG for their invaluable opinions on the terms discussed in this chapter: Drs Jacques Abramowicz, Reem S Abu-Rustum, Kazunori Baba, Beryl Benacerraf, Bernard Benoit, Harm-Gerd Blaas, Liat Gindes, Davor Jurkovic, Wesley Lee, Eberhard Merz, Larry Platt, Dolores Pretorius, Ralf Schild, Ilan Timor-Tritsch, Stefania Tudorache, Boris Tutschek, Mingxing Xie, Aly Youssef et al.

REFERENCES

1. Baba K, Okai T, Satoh K. Development of scan head position indicator for ultrasonic fetal three-dimensional reconstruction. Jpn J Med Ultrasonics. 1986;13(Suppl. 1): 121-2.
2. Merz E, Macchiella D, Bahlmann F, et al. Fetale Fehlbildungs diagnostik mit Hilfe der 3D-Sonographie. Ultraschall Klin Prax. 1991;6:147.
3. Lees WR, Gardener JE, Gillams AR. Three-dimensional ultrasound of the fetus. Radiology. 1991;181(P):132-2.
4. von Ramm OT, Smith SW. Real time volumetric ultrasound imaging system. J Digit Imaging. 1990;3(4):261-6.
5. Nelson TR, Pretorius DH, Sklansky M, et al. Three-dimensional echocardiographic evaluation of fetal heart anatomy and function: acquisition, analysis, and display. J Ultrasound Med. 1996;15(1):1-9.
6. Deng J, Gardener JE, Rodeck CH, et al. Fetal echo-cardiography in three and four dimensions. Ultrasound Med Biol. 1996;22(8):979-86.
7. Merz E, Abramowicz J, Baba K, et al. 3D imaging of the fetal face - recommendations from the International 3D Focus Group. Ultraschall Med. 2012;33(2):175-82.
8. Carvalho JS, Allan LD, Chaoui R, et al. ISUOG Practice Guidelines (updated): sonographic screening examination of the fetal heart. Ultrasound Obstet Gynecol. 2013; 41(3):348-59.
9. DeVore GR, Satou G, Sklansky M. 4D fetal echocardio-graphy-An update. Echocardiography. 2017;34(12):1788-98.
10. Mabrouk M, Raimondo D, Del Forno S, et al. Pelvic floor muscle assessment on three- and four-dimensional transperineal ultrasound in women with ovarian endo-metriosis with or without retroperitoneal infiltration: a step towards complete functional assessment. Ultrasound Obstet Gynecol. 2018;52(2):265-8.
11. Benacerraf BR, Abuhamad AZ, Bromley B, et al. Consider ultrasound first for imaging the female pelvis. Am J Obstet Gynecol. 2015;212(4):450-5.
12. Baken L, Benoit B, Koning AHJ, et al. First-Trimester Crown-Rump Length and Embryonic Volume of Fetuses with Structural Congenital Abnormalities Measured in Virtual Reality: An Observational Study. Biomed Res Int. 2017;2017:1953076.
13. Tutschek B, Blaas HK, Abramowicz J, et al. Three-dimensional ultrasound imaging of the fetal skull and face. Ultrasound Obstet Gynecol. 2017;50(1):7-16.
14. Barisic LS, Stanojevic M, Kurjak A, et al. Diagnosis of fetal syndromes by three- and four-dimensional ultrasound: is there any improvement? J Perinat Med. 2017;45(6): 651-65.
15. Deng J. P04 17: Prevalence of 3D/4D articles published in Ultrasound in Obstetrics & Gynecology and preference for 3D/4D terms used. Ultrasound Obstet Gynecol. 2013;42(Suppl. 1):127-8.
16. Deng J. Terminology of three-dimensional and four-dimensional ultrasound imaging of the fetal heart and other moving body parts. Ultrasound Obstet Gynecol. 2003;22(4):336-44.
17. Vinals F. Current experience and prospect of internet consultation in fetal cardiac ultrasound. Fetal Diagn Ther. 2011;30(2):83-7.
18. Houck RC, Cooke J, Gill EA. Three-dimensional echo: transition from theory to real-time, a technology now ready for prime time. Curr Probl Diagn Radiol. 2005;34(3): 85-105.
19. Sklansky MS, DeVore GR, Wong PC. Real-time 3-dimensional fetal echocardiography with an instan-taneous volume-rendered display: early description and pictorial essay. J Ultrasound Med. 2004;23(2):283-9.
20. Deng J. 3D/4D specific artefacts: how to recognise, minimise and avoid them. 3D Workshop at the 27th World Congress on Ultrasound in Obstetrics and Gynecology; Vienna, Austria; 2017.
21. Sur SD, Jayaprakasan K, Jones NW, et al. A novel technique for the semi-automated measurement of embryo volume: an intraobserver reliability study. Ultrasound Med Biol. 2010;36(5):719-25.
22. Hata T, Kanenishi K, Nitta E, et al. HDlive Flow with HDlive silhouette mode in diagnosis of molar pregnancy. Ultrasound Obstet Gynecol. 2018;52(4):552-4.
23. Chaoui R. Three-dimensional ultrasound assessment of the fetal heart. In: Chiappa E, Cook AC, Botta G, Silverman NH, (Eds). Echocardiographic Anatomy in the Fetus. Berlin, Germany: Springer Science & Business Media; 2009.
24. Deng J, Hall-Craggs MA, Pellerin D, et al. Real-time three-dimensional ultrasound visualization of erection and artificial coitus. Int J Androl. 2006;29(2):374-9.
25. Deng J, Crouch NS, Creighton SM, et al. Minimally-compressive, three- and four-dimensional ultrasound imaging of the clitoris: A feasibility study. Ultrasound Med Biol. 2006;32(10):1479-84.

26. Chatterjee R, Deng J, Pellerin D, et al. Feasibility of dynamic 3-D color Doppler ultrasound for imaging penile vascular change in renal transplant patients with erectile dysfunction responding to sildenafil. Ultrasound Med Biol. 2008;34(6):885-91.

27. Burton P, Deng J, McDonald D, et al. Real-time 3D ultrasound imaging of infant tongue movements during breast-feeding. Early Hum Dev. 2013;89(9):635-41.

28. Baba K, Okai T, Kozuma S, et al. Real-time processable three-dimensional US in obstetrics. Radiology. 1997; 203(2):571-4.

29. Kozuma S, Baba K, Okai T, et al. Dynamic observation of the fetal face by three-dimensional ultrasound. Ultrasound Obstet Gynecol. 1999;13(4):283-4.

30. Campbell S. 4D, or not 4D: that is the question. Ultrasound Obstet Gynecol. 2002;19(1):1-4.

31. Kuno A, Akiyama M, Yamashiro C, et al. Three-dimensional sonographic assessment of fetal behavior in the early second trimester of pregnancy. J Ultrasound Med. 2001;20(12):1271-5.

32. Benoit B, Hafner T, Kurjak A, et al. Three-dimensional sonoembryology. J Perinat Med. 2002;30(1):63-73.

33. Kurjak A, Vecek N, Hafner T, et al. Prenatal diagnosis: what does four-dimensional ultrasound add? J Perinat Med. 2002;30(1):57-62.

34. Timor-Tritsch IE, Platt LD. Three-dimensional ultrasound experience in obstetrics. Curr Opin Obstet Gynecol. 2002;14(6):569-75.

35. Deng J. Start of the art of the heart. Ultrasound Obstet Gynecol. 2001;18(4):405-6.

36. Wang XF, Xiao JP. [Fetal echocardiography—a method for pregnancy diagnosis]. Chinese J Obstet Gynecol. 1964;10:267-9.

37. Campbell S. An improved method of fetal cephalometry by ultrasound. J Obstet Gynaecol Br Commonw. 1968; 75(5):568-76.

38. Allan LD, Tynan MJ, Campbell S, et al. Echocardiographic and anatomical correlates in the fetus. Br Heart J. 1980,44(4):444 51.

39. DeVore GR, Donnerstein RL, Kleinman CS, et al. Real-time-directed M-mode echocardiography: a new technique for accurate and rapid quantitation of the fetal preejection period and ventricular ejection time of the right and left ventricles. Am J Obstet Gynecol. 1981;141(4):470-1.

40. Baba K, Satoh K, Sakamoto S, et al. Development of an ultrasonic system for three-dimensional reconstruction of the fetus. J Perinat Med. 1989;17(1):19-24.

41. Wikipedia. Persistence of vision. [online] Available from https://en.wikipedia.org/wiki/Persistence_of_vision [Accessed December, 2018].

42. Deng J, Yates R, Demetrescu C, et al. Impact of live 4D ultrasound volume rate on recognition of fetal cardiac structures in reformatted 2D views. Ultrasound Obstet Gynecol. 2010;36(Suppl. 1):3.

43. Deng J. How to optimise 4D settings for fetal echo: from theoretical to technical considerations. 3D Workshop at the 26th World Congress on Ultrasound in Obstetrics and Gynecology: Rome, Italy; 2016.

44. Youssef A, Montaguti E, Sanlorenzo O, et al. Reliability of new three-dimensional ultrasound technique for pelvic hiatal area measurement. Ultrasound Obstet Gynecol. 2016;47(5):629-35.

45. Tudorache S, Florea M, Dragusin R, et al. 3D Ultrasound Assessment of the Uterus: Why an Accuracy Study for Mullerian Congenital Anomalies is not Feasible, while Screening Already is, and should be done. J Clin Diagn Res. 2017;5:134.

46. Deng J, Ruff CF, Linney AD, et al. Simultaneous use of two ultrasound scanners for motion-gated three-dimensional fetal echocardiography. Ultrasound Med Biol. 2000;26(6):1021-32.

47. Deng J, Rodeck CH. Current applications of fetal cardiac imaging technology (invited review). Curr Opin Obstet Gynecol. 2006;18(2):177-84.

48. Goncalves LF, Espinoza J, Lee W, et al. A new approach to fetal echocardiography: digital casts of the fetal cardiac chambers and great vessels for detection of congenital heart disease. J Ultrasound Med. 2005;24(4): 415-24.

49. Paladini D, Vassallo M, Sglavo G, et al. Assessment of cardiac function impairment by four-dimensional echocardiography with inversion mode rendering in fetal congenital heart disease. Ultrasound Obstet Gynecol. 2005;26(4):346.

50. Dindoyal I, Lambrou T, Deng J, et al. 2D/3D fetal cardiac dataset segmentation using a deformable model. Med Phys. 2011;38(7):4338-49.

51. Cao HY, Wang Y, Hong L, et al. Morphological features of complex congenital cardiovascular anomalies in fetuses: as evaluated by cast models. J Huazhong Univ Sci Technolog Med Sci. 2017;37(4):596-604.

52. Kurjak A, Hafner T, Kupesic S, et al. Three-dimensional power Doppler in study of embryonic vasculogenesis. J Perinat Med. 2002;30(1):18-25.

53. Chaoui R, Kalache KD, Hartung J. Application of three-dimensional power Doppler ultrasound in prenatal diagnosis. Ultrasound Obstet Gynecol. 2001;17(1):22-9.

54. Deng J, Yates R, Sullivan ID, et al. Dynamic three-dimensional colour Doppler ultrasound of human fetal intracardiac flow. Ultrasound Obstet Gynecol. 2002;20(2): 131-6.

55. Gindes L, Hegesh J, Weisz B, et al. Three and four dimensional ultrasound: a novel method for evaluating fetal cardiac anomalies. Prenat Diagn. 2009;29(7): 645-53.

56. Pooh RK, Korai A. B-flow and B-flow spatio-temporal image correlation in visualizing fetal cardiac blood flow. Croat Med J. 2005;46(5):808-11.

57. Wikipedia. Wagon-wheel effect. [online] Available from https://en.wikipedia.org/wiki/Wagon-wheel_effect [Accessed December, 2018].

Direct Volume Scan or Indirect Volume Scan: Four Relativity Issues in Four-dimensional Ultrasonography (Applicable to Other Multidimensional Imaging Modalities)

Jing Deng

INTRODUCTION

In Chapter 6 on Nomenclature, we introduced two new terms/concepts for dynamic 3D (4D) imaging of a moving organ or body parts—*direct volume scan* and *indirect volume scan*. A direct volume scan refers to any volume scan in which a volume of interest (VOI) is scanned (1) in an instant (i.e., with sufficient temporal resolution), (2) in detail (i.e., with sufficient spatial resolution), (3) in totality (i.e., with sufficient VOI coverage), and (4) in a fitting environment (i.e., with sufficient functional freedom). If any of the above four conditions is not met, it is defined as an indirect volume scan.

Fundamental Difference between a "Real-time" 3D Volume Scan and a Direct or Indirect Volume Scan: Subjective versus Objective Concepts

In terms of real-time 3D imaging (see the Section: Real-timeness in Chapter 6), it concerns only whether or not a 3D ultrasound system is capable of providing an imaging volume at a cinematic rate (i.e. approximate 25 imaging volumes/second, vps). If yes, this creates

persistence of vision in the human brain;[1,2] thus, it is an observer's subjective concept.

In medical imaging, however, what matters is the ability to distinguish and analyze an anatomy's dynamic events, rather than to see it moving continuously in our mind. The unreliability (and potential risk if in a clinical situation) of the latter is analogs to the "wagon-wheel effect" illusion: the wheels of a car running forward too quickly are perceived by us as rotating in reverse due to temporal aliasing artifact.[3] Hence, there is a need for introducing objective terms to describe whether a scanning system is capable of achieving what really matters. The two new concepts consider the relativity between volumetric imaging speed (volume rate) and VOI moving speed. They also deal with at least three other relativity issues of clinical significance (**Table 7.1**).

Four Essential Questions about Four Relativity Issues between Technical/Operative Capability of an Imaging System and Morphophysiology of a Volume of Interest

The two concepts are complex for 4D imaging using ultrasound or any other modalities, but important when

Table 7.1: Direct or indirect volume scan. Four relativity issues that need to be considered during 4D ultrasound or other medical imaging.

Key word	Technical question	Relativity issue between		
		3D/4D ultrasonograph	and	Organ/body part
Fast	How fast is fast enough?	Imaging temporal resolution	and	Time scale of interest
Fine	How fine is fine enough?	Imaging spatial resolution	and	Structural scale of interest
Full	How full is full enough?	Imaging volume	and	Inseparable volume of interest (VOI)
Free	How free is free enough?	Maximal facilitation of 4D scanning	and	Minimal restriction on VOI functioning

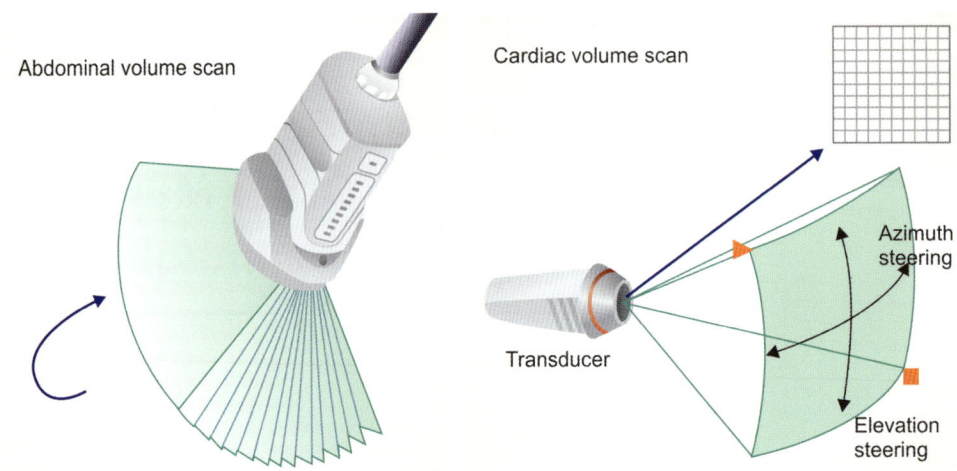

Fig. 7.1: Four-dimensional (4D) data acquisition methods. Left: Using slice (or subvolume)-reconstructed 3D scan, the transducer sweeps over a volume, e.g. 15 ~ 30° for 5 ~ 10 s (second) during 15 ~ 30 cardiac cycles. Cardiac gating must be applied to remove motion artifact (see Fig. 7.2 for reasons). Right: A matrix-array transducer-based system forms an imaging volume in the first place. If its temporal resolution is 25 Hz (imaging volumes/s), motion gating is usually, but not always, unnecessary for general studies. For more detailed imaging of the fetal anatomy and function (Fig. 7.3), gating may become necessary. This is because, at 25 Hz, it takes 40 ms (millisecond) to form an imaging volume by steering scan lines from the orange (▶) to (■), a scanning time much longer than fetal cardiac isovolumetric contraction (about 20 ms) and relaxation (about 25 ms) periods.

it comes to determine if a 4D system is fit or not for research and/or clinical purposes. Therefore, we discuss them in detail in this chapter. Before a 4D investigation of a moving organ such as the fetal heart,[4] or a dynamic body part, such as pelvic muscles,[5] investigators should ask themselves four simple questions listed in **Table 7.1**. These are whether a 3D ultrasound system (or any other modalities) can provide: (1) sufficiently **F**ast temporal resolution (i.e. volumetric, not cross-sectional, imaging speed), (2) sufficiently **F**ine spatial resolution, (3) a sufficiently **F**ull imaging volume, and (4) a sufficiently **F**ree imaging environment.

Simplicity Consideration and Current Inadequate Consideration of the Fourth F-issue

For simplicity, these four issues are discussed separately. But during a real scan, they are usually interactively affected and, therefore, should be considered all together, or at least the first three together, in order to succeed in your usual 3D/4D applications (*see* further sections in this chapter). When 3D/4D ultrasound is extended to currently unusual and delicate areas,[5-9] investigators should also become aware of the fourth **F**-issue (*see* the Section: Relativity Between Maximal Facilitation of 4D Scanning and Minimal Restriction on the VOI Functioning) that is insufficiently considered at present.

Four-dimensional Acquisition Methods with or without Motion Gating

The main interest of this chapter is dynamic volumes such as the fetal heart or other moving body parts. Hence, to image the fourth, temporal dimension as well as the three spatial dimensions of a VOI, 4D, rather than only 3D, techniques must be used. To this end, three main methods are currently in practice: (1) motion-gated slice-reconstruction 3D method, (2) motion-ungated, matrix-array-transducer-based real-time 3D method **(Fig. 7.1)**, and (3) a mix of methods (1) and (2), i.e. motion-gated, subvolume-reconstructed 3D method.

RELATIVITY BETWEEN TEMPORAL RESOLUTION AND TIME SCALE OF INTEREST—HOW FAST IS FAST ENOUGH?

What is an Instant? Rapidly Changing Opera Faces versus Fetal Cardiac Phases

Up to date, any ultrasound imaging volume, no matter how fast it can be formed, such as by matrix-array transducer technology, is built up by many (several hundreds to several thousands) scan lines similar to those forming an imaging plane. There is a time interval, no matter how short it is, between the first and the last scan lines being transmitted/received to build up an imaging volume

(Fig. 7.1). In the definition of *direct volume scan* above, *an instant* denotes a time interval so short that during this period the spatial movement of a VOI is negligible. It does not have an absolute, but a relative, time length because it depends on the volume scanning speed and the VOI's moving speed (as well as other motion features). This can be illustrated, by analogy, the relativity between the camera shutter speed and the face-changing speed **(Fig. 7.2)**.

Clinical Exemplars: Direct versus Indirect Volume Scans

Clinical exemplars are listed in **Table 7.2**. Take for instance, a fetal face that can stay still for at least 10 seconds from the start of a 3D scan (in reality, the stationary period needs to be longer as the operator cannot predict when the face will start moving, positively such as yawning or sucking, and/or passively such as changing its position with body movement). A facial volume scan can be

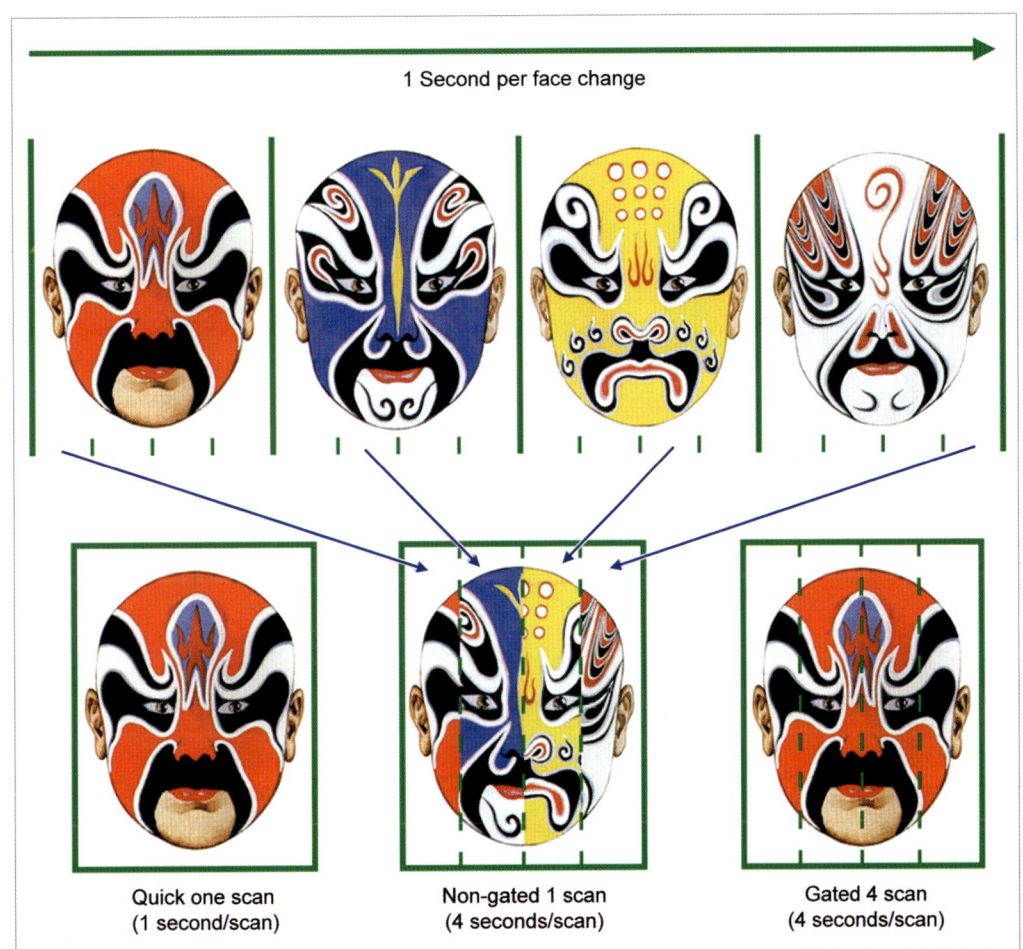

Fig. 7.2: Target speed, scanning speed, motion artifact, and motion gating. Some Chinese opera actors are very skilled at changing faces—altering facial masks in a blink. Imagine an actor can change one face per second and cyclically makes four changes (upper panel). If a camera scans the actor's head from the reader's left to right, and the scanning speed is 1 s per head-width, it is possible (though not necessary) for every scan to capture an entire face (lower panel, left). If the scanning speed is 4 s per head-width, one scan can only capture a quarter of each of the four faces, e.g. the 1st, 2nd, 3rd, and 4th quarters of the four faces, respectively, causing distortion (motion artifact) in the resulting photograph (lower panel, middle). However, a 4-s scan can be synchronized (gated) with the face changing, e.g. starting the first scan with the red-cheeked face through to the white-cheeked face, then moving the camera right for a quarter of a head-width and repeating the scan, and repeating this process twice more. Four non-distorted faces can then be reconstructed; shown here is only the red-cheeked face from the 1st, 2nd, 3rd, and 4th quarters of the 1st, 2nd, 3rd, and 4th scans, respectively (lower panel, right). This gating principle for the actor changing faces applies similarly in cardiac gating as the heart changes faces (phases), too. (Peking Opera face paintings by ML Zhao). *Courtesy*: http://www.jingjuok.com.

Table 7.2: Relativity between temporal resolution and time scale of interest in clinical 3D/4D studies.[†]

3D/4D acquisition methods	Exemplar volume of interest (VOI)	Direct or indirect volume scan
Slice-reconstruction 3D, at 10 s/vol	Fetal face stationary for at least 10 s	Direct, with higher resolution[10]
Real-time 3D, at 40 ms/vol (25 Hz[‡])	Fetal face stationary for at least 10 s	Direct, with lower resolution
Slice-reconstruction 3D, at 10 s/vol	Slow moving fetal face	Indirect, with motion artifact
Slice-reconstruction power Doppler 3D, at 10 s/vol	Peripheral vasculature	Direct, with higher resolution[36,39]
Real-time 3D, at 40 ms/vol (25 Hz[‡])	Peripheral vasculature	Direct, with lower resolution
Real-time 3D, at 40 ms/vol (25 Hz[‡])	Slow moving fetal face	Direct, without motion artifact
Real-time 3D, at 40 ms/vol (25 Hz[‡])	Beating fetal heart (if only interested in long cardiac phases)*	Direct, able to resolve long fetal cardiac systolic/diastolic phases
Real-time 3D, at 40 ms/vol (25Hz[‡])	Shortest fetal cardiac phase (20 ms)*	Indirect, unable to resolve short fetal cardiac phase (20 ms)
Real-time 3D, ≤ 10 ms/vol (100 Hz)	Shortest fetal cardiac phase (20 ms)*	Direct, able to resolve short fetal cardiac phase (20 ms)

*See Figure 7.3
[†]Providing all other three F-conditions also met (see text)
[‡]Hz: Imaging volumes per second (vps), i.e. the reciprocal of 1000 ms/vol

completed either with a slice-reconstruction 3D system capable of forming an imaging volume even over 10 seconds or with a real-time 3D system capable of forming an imaging volume in only 40 ms. Both scans can be regarded as direct volume scans and there are no motion artifacts in the resultant 3D images. But because the former method can provide much higher spatial resolution than the latter does, the former should be preferred in order to obtain more facial details for more reliable clinical assessment.[10-12]

Temporal Resolution of Imaging Volume: Long versus Short Cardiac Phases

Although a 10-second/volume, slice-reconstruction 3D method may complete a direct volume scan of a stationary fetal face, it cannot complete a direct volume scan of a beating fetal heart because the heart also changes "faces" (phases) and even the longest period of the cardiac phase—rapid filling of approximate 95 ms is much shorter than the 10-second/volume-imaging time **(Fig. 7.3)**. Hence, gating is necessary, and a clinical research result is shown in **Figure 7.4**.

So far, the majority of 4D fetal echocardiographic studies are focused on structural abnormalities and gross functionalities. This makes genuine real-time 3D systems (i.e. with a volume rate of approximate 25 Hz or higher) potentially qualify for direct volume scanning the fetal heart, because each imaging volume takes only 40 ms to form, able to resolve the four long cardiac phases (i.e. rapid and reduced ejection, rapid and reduced filling) of at least 80 ms each **(Fig. 7.3)**. It is usually unnecessary to perform motion gating of other structures moving not as rapidly as the fetal heart (Fig. 6.5), provided that the answers to other three **F**-questions are affirmative **(Table 7.1)**.[13]

However, if our interest is to study the intrinsic contractility of the fetal heart, represented by the short, isovolumetric contraction (IVC) and isovolumetric relaxation (IVR) phases **(Fig. 7.3)**, a volume scan using a real-time 3D system at a volume rate of 25 Hz can no longer be regarded as a direct volume scan. This is because the real-time method needs 40 ms to build up an imaging volume, a time much longer than (thus unable to resolve) the IVC phase (20 ms) and IVR phase (25 ms). In other words, even if the first scan line of the imaging volume (the orange triangle in **Figure 7.1**) starts exactly as the IVR phase starts (the two left arrows in **Figure 7.3**), the phase finishes much earlier (right white arrow) than the last scan line to build up the volume (right black arrow), resulting in one imaging volume with mixed IVR and rapid filling morphophysiological information. As we know from **Figure 7.2**, if an imaging speed is slower than the motion of the target, motion artifact will arise when the motion is not gated, therefore, it is an indirect volume scan.

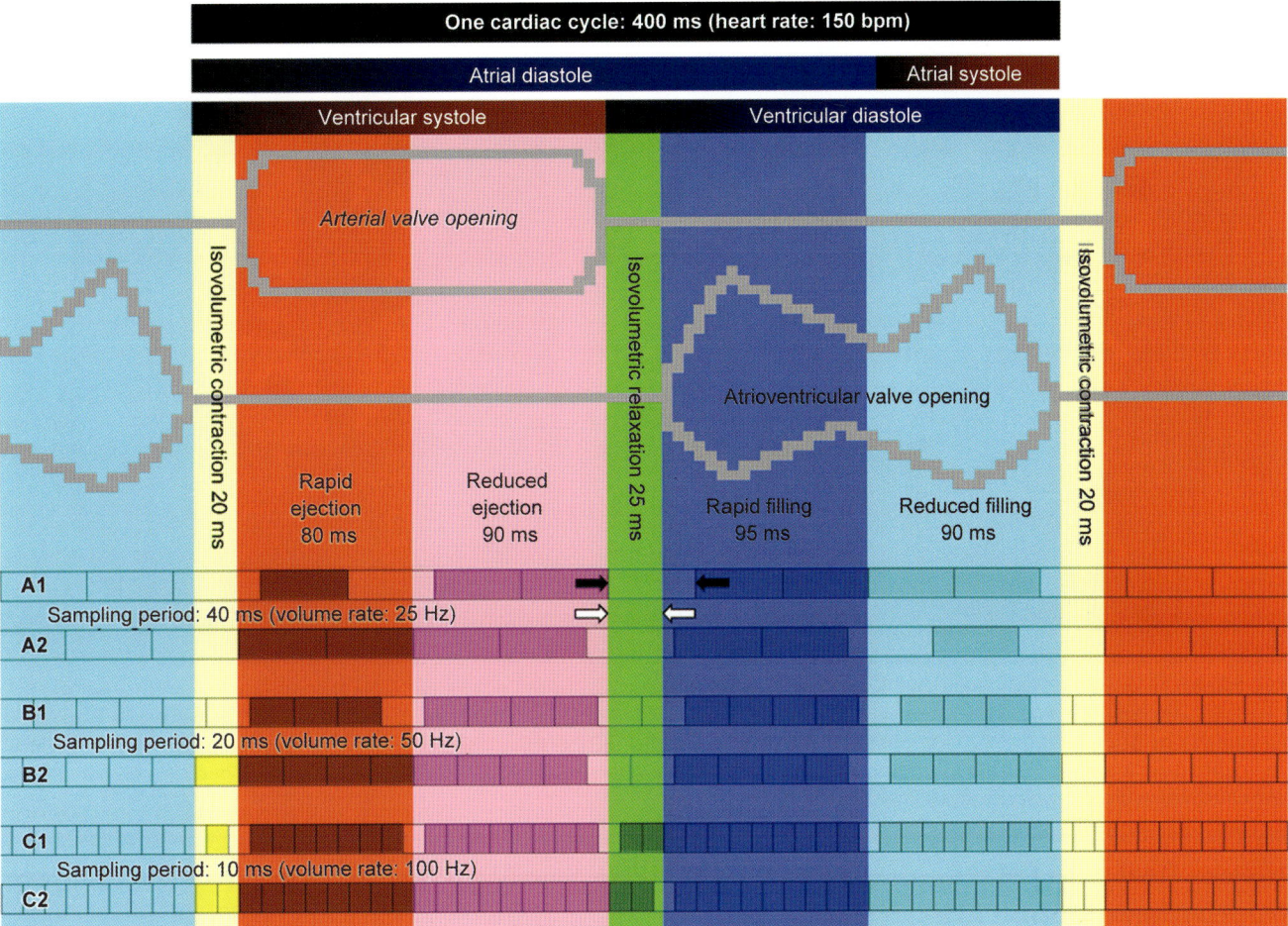

Fig. 7.3: Schematic estimation of sufficiency of various temporal resolutions for distinguishing dynamic events of different time scales. In rows A1 through to C2, each block length represents the time interval needed to form an imaging volume, and in each colored column, darker blocks indicate the number of the samples acquired. At a 25-Hz volume rate, each of the four long fetal cardiac phases, i.e. the rapid and reduced ejection (red and pink columns), and the rapid and reduced filling (blue and turquoise columns) can be fully sampled at least once and most likely twice (A1, A2). This makes long dynamic events distinguishable during imaging. But it takes 40 ms to form an imaging volume at a 25-Hz volume rate (between black arrows), an interval much longer than the two short phases, i.e. isovolumetric contraction (IVC, yellow column) and isovolumetric relaxation (IVR, green column, between white arrows). This means even if the first scan line of the imaging volume starts exactly as the IVR starts (two left arrows), the phase finishes much earlier (right white arrow) than the last scan line to build up the volume (right black arrow, see also Figure 7.1), resulting in one imaging volume with mixed both IVR (green) and rapid filling (blue) morphophysiological information. At 50 Hz, the short phases may happen to (B2 during IVC) or may not (B1 and B2 during IVR) be fully sampled once, resulting in the phases not necessarily being recognizable in images. At 100 Hz, the short phases can be fully sampled at least once (C1 during IVC) and maximally twice (C1 and C2 during IVR), allowing their existence to be depicted during a cardiac cycle. However, the accuracy for measuring the isovolumetric contraction time will only be about 50% at this rate.

Other Movements that can Cause Motion Artifacts

Table 7.2 only lists fetal motions as exemplars. However, in terms of *negligible movement* in clinical practice, the following motions should also be considered (and if possible, avoided or minimized): (1) maternal (such as mother's respiration or body movement), (2) operational (such as manual movement of the transducer or its compression deforming the maternal abdominal wall and displacing the fetal position, and/or (3) environmental (such as an unsteady scanning couch), particularly when motion/deformation caused by any of these factors is greater than the motion of interest such as the fetal cardiac contraction.

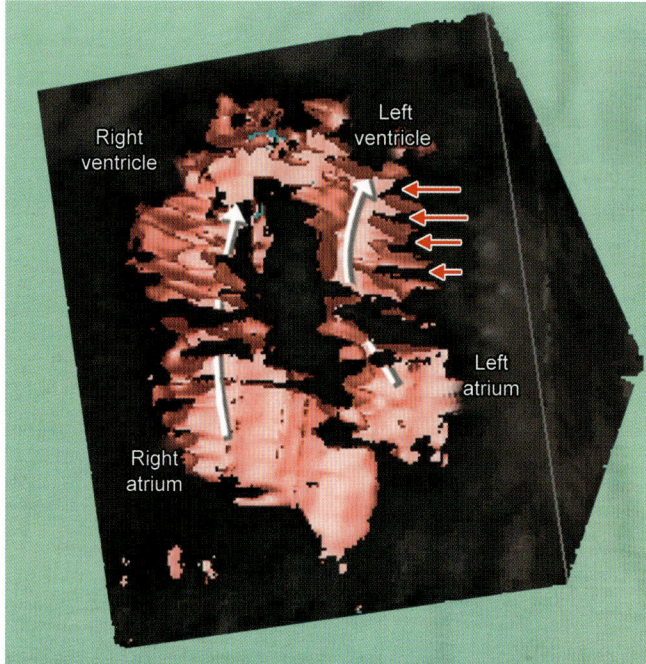 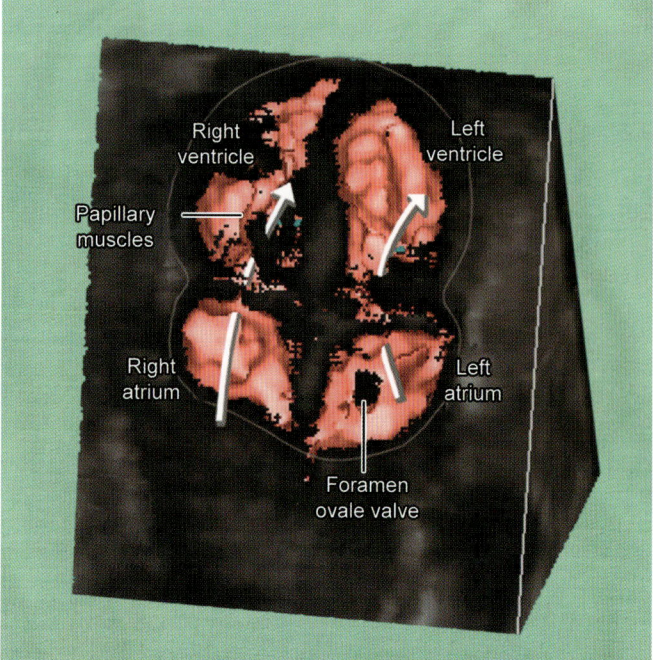

Fig. 7.4: 3D images of a 22-week-old fetal heart. The dark gray cube is part of the thorax, cut open by "image surgery" to reveal the four chambers with internal surfaces displayed in pink (thin light gray lines indicate the external borders of the heart). The left image is analog to non-gated one scan in Figure 7.2, and motion artifacts as evidenced by the spikes (red arrows) make reliable assessments impossible. The right image is analog to gated four scans. As motion artifacts are removed, detailed structures are revealed. Video clips on our website: *www.medphys.ucl.ac.uk/mgi/jdeng* under Fetal Heart > Album 2 entry.

How to Deal with Fetal Cardiac and Nonrhythmic Motion Artifacts?

Four-dimensional echocardiography in children and adults uses ECG to provide cardiac cyclical information for motion gating. Due to the nonavailability of good fetal ECG signals, many other methods have been investigated for fetal cardiac gating. However, only those utilizing the fetal cardiac cyclical information from its own M-mode waveforms including spatiotemporal image correlation (STIC)[14,15] have been succeeded into clinical use.[16-20] Though, even these methods need further refinement.

Gating noncardiac rhythmic motion, such as lip pouting can be found in this study.[21]

For body parts with nonrhythmic motion, such as the milk-sucking tongue, contracting pelvic muscles and more delicate morphophysiologies to be mentioned in the Section: Relativity Between Maximal Facilitation of 4D Scanning and Minimal Restriction on the VOI Functioning, real-time 3D imaging with a direct volume scan is probably the only solution.

Fortunately, most noncardiac anatomies move considerably slower than the fetal heart. This makes most real-time 3D scans (i.e. with a volume rate of approximate 25 Hz or higher) fall into the category of direct volume scan. It may be unnecessary to perform motion gating **(Fig. 7.5)**, provided that the answers to other three **F**-questions are affirmative **(Table 7.1)**.

Balance between Temporal and Spatial Resolution

As mentioned earlier, we must take at least the first three **F**-issues into consideration when imaging the fetal heart, and increasing temporal resolution would not necessarily result in improved cardiac images. A balance can be found in a study examining the impact of matrix-array transducer-based volume rate on recognition of fetal cardiac gross or fine structures (Table 6.2) in reformatted cross-sectional views.[22]

A total of 144 datasets were reformatted; 48 sets in each of three volume rate ranges (<15, 20 ~ 30, >35 vps) **(Table 7.3)**. The recognition rate for identifying all the gross and fine structures was 91.3% (39/48) and 60.4% (29/48), respectively, at 20 ~ 30 vps. If all the gross and fine structures could be recognized in a fetus, regardless

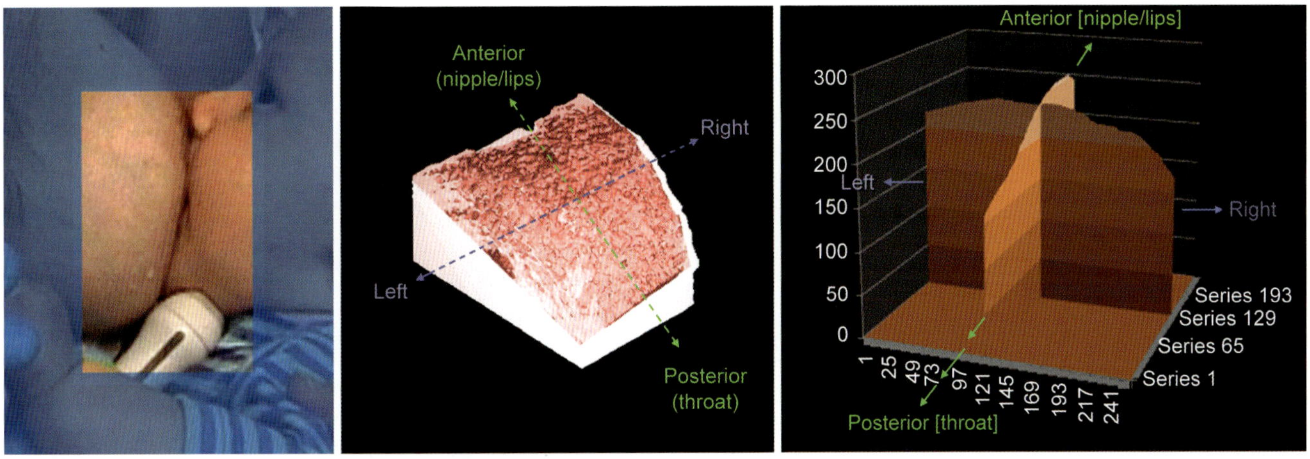

Fig. 7.5: Left: Real-time 3D scan with minimal restriction on the volume of interest—a large part of the baby's tongue (middle), with sufficient spatial and temporal resolution, revealing the morphophysiology of various tongue motion patterns during breastfeeding, and addressing current controversy surrounding the milk-intake mechanism (right; for more detail see the section: Tongue and Infant Feeding). Video clips on our website: *www.medphys.ucl.ac.uk/mgi/jdeng* under Baby Breast/Bottle Feeding entry.

Table 7.3: Impact of matrix-array transducer-based 4D echocardiographic volume rate on recognition of fetal cardiac gross or fine structures from a grand total of 144 4D datasets (see Table 6.2 for definitions of gross and fine structures).

Volume rate range	Number of datasets with recognizable structures out of a subtotal of 48 datasets		Number of fetuses with recognizable structures out of all 12 fetuses	
vps	Gross (%)	Fine (%)	Gross (%)	Fine (%)
< 15	16 (33)	10 (21)	6 (50)	4 (33)
20 ~ 30	39 (91)^*	29 (60)^*	12 (100)^*	10 (83)^*
> 35	20 (42)	13 (27)	06 (50)	5 (42)

^$p < 0.01$ between < 15 and 20 ~ 30 ranges; *$p < 0.01$ between 20 ~ 30 and > 35 ranges

from which datasets from which imaging windows, the recognition rate was 100% (12/12) and 83.3% (10/12), respectively, at 20~30 vps. These recognition rates were all significantly higher than the corresponding rates in the < 15 and > 35 vps groups.

These findings confirmed the above seemingly theoretical, but actually clinically relevant considerations. Too low volume rates, which may improve spatial resolution, do not result in better recognition of either gross or fine structures. This is because it is no longer a genuine direct volume scan, leading to motion artifact. Too high volume rate, which may theoretically remove motion artifact, could actually reduce the recognition of the cardiac structures, in particular fine structures, due to reduced spatial resolution. For the 18~28 gestational weeks studied, a volume rate range between 20 vps and 30 vps can achieve satisfactory recognition of both gross and fine cardiac structures when using the latest, state-of-the-art matrix-array 4D systems.

However, if we further 4D research into detailed fetal cardiovascular hemodynamics, we must equip ourselves with better scanners. To maintain a real-time volume rate, we must also bear in mind whether the spatial resolution and imaging volume size are still sufficient for the VOI under investigation.

RELATIVITY BETWEEN SPATIAL RESOLUTION AND STRUCTURAL SCALE—HOW FINE IS FINE ENOUGH?

Types of Spatial Resolution: Slice-reconstruction 3D versus Real-time 3D Scans

The importance of spatial resolution is easy to understand. In two-dimensional (2D) ultrasound, spatial resolution is further divided into axial resolution and lateral resolution **(Fig. 7.6)**. Ultrasound transducers for cross-

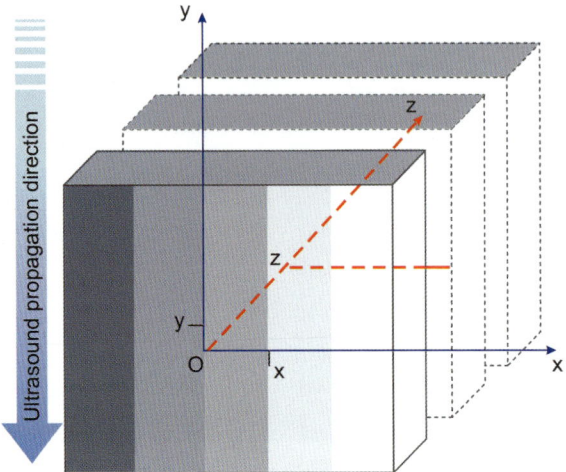

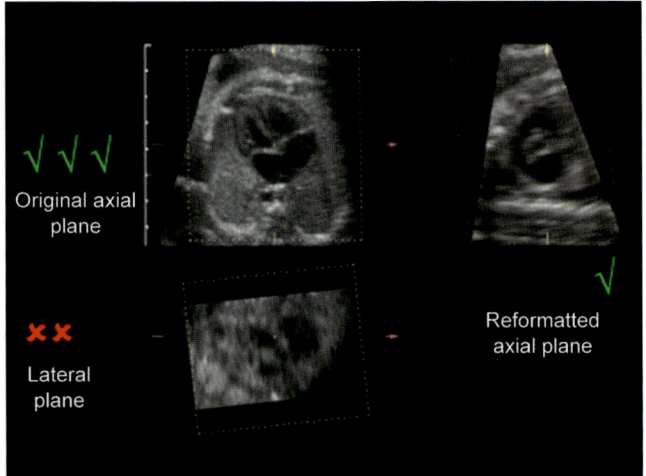

Fig. 7.6: An illustration showing why during a slice-reconstructed volume scan, the spatial resolution varies in different planes. 3D data are collected by moving the imaging plane (block) along z-axis. The y-axis is the ultrasound beam propagation direction with the distance O-y schematically showing axial resolution, i.e. 1 unit). The imaging plane is formed by many ultrasound beams (gray shadings) scanning along the x-axis, with the distance O-x showing lateral resolution, which equals one beam width (i.e. 3 units) as lateral resolution is usually 3 times (i.e. poorer than) the corresponding axial resolution. Although the beam width is identical along both the x-axis and z-axis (which is the thickness of one block), the third resolution in a 3D dataset is mainly determined by the spatial interval (O-z) between two consecutive planes. With mechanical parallel-moving or fan-sweeping the imaging plane, the O-z value is usually larger than the O-x value, i.e. with even poorer resolution (i.e. 4 units) than the lateral resolution.

Fig. 7.7: Different resolution results in different image quality of reformatted three-orthogonal 2D views from a slice-reconstructed 3D scan with STIC: Upper left: The four-chamber view with best quality within the original scanning plane, i.e. corresponding to plane x-y in Figure 7.6 (also called plane A). Lower left: The worst image quality in the plane corresponding to plane x-z (also called plane C), showing unclearly the right atrium and the aortic root. Upper right: The arterial-duct view with intermediate quality in the plane corresponding to plane y-z (also called plane B). When compared with real-time 3D axial resolution (Fig. 6.6), slice-reconstructed 2D/3D/4D images have better in-original-scanning-plane quality but worse off-plane quality.
Courtesy: Drs LF Gonçalves and W Lee.

sectional imaging normally run at a receiving frequency range between 5.0 MHz and 10.0 MHz (transmitting frequency range between 2.5 MHz and 5.0 MHz if in harmonic mode) with sufficient penetration to the in utero heart and provide an axial resolution (along y-axis) of approximate 0.30~0.15 mm. The lateral resolution (beam width, along x-axis) is usually poorer, typically 3 ~ 4 times of axial resolution numbers.

If a (2D) imaging plane, rather than a (3D) imaging volume, is used to obtain serial 2D slices and then stack (reconstruct) them into a volumetric dataset (e.g. during a slice-reconstruction 3D acquisition), there is a third spatial resolution involved. It is determined by the spatial interval between any two consecutive slices along the z-axis, i.e. along the transducer/plane moving direction. The interval is usually approximately 0.5~2 mm, often resulting in resolution even poorer than the lateral resolution **(Fig. 7.6)**.

To simplify the theoretical consideration, we presume resolutions of a slice-reconstruction 3D acquisition to be 0.15 ~ 0.30 mm (y-axis) × 0.45 ~ 1.20 mm (x-axis) × 0.50~2.00 mm (z-axis) **(Fig. 7.6)**. Ultrasound systems with slice-reconstruction 3D mode (including STIC) for indirect volume scanning[16-20] are able to resolve almost all the structures in plane x-y (the original imaging plane), but are unlikely to resolve most fine structures in plane x-z (also called plane C, which is perpendicular to ultrasound propagation direction and reformatted from the 3D dataset), and may or may not resolve some of the gross and/or fine structures in plane y-z. **Figure 7.7** is a typical clinical case of three-orthogonal views reformatted from a slice-reconstructed 3D scan (an indirect volume scan with STIC motion gating), showing the impact of the three different resolutions on image quality. For gross and fine structure classification, *see* Table 6.2.

Ultrasound systems using matrix-array transducers for real-time 3D scanning offer a resolution pattern different from slice-reconstructed 3D approaches. Here, the interslice resolution along z-axis is replaced with another lateral resolution, identical to that along x-axis.

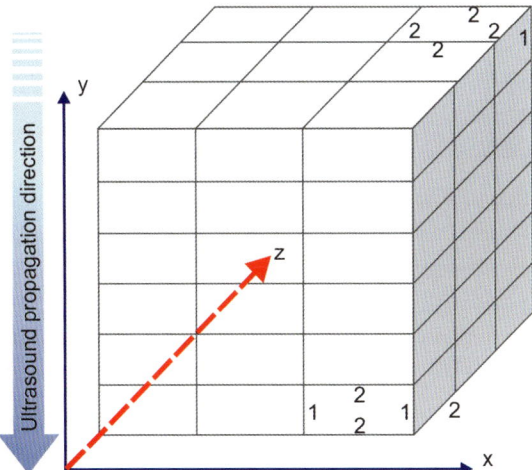

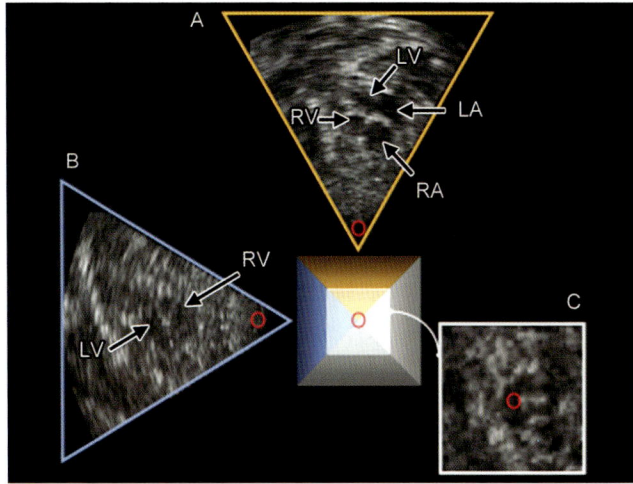

Fig. 7.8: In ultrasound imaging, resolution along the y-axis (i.e. along the sound propagation direction) is better (say 1 unit for simplicity) than lateral resolution (say 2 units) along the x-axis or z-axis (i.e. perpendicular to the direction). Therefore, images on plane x-y (also called plane A) and plane y-z (plane B) are made up of pixels of 1 × 2 resolution while plane x-z (plane C) are made up of pixels of 2 × 2 resolution, resulting in poorer images than those on plane A or B.

Fig. 7.9: Images of a 22-week-old fetal heart from a sparse matrix-array 4D dataset from the right subcostal window. Two simultaneously imaged planes in (A) and (B) are both in parallel to ultrasound propagation direction (and also perpendicular to each other). Due to better axial resolution, major structures, such as the right and left atria (RA, LA), right and left ventricles (RV, LV), are more or less visualized. Due to poorer lateral resolution, simultaneously imaged plane (C) perpendicular to the sound direction shows no identifiable structures. On corresponding video clip, the normal fine structures, such as the foramen valve, interatrial and interventricular septa, and the tricuspid and mitral valves appear to be much thicker than normal because of insufficient spatial resolution and because the structures are perpendicular to the sound direction. Therefore, both ventricular cavities are not properly visualized as with adequate empty space.

In fact, the pattern is that plane x-y and plane y-z have virtually identical axial and lateral resolution combination **(Figs. 7.8 and 7.9)**. So are the image quality in the three-orthogonal views reformatted from a direct volume scan (without gating), showing identical, good imaging quality in plane x-y and plane y-z, in fact, virtually identical resolution in all reformatted planes about the Y-axis [Fig. 6.1 (left 2 images) and Fig. 6.6]. Like in slice-reconstructed 3D images, the resolution in plane x-z is of poor quality.

It is worth noting that none of the three resolutions is evenly distributed along x-, y- or z-axis. For example, obstetric and gynecologic 3D studies often use convex- or vector-array, rather than linear array, transducers, resulting in an imaging plane (and subsequently a reconstructed imaging volume) with dense scan lines in the near-field and sparse lines in the far field, degrading imaging resolution further away from the probe. With beam focusing, the lateral resolution is usually finest in the focal zone. Although the theoretical axial resolution remains the same along the y-axis, the deeper the ultrasound transmission, the weaker their reflection and displayable resolution.

Sparse versus Dense Matrix-array Transducer-based Real-time 3D Imaging

The earliest ultrasound system capable of "real-time" 3D scanning in 1990s ran at 2.5–3.5 MHz frequencies and had a sparse matrix-array with only 256–512 elements, offering about 1 ~ 2 mm lateral resolution at best.[23,24] It was, therefore, possible to use the transducers to visualize the gross structures of the fetal heart, but its fine structures were expectedly not resolved **(Fig. 7.9)**.[25,26] Because it is not fine enough, the sparse real-time 3D cannot be genuinely called a direct volume scan.

Technology has advanced rapidly over the last three decades, making clinically available 3D ultrasound systems with increasingly denser matrix-array transducer with increased number of elements (3,600 in around 2000s,[6-8,27,28] 6,000–8,000 elements in around 2010s,[8] and 10,000 elements most likely in around 2020s).[25] It now provides real-time (about 25 Hz, or volumes/s) temporal resolution with much improved spatial resolution **(Fig. 7.10)**,[22,29] allowing it to be practically used in clinics.[19] They should be regarded as direct volume scan (again, if research or clinical interests do not require resolving every single fine structure of the fetal heart and its short cardiac phases). Even freehand probe movement during 4D acquisition does not cause visible motion artifact[13] (video clips for **Figs. 7.10 and 6.5**).

Similar Improvement has been Made in 4D Color Doppler Spatial and Temporal Resolutions

In early studies, detailed annotations had to be used to indicate each of the intracardiovascular flows in order to help readers to comprehend 4D intracardiovascular color flow images of the fetus **(Fig. 7.11)**.[30] Now, the state-of-the-art ultrasonography can produce self-explanatory 4D color Doppler views of the cardiovasculature **(Fig. 7.12)**.

Now, with sufficient temporal and spatial resolution, we need to consider at least one more **F**-issue—relativity between imaging volume and VOI size, to classify whether a 4D scan is a direct or indirect volume scan.

RELATIVITY BETWEEN IMAGING VOLUME AND INSEPARABLE ENTIRETY OF THE VOLUME OF INTEREST—HOW FULL IS FULL ENOUGH?

The size of a 3D imaging volume varies between different ultrasound systems and between different transducers. Even with a given system with a given transducer, it also varies with different settings. Mainly, the higher the spatial and/or temporal resolutions (the first two **F**s: **F**ineness and **F**astness), the smaller the imaging volume size.

To be "Full Enough" Does not Necessarily Mean to Embrace the Entire Organ of Interest, but the Volume of Interest of the Organ

For a given sized imaging volume with sufficient spatial and temporal resolutions, if it can embrace the entire VOI, it is what the concept of *direct volume scan* means. It needs to be pointed out that the entire VOI means not

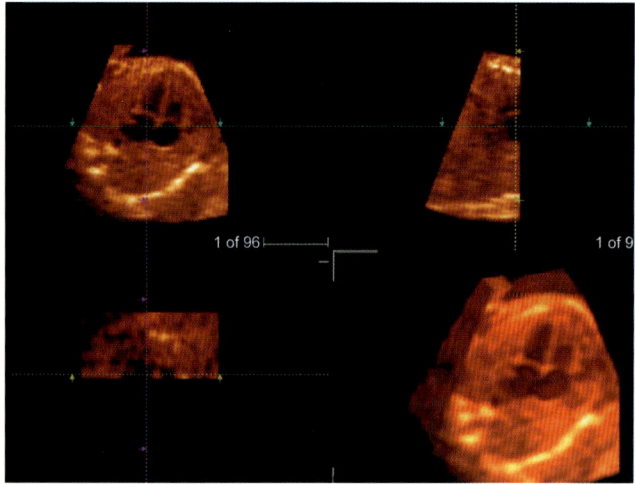

Fig. 7.10: Direct volume scan of a 23-week-old fetal heart with a 5 MHz dense matrix-array transducer (Philips IE33). It provides real-time temporal resolution of about 25 Hz (volumes/s), and much improved spatial resolution (along both x-axis and z-axis), compared with that of earlier sparse matrix-array systems (Fig. 7.9), allowing it to be practically used in clinics. (Video clips on our website: *www.medphys.ucl.ac.uk/mgi/jdeng* under Fetal Heart > Album 5 entry).

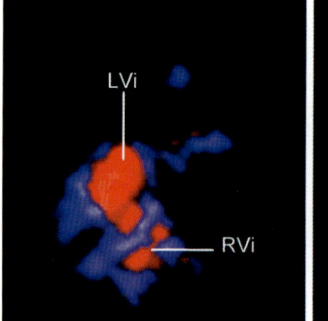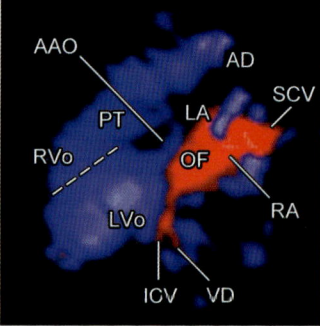

Fig. 7.11: Four-dimensional (4D) intracardiovascular flow from a 15-frame movie of a 4D color Doppler dataset from a 32-week-old fetal heart, viewed left-inferioposteriorly. Red and blue show flows toward and away from the probe located "behind" this page (Left). The reds are diastolic flows filling the right and left ventricular inlets (RVi and LVi). The surrounding blues are probably the flows bounced back from the ventricular walls, which may reflect the elasticity/compliance of the cardiac wall and surrounding tissues (Right). The red indicates flows from the superior and inferior caval veins (SCV and ICV) returning to the right atrium (RA), with partial flow through the oval foramen (OF) into the left atrium (LA). The blues are systolic flows from the right and left ventricular outlets (RVo and LVo) into the pulmonary trunk (PT) and ascending aorta (AAO, mostly obscured by the red), correspondingly. The blues in the two ventricles appear to merge along the dotted line due to color smearing artifacts. (AD: arterial duct; VD: venous duct). *Source*: Reprinted with permission from John Wiley & Sons. Ref. DOI: http://dx.doi.org/10.1046/j.1469-0705.2002.00752.x

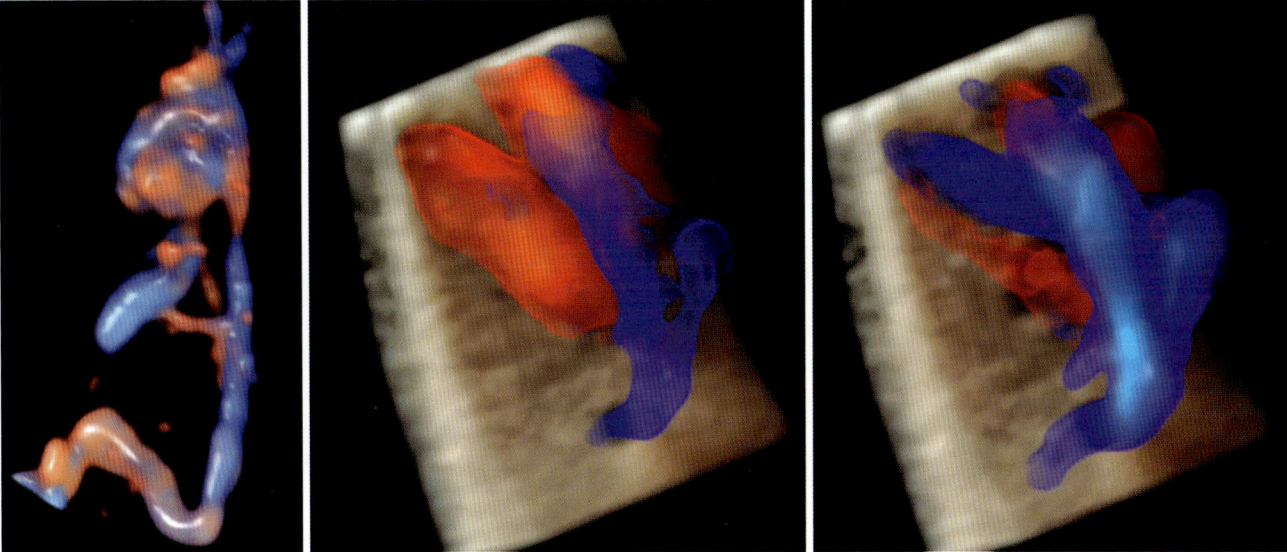

Fig. 7.12: Virtually self-explanatory, 4D color Doppler views of the fetal heart and major blood vessels, obtained using state-of-the-art STIC 4D ultrasound system. Left image: the thoracic, abdominal and umbilical cardiovasculature (*Courtesy*: Professor Greggory DeVore). Middle and right images: the heart viewed from above with the biventricular filling (in red) during diastole and the crossing of the great vessels (in blue) during systole. The systolic filling of the left and right ventricular outflow tracts and the joining of the arterial duct to the descending aorta are also visualized (*Courtesy*: Professor Rabih Chaoui).

necessarily the entire organ of interest, but inseparable entirety of the whole or part of the organ, as long as structural dynamics of interest is fully embraced by a single imaging volume. Take for example the 3D measurement of the left ventricle stroke volume (LVSV = the end-diastolic LV volume—the end-systolic LV volume). Now the interest is the LV volumetric change (rather than the entire heart) through a cardiac cycle. As long as the imaging volume is sufficiently large (full enough) to embrace the largest LV boundary at all times during a cardiac cycle, it is a direct volume scan, regardless whether or not the cardiac atria and great blood vessels can be embraced.

What about if the imaging volume is not full enough, resulting in part of the LV boundary not captured in the 4D dataset, or if clinical interest has become in the volumetric change of the entire heart and connecting great vessels and their branches? If increasing the imaging volume would degrade temporal and/or spatial resolution, an alternative approach must be used. A usual solution is to use multiple imaging subvolumes, each small enough with sufficient temporal and spatial resolution. Through several cardiac cycles, the subvolumes can build up (stitch together) a full imaging volume (i.e. subvolume-reconstructed 3D method), and hopefully, the full volume would be large enough to cover the entire VOI.[4,27]

As long as subvolume-reconstructed 3D acquisition is used through more than one cardiac cycle, the scan is no longer a direct volume scan, but an indirect volume scan, and a gating method must be employed to tackle motion artifact (**Figs. 7.2 and 6.3**).

Difficulty in and Even Impossibility of Performing a Clinically Useful Direct Volume Scan of the Fetal Heart in the Late Gestation

While the above consideration applies to the heart before and after birth, there is a particular difficulty in performing a direct volume scan in the late second and the entire third trimesters due to bony acoustic shadowing.

The fetal skeleton initially develops as (ultrasound penetrable) cartilage and gradually undergoes increasing ossification (with reduced ultrasound penetrability) throughout pregnancy. This leads to increased acoustic shadowing of the vertebrae, ribs, and upper limb bones extensively obscuring ultrasound view of the fetal heart within the thoracic cage from the second half of gestation onward.

In an adult subvolume-reconstructed 3D scan, it is often possible to obtain a sufficiently large full volume by placing a matrix-array transducer with a small footprint on the chest wall in an apical intercostal space, either by

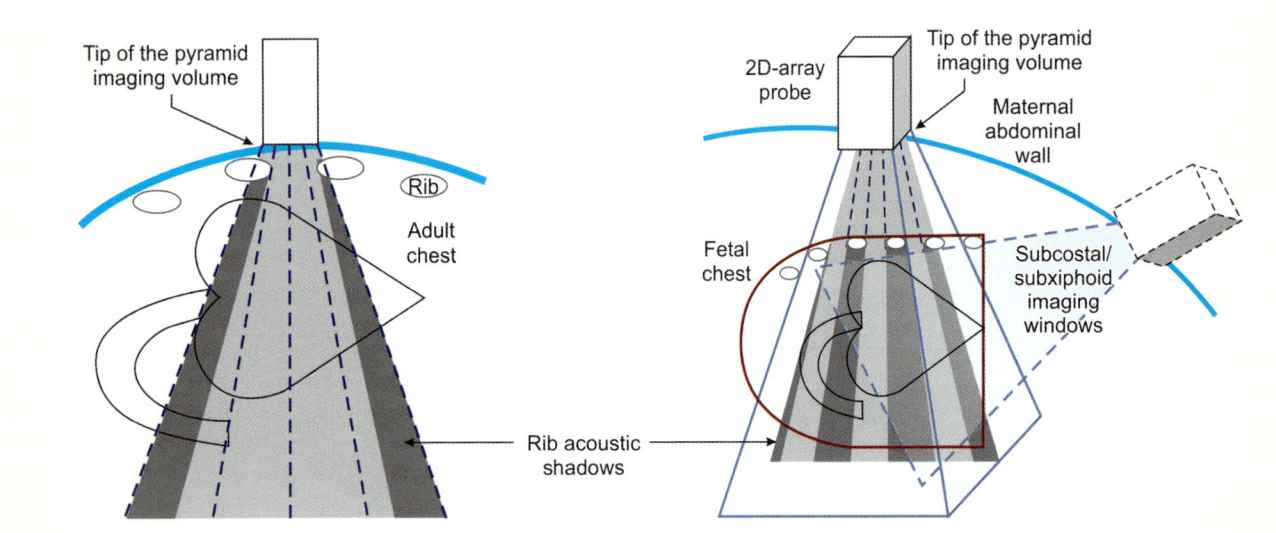

Fig. 7.13: With a larger intercostal space and a shorter transducer-to-heart distance in the adult (left) than in the fetal (right) cardiac imaging, a matrix-array transducer can obtain a wider imaging angle (light gray areas), subsequently a larger imaging volume without being obscured by the rib acoustic shadowing (dark gray areas). When keeping the transducer immobile, an even larger imaging volume can be built up by electronic-steering of several sub-imaging-volumes (between dotted lines in the right drawing) with high temporal and spatial resolutions and with ECG gating in adult studies. This is difficult or even impossible in subvolume-reconstructed 4D acquisition of the fetal heart in the second half of gestation. Because the heart in utero is some distance away from the tip of the pyramid imaging volume on the maternal abdominal wall, the fetal calcified ribs, as well as other calcified structures such as the arms, will cause acoustic shadowing through most imaging windows unless through those non- or less-calcified imaging windows shown in Figure 7.14. If the matrix-array transducer's temporal resolution is fast enough, no gating is necessary for imaging the cardiac structures not in the shadows. But if the VOI is wider than that of the intercostal acoustic gap, subvolume-reconstructed 4D acquisition is not as easy as in adult study. The reason is that, if the transducer has to be moved (say, tilted about a fetal intercostal space) to reveal more structures previously in the shadows, tracking its spatial movement and gating the cardiac motion become essential for reliable volumetric assessment.

means of electronic steering or of manual tilting about the skin spot the footprint is on. However, this is virtually impossible because the fetal chest wall is considerably away from the probe on the maternal abdominal wall **(Fig. 7.13)**. If the transducer has to be moved (say, tilted) to reveal structures previously in the shadows, it has to either be moved to another intercostal space, or be tilted about the FETAL intercostal space. As long as the probe moves during a subvolume-reconstructed 4D scan, it becomes necessary not only to gate the heart motion (temporal gating), but also to track the probe position (spatial tracking) for reliable volumetric assessment.[26,31,32] Both motion gating and position tracking are beyond the scope of this chapter, please refer to the references 14, 15, 31 and 32 for details.

Fortunately, the ventral ends of the fetal ribs remain as the costal cartilage even in the third trimester, particularly helpful to allow direct volume scan and even subvolume-reconstructed 3D scan (indirect volume scan)

of the fetal heart with the possibility of embracing its entirety in late gestation **(Figs. 7.14 and 6.3)**.

Research-claimed 4D Potential and Day-to-day Clinical Reality

The two main potential benefits of 4D ultrasound for off-line assessment of the fetal heart (or any other VOIs) are its ability (1) to scan the fetal heart in its totality, and (2) to display the cardiac structures in any desired orientations/planes. These are highly claimed in research articles, but infrequently realized in clinical practices, due to the acoustic shadowing just mentioned in **Figure 7.13** and the fact that most reformatted views, if not within original scanning planes, have poorer image quality, with the worst on plane C as illustrated in **Figure 7.8** and demonstrated in real cases in **Figure 7.7, Figure 7.9, and Figure 7.10**, and Figure 6.6.

Subsequent claims are that 2D reformatting reduces scanning time that a conventional ultrasound study would

Table 7.4: Impact of imaging angle on image quality (patient number = 16).

Data pairs = 25	Imaging angles	Ant. chest	Apex	Right-ant. chest	Subxiphoid
Gross Structures (Table 6.2)	RA	2.0	2.0	2.0	2.0
	RV	2.0	2.0	2.0	2.0
	LA	2.0	2.0	2.0	2.0
	LV	2.0	2.0	2.0	2.0
	SVC	2.0	1.5	1.0*	2.0
	IVC	1.5	1.5	2.0	2.0
	Ao root	2.0	1.0**	2.0	1.0*
	PA trunk	1.5	1.5	1.5	2.0
Fine Structures (Table 6.2)	Oval valve	0.5*	1.0*	2.0	1.5
	MV	2.0	2.0	2.0	2.0
	TV	2.0	2.0	2.0	2.0
	MV–TV off-set	2.0	2.0	0.5*	1.5
	mIVS	2.0	0.5*	2.0	1.5

*$p < 0.01$ and **$p < 0.05$, when compared with optimal imaging angles (score 2)
(RA and RV: right atrium and ventricle; LA and LV: left atrium and ventricle; SVC and IVC: superior and inferior vena cava; Ao: aortic; PA: pulmonary artery; MV and TV: mitral and tricuspid valve; mIVS: membranous interventricular septum).

take and avoid unnecessary scan repetition. Considering the above drawbacks, the time-saving assumptions can only be true when 4D data can be acquired with high spatial resolution also in non-original scanning plane and with a sufficiently large volume free of various artifacts, in particular, of motion and shadowing artifacts.

A study examined whether different imaging angles could hinder achieving the benefits fully.[29] Retrospectively analyzed were 368 real-time 3D datasets from 45 fetuses. 25 dataset pairs from 16 fetuses (18–24 weeks) were selected based on different imaging angles (**Table 7.4**). All other settings for the scans were identical and a full coverage of the heart was achieved without severe acoustic shadowing using the preferred imaging windows (**Fig. 7.14**). Structures were assessed at gross and fine levels (**Table 7.1**). Image quality was scored as 0 = poor, 1 = fair, and 2 = clear visualization of the structures with quality between each of the two consecutive scores marked as 0.5 or 1.5, respectively. Statistical difference was analyzed using χ^2 test. The time used in viewing a dataset was approximately noted.

The results showed that most of the structures received an average score ≥ 1.5, suggesting that changing imaging angle did not significantly affect assessment. Some gross structures (such as the aortic root and superior vena cava) had a score of 1 with $p < 0.01$ and < 0.05, indicating that changing the imaging angle did have an adverse impact.

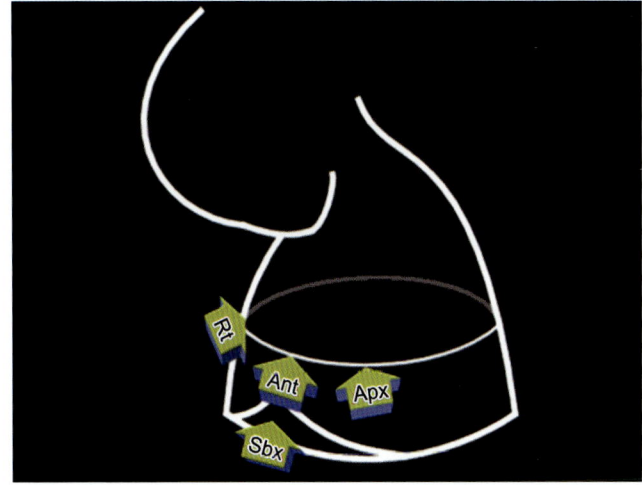

Fig. 7.14: Optimal windows for 4D acquisition of the entire or a large volume of the fetal heart when the rib cage has become significantly calcified with acoustic shadowing.
(Ant: anterior window; Apx: (left) apical window; Rt: right anterior window; Sbx: subxiphoid window).

Fine structures were very significantly affected by this, in particular the oval valve, the thin (membranous) interventricular septum and the offset between the mitral and tricuspid insertion to the septum (**Fig. 7.15**). It also found that identification of structures with score ≤ 1 required 10 minutes longer than those with score > 1.

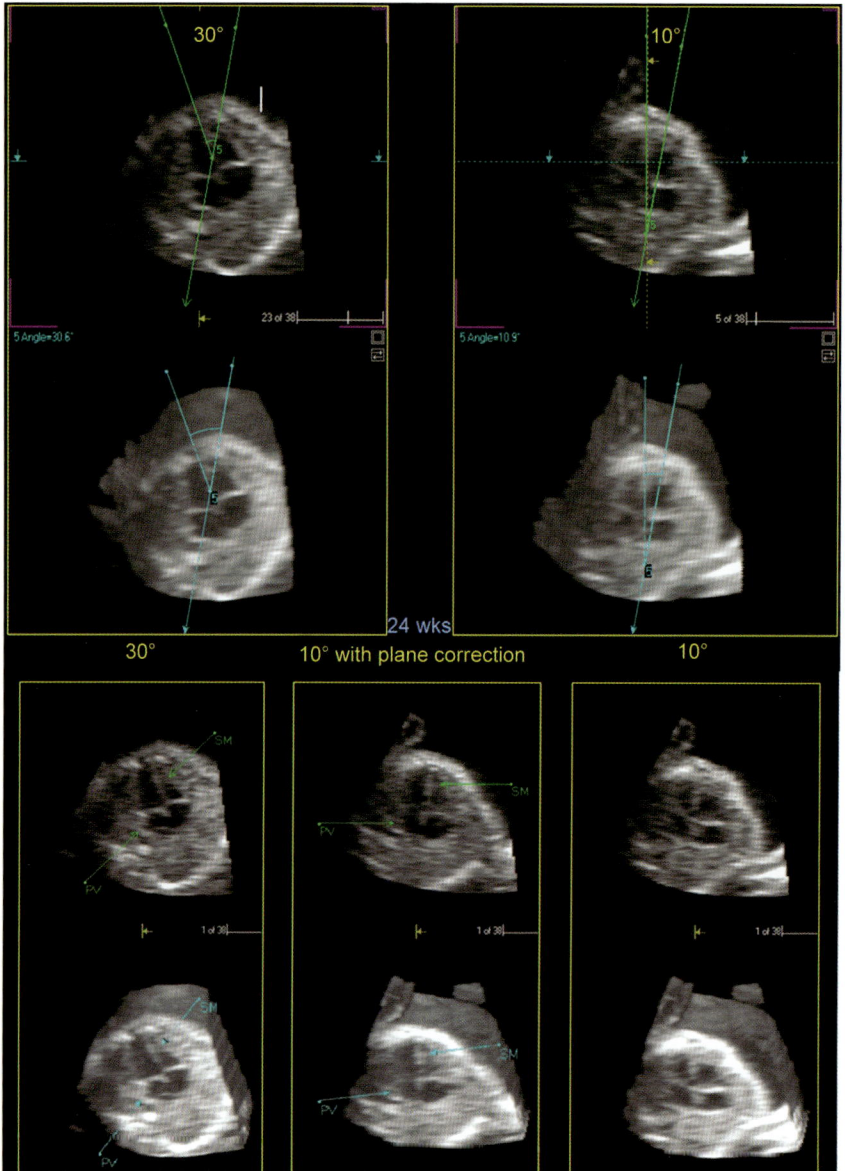

Fig. 7.15: Four-dimensional (4D) depiction of gross and fine fetal cardiac structures (Table 6.2) from different imaging angles with otherwise identical setting. Gross anatomies such as the four chambers are clearly visualized from all angles. Upper and lower left panels: Some fine structures are convincingly depicted with an approximate 30° angle between the interventricular septum and ultrasound insonation, such as the septomarginal trabeculation (SM) and pulmonary veins (PV), the offset (arrow) between the septal insertion of the mitral and tricuspid valves (MV, TV). Upper and lower right: Those fine features are virtually not imaged from an angle of about 10°. Lower middle: After off-line angle-correction to the 30°-acquired view, some fine structures have improved visualization such as the SM and the PV, but the insertion and the existence of membranous interventricular septum (mIVS) remain less convincing. Video clips on our website: *www.medphys.ucl.ac.uk/mgi/jdeng* under Fetal Heart > Album 7 entry.

It concluded that detailed assessment of cardiac structures is not always achievable by reviewing just a single 4D dataset even if the imaging volume embraces the entire heart with connecting great vessels. This is because of the angle dependency in 3D (or any dimensional) ultrasound imaging and because of the worse lateral than axial resolution. The time supposedly to be saved in acquiring fewer 4D datasets should be balanced against inconclusive "full" assessment using those datasets, which give rise to extra time to be required for additional scans or even repeated hospital visits.

> **Box 7.1:** Recommendation on how to acquire as many and detailed as possible fetal cardiac structures during direct volume scanning for maximal 4D data quality with minimal acquisition time and skill.
>
> - Locate imaging windows without significant acoustic shadowing, such as those suggested in **Figure 7.14**
> - Record two to four 4D datasets:
>   - From at least 2 windows/angles, and between them
>   - There should be an angle difference of around 90°, and at each angle
>   - Cover a minimum of four cardiac cycles, and during the cycles
>   - Tilt the probe in slightly different directions

Important Recommendation on Direct Volume Scans for 4D Datasets to be Evaluated Offline or via Telemedicine

In order to attain highest quality 4D datasets with minimal acquisition time (subsequently reducing data Intranet or Internet transfer time), we have to consider the first three **F**-issues as summarized in **Table 7.1**, with particular consideration on how to avoid disadvantage of acoustic shadowing and acoustic dropout. The latter is equivalent on how to take advantages of axial resolution superior to lateral resolution so that structural interfaces perpendicular to ultrasound propagation direction are better resolved. This is especially important if the 4D datasets are to be evaluated by offline internal or inter-institutional colleagues (i.e. via telemedicine).[33] Our recommended protocol is shown in **Box 7.1**.

RELATIVITY BETWEEN MAXIMAL FACILITATION OF 4D SCANNING AND MINIMAL RESTRICTION ON THE VOI FUNCTIONING—HOW FREE IS FREE ENOUGH?

When imaging internal genital organs or the fetus, the maternal abdomen, vagina/uterus, and/or the amniotic fluid provide sufficient buffers against the pressure from the ultrasound transducer. This allows acquiring 3D/4D data of VOIs, such as slow volume changing ovaries[34-36] or the rapidly beating fetal heart, without deforming their shapes and constraining their functions.

However, when extending 3D/4D ultrasound from the above internal anatomies to external body parts such as the penis and the clitoris and newborn tongue and lips,[5-9] direct application of a hard 3D/4D transducer to those soft and delicate VOIs would not only deform their shapes, but also restrict their functions. Strictly speaking, this cannot be regarded as direct volume scan as defined in the "Introduction" of this chapter.

There has been increasingly clinical need for better understanding of those structures in 4D during physiological or pathological processes. Here are a few clinical examples and encouraging 4D ultrasound solutions to address the issues.

Penis and Erectile Dysfunction

Nowadays, more patients survive chronic and serious diseases, but they have a high incidence of erectile dysfunction (ED), e.g. in 40–80% of renal transplantation recipients (RTRs). At UCL Hospitals, these patients are seen by doctors in Reproductive Medicine Unit, Institute for Women's Health. The pathophysiology of ED is often poorly understood, being multifactorial with organic and psychosomatic interactions. Thus, the majority of RTRs with ED remains undiagnosed and untreated or partially treated with significant effect to their quality of life.[28]

From the dynamic morphologic point of view, erection is caused by rapid changes in penile vasculature and musculature. Hence, an ideal modality for imaging erection should be able to visualize a sufficient anatomical volume containing at least the hemodynamic changes within a short period of time. These cannot be assessed fully by conventional, cross-sectional ultrasound imaging of the anatomy and point-based spectral Doppler sampling of blood flow, but recent studies have shown the feasibility of using 4D color Doppler to achieve this.[7,28]

An artificial vagina has been designed for *minimally restraining* the penis during a 4D scan. In fact, the friction between the penis and the "vagina" can help initiate and maintain the erection, *maximally facilitating* the 4D scan **(Figs. 7.16, 7.17 and Table 7.1)**. Of course, the most ideal setting should allow 4D scanning real osculation to be carried out by a couple themselves to minimize psychological impact of a clinical environment on the patients, attaining undisturbed physiological or pathological information. This has been successfully tried on a limited healthy couples (video clips on our website: www.medphys.ucl.ac.uk/mgi/jdeng under Body Parts > Erecting Penis).

Differentiation of penile vasculogenic impotence from other causes is important for treatment. Conventional

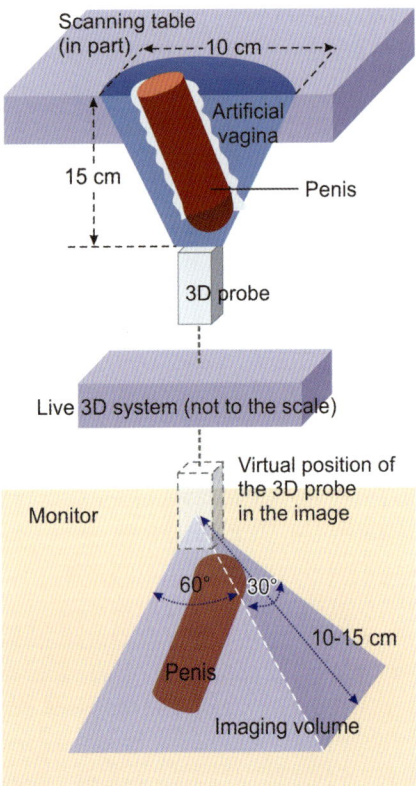

Fig. 7.16: Diagram of the minimally compressive scan setting and the real-time 3D imaging volume. The acoustic vagina not only avoids direct contact/deformation of the penis, but also helps initiate and maintain erection.
Source: Reprinted with permission from John Wiley & Sons. Ref. 7. DOI: http://onlinelibrary.wiley.com/doi/10.1111/j.1365-2605.2005.00617.x/full.

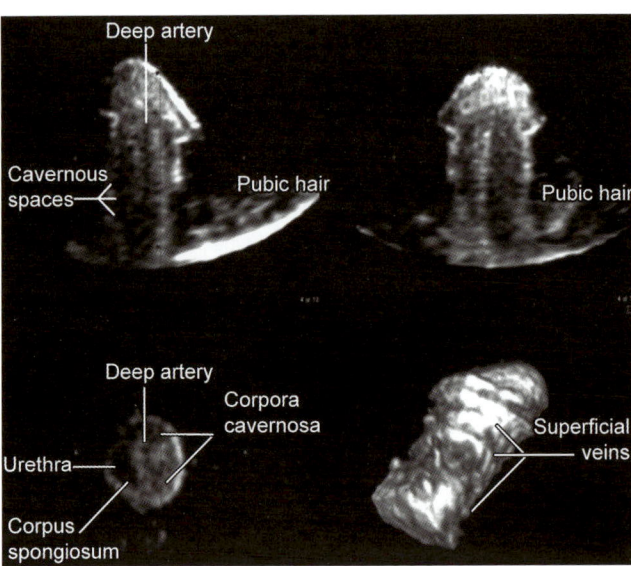

Fig. 7.17: Four-dimensional (4D) imaging of penile erection. The lower right image is a 3D surface view, not only showing the penile body and glans but also the dilated superficial veins. The remaining three images are 2D views reformatted from the 4D dataset. Upper left, right, and lower left are sagittal, transverse and coronal views, respectively. Note that, in this single 4D image acquired over a few seconds, almost all erectile information is displayed. These are, in approximate physiological order of erection: (1) Dilated deep arteries to increase penile inflow. (2) Increased cavernae to retain the inflow. (3) Strengthened and straightened tunica albuginea to help block outflow. (4) Blocked venous drainage. These result in (5) increased penile volume. (6) Dilated urethra to open the pathway to ejection. Video clips on our website: *www.medphys.ucl.ac.uk/mgi/jdeng* under Body Parts > Erecting Penis.
Source: Reprinted with permission from John Wiley & Sons. Ref. 7. DOI: http://onlinelibrary.wiley.com/doi/10.1111/j.1365-2605.2005.00617.x/full.

2D color Doppler assessment with the transducer directly in contact with the penis after intracavernosal stimulant injection often fails to produce reliable results because of limited views by the cross-sectional imaging and the painful procedure. By using real-time 3D ultrasound and dynamic 3D color Doppler with artificial vaginas, cavernosal vascular hemodynamics was only reliably detected in one of the eight RTRs with ED before oral sildenafil in a study. After sildenafil, however, all had reliably detectable flow with grades II to III erection. By the way, the scans were carried out with an imaging volume smaller than the entire penis in order to keep sufficient temporal color Doppler resolution. The findings met the VOI, which was to reveal whether or not there was brief blood flow enhancement of the deep arteries upon sildenafil, they were therefore regarded as direct volume scans.[26]

Clitoris and Female Erection

The clitoris is a poorly understood structure, both in terms of anatomy and physiology.[37] Information about its morphology has been derived from nonphysiological data obtained by intraoperative and postmortem observation, the latter being mainly from elderly postmenopausal women. Surgery to the clitoris has traditionally been recommended for those born with ambiguous genitalia. This policy has become increasingly controversial, with many patients unhappy with the treatments they have received. To date, the only known role for the clitoris is in mediating sexual pleasure, a role which may be compromised by surgery. Further understanding about this organ will provide information for both patients and clinicians when considering treatment options. However, data on the dynamic morphology of the clitoris are scant.

Among available noninvasive medical imaging modalities, mainly ultrasound and magnetic resonance imaging, only ultrasound is able to offer true real-time imaging. However, conventional real-time 2D ultrasound is performed with the transducer in direct contact with the target, coupled either by a thin layer of gel or a jelly offset pad. Consequently, the deformable erectile tissue may become compressed and movements are disturbed or even disabled during scanning. Therefore, the conventional approach cannot show "natural" morphologic changes of superficial structures when its movements are impeded. This limits the use of an excellent imaging technique that would otherwise be capable of providing important information about dynamic morphology.

To overcome those difficulties, a matrix-array transducer was positioned in front of and about 3 cm away from the clitoris, with a gel pad or water pad being placed in between. The pads allowed the delicate structures to be imaged without noticeable deformation **(Fig. 7.18)**. Facilitated by the minimally compressive scanning techniques (Deng et al. 2000), a study established the use of real-time 3D ultrasound for visualization of the organ in its entirety (the glans, body and cruses) using subvolume-reconstruction 3D acquisition (indirect volume scan)

at the peak of orgasm **(Figs. 7.19A and B)** and in part (the clitoral glans and body) undergoing arousal (direct volume scan), without deforming the soft tissue. Quality

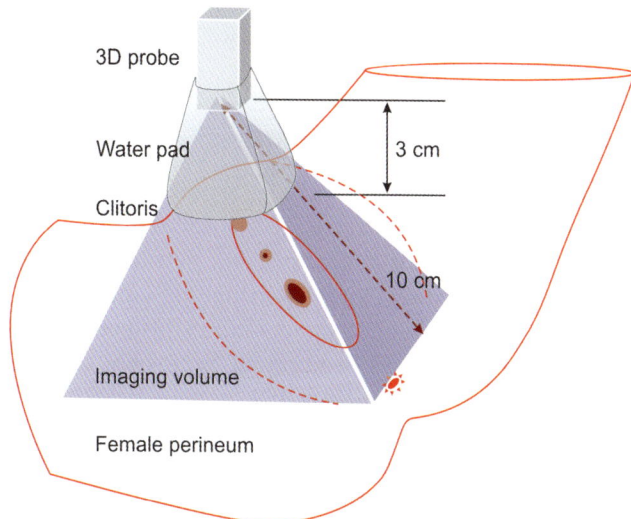

Fig. 7.18: Diagram of the live 3D imaging volume and the minimally compressive scanning setting. (A supporting plastic wrap around the pad sidewall is not shown here. See text for more information). *Source*: Reprinted with permission from Elsevier. Ref. 6. DOI: http://dx.doi.org/10.1016/j.ultrasmedbio.2006.06.006.

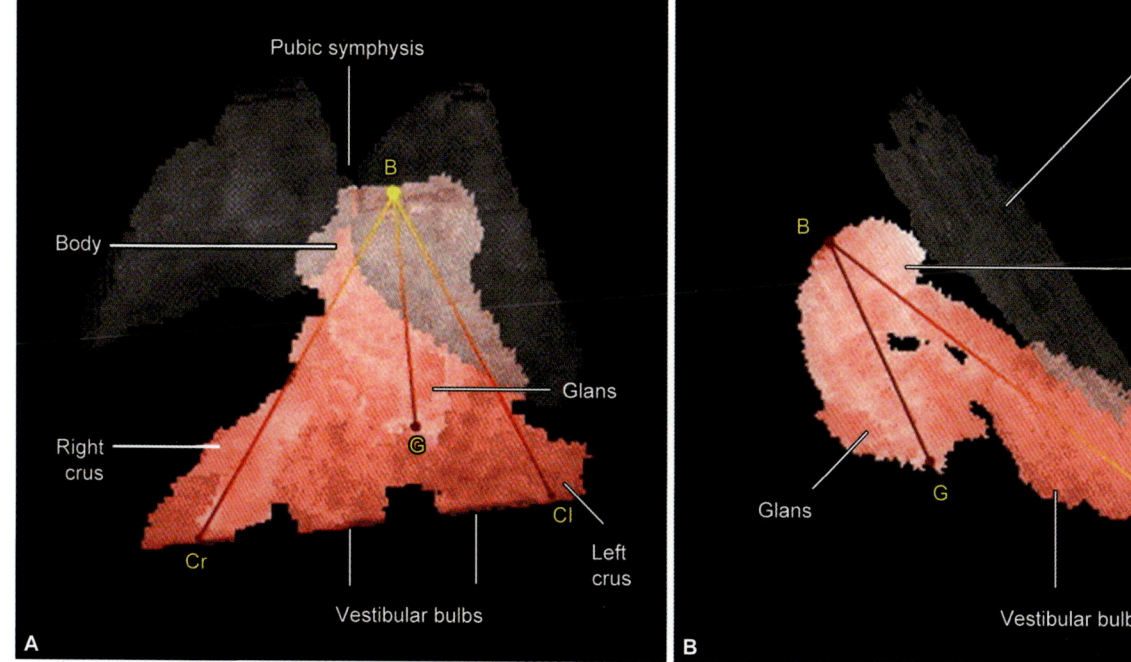

Figs. 7.19A and B: The 3D images are reconstructed from a full volume scan. Nonerectile tissues except for the background bones are removed by image editing and virtually the whole clitoris is revealed. (A) front view; and (B) left side view. Illustrative measurements: distances (mm) between the body top and glans bottom (B–G) = 12, between the body top and right crus (B–Cr) = 31, between the body top and left crus (B–Cl) = 29; angle between the crura to the body top (Cr–B–Cl) = 52°; volume of the complex = 2.74 mL. Video clips on our website: *www.medphys.ucl.ac.uk/mgi/jdeng* under Body Parts > Arousal Clitoris entry. Elsevier. Ref. 6. DOI: http://dx.doi.org/10.1016/j.ultrasmedbio.2006.06.006

3D and 4D images of the clitoral structures could be obtained in all patients (from 71% of a total of 51 datasets). The imaging volume was large enough to cover the clitoral glans and body simultaneously, allowing real-time 3D visualization. Hence, the preparatory study has paved the way for further normative studies and pathological examinations.

Tongue and Infant Feeding

Whether the infant tongue moves by peristaltic action for milk removal from the breast is controversial, with 2D ultrasound studies suggesting non-peristaltic tongue movement, with milk intake relying on oral vacuum (showing up-and-down tongue motion instead). Real-time 3D ultrasound has been found decisive to address the controversy and demonstrated its potential for perinatal study. A small matrix-array 7 MHz transducer (designed for pediatric cardiac studies) can be used for submental imaging of the mouth (tongue and hard–soft palates) during breastfeeding with minimal, if any, constraint on their functioning while covering a sufficiently large part of the tongue with sufficient temporal and spatial resolution, i.e. with a direct volume scan) **(Fig. 7.5)**.

Results from a preliminary study have shown both peristalsis in 2D views reformatted along the genuine medial plane and up-and-down motion in 2D views perpendicular to the medial plane. Ambiguous motion patterns are seen in 2D views reformatted from the planes inbetween the above two planes. The more the 2D views are reformatted off the medial plane, the more the up-and-down motion are clearly observed.[8,38,39] Although a study with a large number of normal babies is needed, our initial finding has discovered, at least part of the cause of the controversy, and paved the way for more comprehensive imaging of normally and abnormally fed neonates and infants, and for more physiological milk-bottle designing.

SUMMARY

The above infant tongue study, together with other exemplary studies mentioned in this chapter, demonstrate the importance of 4D imaging in revealing the fundamental morphophysiology of the human body that would otherwise be difficult or even impossible to discover without employing a direct volume scan with careful consideration of the 4Fs summarized in **Table 7.1**.

In brief, when imaging in 4D, think of 4Fs!

ACKNOWLEDGMENTS

I am deeply indebted to my supervisors and colleagues, with their names listed or not (yet) listed in our publications among the references. They have supported multiple 4D imaging projects at the University College London (UCL) and UCL Hospitals, including Institute for Women's Health, Institute of Child Health and GOS Children's Hospital, and Department of Medical Physics over the past 25 years, and now at Barts Heart Centre. Part of this chapter is based upon the author's PhD thesis, supervised by Professors Charles Rodeck and Alfred Linney, and examined by Professors Stuart Campbell and the late Peter Wells.

REFERENCES

1. Wikipedia. Persistence of vision. [online] Available from https://en.wikipedia.org/wiki/Persistence_of_vision [Accessed december, 2018].
2. Deng J. How to optimise 4D settings for fetal echo: from theoretical to technical considerations. 3D Workshop at the 26th World Congress on Ultrasound in Obstetrics and Gynecology: Rome, Italy; 2016.
3. Wikipedia. Wagon-wheel effect. [online] Available from https://en.wikipedia.org/wiki/Wagon-wheel_effect [Accessed December, 2018].
4. Deng J. Terminology of three-dimensional and four-dimensional ultrasound imaging of the fetal heart and other moving body parts. Ultrasound Obstet Gynecol. 2003;22(4):336-44.
5. Youssef A, Montaguti E, Sanlorenzo O, et al. Reliability of new three-dimensional ultrasound technique for pelvic hiatal area measurement. Ultrasound Obstet Gynecol. 2016;47(5):629-35.
6. Deng J, Crouch NS, Creighton SM, et al. Minimally-compressive, three- and four-dimensional ultrasound imaging of the clitoris: a feasibility study. Ultrasound Med Biol. 2006;32(10):1479-84.
7. Deng J, Hall-Craggs MA, Pellerin D, et al. Real-time three-dimensional ultrasound visualization of erection and artificial coitus. Int J Androl. 2006;29(2):374-79.
8. Burton P, Deng J, McDonald D, et al. Real-time 3D ultrasound imaging of infant tongue movements during breastfeeding. Early Hum Dev. 2013;89(9):635-41.
9. Oversand SH, Atan IK, Shek KL, et al. Association of urinary and anal incontinence with measures of pelvic floor muscle contractility. Ultrasound Obstet Gynecol. 2016;47(5):642-5.
10. Merz E, Welter C. 2D and 3D Ultrasound in the evaluation of normal and abnormal fetal anatomy in the second and third trimesters in a level III center. Ultraschall Med. 2005;26(1):9-16.
11. Merz E, Abramowicz J, Baba K, et al. 3D imaging of the fetal face–recommendations from the International 3D Focus Group. Ultraschall Med. 2012;33(2):175-82.

12. Tutschek B, Blaas HK, Abramowicz J, et al. Three-dimensional ultrasound imaging of the fetal skull and face. Ultrasound Obstet Gynecol. 2017;50(1):7-16.

13. Deng J. 3D/4D specific artefacts: how to recognise, minimise and avoid them. 3D Workshop at the 27th World Congress on Ultrasound in Obstetrics and Gynecology: Vienna, Austria; 2017.

14. Nelson TR, Pretorius DH, Sklansky M, et al. Three-dimensional echocardiographic evaluation of fetal heart anatomy and function: acquisition, analysis, and display. J Ultrasound Med. 1996;15(1):1-9.

15. Deng J, Gardener JE, Rodeck CH, et al. Fetal echocardiography in three and four dimensions. Ultrasound Med Biol. 1996;22(8):979-86.

16. Goncalves LF, Espinoza J, Romero R, et al. Four-dimensional fetal echocardiography with spatiotemporal image correlation (STIC): a systematic study of standard cardiac views assessed by different observers. J Matern Fetal Neonatal Med. 2005;17(5):323-31.

17. Espinoza J, Lee W, Comstock C, et al. Collaborative study on 4-dimensional echocardiography for the diagnosis of fetal heart defects: the COFEHD study. J Ultrasound Med. 2010;29(11):1573-80.

18. Carvalho JS, Allan LD, Chaoui R, et al. ISUOG Practice Guidelines (updated): sonographic screening examination of the fetal heart. Ultrasound Obstet Gynecol. 2013;41(3):348-59.

19. DeVore GR, Satou G, Sklansky M. 4D fetal echocardiography-An update. Echocardiography. 2017;34(12):1788-98.

20. Yeo L, Luewan S, Romero R. Fetal Intelligent Navigation Echocardiography (FINE) Detects 98% of Congenital Heart Disease. J Ultrasound Med. 2018;37(11):2577-93.

21. Deng J, Newton NM, Hall-Craggs MA, et al. Novel technique for three-dimensional visualisation and quantification of deformable, moving soft-tissue body parts. Lancet. 2000;356(9224):127-31.

22. Deng J, Yates R, Demetrescu C, et al. Impact of live 4D ultrasound volume rate on recognition of fetal cardiac structures in reformatted 2D views. Ultrasound Obstet Gynecol. 2010;36(Suppl 1):3.

23. Smith SW, Trahey GE, von Ramm OT. Two-dimensional arrays for medical ultrasound. Ultrason Imaging. 1992;14(3):213-33.

24. Houck RC, Cooke J, Gill EA. Three-dimensional echo: transition from theory to real-time, a technology now ready for prime time. Curr Probl Diagn Radiol. 2005;34(3):85-105.

25. Sklansky MS, Nelson T, Strachan M, et al. Real-time three-dimensional fetal echocardiography: initial feasibility study. J Ultrasound Med. 1999;18(11):745-52.

26. Deng J, Sullivan ID, Yates R, et al. Real-time three-dimensional fetal echocardiography—Optimal imaging windows. Ultrasound Med Biol. 2002;28(9):1099-105.

27. Wang XF, Deng YB, Nanda NC, et al. Live three-dimensional echocardiography: imaging principles and clinical application. Echocardiography. 2003;20(7):593-604.

28. Chatterjee R, Deng J, Pellerin D, et al. Feasibility of dynamic 3-D color Doppler ultrasound for imaging penile vascular change in renal transplant patients with erectile dysfunction responding to sildenafil. Ultrasound Med Biol. 2008;34(6):885-91.

29. Deng J, Yates R, Sullivan ID, et al. OC131: Impact of imaging angle on reviewers' confidence in assessment of 4D fetal echocardiographic datasets. Ultrasound Obstet Gynecol. 2006;28(4):397.

30. Deng J, Yates R, Sullivan ID, et al. Dynamic three-dimensional colour Doppler ultrasound of human fetal intracardiac flow. Ultrasound Obstet Gynecol. 2002;20(2):131-6.

31. Baba K, Okai T. Basis and principles of three-dimensional ultrasound. In: Baba K, Jurkovic D, (Eds). Three-Dimensional Ultrasound in Obstetrics and Gynecology. London: Parthenon; 1997. pp. 1-19.

32. Deng J. PhD Thesis on Dynamic three-dimensional fetal echocardiography. London: University of London; 2003.

33. Vinals F. Current experience and prospect of Internet consultation in fetal cardiac ultrasound. Fetal Diagn Ther. 2011;30(2):83-7.

34. Kupesic S, Kurjak A. Predictors of IVF outcome by three-dimensional ultrasound. Hum Reprod. 2002;17(4):950-5.

35. Raine-Fenning N, Jayaprakasan K, Deb S, et al. Automated follicle tracking improves measurement reliability in patients undergoing ovarian stimulation. Reprod Biomed Online. 2009;18(5):658-63.

36. Kurjak A, Kupesic S, Anic T, et al. Three-dimensional ultrasound and power doppler improve the diagnosis of ovarian lesions. Gynecol Oncol. 2000;76(1):28-32.

37. Crouch NS, Minto CL, Laio LM, et al. Genital sensation after feminizing genitoplasty for congenital adrenal hyperplasia: a pilot study. BJU Int. 2004;93(1):135-8.

38. Deng J, Burton P, McDonald D, et al. Real-time 3D ultrasound of tongue movements during breast-feeding—would the findings lead to prenatal studies? Ultrasound Obstet Gynecol. 2011;38(Suppl 1):245-6.

39. Hartung J, Heling KS, Rake A, et al. Detection of an aneurysm of the vein of Galen following signs of cardiac overload in a 22-week old fetus. Prenat Diagn. 2003;23(11):901-3.

Three-dimensional/ Four-dimensional Pelvic Floor Ultrasound

Hans Peter Dietz

INTRODUCTION

Ultrasound is the primary imaging method in gynecology, and it is also widely used in urology and colorectal surgery. This makes the modality increasingly popular in the imaging assessment of pelvic floor anatomy, a field that all three specialties are routinely involved with. This development is long overdue, especially as pathophysiology and etiology of most pelvic floor conditions are still poorly understood. The advent of three-dimensional (3D) ultrasound allows access to the axial plane and arbitrarily definable parasagittal and oblique planes which has greatly facilitated the assessment of the levator ani muscle, the anal sphincter, and of paraurethral abnormalities, such as urethral diverticula. At least as importantly, four-dimensional (4D) ultrasound enables the observation of function in the form of maneuvers, such as cough, Valsalva, and pelvic floor muscle contraction.

While 3D imaging has also been used with techniques such as endovaginal and endoanal ultrasound, its main utility lies in exoanal, translabial, or transperineal ultrasound which allows assessment of the entire pelvic floor in a very few volume data sets. The author terms this modality "pelvic floor ultrasound".[1] It is unique in that it allows a comprehensive assessment of pelvic floor structures in one single, noninvasive investigation of less than 10 minutes duration. The modality replaces a number of other, more expensive, invasive, and/or costly methods, such as videocystourethrography, magnetic resonance imaging (MRI), defecation proctography, and endoanal ultrasound, using systems almost universally available. Indications are given in **Box 8.1**.

Box 8.1: Indications for three-dimensional (3D)/four-dimensional (4D) pelvic floor ultrasound.

- Urinary incontinence
- Recurrent urinary tract infections
- Persistent dysuria
- Symptoms of voiding dysfunction
- Symptoms of pelvic organ prolapse
- Obstructed defecation
- Anal incontinence
- Vaginal discharge or bleeding after pelvic floor surgery
- Pelvic or vaginal pain after pelvic floor surgery
- Dyspareunia
- Vaginal or perineal cysts or masses
- Synthetic implant visualization (slings, meshes, and bulking agents)
- Levator ani muscle assessment after childbirth
- Obstetric perineal or anal sphincter injuries (OASIs).

The growing interest in imaging of pelvic floor structures is attributable to a number of factors. Most importantly, pelvic floor dysfunction is increasingly prevalent in aging populations. The estimated lifetime risk for prolapse or urinary incontinence surgery is 10–20% in developed societies.[2,3] Our understanding of the pathophysiology of those conditions, however, is limited. This is nowhere more true than in the treatment of female pelvic organ prolapse (POP), with about one-third of all procedures being reoperations.

The International Urogynecological Association (IUGA) now offers a six-module online learning system with individual teaching by preceptors able to provide feedback in seven languages currently (https://www.iuga.org/tools/pfic/pfic-overview). Standardization efforts through IUGA and the American Institute of Ultrasound in Medicine (AIUM) are also going to support clinical practice in this field.

BASIC TECHNIQUE

The basic requirements for pelvic floor imaging include a B-mode capable two-dimensional (2D) ultrasound system with cine-loop function, a 3.5–6 MHz curved array transducer, and a videoprinter. However, to allow for the full scope of diagnostic capabilities, 3D/4D imaging is indispensable. Any 4D capable system with abdominal 4D transducers, such as those used for obstetric imaging is suitable, provided the aperture angle (field of view) is 70° or higher, and the acquisition angle of the volume transducer can be set to at least 70°. For severe prolapse and hiatal ballooning, aperture and acquisition angles of 80–90° are sometimes necessary.

The examination is performed with the patient in dorsal lithotomy, with hips flexed and slightly abducted, or in the standing position if necessary. A full bladder or bowel may prevent full development of POP.[4] Therefore, imaging is best performed after bladder emptying. Catheterization may be necessary if postvoid residuals are over 50 mL.

The probe is covered with a powder-free glove, condom, or thin plastic wrap after spreading ultrasound gel on the transducer surface, avoiding the trapping of air bubbles between transducer surface and glove. The probe is placed on the perineum after parting the labia, producing a typical mid-sagittal view as seen in **Figures 8.1A and B**, defined by the simultaneous depiction of both urethra anteriorly and anorectum posteriorly

(Figs. 8.1A and B). The symphysis pubis provides a bony point of reference anteriorly. Tissue hydration and scar tissue may affect visibility, but obesity is virtually never a problem provided the labia are parted. Conditions are optimal in pregnancy, and poorest in the senium due to varying degrees of tissue hydration.

The transducer can usually be placed quite firmly without causing discomfort, unless there is marked atrophy or vulvitis. On the other hand, during a Valsalva, it is essential not to exert undue pressure to allow pelvic organ descent to occur to its full extent. After the examination, the probe is mechanically cleaned, followed by treatment with alcoholic wipes or other forms of disinfection.

While there is no consensus on image orientation, the first published translabial images had the perineum at the top and the symphysis pubis on the left, which is still the most commonly used orientation. It is particularly convenient when using 3D/4D systems as shown in **Figures 8.2A to D**. The top left image represents the mid-sagittal or "A" plane, the top right is the coronal or "B" plane, and the bottom left is the axial or "C" plane. The bottom right shows a rendered volume of the levator hiatus.

The development of 3D/4D imaging has given clinicians simple access to the axial plane. Translabial 3D/4D allows imaging of the levator hiatus **(Figs. 8.2A to D)**, the central opening in the levator plate, in the axial or "C" plane. The levator hiatus is the largest potential hernial portal in the human body[5] and the most crucial soft tissue component of the birth canal. POP is best understood as a hernia through the levator hiatus. In childbirth, the hiatus has to stretch very substantially and over a short period of time,[6] putting strain on the

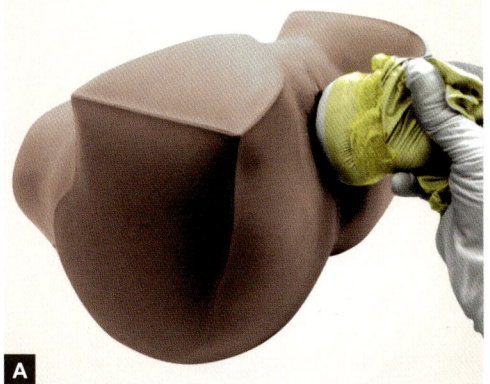

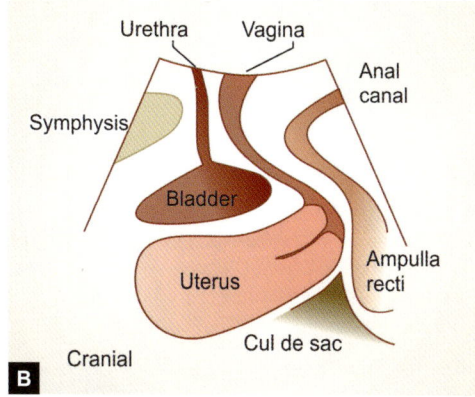

Figs. 8.1A and B: (A) Transducer placement on the perineum; (B) Schematic representation of the resulting mid-sagittal field of vision. *Source*: Right image adapted with permission from Dietz HP. Ultrasound imaging of the pelvic floor: Part 1: two-dimensional aspects. Ultrasound Obstet Gynecol. 2004;23(1):80-92.

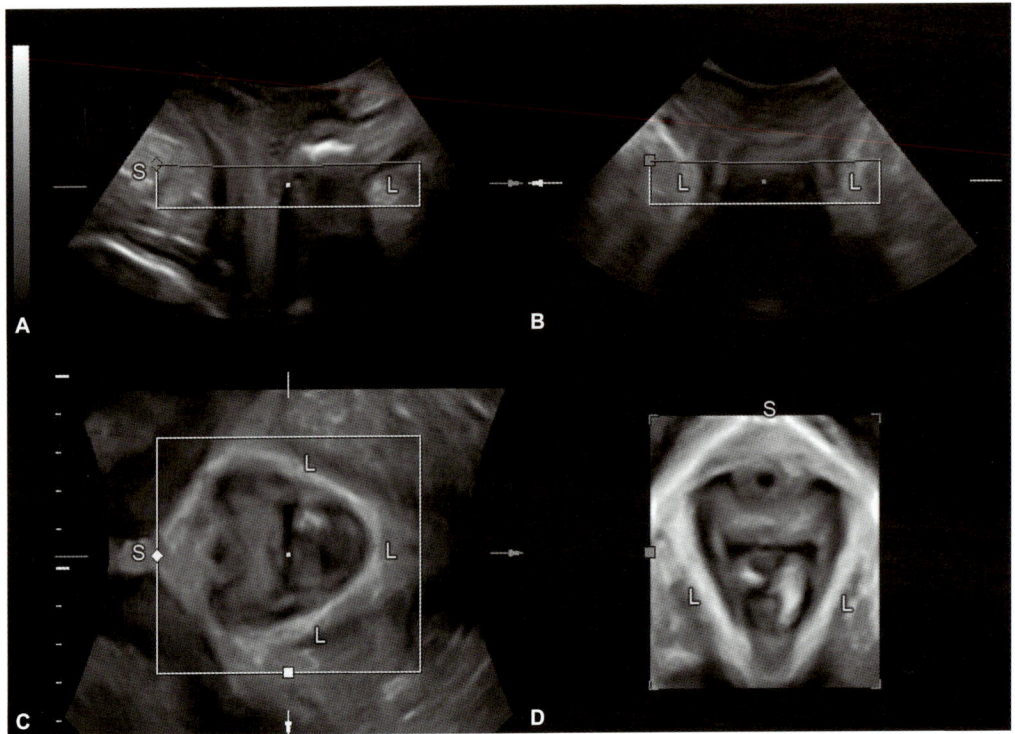

Figs. 8.2A to D: Standard representation of female pelvic floor structures on translabial/perineal ultrasound. The mid-sagittal plane is shown in (A), the coronal in Figure B, and the axial in Figure C. A rendered volume (i.e. the semitransparent representation of all pixels in the "region of interest", the box seen in Figures A to C) in the axial plane is given in Figure D. Often, Figures A and D are of the most interest and are combined, leaving out B and C. In Figure D, the patient's right hand side is represented on the left, as if the pelvic floor was viewed from below.
Source: Reproduced with permission from Dietz HP. Pelvic floor ultrasound. In: Fleischer AC (Ed). Sonography in Obstetrics and Gynecology: Principles and Practice. New York: Tata McGraw Hill; 2017.

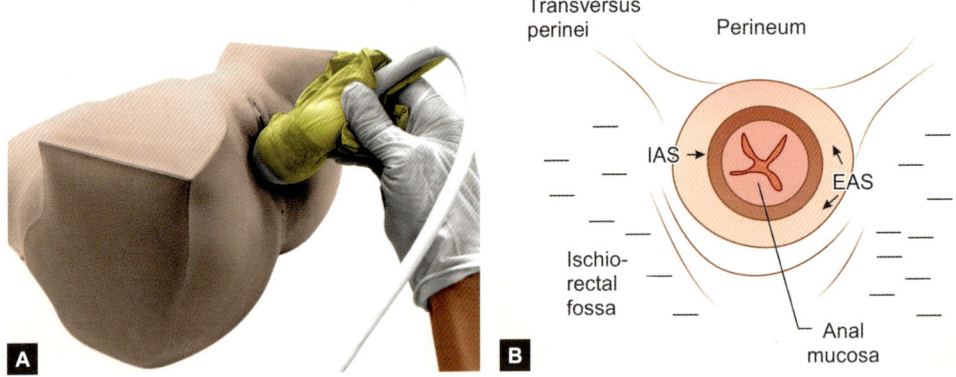

Figs. 8.3A and B: (A) Transducer placement for exoanal sphincter imaging; (B) Schematic illustration of imaged structures in the resulting coronal or transverse plane. (EAS: external anal sphincter; IAS: internal anal sphincter)
Source: Reproduced with permission from Dietz HP. Pelvic floor ultrasound. In: Fleischer AC (Ed). Sonography in Obstetrics and Gynecology: Principles and Practice. New York: Tata McGraw Hill; 2017.

muscle itself and its insertion on the inferior pubic ramus. Not surprisingly, permanent damage is common.[7]

The coronal plane is of increasing interest as it provides views of the anal sphincter complex, with volume acquisition best performed in this plane, as shown in **Figures 8.3A and B**. The increasing focus on anal sphincter trauma makes the development of this method particularly timely and important.[8]

ANTERIOR COMPARTMENT PATHOLOGY

Residual Urine and Bladder Wall

The first step in a pelvic floor ultrasound assessment usually is the determination of postvoid residual urine. The residual volume (in mL) can be estimated using the formula X cm × Y cm × 5.6,[9] with X and Y denoting the largest dimensions of the bladder, obtained perpendicular to each another, in the mid-sagittal plane. Volumes over 50 mL are regarded as abnormal and should be confirmed after at least one more void. Occasionally, incidental foreign bodies or bladder tumors may be detected. Detrusor wall thickness of more than or equal to 5 mm (detrusor hypertrophy) seems associated with urge of urinary incontinence and detrusor overactivity. Detrusor hypertrophy can be variable depending on location, with the dome often thicker than the posterior bladder base beyond the trigone, especially in women with cystocele **(Fig. 8.4)**. As a result, DWT is not in fact a good test.[10] Unlike the situation in the male bladder, DWT may not be predictive of voiding difficulty in women.[11] Occasionally, a trigonal cystic structure may be observed, the differential diagnosis being ureterocele and nabothian follicle.

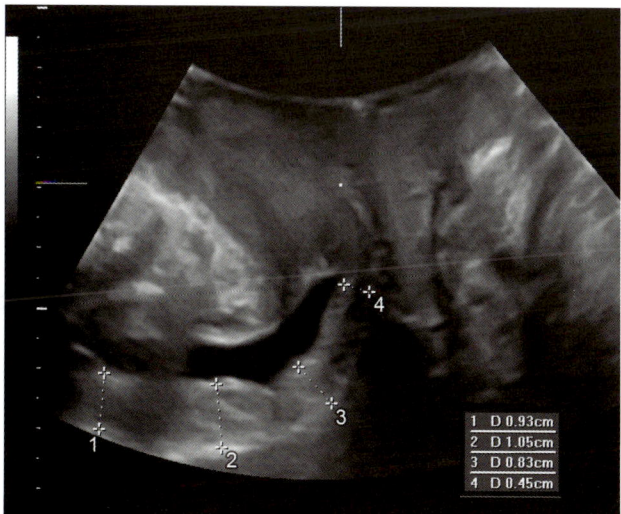

Fig. 8.4: Detrusor hypertrophy seen in the mid-sagittal plane in a patient with urodynamic detrusor overactivity.
Source: Reproduced with permission from Dietz H. Pelvic floor ultrasound: abnormal findings. In: Merz E (Ed). Atlas of 3D/4D Ultrasound in Obstetrics and Gynecology. Stuttgart: Thieme Medical Publishers; 2018.

ANATOMY OF STRESS URINARY INCONTINENCE

In women suffering from stress urinary incontinence or urodynamic stress incontinence, the proximal urethra commonly rotates posteroinferiorly on Valsalva maneuver as urethra and anterior vaginal wall are tethered to the symphysis pubis and the pelvic sidewall. In essence, the symphysis acts as a fulcrum around which the entire anterior compartment rotates. Points of reference for measurements of bladder neck mobility are either the central axis of the symphysis pubis or its inferior-posterior margin. Bladder neck mobility can be determined in a highly repeatable fashion **(Figs. 8.5A and B)**.[12] The difference between values at rest and on maximal Valsalva yields a numerical value for bladder neck descent (BND). Funneling of the internal urethral meatus is often observed on Valsalva in women suffering from stress urinary incontinence. Funneling is commonly, but not always, seen at the time of urine leakage.

ANTERIOR COMPARTMENT PROLAPSE

Descent of the anterior vaginal wall or "cystocele" does indeed usually mean descent of the bladder. However, occasionally a urethral diverticulum or other cystic structures of the anterior vaginal wall, such as Gartner duct cysts may be responsible. Urethral diverticula are commonly overlooked in women with lower urinary tract symptoms, resulting in substantial delays in treatment. Small diverticula may appear as a mostly hyperechogenic irregularity of the urethra, although most show a clearly cystic or solid-cystic appearance.[13] Any spatially circumscribed paraurethral abnormality is better appreciated in the sectional planes, which are useful in differentiating other cystic or mixed solid-cystic structures from a urethral diverticulum. Sectional imaging can help with surgical planning, especially with more complex diverticula. **Figures 8.6A to H** show typical appearances of four very different, urethroscopically confirmed urethral diverticula in the mid-sagittal and coronal planes.

Most often, however, a clinical "cystocele" is indeed a prolapse of the bladder. Historically, two types of cystoceles have been described, and they have rather distinct functional implications.[14] A cystourethrocele is associated with stress urinary incontinence and normal voiding, a cystocele with intact retrovesical angle is often found in women with voiding dysfunction and symptoms

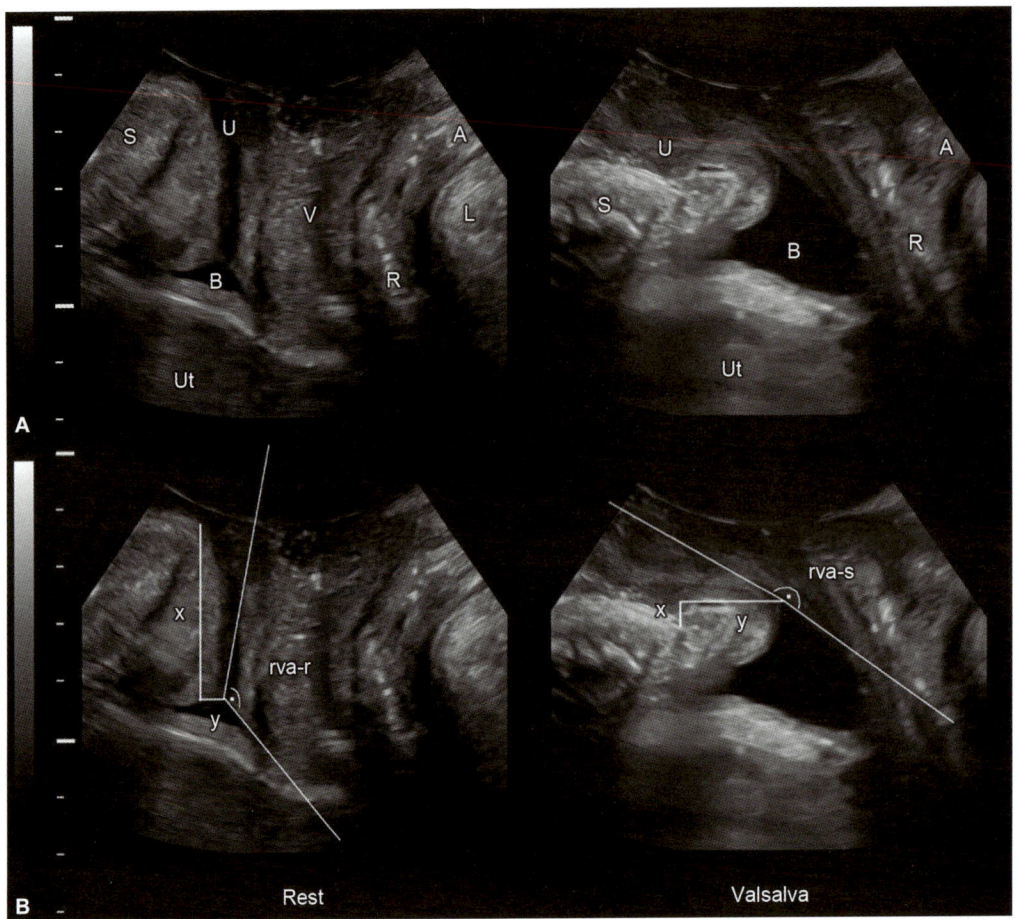

Figs. 8.5A and B: Determination of bladder neck descent and retrovesical angle: ultrasound images show the mid-sagittal plane at rest (A) and on Valsalva (B). The lower images demonstrate the measurement of distances between inferior symphyseal margin and bladder neck (vertical, X and horizontal, Y) and the retrovesical angle at rest (RVA-R) and on Valsalva. (A: anal canal; B: bladder; L: levator ani; R: rectal ampulla; S: symphysis pubis, U: urethra; Ut: uterus; V: vagina)
Source: Reproduced with permission from Dietz HP. Pelvic floor ultrasound in incontinence: What's in it for the surgeon? Int Urogynecol J. 2011;22(9):1085-97.

of prolapse. The latter is associated with avulsion of the levator ani, as opposed to a cystourethrocele, which argues against a traumatic pathogenesis for the latter condition. Sometimes, a severe cystocele may result in inversion of the bladder neck, that is, rotation of the bladder neck through up to 180° on Valsalva and up to 6 cm of BND, and marked urethral kinking, as in **Figures 8.7A and B**. It is not surprising that such women often suffer from substantial voiding dysfunction.

CENTRAL COMPARTMENT

The uterus is harder to see than the anechoic bladder as it is isoechoic and similar in echotexture to the vagina.

In those women with uterine descent, a specular (mirror-like) echo commonly indicates the leading edge of the cervix. Nabothian follicles may help distinguish the cervix from vaginal wall. **Figure 8.8** shows quantification of pelvic organ descent in a patient with three compartment prolapse, with the cervix containing two small nabothian follicles.

Occasionally, imaging will show a retroverted uterus compressing the urethra and/or bladder neck, explaining problems with bladder emptying. On the other hand, a low anteverted uterus may result in rectal intussusception in women with symptoms of obstructed defecation, a condition termed a colpocele on defecation procto-graphy (**Figs. 8.9A and B**).

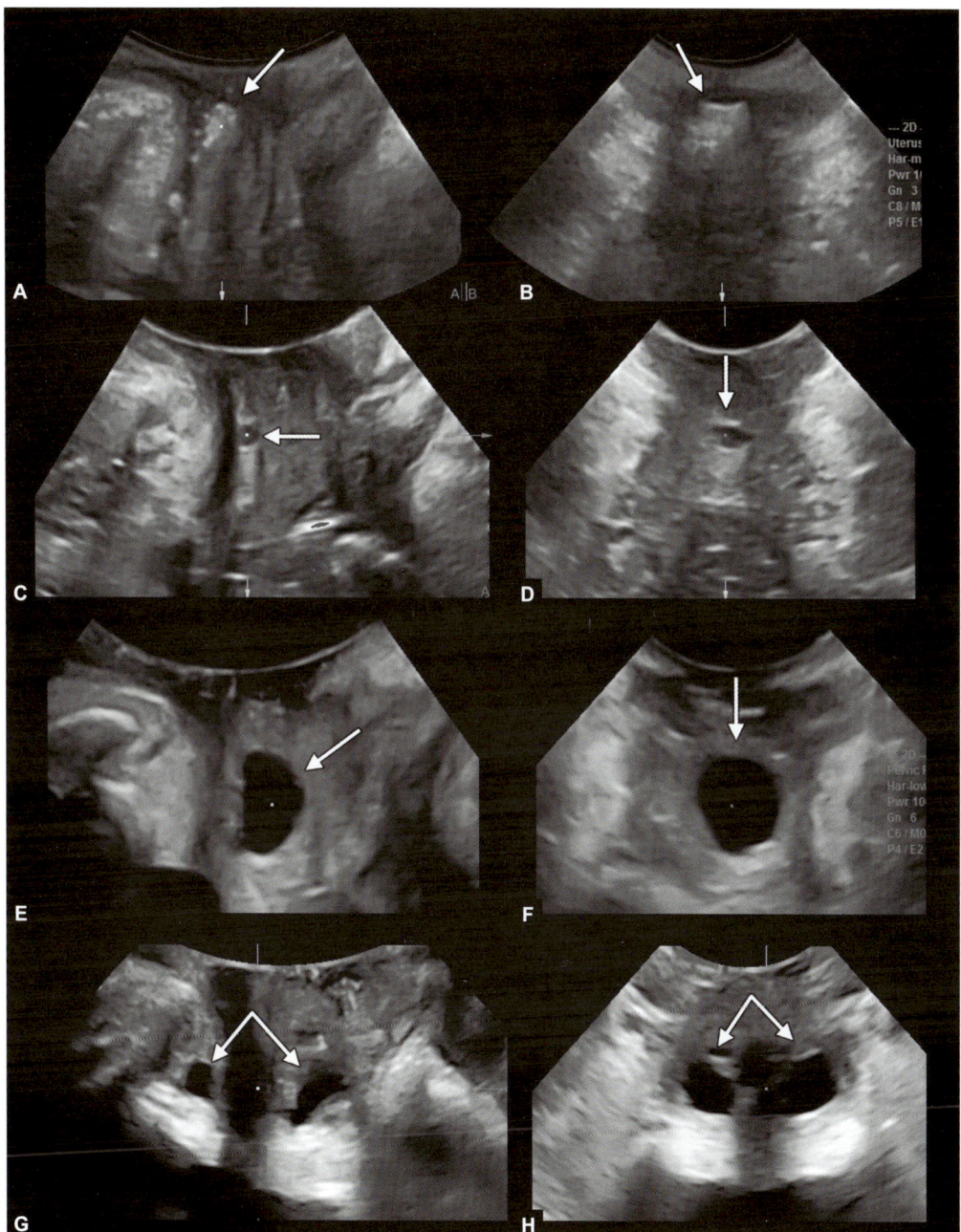

Figs. 8.6A to H: Urethral diverticula (confirmed by urethroscopy) seen in the mid-sagittal (A, C, E, and G) and coronal planes (B, D, F, and H). A/B shows a small diverticulum that appears as a largely hyperechogenic abnormality. C/D is a very small, exclusively anechoic diverticulum. E/F is the typical appearance of a symptomatic posterior diverticulum while G/H illustrates a large, near-circumferential, horseshoe-shaped diverticulum.

POSTERIOR COMPARTMENT

A clinical "rectocele", or more accurately, descent of the posterior vaginal wall, can be due to several distinct anatomical abnormalities with different therapeutic implications. Even digital rectal examination (which needs to be performed on Valsalva to demonstrate true rectocele and intussusception) is not routinely employed, hence those different entities tend to be comprehensively ignored by those who do not use imaging in such patients.

The link between anatomical abnormality and obstructed defecation (incomplete bowel emptying, straining at stool and digitation),[15] is not fully appreciated by gynecologists, and sometimes not even by colorectal

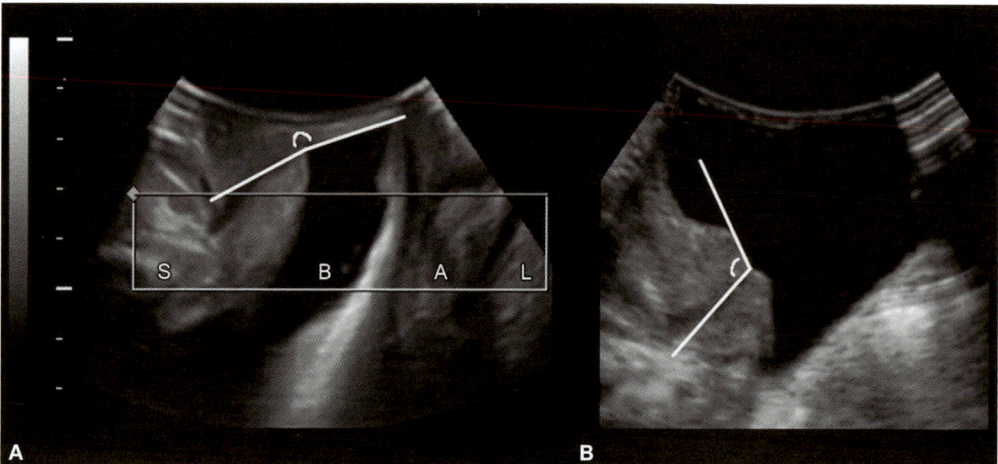

Figs. 8.7A and B: Cystocele types as seen on maximal Valsalva in the mid-sagittal plane. Figure A shows a cystocele with open retrovesical angle of over 180° (RVA, indicated by lines placed through the trigone and the proximal urethra). Figure B is a typical large cystocele with intact retrovesical angle of about 110°. (A: anal canal; B: bladder; L: levator ani; S: symphysis pubis)

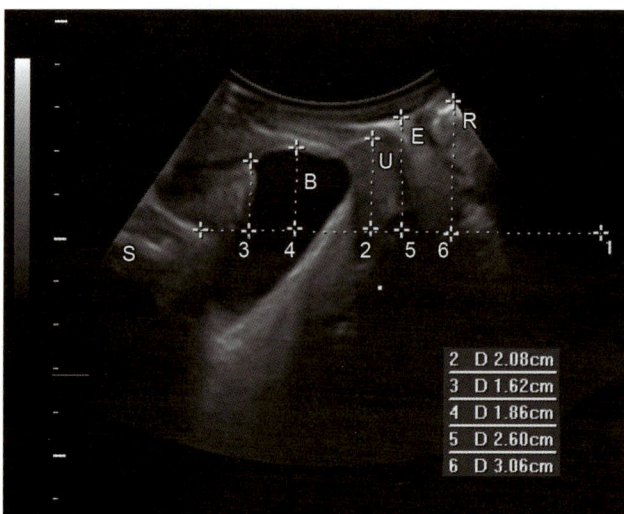

Fig. 8.8: On Valsalva in the mid-sagittal plane, prolapse is quantified against a horizontal line placed through the inferoposterior symphyseal margin, as in this patient with three-compartment prolapse. There is descent of the bladder neck to 16 mm below the symphysis, of the bladder to 19 mm below, of the uterus to 21 mm below, of an enterocele to 26 mm below, and of the rectal ampulla to 31 mm below the reference line. There are two small nabothian follicles below the "2" and above the "5". (B: bladder; E: enterocele; R: rectal ampulla; S: symphysis pubis; U: uterus)
Source: Reproduced with permission from Dietz H. Pelvic floor ultrasound: abnormal findings. In: Merz E (Ed). Atlas of 3D/4D Ultrasound in Obstetrics and Gynecology. Stuttgart: Thieme Medical Publishers; 2018.

surgeons. Defecation proctography, the diagnostic gold standard, is invasive, expensive, and not commonly available. Pelvic floor ultrasound, on the other hand, is cheaper, noninvasive, and much better accepted by the patient and entirely capable of replacing all other diagnostic modalities, even without 3D/4D imaging. The latter allows an appreciation of the role of hiatal ballooning and the resulting perineal hypermobility, a phenomenon that is often incompletely appreciated and clearly associated with rectal intussusception.[16]

Most commonly, however, posterior compartment descent on clinical examination is due to a "true" or radiological rectocele on imaging: a defect of the rectovaginal septum (RVS) that results in herniation of the anterior wall of the rectal ampulla into the vagina.[17] On translabial imaging, the RVS is often not easy to visualize unless one uses endovaginal imaging, but direct assessment of the RVS on static ultrasound seems to be of very limited clinical utility.[18] Diagnosis of a "true" rectocele relies on the demonstration of a diverticulum, i.e. a discontinuity of the anterior anal muscularis on Valsalva **(Figs. 8.10A to D)**. An abnormally distensible, intact RVS results in descent of the rectal ampulla without the formation of a diverticulum; hence such patients are often spared symptoms of obstructed defecation.[15]

Other causes of a clinical "rectocele" include a combined rectoenterocele, an isolated enterocele, rectal intussusception **(Figs. 8.11A to C)**, or a deficient perineum giving the impression of a "bulge". Rectal intussusception is an early stage of rectal prolapse where rectal mucosa and muscularis enters the proximal anal canal, changing it to a "martini glass" configuration **(Figs. 8.11A to C)**.[19] This condition, not uncommon but rarely diagnosed by

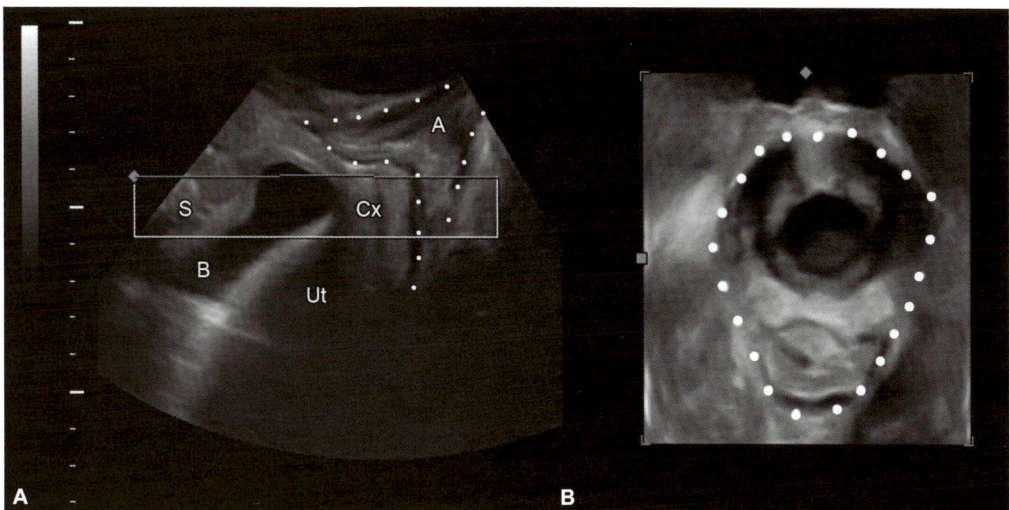

Figs. 8.9A and B: (A) A colpocele, i.e. a rectal intussusception propelled by the cervix of a low uterus. This usually is due to the cervix (as in this patient), but very occasionally an acutely retroverted uterus can result in a colpocele caused by the fundus. The anal canal and anterior rectal wall are shown by the dotted line, with the cervix inverting the anterior wall of the rectal ampulla; (B) The dotted line shows hiatal area. (A: anal canal; B: bladder; Cx: cervix; S: symphysis pubis; Ut: uterus)
Source: Reproduced with permission from Dietz H. Pelvic floor ultrasound: abnormal findings. In: Merz E (Ed). Atlas of 3D/4D Ultrasound in Obstetrics and Gynecology. Stuttgart: Thieme Medical Publishers; 2018.

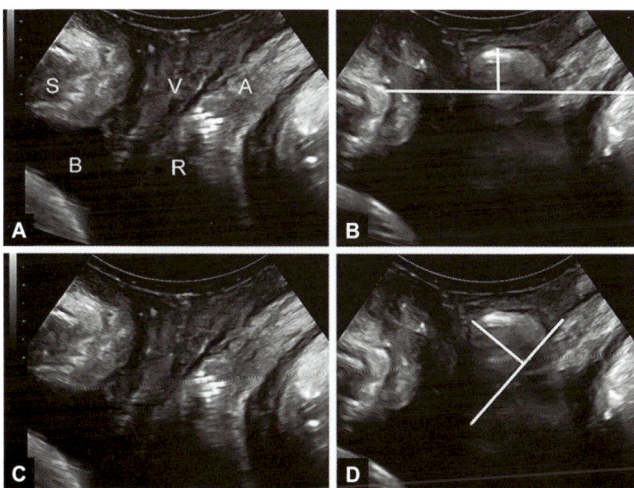

Figs. 8.10A to D: Translabial ultrasound images in the mid-sagittal plane. A and C are images at rest, B and D are obtained on maximal Valsalva. B shows rectocele descent against a reference line placed through the inferoposterior symphyseal margin; D shows rectocele depth measured against a reference line placed through the ventral aspect of the internal anal sphincter. (A: anal canal; B: bladder; R: rectal ampulla; S: symphysis pubis; V: vagina)
Source: Reproduced with permission from Zhang X, Shek KL, Dietz HP. How large does a rectocele have to be to cause symptoms? Int Urogynecol J. 2015;26(9):1355-9.

gynecologists, is strongly associated with abnormalities of the levator ani muscle and hiatus which require 3D/4D imaging for diagnosis (see here).[16]

The omission of a proper diagnostic workup in women with posterior compartment prolapse and obstructed defecation can have substantial therapeutic consequences. The overwhelming majority of women with "rectocele" are treated with a posterior colporrhaphy, creating a scar plate between vagina and anorectum, distorting and compressing a true rectocele, enterocele, or intussusception, without addressing the actual underlying abnormality. This also applies to mesh use in the posterior compartment which commonly hides the problem by preventing the development of a rectocele or intussusception into the vagina. This does not mean that the problem is gone: it is hidden from view, and rectocele or intussusception now develop into the perineum rather than the vagina **(Figs. 8.12A to C)**. Of course, symptoms of obstructed defecation remain and may even get worse. Appropriate surgical approaches result in the disappearance of the original anatomical abnormality, and such approaches do in fact exist in the Richardson technique of defect-specific rectocele repair,[20] and in rectopexy in cases of intussusception.

Figures 8.13A to C demonstrate the appearance of a typical isolated enterocele which most commonly manifests as posthysterectomy vault prolapse, but often rectocele and enterocele coexist, even in those with an intact uterus. The contents of an enterocele are often small bowel and/or omentum which appear isoechoic

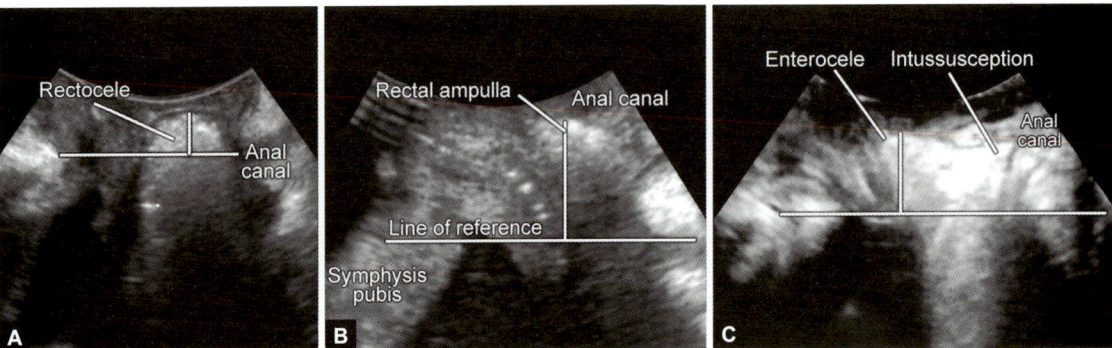

Figs. 8.11A to C: Anatomical abnormalities of the posterior vaginal compartment associated with symptoms of obstructed defecation, showing (A) "true rectocele", i.e. a defect of the rectovaginal septum; (B) Descent of the rectal ampulla without rectocele (perineal hypermobility); and (C) Rectal intussusception.

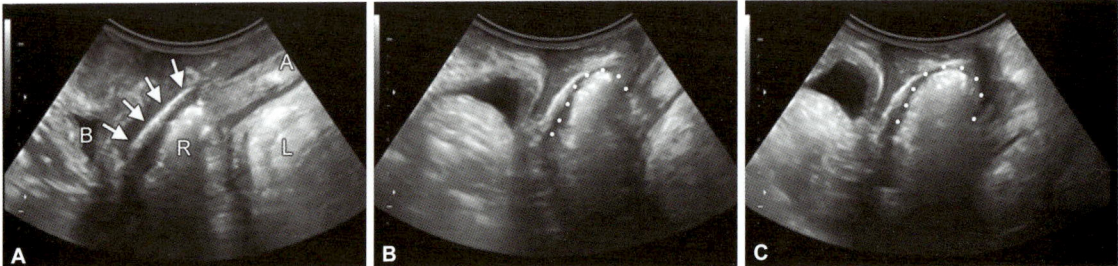

Figs. 8.12A to C: Posterior mesh repair (small arrows) usually "cures" the vaginal manifestation of rectocele. However, sometimes the rectocele itself, i.e. the diverticulum of the rectal ampulla, is still sufficiently large to cause symptoms, developing into the perineum rather than the vagina (arrow, outlined by dots).

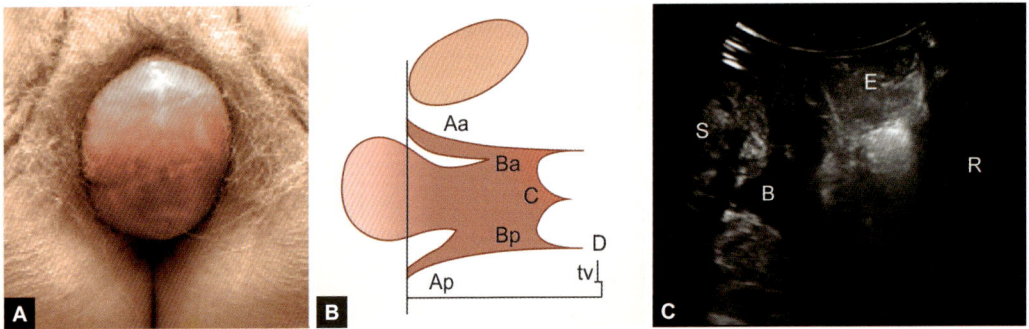

Figs. 8.13A to C: (A) Vault prolapse/enterocele on clinical photograph; (B) Representation on POP-Q (Ba = –3, D = +2.5, and Bp = –1); and (C) Appearances on imaging. (B: bladder; E: enterocele; R: rectal ampulla; S: symphysis pubis).
Source: Reproduced with permission from Dietz HP. Pelvic organ prolapse—a review. Aust Fam Physician. 2015;44(7):446-52.

and homogeneous, less commonly sigmoid colon which tends to be more inhomogeneous with hypoechogenic aspects indicating bowel wall.

ANAL SPHINCTER

To date, the anal canal has usually been examined with endoanal ultrasound[21] and MRI,[22] e.g. after obstetric anal sphincter injury (OASI). Both techniques are invasive: distortion of the anatomy is inevitable, and imaging on contraction to enhance tissue discrimination is impossible. Exoanal ultrasound[23] does not have these disadvantages and is better tolerated.[24] The method is now widely used, either with endovaginal or transabdominal probes providing volume data acquisition and hence a multislice or tomographic representation of external and internal anal sphincters (IASs).[8] We use a curved array obstetric volume transducer perpendicular to the anal canal, that is, in the coronal plane **(Figs. 8.3A and B)**. The probe is inclined from ventrocaudal to dorsocranial and adjusted in the ventrodorsal direction to make sure that the region of interest is sufficiently distant from the transducer surface to be in a single focal zone. Additional application of gel in the midline can help by filling the fourchette or perineum. Imaging is performed on pelvic floor muscle contraction which enhances the definition of muscular defects and may reduce false-positives.

Figure 8.14 shows typical findings in a nulliparous patient with intact anal sphincter and perineum. The dark ring structure represents the IAS, the hyperechogenic ring is the external anal sphincter. Sphincter defects (that is, breaks in those ring structures), detected on exoanal 4D ultrasound, are associated with anal incontinence, both after primary repair[25,26] and later in life.[27] To quantify

defects, we determine the number of abnormal slices, with at least 4/6 slices required for the diagnosis of a "residual defect",[27] analogous to the definition of residual defects on endoanal ultrasound.[28] This is usually combined with measurement the defect angle as in **Figure 8.15**, which shows an undiagnosed 3D tear after episiotomy, with the EAS trauma overlooked by the obstetric attendant. A cutoff has empirically been set at 30°, again analogous to endoanal imaging.[28]

While pain, edema and the presence of suture material makes imaging difficult shortly after childbirth, exoanal imaging is feasible within very few days, although findings show substantial change over time, with suture material disappearing and edema receding. Follow-up after 2–3 months, once neuropathy has had a chance to recover, allows an assessment of the quality of both diagnosis and treatment in delivery suite. Establishment of postnatal imaging services in the context of "perineal clinics" is well overdue. Maternal trauma is commonly

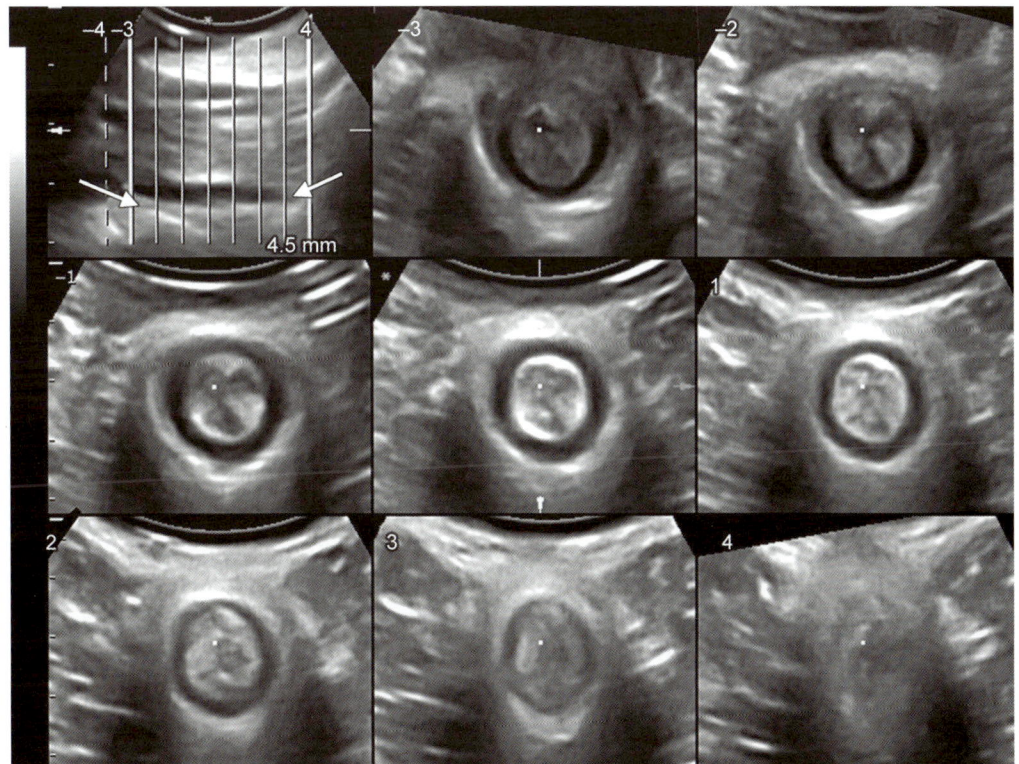

Fig. 8.14: Tomographic imaging of the anal sphincters, normal findings. The top left hand image represents a mid-sagittal reference plane, with vertical lines indicating the location of the remaining eight coronal plane slices. These latter eight slices bracket the anal canal from above (left) of the external sphincter to below (right) of the internal sphincter. The dark ring structure represents the internal anal sphincter, the hyperechogenic ring is the external anal sphincter.
Source: Reproduced with permission from Shek KL, Zazzera VD, Atan IK, et al. The evolution of transperineal ultrasound findings of the external anal sphincter during the first years after childbirth. Int Urogynecol J. 2016;27(12):1899-1903.

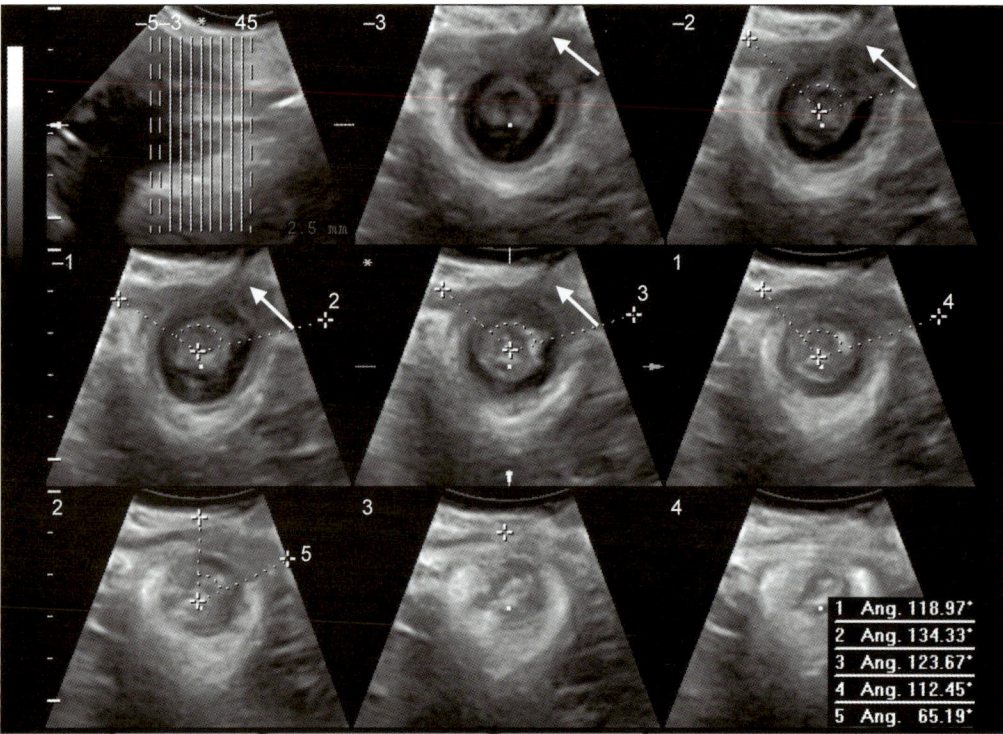

Fig. 8.15: Overlooked, unrepaired 3b tear with well-repaired episiotomy. The angle measurements illustrate quantification of this tear which measures well over 30° in 5/6 slices.
Source: Reproduced with permission from Dietz HP. Exoanal Imaging of the Anal Sphincters. J Ultrasound Med. 2018;37(1):263-80.

overlooked after childbirth, with personnel experience the main factor,[29] and primary repair is clearly insufficient in many cases.[25-27]

Figures 8.16 to 8.18 show residual anal sphincter trauma after vaginal births: a fair result after end-to-end repair (**Fig. 8.16**), a fair reconstructive result after an overlap repair (**Fig. 8.17**), and a rectovaginal fistula after a poorly repaired fourth-degree tear (**Fig. 8.18**). Due to increasing medicolegal and public pressure, maternal trauma will likely become a key performance indicator of maternity services in developed countries, although there will be substantial political resistance in some jurisdictions.[30] As regards to antenatal and intrapartum clinical research, future obstetric intervention trials should include modern 3D/4D imaging as an outcome measure since maternal trauma is clearly the most common major adverse consequence of vaginal childbirth.

On a final note, occasionally the clinician will encounter incidental findings that can interfere with identification of the caudal margin of the IAS and hence complicate reproducible slice placement. **Figure 8.19** is a symptomatic hemorrhoid while **Figure 8.20** shows an

(iatrogenic) defect of the IAS after hemorrhoidectomy. However, IAS abnormalities may be found in asymptomatic women without previous surgery.

SYNTHETIC IMPLANTS

Synthetic implants have become popular for the surgical treatment of stress urinary incontinence since the mid-90s, and more recently also for POP. Complications such as chronic pain and erosion have resulted in substantial adverse publicity on social media and in the lay press. This is leading to an increasing number of referrals for imaging of slings and meshes.

Biological materials, such as Surgisis or Permacol degrade over time and do not remain visible on any imaging modality, but this is not the case for implants made of polypropylene and similar synthetic materials. These are virtually invisible on MR, CT, and conventional X-ray, but highly echogenic. Ultrasound can confirm the presence of suburethral slings and meshes (**Figs. 8.21 to 8.25**) and distinguish different types of implants.[12] Polypropylene suburethral slings have a characteristic sonographic

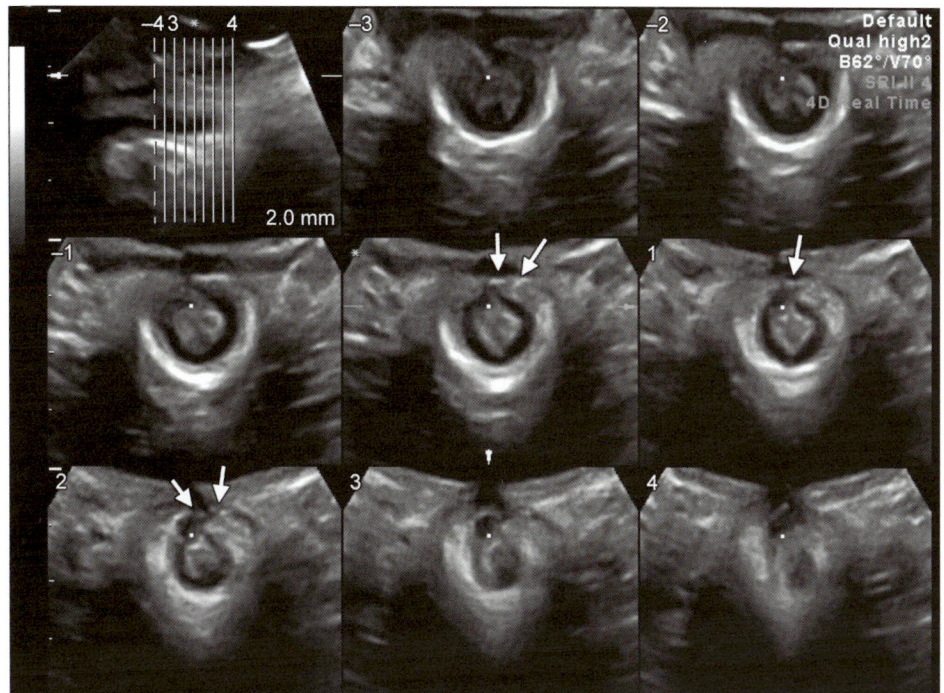

Fig. 8.16: Fair reconstructive result after end-to-end repair of a 3c tear after forceps delivery [defects indicated by (*)].
Source: Reproduced with permission from Dietz HP. Exoanal Imaging of the Anal Sphincters. J Ultrasound Med. 2018;37(1):263-80.

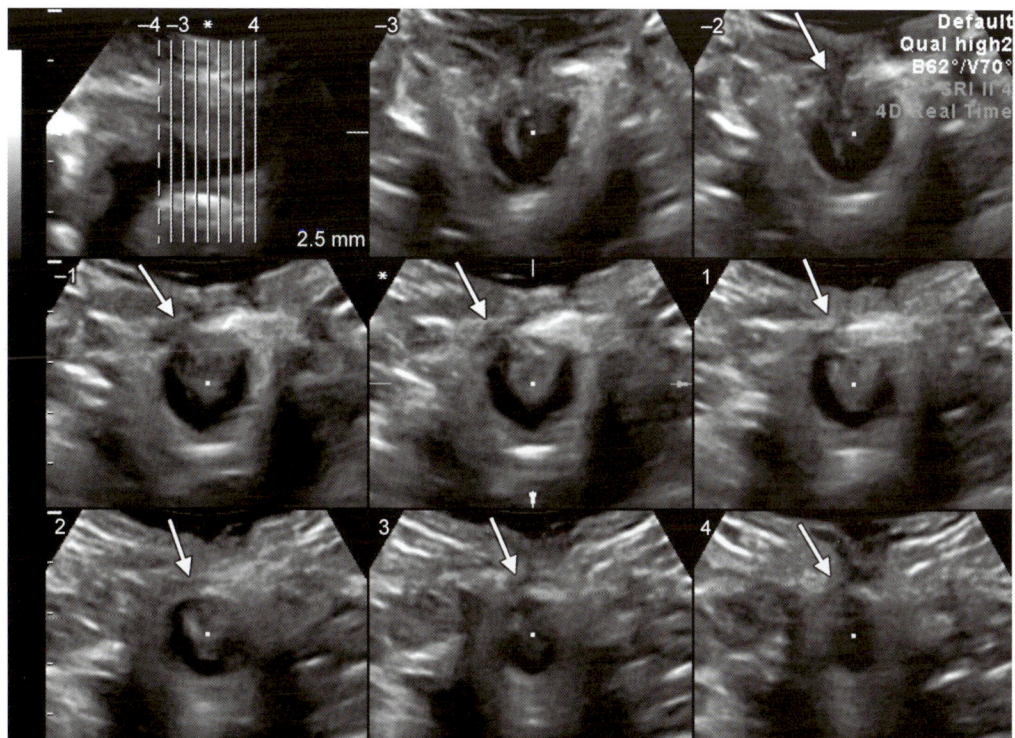

Fig. 8.17: Status after overlap repair of a 3c tear, with arrows indicating the site of the repair. Appearances are those of an average overlap repair.

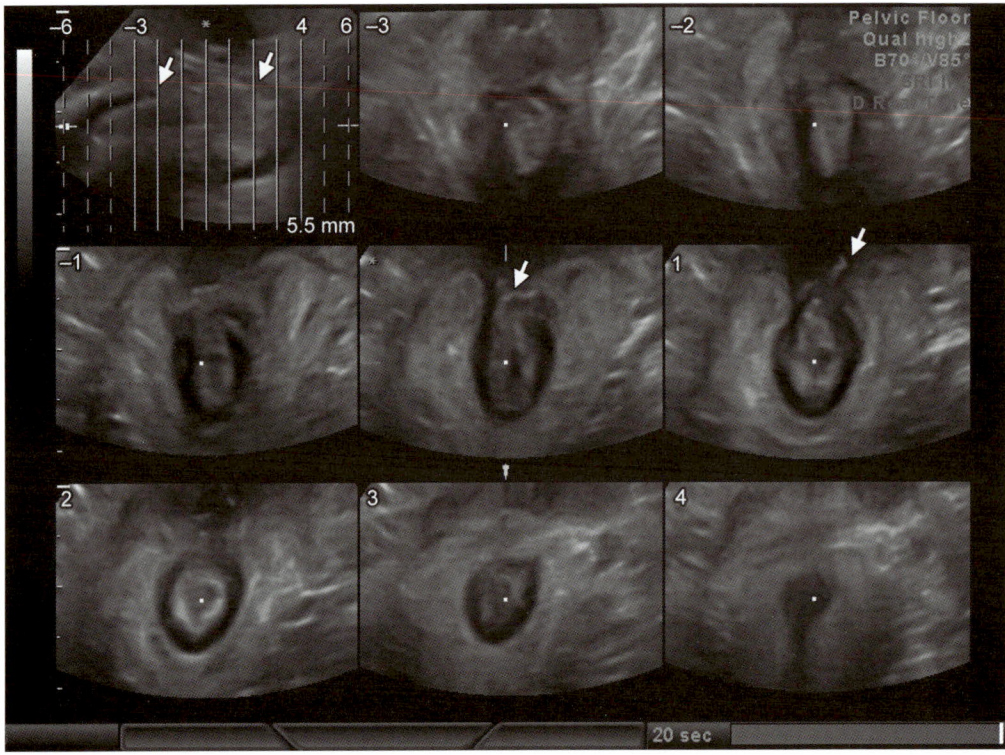

Fig. 8.18: Small rectovaginal fistula 3 months after insufficiently repaired 3c tear. The fistula is a small filiform echogenic line, indicated by arrows in two central slices. The two arrows in the top left hand image indicate the longitudinal extent of the internal anal sphincter defect. *Source*: Reproduced with permission from Dietz HP. Exoanal Imaging of the Anal Sphincters. J Ultrasound Med. 2018;37(1):263-80.

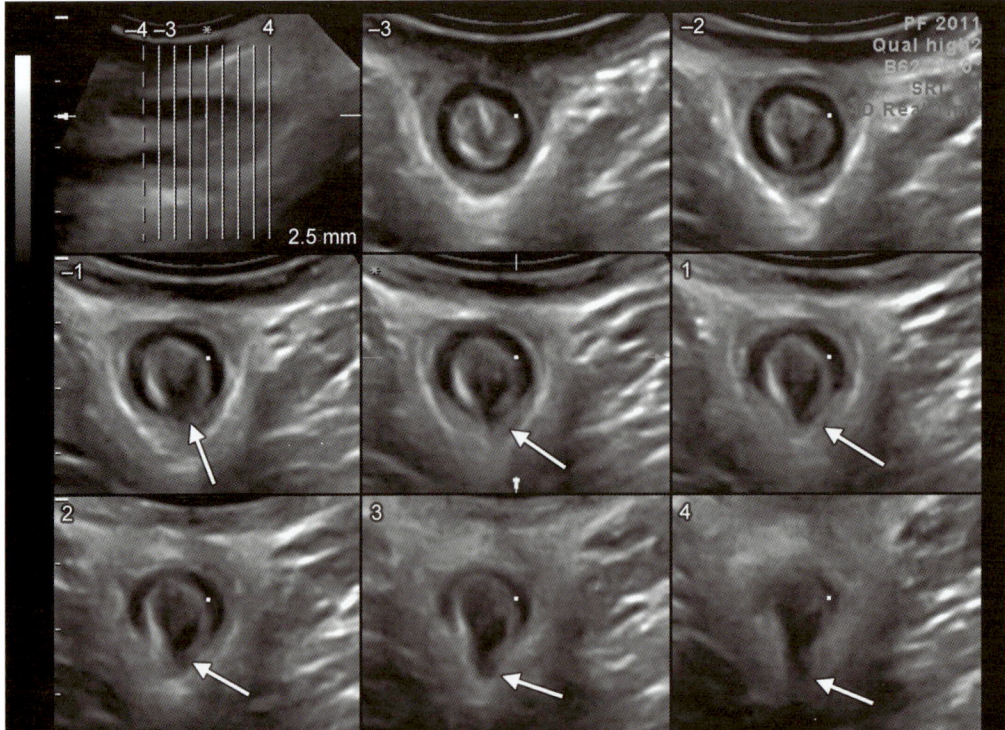

Fig. 8.19: Symptomatic hemorrhoid on tomographic imaging, indicated by arrows. Hemorrhoids can obscure the distal aspect of the internal anal sphincter and sometimes even the external anal sphincter (EAS), interfering with the assessment.

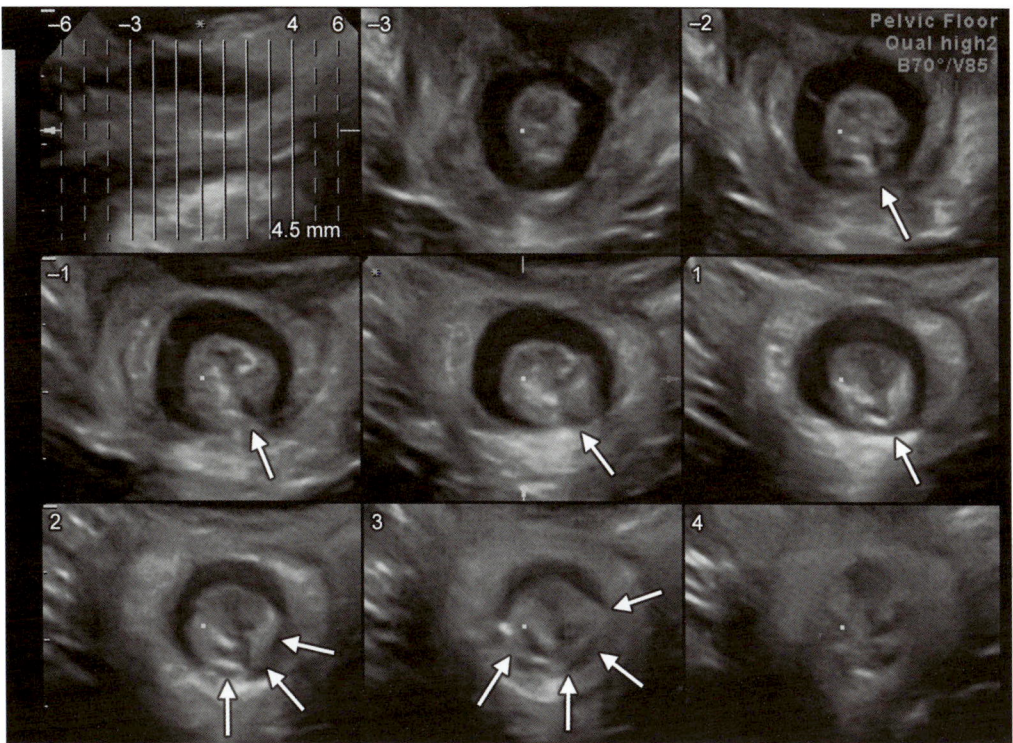

Fig. 8.20: Status after hemorrhoidectomy in a 60-year-old patient with mild anal incontinence. The internal anal sphincter is invisible between 4 o'clock and 7 o'clock in most slices and thickened over the remaining circumference, indicating iatrogenic trauma.
Source: Reproduced with permission from Dietz HP. Exoanal Imaging of the Anal Sphincters. J Ultrasound Med. 2018;37(1):263-80.

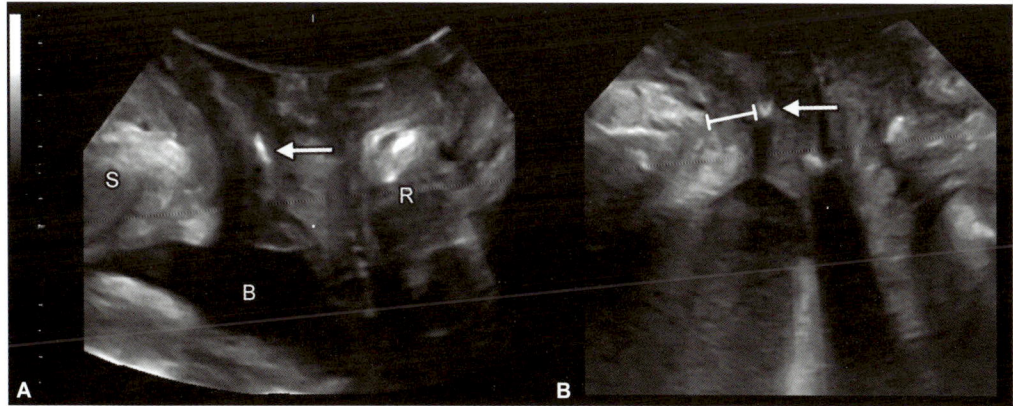

Figs. 8.21A and B: Appearance of a typical suburethral sling (arrow) in the mid-sagittal plane at rest (A) and on maximal Valsalva (B). The line in "B" demonstrates measurement of the sling-pubis gap.

appearance that changes on Valsalva or coughing as the implant is deformed by interaction with surrounding tissues. Sectional planes generated from volume data are highly useful in defining course and type of an implant, while a cine-loop of volumes obtained during a Valsalva maneuver will allow review of the implant under different insonation angles, helping to optimize visualization.

Suburethral slings act by direct, dynamic compression visible on imaging, with the sling commonly changing from a linear to a C- shape **(Figs. 8.21A and B)**.[31] Complications, such as voiding dysfunction or de novo symptoms of urgency and/or urge incontinence often are associated with a sling that appears as a tightly curled band with a low "sling-pubis gap" **(Figs. 8.21A and B)**. A gap of

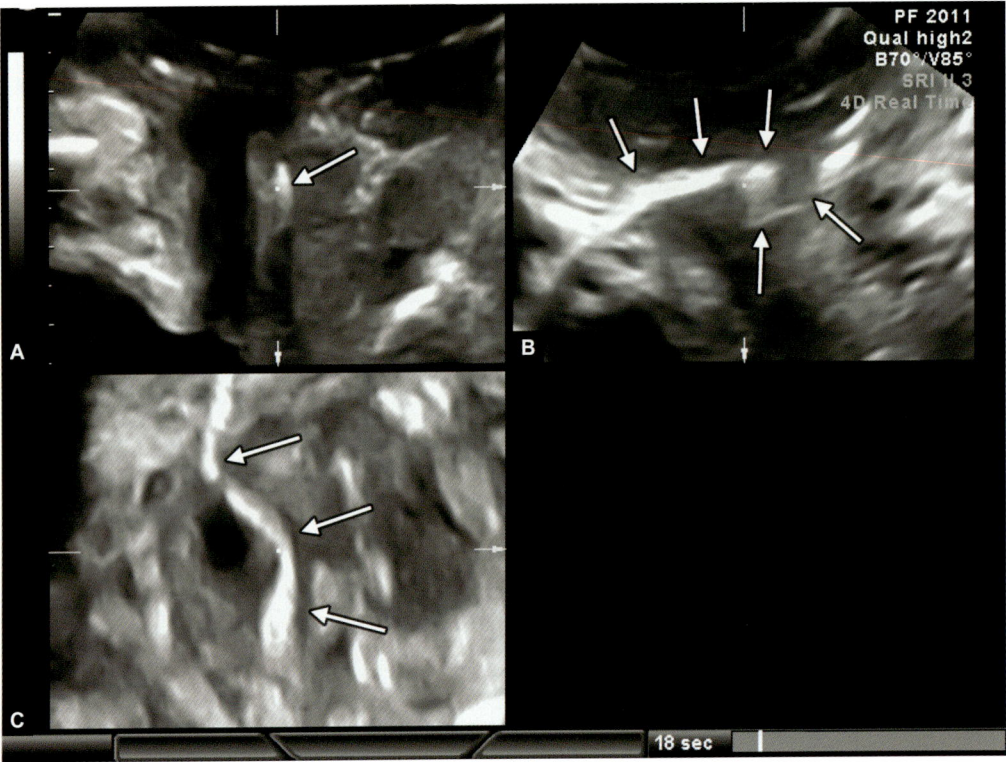

Figs. 8.22A to C: "Tethered" suburethral sling in the (A) mid-sagittal; (B) coronal; and (C) axial plane. The tape (arrows) looks normal in Figure A, but in Figures B and C, it is evident that it perforates the urethral rhabdosphincter. The urethroscopy was normal. Such placement is due to surgical error and may be asymptomatic.

8–14 mm on maximal Valsalva can be rated as "normal".[31] An implant that is rigid and highly compressive, with a sling-pubis gap of less than 8 mm, may indicate the need for either dilatation/stretching of the sling if identified within the first week or 10 days, or sling division at a later stage.

In some instances, slings appear to be "tethered", i.e. placed deep to the fascia of the urethral rhabdo-sphincter and, therefore, through the muscle rather than outside it, as shown in **Figures 8.22A to C**. Occasion-ally, imaging will suggest perforation and/or stenosis **(Figs. 8.23A to D)**. Sling division, a minor procedure that can be performed under local anesthetic, usually results in a gap of 5–10 mm between mesh arms documenting successful division. Rarely, faulty sling placement will result in perforation and even transection of the urethra, and ultimately the implant may be found in the space of Retzius **(Figs. 8.24A to C)**.

Mesh implants used in prolapse surgery are another increasingly common indication for 3D/4D imaging **(Figs. 8.25 to 8.30)**. In the anterior compartment, mesh is commonly situated posterior to the bladder neck, adjacent to the trigone and the posterior bladder wall, and the posterior bladder wall, visible as an echogenic linear or curvilinear structure.[32-34] Mesh can be identified in the three orthogonal planes **(Figs. 8.25A to C)** and also in rendered volumes **(Figs. 8.26A and B)**.

A Valsalva maneuver improves visualization and usually shows anterior compartment mesh rotating dor-socaudally around the fulcrum of the symphysis pubis. More caudally placed transobturator meshes can act like a large bladder neck sling. Persistent or recurrent pro-lapse of the central or posterior compartment can impair visualization by translabial imaging. So-called "mesh shrinkage" is a common misconception and due to poor surgical technique and/or an excess of material, resulting in mesh folds during implantation or immediately after closure, rather than an active biological process.[33,34]

While anterior compartment mesh clearly reduces recurrence (overview[35]), recurrence after mesh use is not that uncommon, especially in women with a highly abnormal levator ani. This can be a particularly vexing

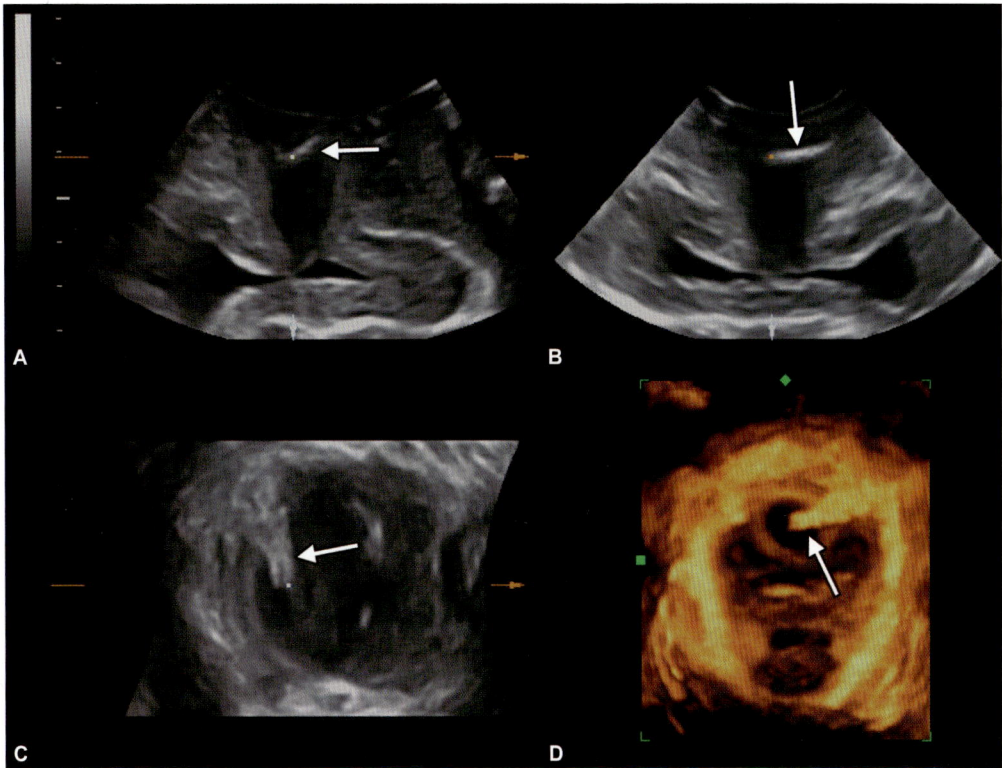

Figs. 8.23A to D: A partially removed TVT that has perforated the urethra (arrows) as imaged in the sectional planes (A to C) and an axial rendered volume (D), indicated by arrow. There is very substantial detrusor hypertrophy, indicating obstruction.

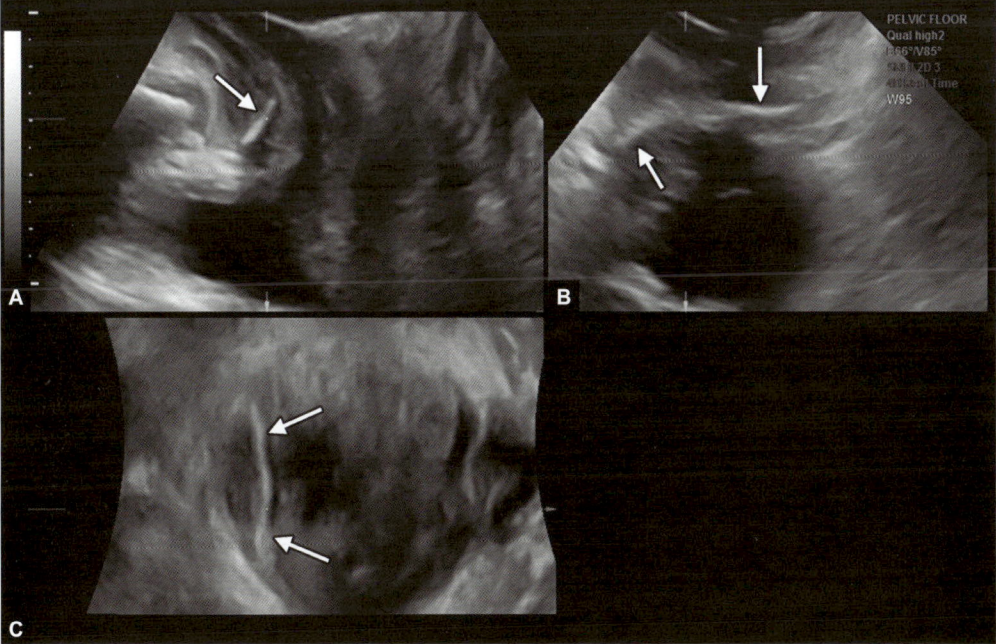

Figs. 8.24A to C: The end result of urethral tape erosion may not necessarily be surgical removal. Occasionally, the tape may erode through the entire urethra. This transobturator tape (arrow), 7 years after implantation, is now situated in the space of Retzius. An orthogonal representation such as this is particularly useful to define the spatial extent of unusual paraurethral findings.
Source: Reproduced with permission from Dietz H. Pelvic floor ultrasound: abnormal findings. In: Merz E (Ed). Atlas of 3D/4D Ultrasound in Obstetrics and Gynecology. Stuttgart: Thieme Medical Publishers; 2018.

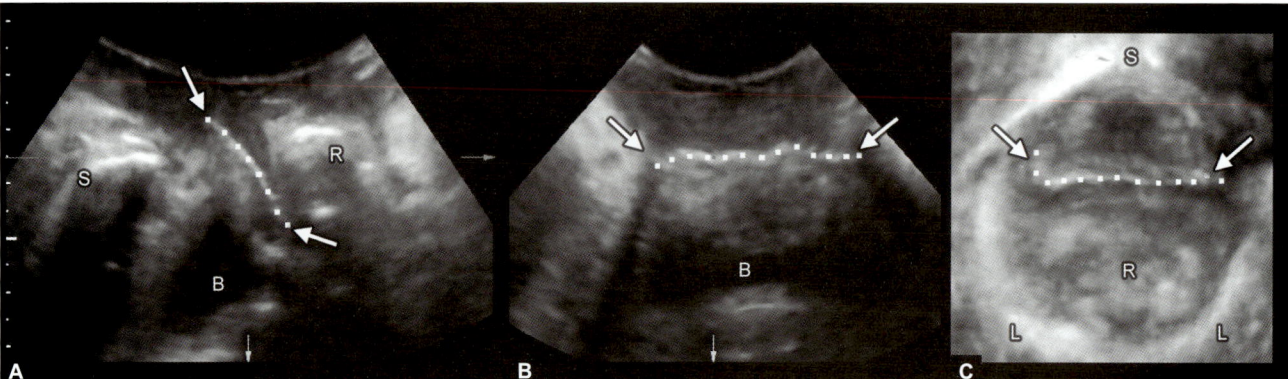

Figs. 8.25A to C: Anterior compartment mesh on Valsalva (A, mid-sagittal plane; B, coronal plane; and C, axial plane). Arrows show mesh length in the mid-sagittal (left) and the coronal plane (center and right). (B: bladder; L: levator ani; R: rectum; S: symphysis)
Source: Reproduced with permission from Dietz HP, Erdmann M, Shek KL. Mesh contraction: myth or reality? Am J Obstet Gynecol. 2011;204(2): 173.e1-4.

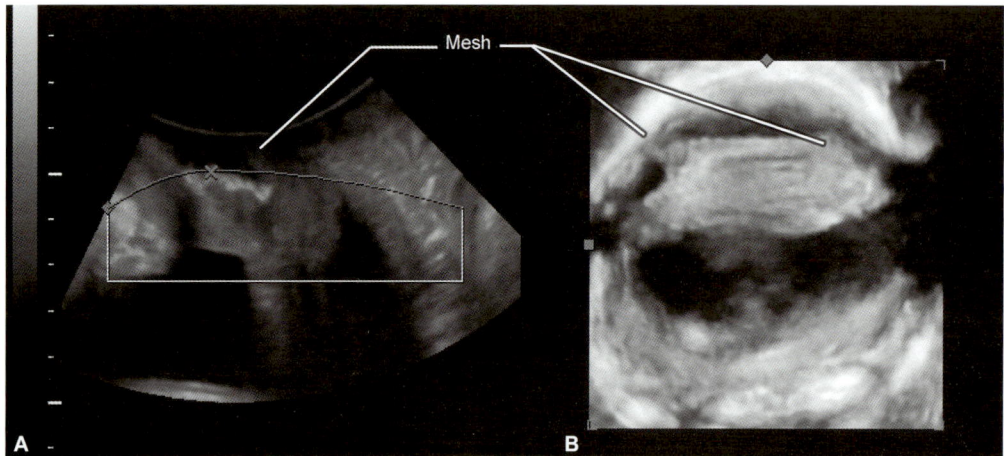

Figs. 8.26A and B: (A) Perigee mesh in the mid-sagittal plane; (B) A rendered volume showing the mesh structure and two of the arms.

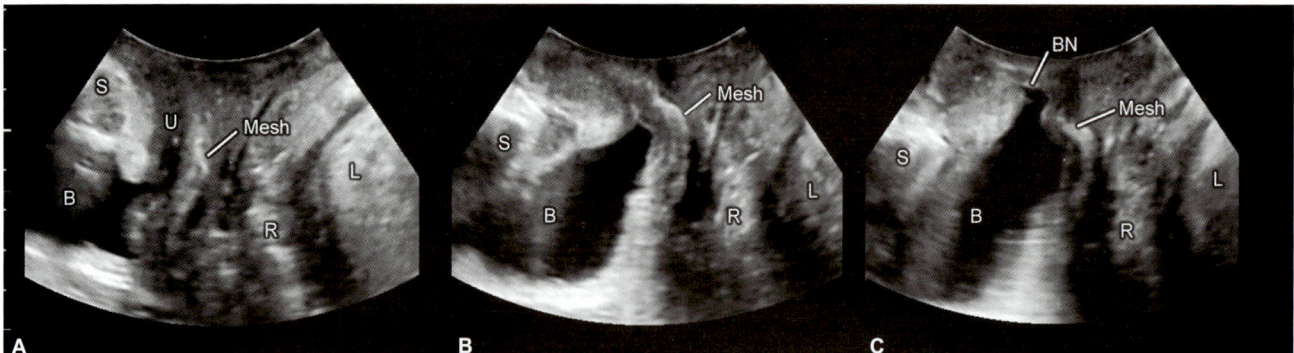

Figs. 8.27A to C: Ultrasound images showing anterior mesh failure: (A) At rest; (B) On submaximal Valsalva maneuver; (C) On maximum Valsalva. Cystocele recurrence ventral and caudal to a well-supported mesh suggests that the caudal aspect of the implant was insufficiently secured to the bladder neck, leading to dislodgement of the mesh from the bladder base. (B: bladder; BN: bladder neck; L: levator ani; R: rectum; S: pubic symphysis; U: urethra)
Source: Reproduced with permission from Shek KL, Wong V, Lee J, et al. Anterior compartment mesh: a descriptive study of mesh anchoring failure. Ultrasound Obstet Gynecol. 2013;42(6):699-704.

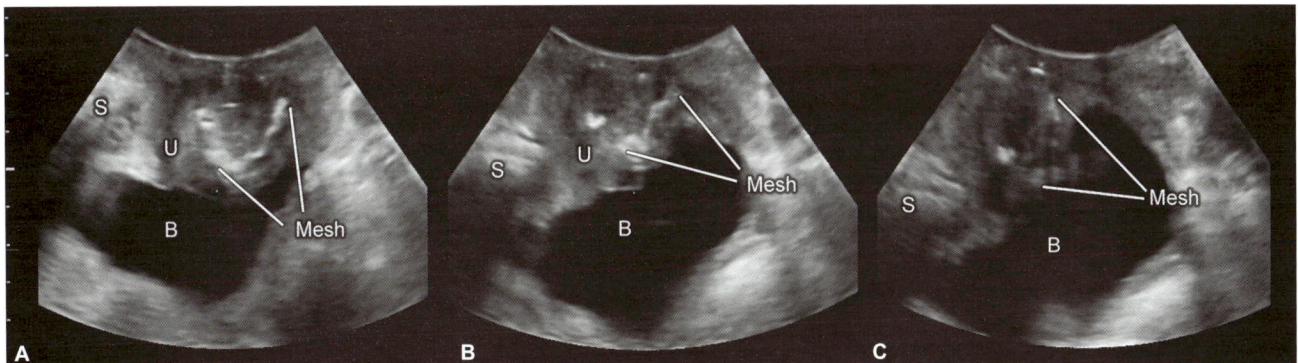

Figs. 8.28A to C: Ultrasound images showing apical mesh failure: (A) At rest; (B) On submaximal Valsalva maneuver; (C) On maximum Valsalva. Cystocele recurrence dorsal to the mesh with high mobility of the cranial mesh aspect suggests dislodgement of apical attachment. (B: bladder; S: pubic symphysis; U: urethra)
Source: Reproduced with permission from Shek KL, Wong V, Lee J, et al. Anterior compartment mesh: a descriptive study of mesh anchoring failure. Ultrasound Obstet Gynecol. 2013;42(6):699-704.

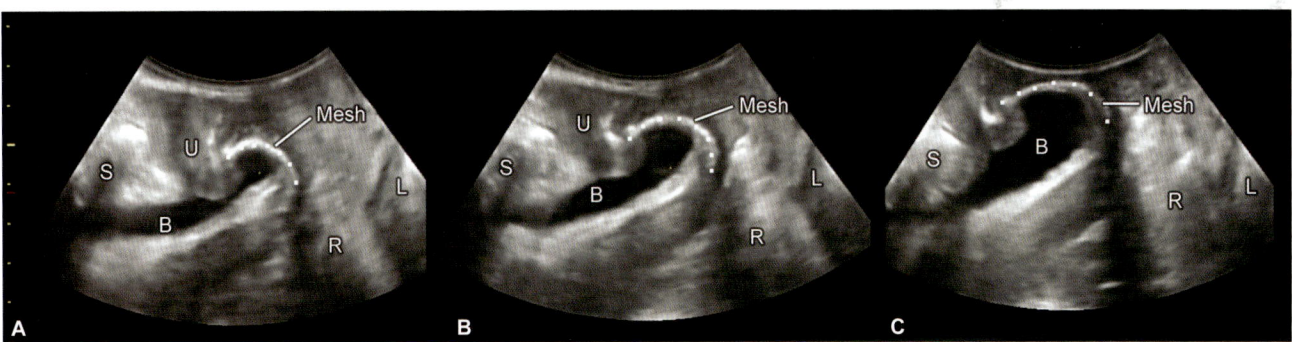

Figs. 8.29A to C: Ultrasound images showing global mesh failure: (A) At rest; (B) On submaximal Valsalva maneuver; (C) On maximum Valsalva. Cystocele recurrence behind the mesh is associated with high mobility of the entire mesh on Valsalva, suggesting dislodgement of both lateral and apical attachments. (B: bladder; L: levator ani; R: rectum; S: pubic symphysis)
Source: Reproduced with permission from Shek KL, Wong V, Lee J, et al. Anterior compartment mesh: a descriptive study of mesh anchoring failure. Ultrasound Obstet Gynecol. 2013;42(6):699-704.

problem. In a study of recurrence after anterior mesh repair,[36] we found three distinct anatomical situations: (1) Anterior failure: Cystocele ventral and caudal to the implant with intact anchoring; (2) Apical failure: Cystocele/anterior enterocele/uterine prolapse dorsal and caudal to the implant with failure of apical anchoring; and finally (3) Global failure: Cystocele with high implant mobility due to failure of both apical and lateral anchoring mechanisms **(Figs. 8.27 to 8.29)**.

Dislodgment of mesh anchoring structures is associated with a large hiatal area on Valsalva; the larger the hiatus, the greater the strain placed on anchoring structures, and the higher the probability of mechanical failure.[36] Hence, dislodgment of anchoring structures is plainly an engineering issue; unfortunately, the poor press of intravaginal mesh is currently impeding further development work in this field.

Anterior compartment meshes result in superior anatomical outcomes, especially in women with major levator tears.[35] However, this does not seem to be the case in the posterior compartment, and fortunately one is much less likely to encounter posterior meshes. **Figures 8.30A to C** demonstrate both the typical appearance of such an implant and the most common form of "failure". While on clinical examination, the posterior compartment prolapse seems cured, the rectal diverticulum that is a "true" rectocele now develops into the perineum, which is associated with recurrent or even worsened symptoms of obstructed defecation.

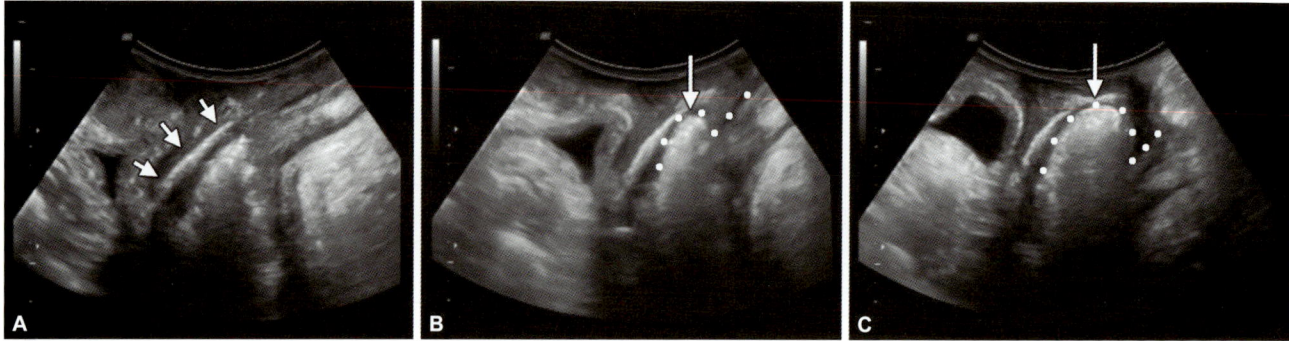

Figs. 8.30A to C: Posterior compartment mesh (small arrows) in patient with recurrent rectocele (large arrow) into the perineum. (A) At rest; (B) submaximal Valsalva; (C) At full Valsalva. The rectocele is outlined by dots. This is a common observation after posterior mesh since the RVS defect is usually not closed by such surgery.

LEVATOR ANI

The introduction of 3D/4D pelvic floor ultrasound has arguably had its greatest impact in the development of simple, inexpensive, and highly repeatable imaging of the levator ani muscle. Translabial ultrasound has confirmed 60-year old, forgotten clinical data[37] and much more recent MRI studies[38] showing that major structural abnormalities of the levator ani muscle are common in vaginally parous women.[39] Population prevalence depends crucially on age at first birth and obstetric practice, with trauma rates as low as 2% in populations with traditional reproductive behavior,[40] 10–15% after normal vaginal delivery in Western populations, 10–20% after vacuum, and 40–60% after forceps delivery, with the highest prevalence after rotational forceps; for an overview of prevalence see reference 41.

A reproducible assessment of the levator ani on sectional imaging requires identification of the plane of minimal dimensions, i.e. the minimal distance between the symphysis and the anorectal angle **(Figs. 8.31A to D)**. This is the reference plane for assessment of the levator hiatus and puborectalis muscle. A complete defect of this muscle, that is, a disconnection of the muscle from its insertion, is defined as "avulsion".

To date, the only known mechanism for avulsion is vaginal childbirth, with the trauma occurring at crowning of the fetal head. Avulsion is almost always occult as the vaginal skin and muscularis layer tend to fail in a different location, together with the perineal body. This leaves the site of avulsion covered by intact vagina and hence occult, even if a hematoma may signal hidden trauma.

Figures 8.32A to C show clinical examination, axial plane ultrasound, and MRI in a patient with unilateral right-sided levator avulsion after an uncomplicated term normal vaginal delivery. While avulsion can be identified by palpation[42] and on 2D parasagittal imaging,[43] tomographic translabial imaging using standard 3D/4D abdominal/obstetric probes is clearly more reproducible,[44-46] and it correlates well with MR for the diagnosis of levator trauma.[47]

The standard methodology for imaging the levator ani is shown in **Figure 8.33** in a nulliparous woman with an unusually thick puborectalis muscle. **Figures 8.34A and B** show a complete right-sided avulsion of the puborectalis on tomographic imaging, a bilateral defect on TUI **(Fig. 8.35)**, and complete on the right and partial on the left. Incomplete defects may not be associated with prolapse or prolapse recurrence[48] which implies that the distinction between incomplete and complete trauma is important. The minimal requirement for the diagnosis of a full avulsion is the finding of a disconnected muscle in at least the plane of minimal dimensions and slices 2.5 mm and 5 mm cranial to this plane.[46] Slice location is of the essence, and it is fortunate that the appearance of the symphysis pubis allows standardization of slice location to within 1 mm: the three central slices should be adjusted to show the symphysis pubis/the inferior pubic rami to be open in the most caudal slice, closing in the central slice, and invisible due to acoustic shadowing in the most cranial if the three slices **(Figs. 8.33 to 8.36)**.

Care has to be taken with identification of the plane of minimal dimensions since insufficient anticlockwise rotation of the A plane will result in false-positive findings

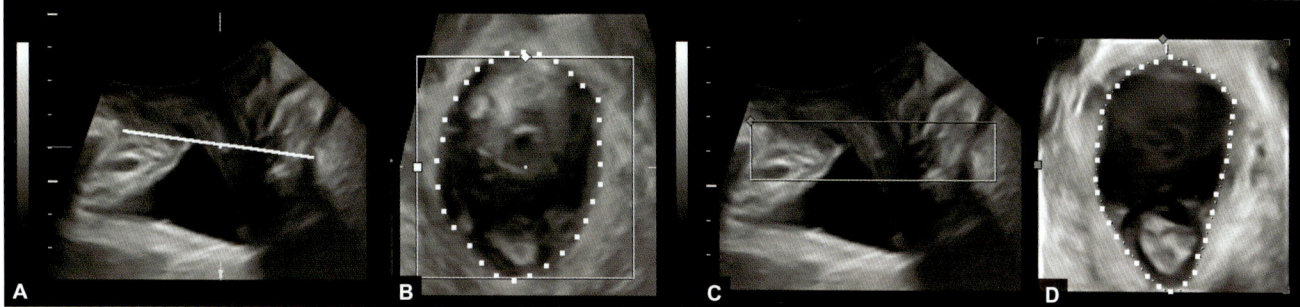

Figs. 8.31A to D: Measuring hiatal dimensions as shown in an oblique single axial plane (A and B) and in a rendered volume (C and D). The determination of hiatal dimensions using a single oblique axial plane is shown in (A) and (B). The mid-sagittal plane on the left (A) demonstrates a line indicating the minimal sagittal diameter of the hiatus, i.e. the location of the oblique axial plane shown in (Figure B). The region of interest (ROI) box in Figure C (in this case approximately 1.8 cm deep) is located between the symphysis pubis and the levator ani posterior to the anorectal angle. Figure D represents a semi-transparent view of all pixels in the ROI box on the left. The dotted line in Figures B and D represent hiatal area measurements [23.05 cm² in (B), 21.77 cm² in (D)].
Source: Reproduced with permission from Dietz HP, Wong V, Shek KL. A simplified method for determining hiatal biometry. Aust N Z J Obstet Gynaecol. 2011;51(6):540-3.

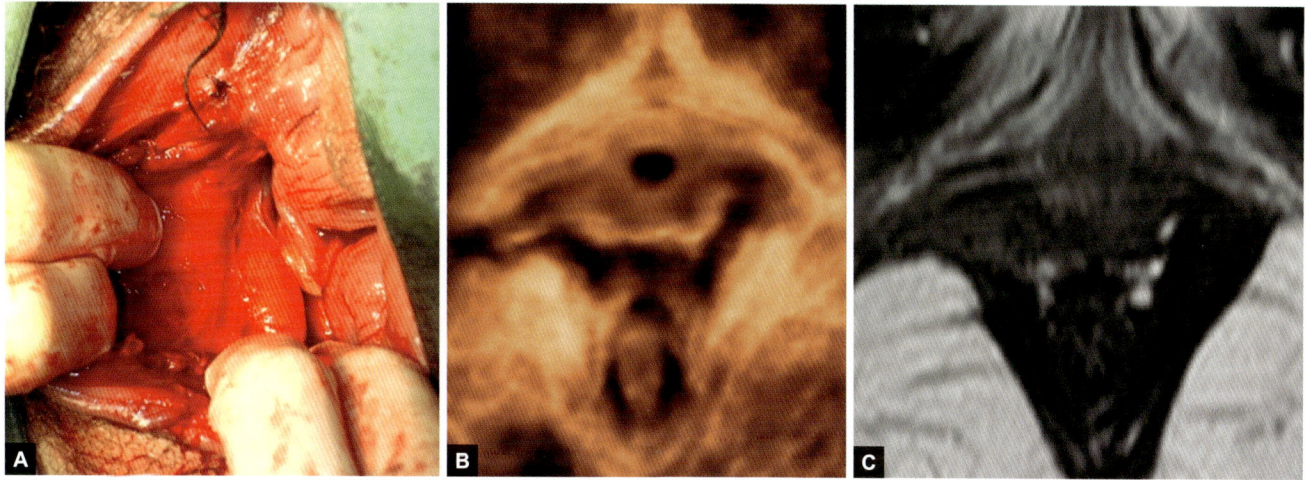

Figs. 8.32A to C: Typical right-sided levator avulsion injury as diagnosed in the delivery suite after a normal vaginal delivery at term, on three-dimensional (3D) ultrasound (center) and on magnetic resonance imaging (right) 3 months postpartum. This patient was asymptomatic apart from deep dyspareunia.
Source: Reproduced with permission from Dietz HP, Gillespie AV, Phadke P. Avulsion of the pubovisceral muscle associated with large vaginal tear after normal vaginal delivery at term. Aust N Z J Obstet Gynaecol. 2007;47(4):341-4.

in caudal slices. This is most likely in women with a strong levator contraction in whom warping of the levator plate from ventrocaudal to dorsocranial may be quite marked.

If findings on TUI are equivocal due to partial trauma, scar tissue, limited image quality, or artifact, the "levator-urethra gap" (LUG) **(Figs. 8.36A to C)** can be of help,[49] although this measurement is of course subject to interethnic and interindividual variation. Different cutoffs for a "normal" LUG have been established for Caucasians (2.5 cm)[49] and East Asians (2.36 cm).[47] While

the examination is usually done on pelvic floor muscle contraction to enhance tissue discrimination, multislice imaging at rest seems to be equally valid.[50]

Avulsion (as well as irreversible overdistension of the levator ani muscle) in childbirth plays a central role in the etiology of female POP. There are bound to be other factors that are much more difficult to investigate, such as altered biomechanics of intact muscle, facial trauma, and neuropathy. However, it is clear that avulsion enlarges the levator hiatus,[51] reduces contractile strength,[52] and is

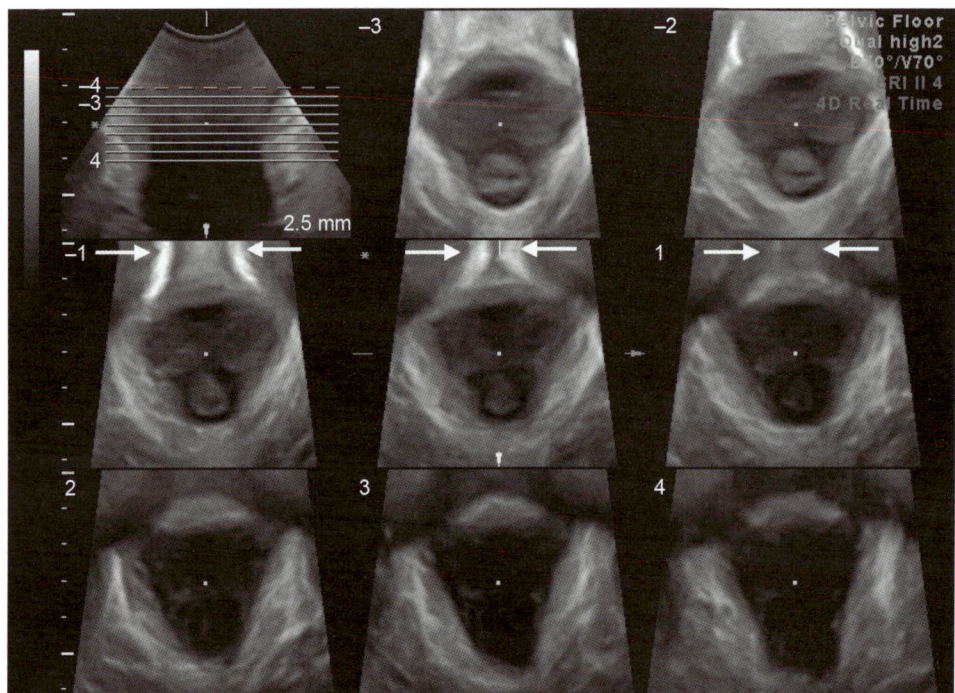

Fig. 8.33: Normal findings on tomographic translabial imaging, axial plane, at an interslice interval of 2.5 mm. For standardization, the symphysis pubis (arrows) is supposed to appear open in the left-central slice, closing in the central slice, and invisible due to acoustic shadowing in the right-central slice.

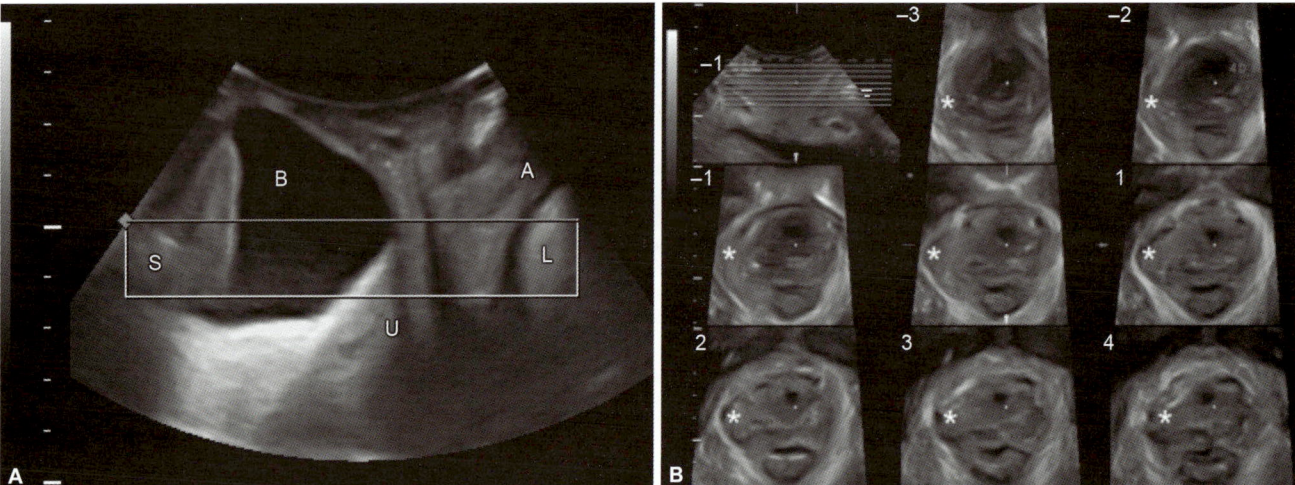

Figs. 8.34A and B: Right-sided avulsion in patient with third-degree cystocele and first-degree uterine prolapse. (A) The mid-sagittal plane shows descent of bladder and uterus on Valsalva; Figure B is a tomographic representation of the puborectalis muscle in the patient obtained on pelvic floor muscle contraction, showing a right-sided complete avulsion (*). The patient's right side is represented on the left side of the slices. (A: anal canal; B: bladder; L: levator ani; S: symphysis pubis, U: uterus)
Source: Reproduced with permission from Dietz H. Pelvic floor ultrasound: abnormal findings. In: Merz E (Ed). Atlas of 3D/4D Ultrasound in Obstetrics and Gynecology. Stuttgart: Thieme Medical Publishers; 2018.

associated with prolapse, especially of the anterior and central compartments.[53,54] Levator defects seem to be the single strongest risk factor for prolapse recurrence after reconstructive surgery.[55]

Another major risk factor for prolapse and prolapse recurrence is the size of the levator hiatus. Axial plane imaging by 4D translabial ultrasound has made us understand that the levator hiatus is the largest potential

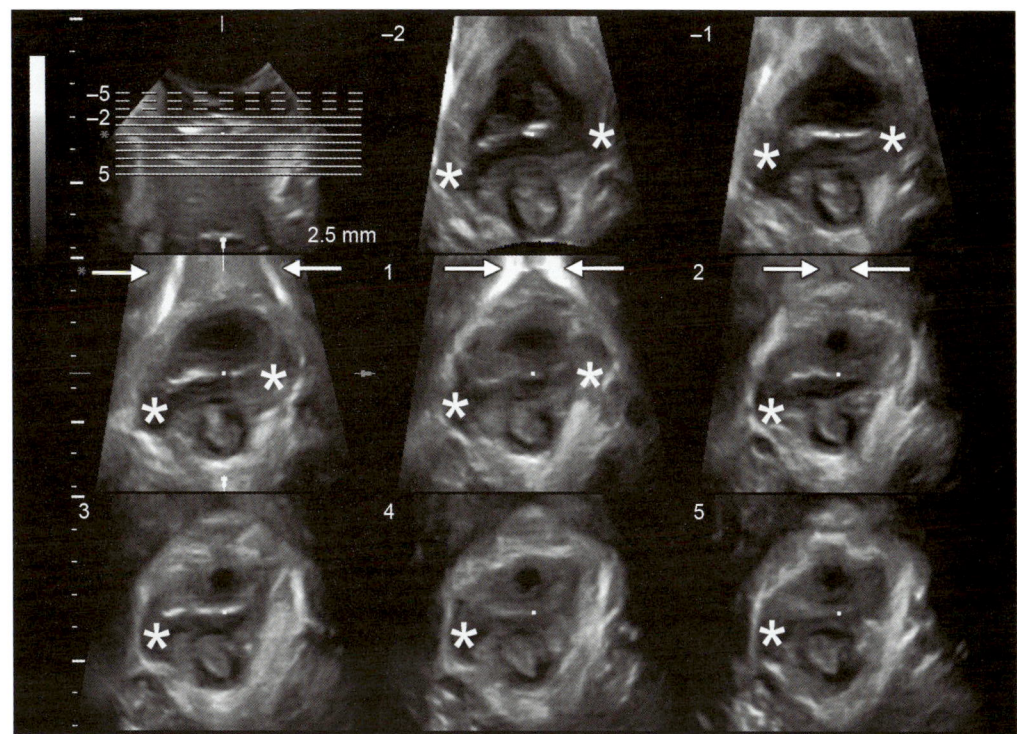

Fig. 8.35: Tomographic imaging of the puborectalis, showing a complete right-sided and partial left-sided avulsion. The required appearance of the symphysis pubis [open on the left-central slice, closing on the central slice, and closed (invisible) on the right-central slice] is shown by the arrows.
Source: Reproduced with permission from Dietz H. Pelvic floor ultrasound: abnormal findings. In: Merz E (Ed). Atlas of 3D/4D Ultrasound in Obstetrics and Gynecology. Stuttgart: Thieme Medical Publishers; 2018.

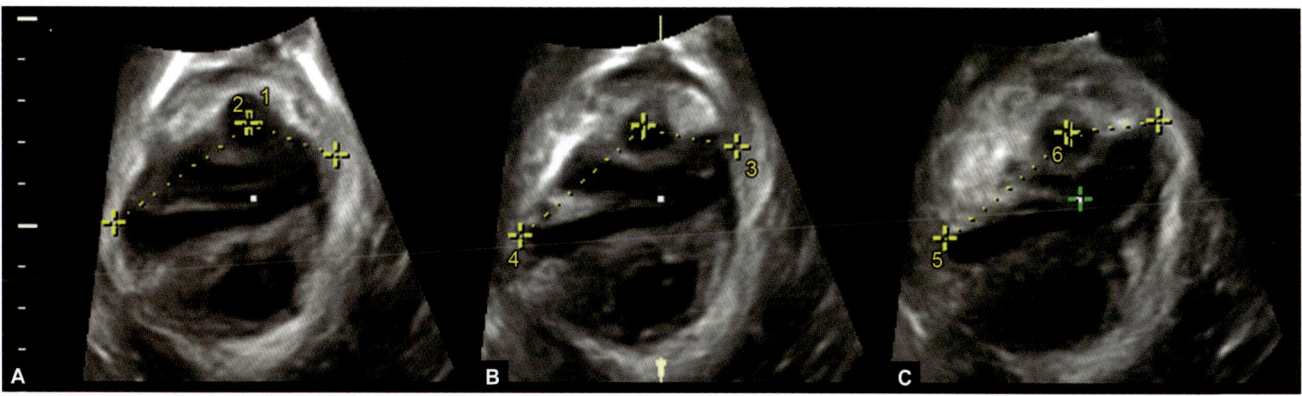

Figs. 8.36A to C: Measurement of the levator-urethra gap (LUG) in the three central slices of a tomographic representation of the puborectalis muscle. All measurements on the left (the patient's right) are clearly abnormal, indicating a complete right-sided avulsion.
Source: Reproduced with permission from Dietz H. Pelvic floor ultrasound: abnormal findings. In: Merz E (Ed). Atlas of 3D/4D Ultrasound in Obstetrics and Gynecology. Stuttgart: Thieme Medical Publishers; 2018.

hernial portal in the human abdominal envelope. Prolapse is a hernia of pelvic organs through the levator hiatus. This triangular opening is the most complex "defect" in the abdominal wall as it is crucial for the function of three vital organ systems—(1) the reproductive tract, (2) the lower urinary tract, and (3) the lower gastrointestinal tract. The pelvic floor in women is a compromise between competing priorities. Reproduction

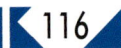

is of course the top priority, and it is not surprising that pelvic floor disorders are common.

Hiatal enlargement to 25 cm² on Valsalva or higher is defined as "ballooning" as it predicts signs and symptoms of prolapse,[56] and on the basis of normative data in young nulliparous women.[57]

Hiatal area can be assessed both in the axial plane of minimal hiatal dimensions or in rendered volumes (*see* **Figures 8.31A to D** for a comparison of the two methods).[58] The degree of distension is strongly associated with prolapse and symptoms of prolapse,[56] and both avulsion and "ballooning" seem to be independent risk factors of female POP and POP recurrence after reconstructive surgery.[55] Hiatal distensibility is also the pathophysiological correlate of "vaginal laxity",[59] a common and often misunderstood complaint that can result in significant bother, especially in younger women in whom it is often the first symptom of prolapse.

CONCLUSION

Three-dimensional/4D imaging has transformed the sonographic evaluation of pelvic floor structures, mainly because this modality allows simple, cheap, and highly reproducible assessment of structures in the axial plane, and the tomographic representation of structures of interest such as levator ani and anal sphincters. The growing availability of both equipment and training will likely make this modality an integral part of any urogynecological investigation.

The use of imaging in pelvic floor medicine will help communication with our patients, but also between the different specialties dealing with those patients. The method will improve not just diagnostic but also therapeutic skills. Tomographic imaging of the anal sphincter and levator ani will enable clinicians to assess maternal birth trauma with unprecedented ease and accuracy, and at minimal cost. Clinical audit and intervention trials will allow not just better treatment, but enable efforts at primary and secondary prevention.

A better understanding of prolapse as a hernia of pelvic organs through the levator hiatus will engender new surgical approaches, such as the direct reconstruction of levator tears and compensatory procedures. Treatment is blind without proper diagnosis. Pelvic floor ultrasound has made us see abnormalities of functional anatomy that have been ignored and misunderstood for far too long.

REFERENCES

1. Dietz HP. Pelvic floor ultrasound. In: Cardozo L, Staskin D (Eds). Female Urology and Urogynecology. Abingdon: Informa Healthcare; 2006.
2. Olsen AL, Smith VJ, Bergstrom JO, et al. Epidemiology of surgically managed pelvic organ prolapse and urinary incontinence. Obstet Gynecol. 1997;89(4):501-6.
3. Smith FJ, Holman CD, Moorin RE, et al. Lifetime risk of undergoing surgery for pelvic organ prolapse. Obstet Gynecol. 2010;116(5):1096-100.
4. Dietz HP, Wilson PD. The influence of bladder volume on the position and mobility of the urethrovesical junction. Int Urogynecol J. 1999;10(1):3-6.
5. Dietz HP, Steensma A. Dimensions of the levator hiatus in symptomatic women. Ultrasound Obstet Gynecol. 2005; 26(4):369-70.
6. Svabik K, Shek KL, Dietz HP. How much does the levator hiatus have to stretch during childbirth? BJOG. 2009;116(12):1657-62.
7. Dietz HP. Classifying major delivery-related pelvic floor trauma. Int Urogynecol J. 2006;17(S2):S124-5.
8. Dietz HP. Exoanal Imaging of the Anal Sphincters. J Ultrasound Med. 2018;37(1):263-80.
9. Dietz HP, Velez D, Shek KL, et al. Determination of post-void residual by translabial ultrasound. Int Urogynecol J. 2012;23(12):1749-52.
10. Lekskulchai O, Dietz HP. Detrusor wall thickness as a test for detrusor overactivity in women. Ultrasound Obstet Gynecol. 2008;32(4):535-9.
11. Lekskulchai O, Dietz HP. Is detrusor hypertrophy in women associated with voiding dysfunction? Aust N Z J Obstet Gynaecol. 2009;49(6):653-6.
12. Dietz HP. Pelvic floor ultrasound in incontinence: What's in it for the surgeon? Int Urogynecol J. 2011;22(9): 1085-97.
13. Guichard P, Gillor M, Dietz HP. Imaging of urethral diverticula by 4D-translabial ultrasound. Int Urogynecol J. 2018. [Epub ahead of print].
14. Eisenberg VH, Chantarasorn V, Shekh KL, et al. Does levator ani injury affect cystocele type? Ultrasound Obstet Gynecol. 2010;36(5):618-23.
15. Dietz HP, Korda A. Which bowel symptoms are most strongly associated with a true rectocele? Aust N Z J Obstet Gynaecol. 2005;45(6):505-8.
16. Rodrigo N, Shek KL, Dietz HP. Rectal intussusception is associated with abnormal levator ani muscle structure and morphometry. Tech Coloproctol. 2011;15(1):39-43.
17. Dietz HP, Steensma AB. Posterior compartment prolapse on two-dimensional and three-dimensional pelvic floor ultrasound: the distinction between true rectocele, perineal hypermobility and enterocele. Ultrasound Obstet Gynecol. 2005;26(1):73-7.
18. Dietz HP. Can the rectovaginal septum be visualised on ultrasound? Ultrasound Obstet Gynecol. 2011;37(4): 348-52.

19. Guzmán Rojas R, Kamisan Atan I, Shek KL, et al. The prevalence of abnormal posterior compartment anatomy and its association with obstructed defecation symptoms in urogynecological patients. Int Urogynecol J. 2016;27(6): 939-44.

20. Guzmán Rojas R, Kamisan Atan I, Shek KL, et al. Defect-specific rectocele repair: medium-term anatomical, functional and subjective outcomes. Aust N Z J Obstet Gynaecol. 2015;55(5):487-92.

21. Sultan AH. Anal incontinence after childbirth. Curr Opin Obstet Gynecol. 1997;9(5):320-4.

22. Stoker J, Rociu E, Bosch JL, et al. High-resolution endo-vaginal MR imaging in stress urinary incontinence. Eur Radiol. 2003;13(8):2031-7.

23. Peschers UM, DeLancey JO, Schaer GN, et al. Exoanal ultrasound of the anal sphincter: normal anatomy and sphincter defects. Br J Obstet Gynaecol. 1997;104(9): 999-1003.

24. Van Gruting I, Arendsen L, Naiu M, Thakar R, Sultan A. Can transperineal ultrasound replace endoanal ultra-sound for the detection of anal sphincter defects? Int Urogynecol J. 2017;27(S1):S51-2.

25. Shek KL, Guzman-Rojas R, Dietz HP. Residual defects of the external anal sphincter following primary repair: an observational study using transperineal ultrasound. Ultrasound Obstet Gynecol. 2014;44(6):704-9.

26. Turel F, Langer S, Shek KL, Dietz HP. Long-term follow-up of Obstetric Anal Sphincter Injury. Dis Colon Rectum 2019 Mar;62(3):348-356. doi: 10.1097/DCR. 0000000000001297.

27. Guzmán Rojas RA, Shek KL, Langer SM, et al. Prevalence of anal sphincter injury in primiparous women. Ultrasound Obstet Gynecol. 2013;42(4):461-6.

28. Roos A, Thakar R, Sultan AH. Outcome of primary repair of obstetric anal sphincter injuries (OASIS): does the grade of tear matter? Ultrasound Obstet Gynecol. 2010;36(3): 368-74.

29. Andrews V, Sultan AH, Thakar R, et al. Occult anal sphincter injuries—myth or reality? BJOG. 2006;113(2):195-200.

30. Dietz HP, Pardey J, Murray H. Maternal birth trauma should be a key performance indicator of maternity services. Int Urogynecol J. 2015;26(2):29-32.

31. Chantarasorn V, Shek KL, Dietz HP. Sonographic appearance of transobturator slings: implications for func-tion and dysfunction. Int Urogynecol J. 2011;22(4):493-8.

32. Shek KL, Rane A, Goh J, et al. OC256: Imaging of the Perigee transobturator mesh and its effect on stress incontinence. Ultrasound Obstet Gynecol. 2007;30(4):446.

33. Dietz HP, Erdmann M, Shek KL. Mesh contraction: myth or reality? Am J Obstet Gynecol. 2011;204(2):173.e1-4.

34. Svabik K, Martan A, Masata J, et al. Ultrasound appearances after mesh implantation—evidence of mesh contraction or folding? Int Urogynecol J. 2011;22(5):529-33.

35. Wong V, Shek KL. The mesh debate: Transvaginal anterior anchored mesh should not be abandoned. Aust N Z J Obstet Gynaecol. 2017;57(1):105-7.

36. Shek KL, Wong V, Lee J, et al. Anterior compartment mesh: a descriptive study of mesh anchoring failure. Ultrasound Obstet Gynecol. 2013;42(6):699-704.

37. Gainey HL. Post-partum observation of pelvic tissue damage. Am J Obstet Gynecol. 1943;45(3):457-66.

38. DeLancey JO, Morgan DM, Fenner DE, et al. Comparison of levator ani muscle defects and function in women with and without pelvic organ prolapse. Obstet Gynecol. 2007;109(2 Pt 1):295-302.

39. Dietz HP, Lanzarone V. Levator trauma after vaginal delivery. Obstet Gynecol. 2005;106(4):707-12.

40. Turel F, Caagbay D, Dietz HP. OP28.04: The prevalence of major birth trauma in Nepali women. J Ultrasound Med. 2017;50(S1):140.

41. Dietz HP, Wilson PD, Milsom I. Maternal birth trauma: why should it matter to urogynaecologists? Curr Opin Obstet Gynecol. 2016;28(5):441-8.

42. Dietz HP, Shek C. Validity and reproducibility of the digital detection of levator trauma. Int Urogynecol J Pelvic Floor Dysfunct. 2008;19(8):1097-101.

43. Dietz HP, Shek KL. Levator defects can be detected by 2D translabial ultrasound. Int Urogynecol J Pelvic Floor Dysfunct. 2009;20(7):807-11.

44. Dietz HP. Quantification of major morphological abnormalities of the levator ani. Ultrasound Obstet Gynecol. 2007;29(3):329-34.

45. Adisuroso T, Shek KL, Dietz HP. Tomographic ultrasound imaging of the pelvic floor in nulliparous women: limits of normality. Ultrasound Obstet Gynecol. 2012;39(6): 698-703.

46. Dietz HP, Bernardo MJ, Kirby A, et al. Minimal criteria for the diagnosis of avulsion of the puborectalis muscle by tomographic ultrasound. Int Urogynecol J. 2011;22(6): 699-704.

47. Zhuang RR, Song YF, Chen ZQ, et al. Levator avulsion using a tomographic ultrasound and magnetic resonance-based model. Am J Obstet Gynecol. 2011;205(3): 232.e1-8.

48. Pilzek A, Havard L, Guzman Rojas R, et al. Recurrence after prolapse surgery: does partial avulsion matter? Ultrasound Obstet Gynecol. 2013;42(S1):37-8.

49. Dietz HP, Abbu A, Shek KL. The levator-urethra gap measurement: a more objective means of determining levator avulsion? Ultrasound Obstet Gynecol. 2008;32(7): 941-5.

50. Dietz HP, Pattillo Garnham A, Guzmán Rojas R. Diagnosis of levator avulsion: Is it necessary to perform TUI on pelvic floor muscle contraction? Ultrasound Obstet Gynecol. 2017;49(3):252-6.

51. Shek KL, Dietz HP. The effect of childbirth on hiatal dimensions: a prospective observational study. Obstet Gynecol. 2009;113(4):1272-8.

52. Dietz HP, Shek C. Levator avulsion and grading of pelvic floor muscle strength. Int Urogynecol J. 2008;19(5): 633-6.

53. Dietz HP, Steensma AB. The prevalence of major abnormalities of the levator ani in urogynaecological patients. BJOG. 2006;113(2):225-30.

54. Dietz HP, Simpson JM. Levator trauma is associated with pelvic organ prolapse. BJOG. 2008;115(8):979-84.

55. Friedman T, Eslick G, Dietz HP. Risk factors for prolapse recurrence—systematic review and meta-analysis. Int Urogynecol J. 2018;29(1):13-21.

56. Dietz HP, Shek C, De Leon J, et al. Ballooning of the levator hiatus. Ultrasound Obstet Gynecol. 2008;31(6):676-80.

57. Dietz HP, Shek KL, Clarke B. Biometry of the pubovisceral muscle and levator hiatus by three-dimensional pelvic floor ultrasound. Ultrasound Obstet Gynecol. 2005;25(6): 580-5.

58. Dietz HP, Wong V, Shek KL. A simplified method for determining hiatal biometry. Aust N Z J Obstet Gynaecol. 2011;51(6):540-3.

59. Dietz HP, Stankiewicz M, Atan IK, et al. Vaginal laxity: what does this symptom mean? Int Urogynecol J. 2018;29(5): 723-8.

9

How to Think in Three Dimensions?

Eldar Volpert, Liat Gindes

INTRODUCTION

Thinking in three dimensions (3D) enables the manipulation of the acquired volume in a manner that results in a meaningful image. The goal of this chapter is to empower the reader to formulate the right questions and to obtain the right answers, using three-dimensional ultrasound (3D US).

The clinical application of the 3D US technique in obstetrics and gynecology is gradually expanding since its introduction three decades ago. The 3D US technology is applied to enhance the diagnosis of fetal embryology[1-5] anatomy[6-15] and malformations.[16-21] In addition, it is also applied as a mainstay tool in the diagnosis of gynecologic problems, including but not limited to uterine malformations adnexal masses and obstetric anal sphincter tears.[22-25] With the introduction of ultrasound machines containing 3D probes in increasing numbers, this exciting technique is becoming more practical than ever before. Due to this increasing availability of 3D US, there is a growing need to train providers in how to master this technique to its full capability. The most important step in learning how to apply 3D US in practice, is learning how to think in 3D.

The acquisition of 3D US data is primarily preformed through the use of specialized probes either mechanical or electronic that allow for a rapid collection of volume data.[22,26-28] Once acquired, the data can be manipulated and displayed using various techniques. The data can be presented as two-dimensional (2D) images that are perpendicular to each other (the multiplanar view). This method shows the three orthogonal planes simultaneously and therefore allows for the data to be presented accordingly. An additional option is to present the 2D images of the volume as sequential serial images, similar to CT or MRI (tomographic ultrasound imaging—TUI, Multi-slice view). The data can also be presented as a 3D image that combines multiple 2D parallel images as a single image (render mode) or as a thin slice in the multiplanar or TUI views (volume contrast imaging or thick slice).

3D AS VOXELS

The information in the volume is composed of voxels.[29] Each voxel has four characteristics: three coordinates on the x-, y-, and z-axis and its color on grayscale. When the data is initially acquired, it forms a 3D structure full of voxels. Slicing through the 3D structure using a 2D plane at different angles results in varying 2D pictures, based on the different voxels included. Each picture can provide a different type of information.

MULTIPLANAR VIEW AND THE REGION OF INTEREST

The most basic and practical tool (multiplanar view) presents the information as three orthogonal planes **(Fig. 9.1A)**. The three planes are presented facing forward as shown in **Figure 9.1B**. Each two planes have a common axis. All three orthogonal planes share a single voxel called the region of interest (ROI). In **Figure 9.1A**, the ROI is at the center, but the ROI can be positioned at any place in the volume. By standing with the cursor on the ROI and moving it from its place, the corresponding perpendicular planes shift to another particular position in the volume.

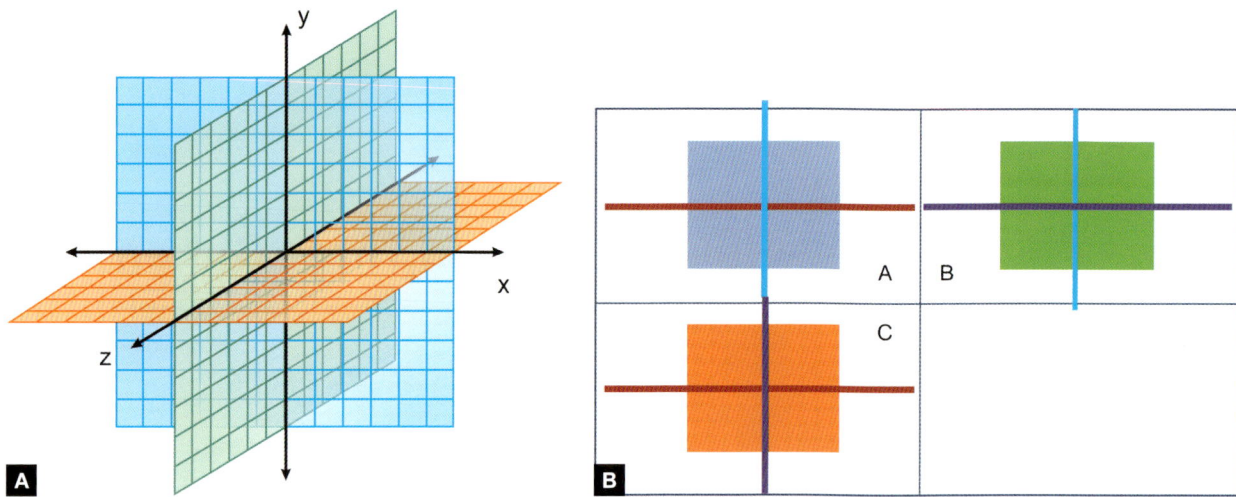

Figs. 9.1A and B: The three orthogonal planes: (A) The intersection of the three orthogonal planes forming the three axes; (B) The three planes as presented on multiplanar view. Note the corresponding colors.

Each of the planes displays a cross-section of the data in a 2D view. Plane A (blue plane on the **Figures 9.1A and B**) is the acquisition plane and is the same as the standard 2D view obtained using the standard 2D probe. Plane B (green in **Figures 9.1A and B**) is perpendicular to plane A. The image obtained on this plane is identical to the image obtained by rotating the transducer by 90°. Plane C (orange in **Figures 9.1A and B**) is also perpendicular to the other planes, however, it cannot be obtained using rotation of the transducer. This plane has a lower resolution in comparison to the other two planes for this reason. The data volume acquired during a scan is now represented as three 2D images that are perpendicular to each other. For practical purposes, in **Figure 9.1**, these planes are attached to each other at the midline of the displayed image, nevertheless this is not mandatory. The ROI is common to all three planes.

Each two planes share one axis line **(Fig. 9.1A)**. The A and C planes share the x-axis. The intersection between these planes is similar to an open laptop: plane A is the screen and plane C is the keyboard **(Fig. 9.2A)**. Similarly, the A and B planes share the y-axis. Just like an open book with the front cover represented by plane A and the back cover by plane B **(Fig. 9.2B)**. The B and C planes share the z-axis. This is less intuitive, but one can compare this view to looking at a chair from the side. The bottom represents plane C while the back represents plane B.

The fetal face can be used as an excellent example of this concept, since it can be grasped intuitively. In the fetal face volume presented in **Figure 9.3**, the data was processed and displayed so that the coronal view of the face is represented in plane A, the sagittal view on plane B, and the axial view on plane C.

MOVEMENT OF THE ROI

The meaning of the special location of the ROI can by explained using the fetal face **(Fig. 9.3)**. By moving the ROI on one plane, significant information will appear on the other planes. In the example of **Figure 9.3** (animated in clip S1), the ROI is placed between the fetal eyes. When the dot moves along one axis, only one plane will change. Moving the ROI along the y-axis (view in clip S1) represented by the blue line in **Figure 9.3**, the image of the fetal face in the coronal view (plane A) and the sagittal view (plane B) remain the same. On the other hand, the display in plane C continuously changes as the data is presented along the changing y-coordinate. Change of the position of the ROI along the y-axis (blue line) in plane A or B will cut through different axial layers of the fetal face in this example. On the level of the hard palate, plane C would show a full axial view of the palate. Moving the ROI along the axis, as explained in this case, can be used to obtain a more detailed display of the fetal palate.

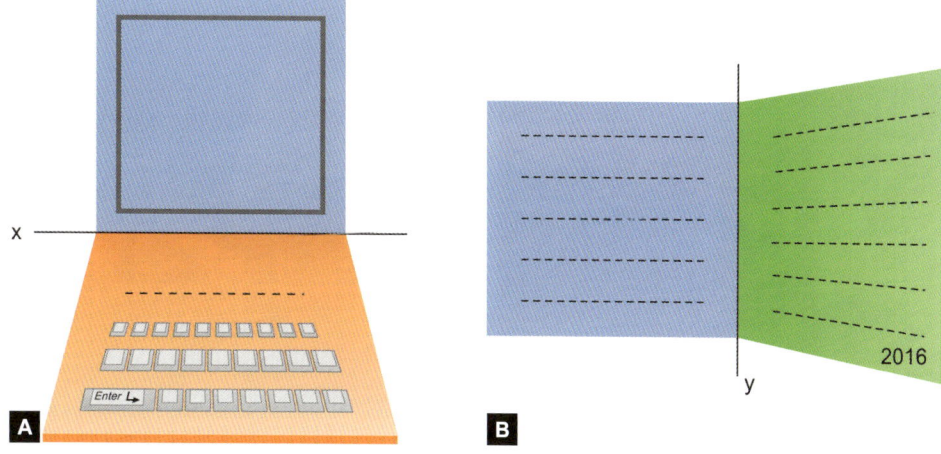

Figs. 9.2A and B: The intersection of two planes sharing a common axis: (A) The intersection of plane A and plane C is similar to a laptop with plane A represented by the screen and plane C by the keyboard; (B) The intersection of plane A and plane B is similar to an open book with plane A representing the front cover and plane B representing the back cover.

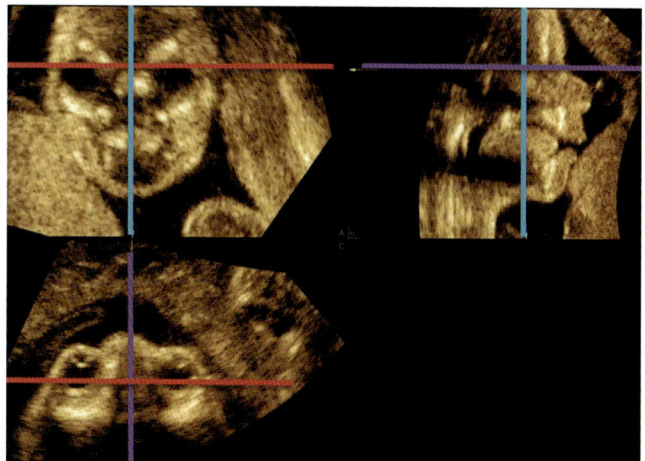

Fig. 9.3: The fetal face in multiplanar view with the coronal view on plane A sagittal view on plane B and axial view on plane C. Note the three axes each with its own distinct color as seen on each of the planes.

This method facilitates the diagnosis of malformations such as cleft palate in challenging cases.[7,12]

Similarly, moving the ROI along one of the other axes (represented in **Figure 9.3** by red and purple lines, clip S1) preserves the coordinates of the other two axes, thus resulting in changes on one plane only. However, when the ROI is moved to another location on the plane, not along one of the axes, the two adjacent planes change. It is recommended to place the ROI in a meaningful location and to move it systematically.

In order to fully master the concept, it is advisable to attempt this process on several datasets before continuing with this chapter. Through repeated experimentation, one can more easily grasp the ideas presented so far and apply them more readily. Do not hesitate to experiment with the dataset as one can always press the "initial" button in order to return to the starting point.

ROTATION OF THE VOLUME AROUND THE X-, Y- OR Z-AXIS

Another tool for the offline analysis of the volume is rotation around one axis—*x, y or z*. To conceptualize the rotation of the y-axis, it is helpful to think of an example of a ballerina swinging on her toe **(Fig. 9.4)**. By rotating the y-axis, the coronal and sagittal planes of the ballerina will appear on plane A and B alternately (seeing her in front and from the side alternatively). Looking at her from plane C is similar to looking at her from below or above. Looking from below, one would see her leg rotating clockwise or counter-clockwise. In plane C the ballerina remains in the same relative position, but the image is turned around.

Rotating the *x*-axis can be compared to a gymnast swinging on a bar **(Fig. 9.5)**. By rotating the x-axis, the coronal and axial planes of the gymnast will appear on planes A and C alternately. Observing from below or in front of the gymnast demonstrates her axial and coronal

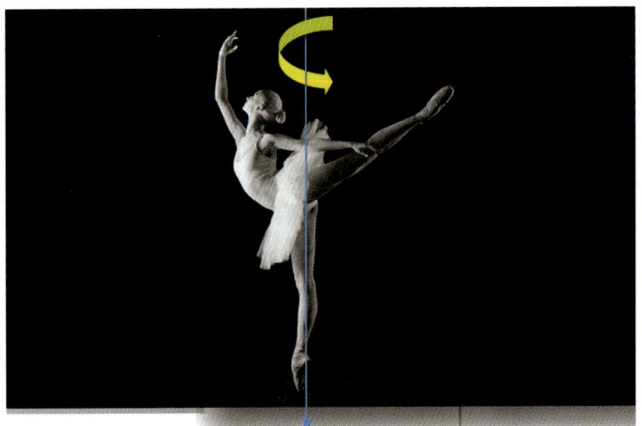

Fig. 9.4: A ballerina swinging on her toe. The axis traversing from head to toe is the y-axis and her movement is similar to the rotation of volume around the y-axis.

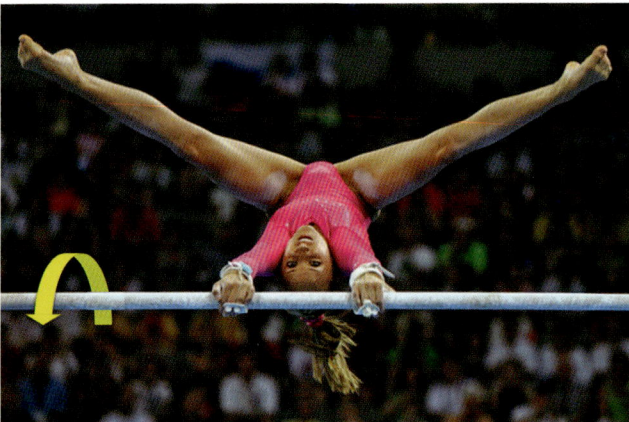

Fig. 9.5: A gymnast swinging on a bar. The axis traversing along the bar is the x-axis. The movement of the gymnast is similar to rotating the volume around the x-axis.

planes alternately. Looking at her on plane B is identical to looking at her from the side. In plane B, she is viewed in the same sagittal plane rotating clockwise or counter-clockwise. The gymnast remains in the same relative position, but the image is turned around.

Rotating the z-axis can be compared to a gymnast preforming a flip-flop **(Fig. 9.6)**. Observing her on plane A, she is facing the audience turning in a clockwise fashion. Looking at her from the side (plane B) or from below (plane C) demonstrates her sagittal and axial planes alternately. Rotation of the volume along one axis changes the image in two planes and makes the image rotate on the third plane.

ALIGNMENT OF THE VOLUME

Our brain does not process oblique images. The combination of two processing tools, moving the ROI and rotating the volume results in alignment of the volume. Therefore, it allows for the composition of meaningful images with relevant information. The movement through the volume should be a result of prior planning. Oblique views do not enable proper evaluation and skew the information resulting in an imprecise interpretation. The key to performing a successful alignment is to find a line or two symmetric organs that can be aligned in at least two planes.

The initial step in performing an alignment is to locate the ROI. The ROI should be positioned along a straight organ (i.e. aorta, endometrial line, falx cerebri,

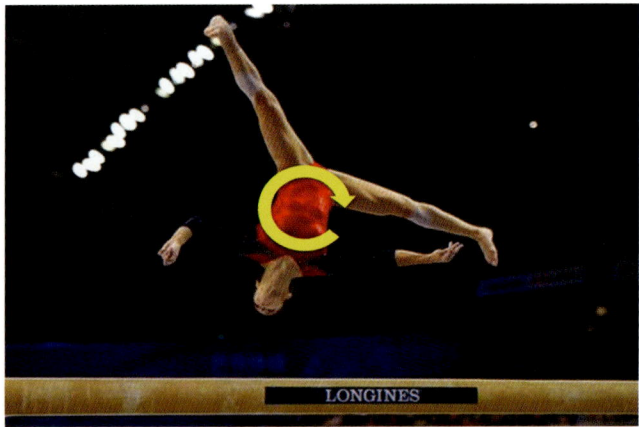

Fig. 9.6: A gymnast preforming a flip-flop. The z-axis traverses through her body from abdomen to back. While performing a flip-flop, her body turns around the z-axis.

long bone, interventricular septum, spine, etc.) or in the middle of two symmetric points (the two eyes). The axis should then be rotated so that the symmetric organs are parallel to the x-, y- or z-axis line and repeated on the next two planes to a point where the straight organ is aligned on at least two planes. It is preferable to initially work with the plane that has the most recognizable view.

PRACTICAL EXAMPLES OF VOLUME ALIGNMENT

The region between the fetal eyes on a coronal view, when examining the fetal face, is a good position for the alignment of face volume (**Fig. 9.3**). Imagining a line transecting through the two orbits, it is possible then to rotate the line so it is parallel at the axial and coronal view. Since the ROI is placed in the middle, between the two orbits, the orbits are not demonstrated on the sagittal plane.

An additional example of how to properly align a 3D data volume may be illustrated when performing a data acquisition in sagittal view of the fetal brain in an attempt to obtain an accurate measurement of the corpus callosum. In **Figure 9.7A**, there is a depiction of an apparent image of the corpus callosum and cavum septi pellucidi. However, this is an oblique or diagonal view which includes a joined portion of the lateral ventricle and portion of the corpus callosum. Using the multiplanar view (**Fig. 9.7B**) unveils the mistake and identifies the spatial location of the ROI in the lateral ventricle. In order to avoid this potential mistake, it is important to first position the ROI on the target organ, in this particular case the corpus callosum in plane B, then the corpus callosum will appear in plane A (**Fig. 9.7C**). Recent studies have demonstrated the feasibility of using multiplanar view in the evaluation of the normally developing fetal corpus callosum and its advantages in the evaluation of the surrounding structures as well as certain anomalies.[30-32]

3D MANIPULATION OF THE FETAL CARDIOVASCULAR SYSTEM

Another example of the use of 3D US in determining spatial arrangement can be demonstrated when using the multiplanar technique to assist in the display of the aortic and ductal arches. The first step in the process is to acquire the volume when the probe is directed at the four-chamber view, which is then presented on plane A (**Fig. 9.8A**). The acquired plane can be an axial or an oblique plane. The next step is to move the ROI in plane A to the descending aorta (**Fig. 9.8B**). The following step is to align the volume on two separate planes, in this case plane B and plane C, using a straight organ (the descending aorta—**Figures 9.8C and D**). Then the ROI is moved cephalad on plane B until the four-chamber view appears on plane A (**Fig. 9.8E**). Continuing in this direction on plane B eventually reveals the 3-vessl view on plane A (**Fig. 9.8F**). Aligning the main pulmonary artery and the descending aorta along the y-axis on plane A using z-axis

rotation results in the display of the ductal arch in the corresponding position on plane B. In order to display the aortic arch, z-axis rotation is performed on plane A to the point where the ascending and descending aorta are aligned along the y-axis. The aortic arch is now on display in plane B (**Fig. 9.8G**). To demonstrate the insertion of the systemic veins into the right atrium, the ROI is moved to the superior vena cava (SVC) on plane A (**Fig. 9.8H**). The SVC, IVC, and right atrium are now in full view on plane B. The same method can be used to demonstrate the trachea.

There are additional techniques that were developed in order to obtain specific views through acquired heart volume, such as the spin technique.[33]

APPLICATION OF MULTIPLANAR VIEW TO IDENTIFY MÜLLERIAN ANOMALIES

Another instance where proper alignment is essential to achieving the correct view is when attempting to obtain a coronal view of the uterus. This is the case when trying to diagnose Müllerian anomalies.[22] In the past, the proper diagnosis of Müllerian anomalies involved surgical exploration of the exterior contour of the uterus through laparotomy or laparoscopy combined with surgical exploration of the uterine cavity through hysteroscopy. Needless to mention that the risks of surgery, costs and recovery make this mode of diagnosis less than optimal. The introduction of 3D US has provided an alternative diagnostic tool with comparable sensitivity and specificity to the former surgical standard. The advantages of a sonographic diagnosis both in risks to the patient and cost of evaluation are significant.

SUMMARY

The 3D US technique enables the acquisition display and processing of data in a fascinating and instrumental fashion. After studying how to use the practical tools of moving the ROI and rotating the volume, it is possible to extend its use beyond multiplanar view and to incorporate the additional available options, including VCI render mode and tomographic ultrasound view. In our experience, the multiplanar view is more user-friendly and quicker to manipulate and thus most advantageous to use in everyday work.

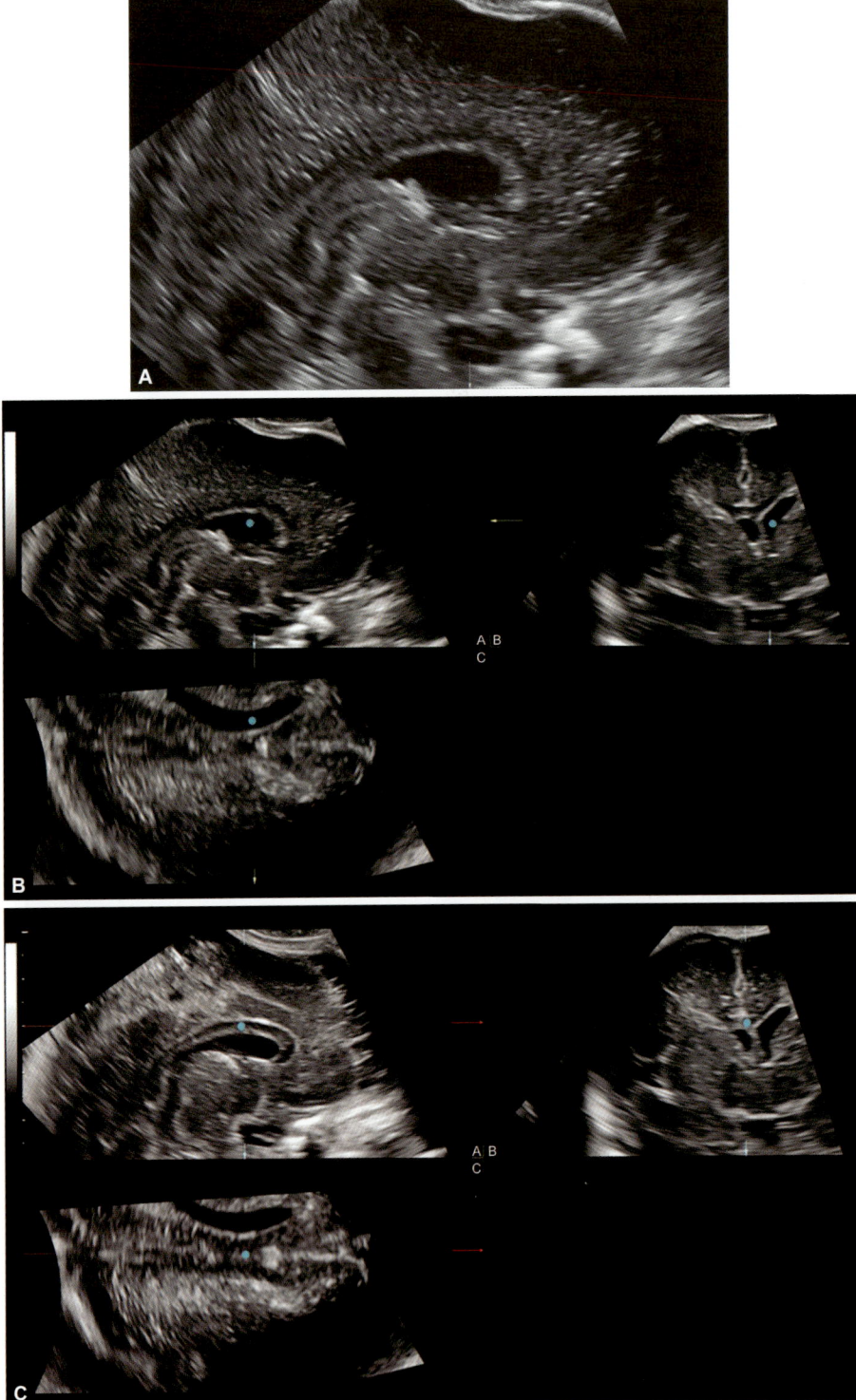

Figs. 9.7A to C: A multiplanar view of the corpus callosum: (A) A sagittal view of the corpus callosum as appears on plane A after volume acquisition. This view is oblique and includes a portion of the anterior horn of the lateral ventricle which is mistaken for part of the corpus callosum when viewed on plane A alone; (B) The multiplanar view reveals the mistake when the ROI is placed at the anterior portion of the presumed cavum septi pelucidi, the corresponding position on plane B and plane C shows the actual location in the anterior horn of the lateral ventricle; (C) Moving the ROI on plane B to the corpus callosum results in a full display of the corpus callosum in sagittal view on plane A.

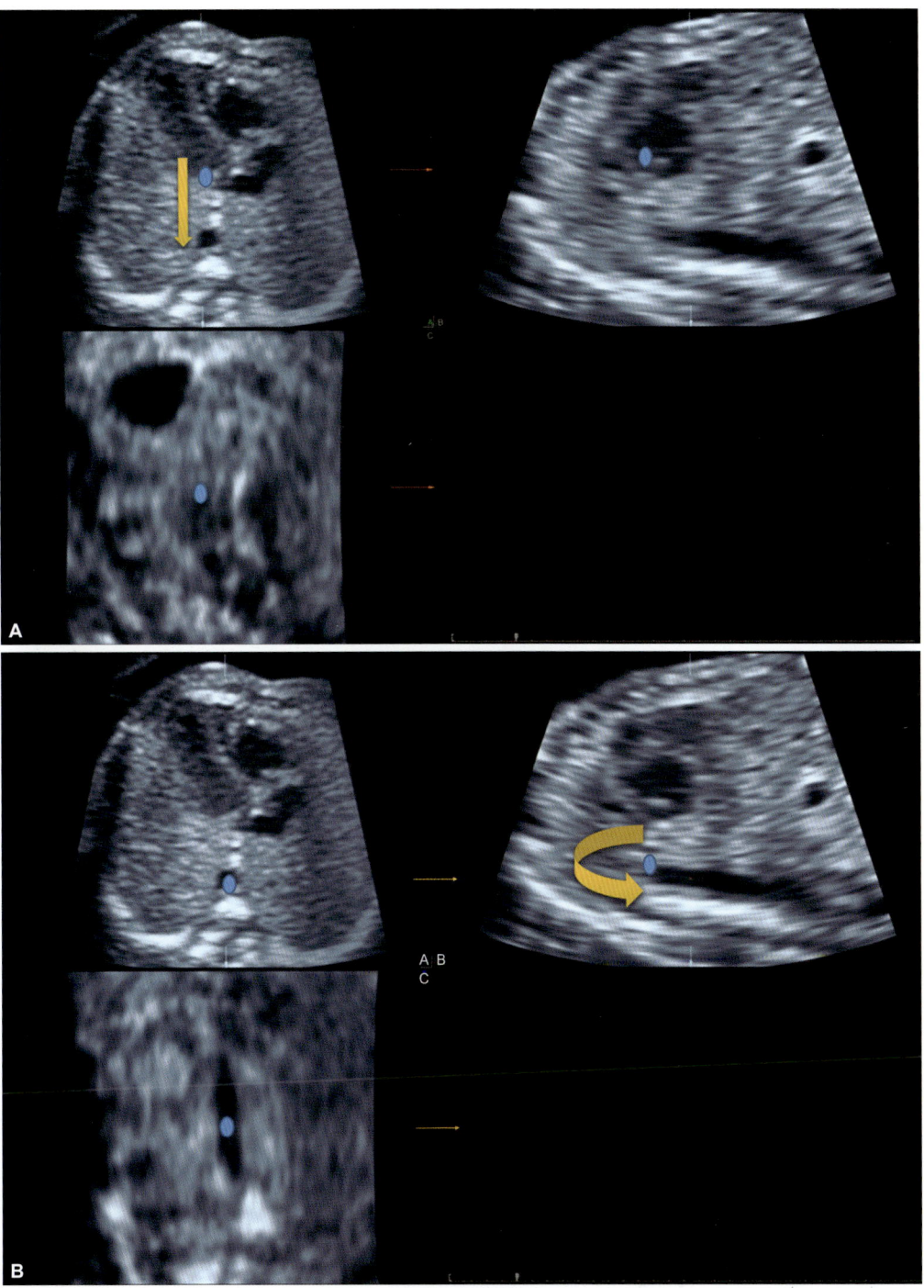

Figs. 9.8A and B

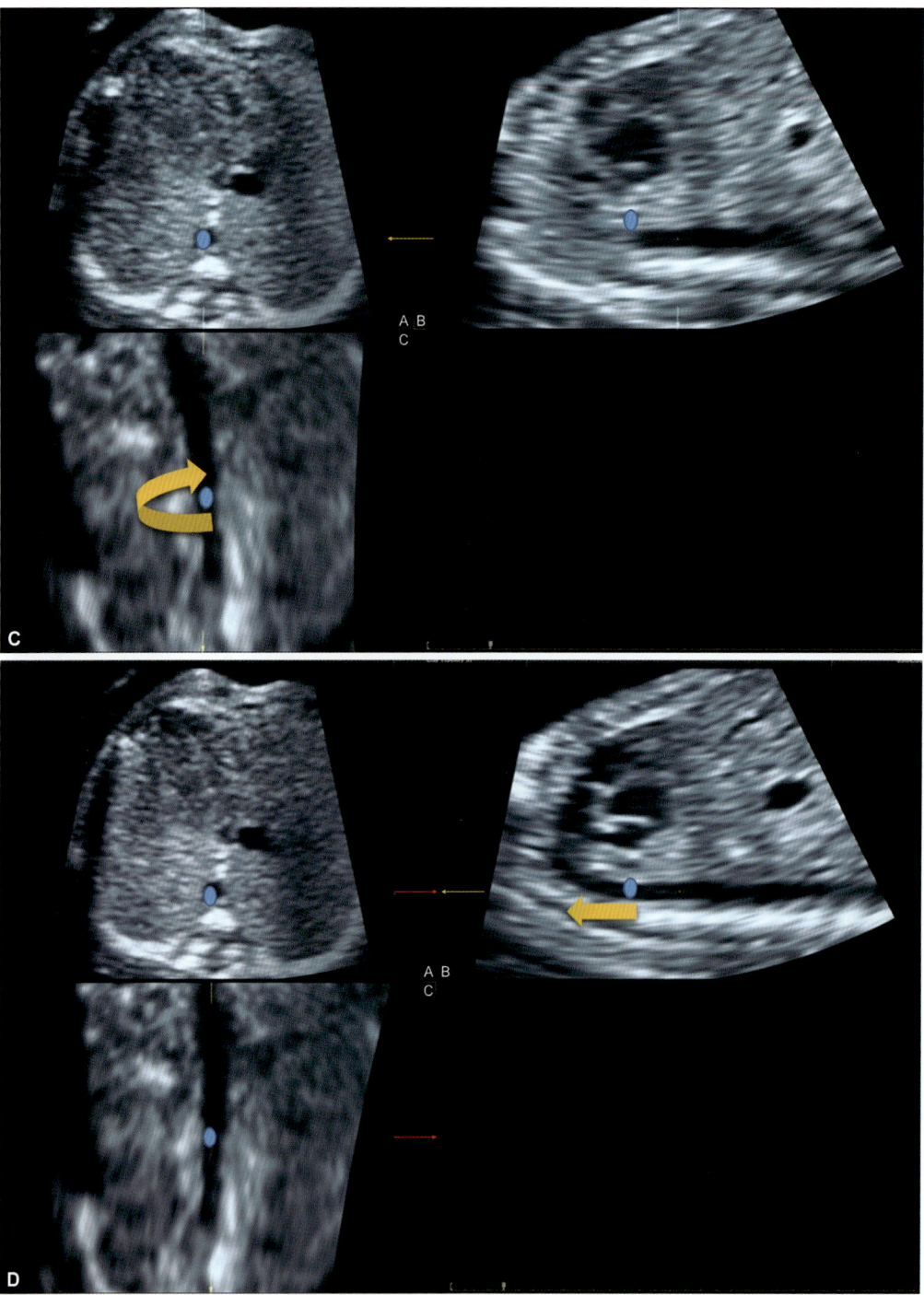

Figs. 9.8C and D

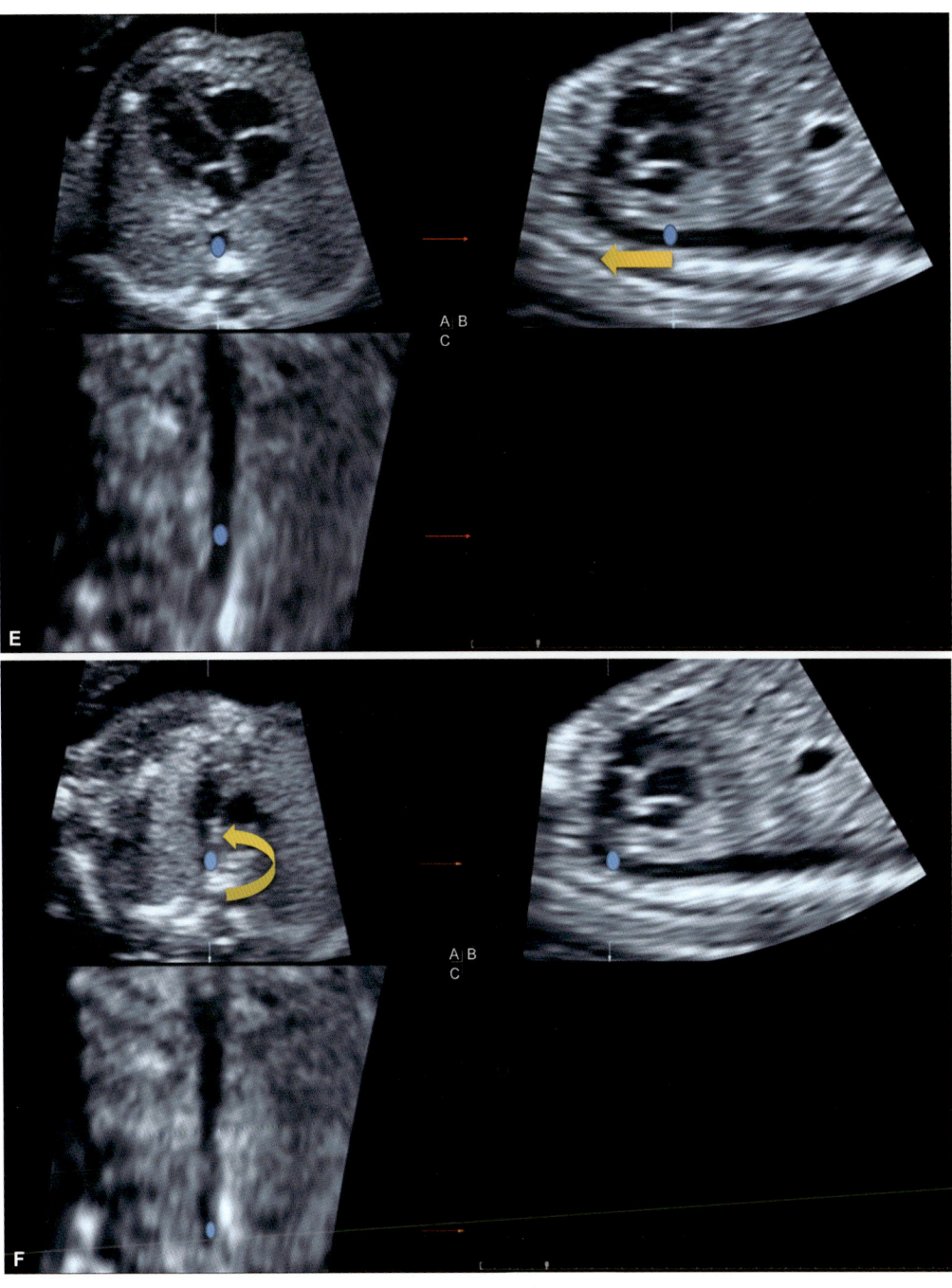

Figs. 9.8E and F

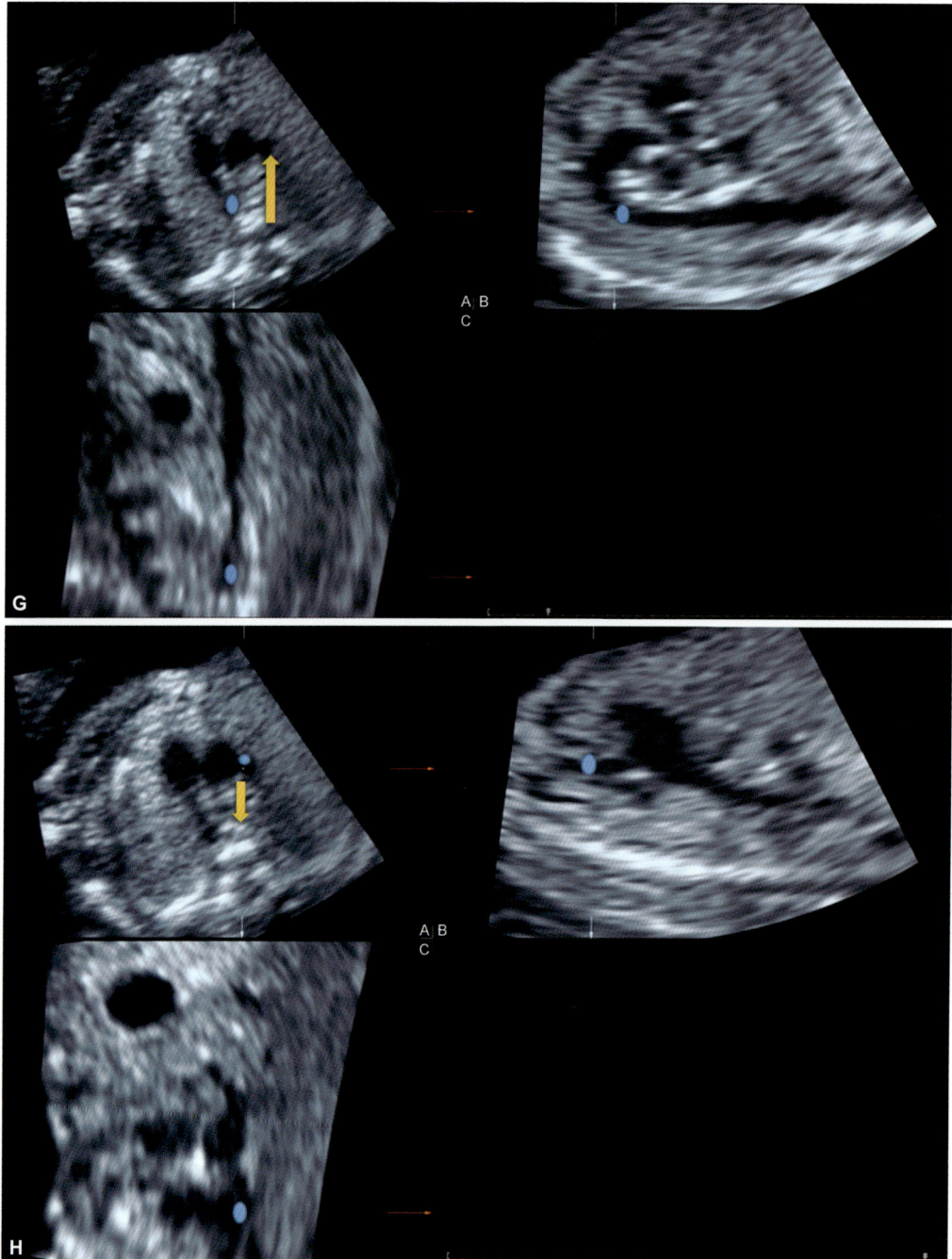

Figs. 9.8G and H

Figs. 9.8A to H: A practical approach to 3D volume manipulation of the fetal cardiovascular system in order to obtain certain hard to view segments. The yellow arrows indicate the direction of the next step action either by moving the ROI or rotation of the axis. (A) A multiplanar view of the fetal heart as acquired with spatiotemporal image correlation (STIC). The acquisition plane can be oblique. In plane A the descending aorta is seen in axial view; (B) The ROI is moved to the aorta in plane A; (C) Working on plane B, the z-axis (of plane B) is rotated so the aorta is parallel to the x-axis; (D) Working on plane C, z-axis rotation of the aorta aligns the organ parallel to the y-axis; (E) The ROI is moved cephalad on plane B to reveal the four-chambered view on plane A; (F) The ROI is moved further cephalad on plane B to reveal the three-vessel view on plane A. In order to demonstrate the ductal arch on plane B, the ROI is positioned on the descending aorta in plane A with the main pulmonary artery and descending aorta aligned along the y-axis; (G) In order to demonstrate the aortic arch on plane B, the z-axis is rotated on plane A to align the ascending and descending aorta along the y-axis; (H) For demonstration of the bicaval view on plane B, the ROI is moved to the superior vena cava on plane A. This process is repeated to view the trachea.

REFERENCES

1. Gindes L, Matsui H, Achiron R, et al. Comparison of ex-vivo high-resolution episcopic microscopy with in-vivo four-dimensional high-resolution transvaginal sonography of the first-trimester fetal heart. Ultrasound Obstet Gynecol. 2012;39:196-202.

2. Blaas HG, Taipale P, Torp H, et al. Three-dimensional ultrasound volume calculations of human embryos and young fetuses: a study on the volumetry of compound structures and its reproducibility. Ultrasound Obstet Gynecol. 2006; 27:640-6.

3. Blaas HG, Eik-Nes SH, Isaksen CV. The detection of spina bifida before 10 gestational weeks using two- and three-dimensional ultrasound. Ultrasound Obstet Gynecol. 2000;16:25-9.

4. Benoit B, Hafner T, Kurjak A, et al. Three-dimensional sonoembryology. J Perinat Med. 2002;30:63-73.

5. Blaas HG, Eik-Nes SH. Sonoembryology and early prenatal diagnosis of neural anomalies. Prenatal Diagnosis. 2009; 29:312-25.

6. Gindes L, Weissmann-Brenner A, Weisz B, et al. Identification of the fetal hippocampus and fornix and role of 3-dimensional sonography. J Ultrasound Med. 2011;30: 1613-8.

7. Tutschek B, Blaas HK, Abramowicz J, et al. Three-dimensional imaging of the fetal skull and face. Ultrasound Obstet Gynecol. 2017;50:7-16.

8. Zajicek M, Achiron R, Weisz B, et al. Sonographic assessment of fetal secondary palate between 12 and 16 weeks of gestation using three-dimensional ultrasound. Prenat Diagn. 2013;33:1-4.

9. Gindes L, Malach S, Weisz B, et al. Measuring the perimeter and area of the Sylvian fissure in fetal brain during normal pregnancies using 3-dimensional ultrasound. Prenat Diagn. 2015;35:1-9.

10. Danon E, Weisz B, Achiron R, et al. Three-dimensional ultrasonographic depiction of fetal brain blood vessels. Prenat Diagn. 2016;36:407-17.

11. Weissmann-Brenner A, Zajicek M, Weisz B, et al. Feasibility of detection of the 3-vessel and trachea view using 3-dimensional sonographic volumes. J Ultrasound Med. 2014;33:681-5.

12. Merz E, Abramovicz J, Baba K, et al. 3D imaging of the fetal face—recommendations from the International 3D Focus Group. Ultraschall Med. 2012;33:175-82.

13. Kivilevitch Z, Gindes L, Deutsch H, et al. In-utero evaluation of the fetal umbilical-portal venous system: two- and three-dimensional ultrasonic study. Ultrasound Obstet Gynecol. 2009;34:634-42.

14. Gindes L, Pretorius DH, Romine LE, et al. Three-dimensional ultrasonographic depiction of fetal abdominal blood vessels. J Ultrasound Med. 2009;28:977-88.

15. Zalel Y, Yagel S, Achiron R, et al. Three-dimensional ultrasonography of the fetal vermis at 18 to 26 weeks' gestation: time of appearance of the primary fissure. J Ultrasound Med. 2009;28:1-8.

16. Gindes L, Weissmann-Brenner A, Zajicek M, et al. Three-dimensional ultrasound demonstration of the fetal palate in high-risk patients: the accuracy of prenatal visualization. Prenat Diagn. 2013;33:436-41.

17. Bertucci E, Gindes L, Mazza V, et al. Vermian biometric parameters in the normal and abnormal fetal posterior fossa: three-dimensional sonographic study. J Ultrasound Med. 2011;30:1403-10.

18. Gindes L, Benoit B, Pretorius DH, et al. Abnormal number of fetal ribs on 3-dimensional ultrasonography: associated anomalies and outcomes in 75 fetuses. J Ultrasound Med. 2008;27:1263-71.

19. Merz E, Pashaj S. Advantages of 3D ultrasound in the assessment of fetal abnormalities. J Perinat Med. 2017;45: 643-50.

20. Schramm T, Gloning KP, Minderer S, et al. 3D ultrasound in fetal spina bifida. Ultraschall Med. 2008;29:289-90.

21. Dyson RL, Pretorius DH, Budorick NE, et al. Three-dimensional ultrasound in the evaluation of fetal anomalies. Ultrasound Obstet Gynecol. 2000;16:321-8.

22. Bega G, Lev-Toaff A, O'Kane P, et al. Three-dimensional ultrasonography in gynecology technical aspects and clinical applications. J Ultrasound Med. 2003;22:1249-69.

23. Weissmann-Brenner A, Haas J, Barzilay E, et al. Added value of 3-dimensional sonography for endometrial evaluation in early puerperium. J Ultrasound Med. 2013; 32:587-92.

24. Lee JH, Pretorius DH, Weinstein M, et al. Transperineal three-dimensional ultrasound in evaluating anal sphincter muscles. Ultrasound Obstet Gynecol. 2007;30:201-9.

25. Alcazar JL, Jurado M. Three-dimensional ultrasound for assessing women with gynecological cancer: A systematic review. Gynecol Oncol. 2011;120:340-6.

26. Abuhamad A. Automated multiplanar imaging. J Ultrasound Med. 2004;23:573-6.

27. Abuhamad A. Standardization of 3-dimensional volumes in obstetric sonography. J Ultrasound Med. 2005;24: 397-401.

28. Merz E, Benoit B, Blaas HG, et al. Standardization of three-dimensional images in obstetrics and gynecology: consensus statement. Ultrasound Obstet Gynecol. 2007;29:697-703.

29. Deng J, Rodeck CH. New fetal cardiac imaging techniques. Prenat Diagn. 2004;24:1092-103.

30. Pashaj S, Merz E. Detection of fetal corpus callosum abnormalities by means of 3D ultrasound. Ultraschall Med. 2016;37:185-94.

31. Pashaj S, Merz E. Prenatal demonstration of normal variants of the pericallosal artery by 3D ultrasound. Ultraschall Med. 2014;35:129-36.

32. Pashaj S, Merz E, Wellek S. Biometry of the fetal corpus callosum by three-dimensional ultrasound. Ultrasound Obstet Gynecol. 2013;42:691-8.

33. DeVore GR, Polanco B, Sklansky MS, et al. The 'spin' technique: a new method for examination of the fetal outflow tracts using three-dimensional ultrasound. Ultrasound Obstet Gynecol. 2004;24:72-82.

Three-dimensional Examination of the Placenta

Erich Hafner

INTRODUCTION

Contrary to two-dimensional (2D) ultrasound, three-dimensional (3D) sonography provides several advantages on what the examination of the placenta is concerned. Basically, the placenta can be described as a nondescript or even bland organ. Consequently, conventional 2D sonography deals only with placental location, length and width, placental thickness, and the occurrence of placental calcifications **(Fig. 10.1)**. 3D placental sonography by contrast allows us a much more integral approach by measuring placental volume and growth as well as placental blood flow in the entire placental mass as well as outside of the placenta in what is called the placental bed. This makes it also possible to appreciate the array of the placental vessels in order to identify placentas with reduced blood flow or even morbidly adherent placentas.

PLACENTAL VOLUME

It is long-standing knowledge that placental and neonatal weights are closely correlated. This led to attempts to estimate placental weight by 2D methods in order to detect fetuses at risk of being growth restricted.[1-3] 3D sonography can much more reliably detect small placentas not only in the 2nd or 3rd trimester,[4] but much more importantly even in the 1st trimester.[5-10] It, thus, enables us to start prophylactic treatment. Both the VOCAL **(Fig. 10.2)** and the multiplanar **(Fig. 10.3)** way of measuring placental volume leads to robust results.[11] A review on 1st trimester 3D placental volumetry, done by Antonia Farina, shows that the performance of detecting small-for-gestational-age (SGA) fetuses was only by 24.7% at a 10% false-positive rate. This can partly be attributed to the great heterogeneity in the way of measuring

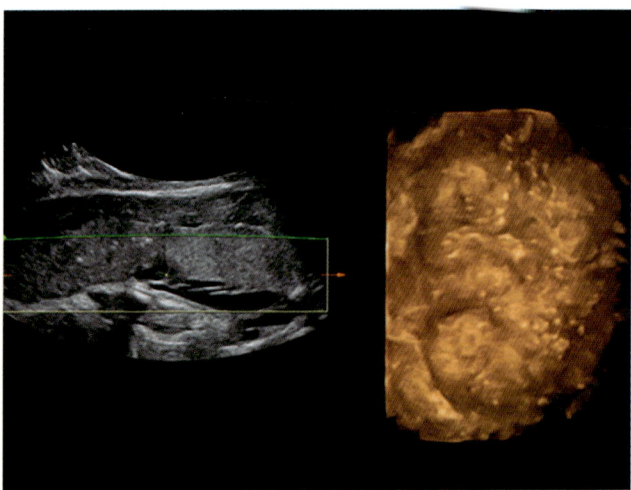

Fig. 10.1: Three-dimensional (3D) rendering of a placenta with multiple calcifications.

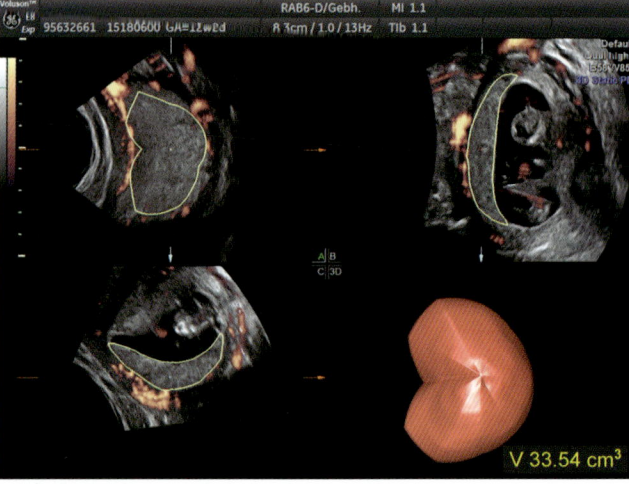

Fig. 10.2: Measurement of the placental volume in the 1st trimester using VOCAL technique.

placental volume as well as evaluating the data.[12] The author proposes nevertheless that 1st trimester placental volume measurement might be integrated into a multivariable screening protocol for the detection of SGA infants. Moreover, several studies show reduced 1st trimester placental volume also to be a risk factor for preeclampsia.[13-16] Another placental disorder leads to an enlargement and increased thickness of the placenta sometimes beginning at the end of the first but more markedly in the 2nd trimester of pregnancy. Because of

its homogeneous appearance given by the ultrasound machines back in the 90s, it has repeatedly been called "jelly-like" placenta.[17-19] With the actual machines, these placentas, instead of having large homogeneous areas, show enlarged lacunae with slow blood flow. This slow blood flow surrounds areas of normal placental tissue but also regions of hematomas as well as fibrin depositions, subchorionic hematomas, and infarctions. Whereas vessels in normal placentas are equally distributed with branching in the secondary and tertiary stem villi **(Figs. 10.4A and B)**, these areas of slow-flowing maternal blood are not color-coded, the stem vessels are crowded together or broadened in caliber with large nonvascular areas, thus being the consequence of widespread placental tissue demise **(Fig. 10.5)**. 3D rendering of this condition shows a bubbly appearance **(Fig. 10.6)**, 3D power Doppler displays the vessels being unequally distributed in the entire placenta, indicating the destruction of large placental areas.

THREE-DIMENSIONAL COLOR DOPPLER ULTRASOUND

As mentioned earlier, color Doppler ultrasound can visualize the number, course, caliber, coiling, and branching of vessels **(Figs. 10.4A and B)**. This 3D approach can add most valuable additional information: the whole picture of the vessel distribution within the placenta as well as in the region of the maternal placental bed. Reduced supply of nutrients and oxygen both in the placental

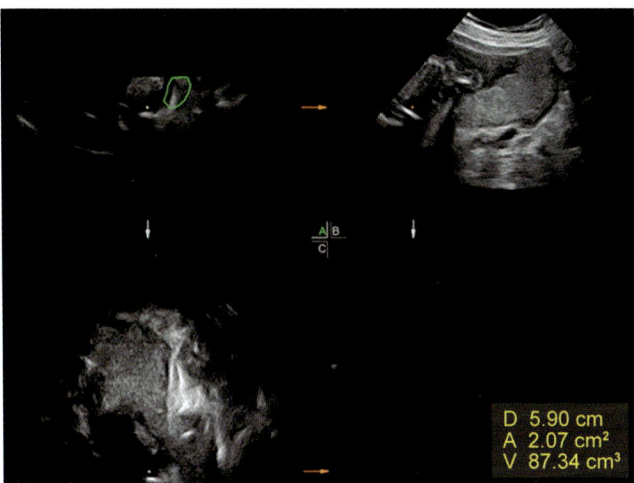

Fig. 10.3: Measurement of a very small placenta at 20 weeks using the multiplanar technique. Note that the placental volume is only 87.34 mL (normal 250 mL). The baby was delivered at 24 weeks after lung maturation but died.

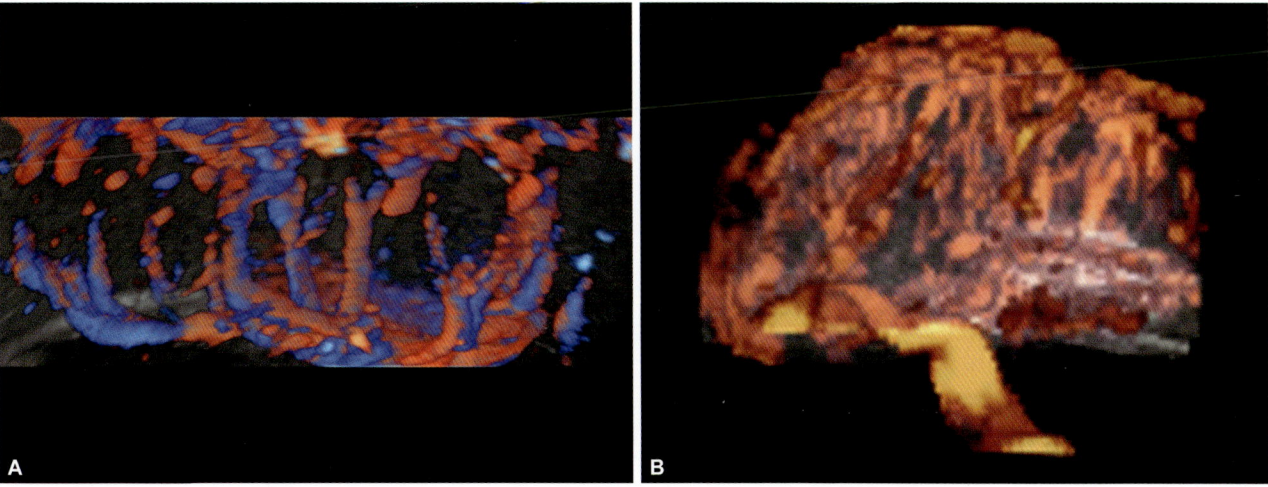

Figs. 10.4A and B: Three-dimensional (3D) placental vessel distribution at (A) 25 weeks and (B) 32 weeks in a normal placenta. Note the high number of parallel, equally distributed primary, secondary, and tertiary stem vessels inside the placenta.

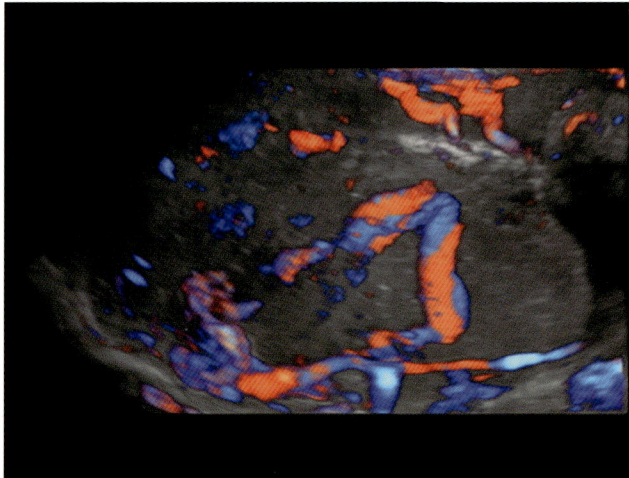

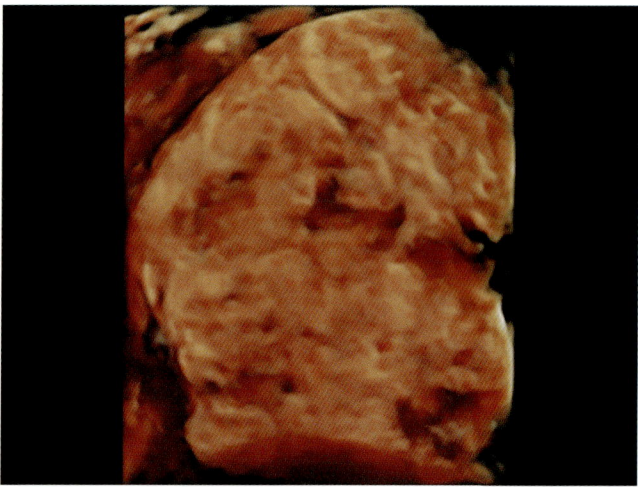

Fig. 10.5: Three-dimensional (3D) color depiction of a thick enlarged "jelly-like" placenta in the 3rd trimester. See the paucity of vessels, partly with broadened calibers, and partly crowded together leaving out large areas.

Fig. 10.6: Three-dimensional (3D) rendering of a "jelly-like" placenta. Note the bubbly appearance.

bed and within the placental tissue will lead to a decrease in the number, distribution, and appearance of these vessels,[20] which can only be shown by using 3D color Doppler.[21-24] This has initially been done using the so-called placental vascular sonobiopsy. For this purpose, the power Doppler window is placed over the placenta, and a spherical 3D volume obtained between the basal and chorionic plate. The grayscale and color values are automatically calculated by VOCAL. A sequence of three placental sections separated by successive rotations of 60° is obtained, and three or four spherical sampling sites are chosen in each plane. This method has the advantage to be applied both in early and in late pregnancy. Its disadvantage, however, is the selection of the regions for the spherical 3D biopsies which appear to be arbitrary.[24,25] This led to inconsistent results on what the development of the vasculature throughout the pregnancy is concerned.[24-28] As the 3D volume box can easily display the entire 1st trimester placenta, this disadvantage could, at least in the 1st trimester, be overcome **(Fig. 10.7)** and led to a number of publications focusing on placental 3D power Doppler perfusion in early pregnancy.[20-22,29-32] This method could be shown to provide already in the 1st trimester valuable information on a woman's risk of developing preeclampsia and fetal growth restriction **(Figs. 10.8 and 10.9)**. Appreciating the distribution, the course and the caliber of placental vessels are also useful in differentiating between normal and invasive placental attachment as it is seen in placenta accreta versus placenta increta **(Fig. 10.10)**.

FUTURE

Three-dimensional volume rendering does not only provide placental volume data but can also be used to appreciate placental shape. We know that women who undergo early problems of placental intrauterine growth and spreading will often end up with differently shaped placentas like bilobate or succenturiate placentas. This can easily be detected by using the 3D VOCAL mode and women can subsequently be observed more precisely **(Figs. 10.11A to C)**.

Placental bed vessels might also be studied more in detail. We know that the number of the placental vessels and their flow is reduced considerably in women at risk of developing preeclampsia and preeclampsia plus fetal growth restriction. This can already be seen in the 1st trimester.[21] 3D color (power) Doppler can also show the vessel distribution on the placental surface. It could be hypothesized that the visibility of those vessels is a matter of spiral artery transformation, thus giving us an idea of whether deep placentation has correctly taken place.[33] It seems that this distribution is different in women a risk for the abovementioned problems in that vessels concentrate in the center of the placental bed. This could lead to reduced supply in the periphery **(Figs. 10.12A and B)**.

Three-dimensional sonography of the placenta gives us a multitude of new insight about the role of the placenta in normal and pathologic pregnancies. We are only at the beginning of a long scientific journey in which 3D placenta will be a most important tool.

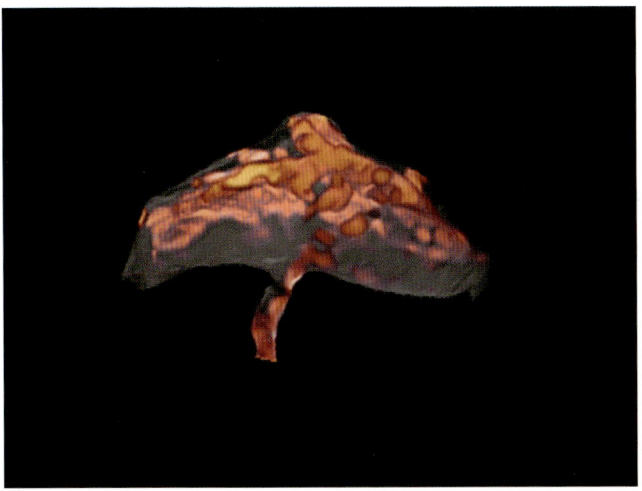

Fig. 10.7: Three-dimensional (3D) power Doppler rendering of a normal placenta in the 1st trimester depicting the entire placenta and the placental bed. Note the huge difference in the number of vessels in the placental bed compared with the actual placenta.

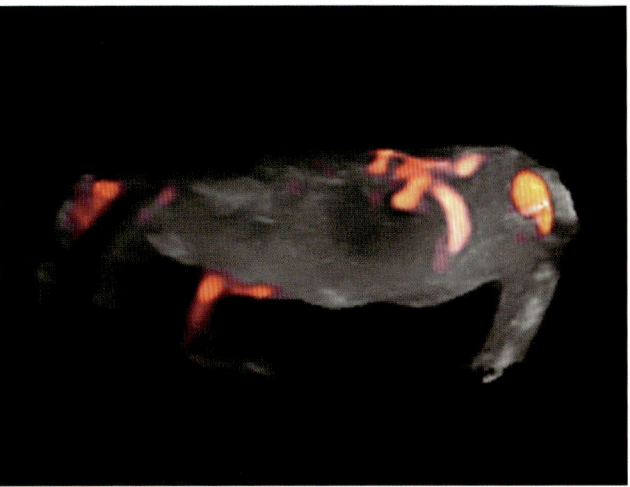

Fig. 10.8: Three-dimensional (3D) power Doppler rendering of a 1st trimester placenta. The woman developed preeclampsia and fetal growth restriction later in pregnancy. Note the scarcity of vessels in the placental bed.

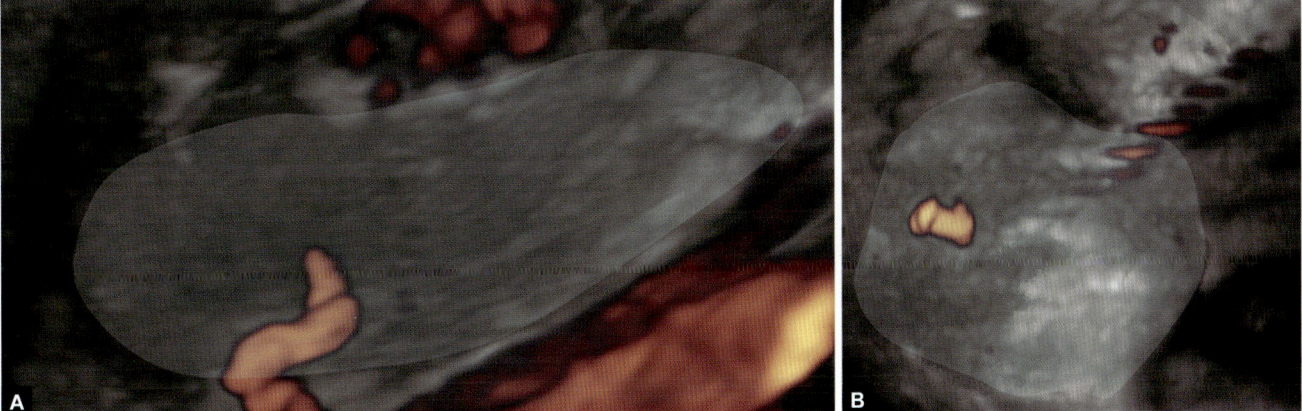

Figs. 10.9A and B: The same placenta as earlier depicted in three-dimensional (3D) power Doppler rendering. Note that there is only one vessel visible in the placental bed: (A) Lateral view; and (B) View from above.

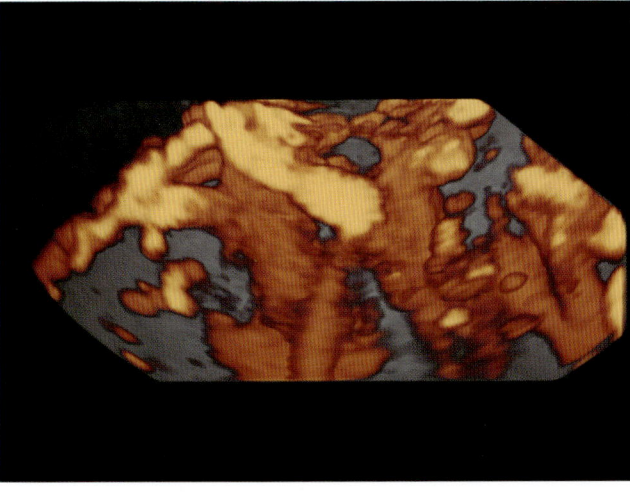

Fig. 10.10: Three-dimensional (3D) rendering of abnormal vessel distribution and large variations of calibers in a placenta accreta.

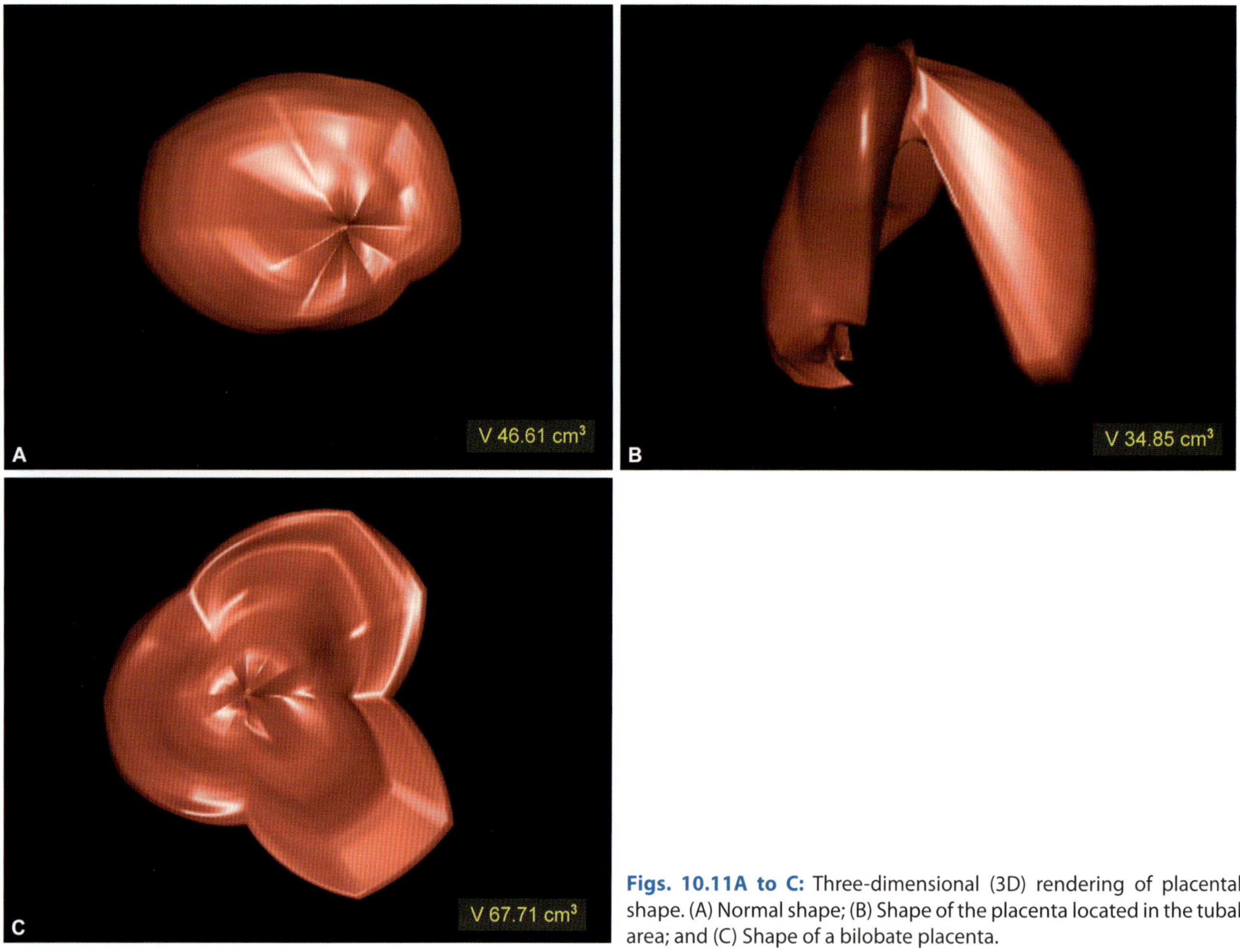

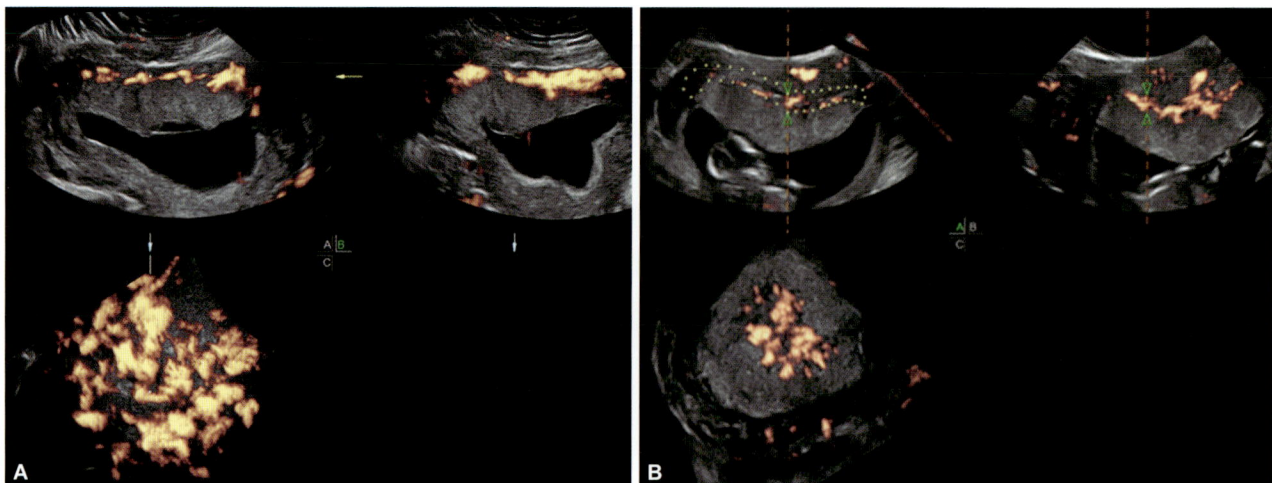

V 46.61 cm³

A

V 34.85 cm³

B

V 67.71 cm³

C

Figs. 10.11A to C: Three-dimensional (3D) rendering of placental shape. (A) Normal shape; (B) Shape of the placenta located in the tubal area; and (C) Shape of a bilobate placenta.

A

B

Figs. 10.12A and B: (A) Three-dimensional (3D) power Doppler of placental bed vessels. Vessels are equally distributed all over the placental surface; and (B) 3D power Doppler of placental bed vessels. Note that most vessels cluster in the center of the placental bed.

CONCLUSION

3D ultrasound is the appropriate way to examine placental volume, thickness, growth, blood flow, placental bed perfusion, etc. It therefore can provide valuable insights on the cause of a particular problem such as severe fetal growth restriction. Thus an adequate therapeutic regime can be chosen and the outcome be improved.

REFERENCES

1. Aherne W. A weight relationship between the human foetus and placenta. Biol Neonat. 1966;10:113-8.
2. Hoogland HJ, de Haan J, Martin CB. Placental size during early pregnancy and outcome: a preliminary report of a sequential ultrasonographic study. Am J Obstet Gynecol. 1980;150:441-3.
3. Jauniaux E, Ramsay B, Campbell S. Ultrasonographic investigation of placental morphologic characteristics and size during the second trimester of pregnancy. Am J Obstet Gynecol. 1994;170:130-7.
4. Hafner E, Philipp T, Schuchter K, et al. Second-trimester measurements of placental volume by three-dimensional ultrasound to predict small-for-gestational-age infants. Ultrasound Obstet Gynecol. 1998;12:97-102.
5. Hafner E, Metzenbauer M, Dillinger-Paller B, et al. Correlation of first trimester placental volume and second trimester uterine artery Doppler flow. Placenta. 2001;22:729-34.
6. Metzenbauer M, Hafner E, Höfinger D, et al. Three-dimensional ultrasound measurement of the placental volume in early pregnancy: method and correlation with biochemical placenta parameters. Placenta. 2001;22:602-5.
7. Hafner E, Metzenbauer M, Höfinger D, et al. Placental growth from the first to the second trimester of pregnancy in SGA-foetuses and pre-eclamptic pregnancies compared to normal foetuses. Placenta. 2003;24:336-42.
8. Placencia W, Akolekar R, Dagklis T, et al. Placental volume at 11-13 weeks' gestation in the prediction of birth weight percentile. Fetal Diagn Ther. 2011;30:23-8.
9. Schwartz N, Sammel MD, Leite R, et al. First-trimester placental ultrasound and maternal serum markers as predictors of small-for-gestational-age infants. Am J Obstet Gynecol. 2014;211:253.e1-8.
10. Arakaki T, Hasegawa J, Nakamura M, et al. Prediction of early- and late-onset pregnancy-induced hypertension using placental volume on three-dimensional ultrasound and uterine artery Doppler. Ultrasound Obstet Gynecol. 2015;45:539-43.
11. Nowak PM, Nardozza LM, Araujo Júnior E, et al. Comparison of placental volume in early pregnancy using multiplanar and VOCAL methods. Placenta. 2008;29:241-5.
12. Farina A. Systematic review on first trimester three-dimensional placental volumetry predicting small for gestational age infants. Prenat Diagn. 2016;36:135-41.
13. Hafner E, Metzenbauer M, Höfinger D, et al. Comparison between three-dimensional placental volume at 12 weeks and uterine artery impedance/notching at 22 weeks in screening for pregnancy-induced hypertension, pre-eclampsia and fetal growth restriction in a low-risk population. Ultrasound Obstet Gynecol. 2006;27:652-7.
14. Rizzo G, Capponi A, Cavicchioni O, et al. First trimester uterine Doppler and three-dimensional ultrasound placental volume calculation in predicting pre-eclampsia. Eur J Obstet Gynecol Reprod Biol. 2008;138:147-51.
15. Plasencia W, González-Dávila E, González Lorenzo A, et al. First trimester placental volume and vascular indices in pregnancies complicated by preeclampsia Prenat Diagn. 2015;35:1247-54.
16. González-González NL, González-Dávila E, Padrón E, et al. Value of Placental Volume and Vasculature Flow Indices as Predictors of Early and Late Preeclampsia at First Trimester. Fetal Diagn Ther. 2018;44:256-63.
17. Jauniaux E, Ramsey B, Campbell S. Ultrasonographic investigations of placental morphologic characteristics during the second trimester of pregnancy. Am J Obstet Gynecol. 1994;170:130-7.
18. Mayhew TM, Charnok-Jones DS, Kaufmann B. Aspects of Human Fetoplacental Vasculogenesis and Angiogenesis. III. Changes in Complicated Pregnancies. Placenta. 2004;25:127-9.
19. Raio L, Ghezzi F, Cromi A, et al. The thick heterogeneous (jellylike) placenta: a strong predictor of adverse pregnancy outcome. Prenat Diagn. 2004;24:182-8.
20. Lyall F, Robson SC, Bulmer JN. Spiral artery remodeling and trophoblast invasion in preeclampsia and fetal growth restriction: relationship to clinical outcome. Hypertension. 2013;62:1046-54.
21. Hafner E, Metzenbauer M, Stümpflen I, et al. First trimester placental and myometrial blood perfusion measured by 3D power Doppler in normal and unfavourable outcome pregnancies. Placenta. 2010;31:756-63.
22. Hafner E, Metzenbauer M, Stümpflen I, et al. Measurement of placental bed vascularization in the first trimester, using 3D-power-Doppler, for the detection of pregnancies at-risk for fetal and maternal complications. Placenta. 2013;10:892-8.
23. Eastwood KA, Patterson C, Hunter AJ, et al. Evaluation of the predictive value of placental vascularisation indices derived from 3-dimensional power Doppler whole placental volume scanning for prediction of pre-eclampsia: a systematic review and meta-analysis. Placenta. 2017;51:89-97.
24. Moran MC, Mulcahy C, Zombori G, et al. Placental volume, vasculature and calcification in pregnancies complicated by pre-eclampsia and intrauterine growth restriction. Eur J Obstet Gynecol Reprod Biol. 2015;195:12-7.
25. Mercé LT, Barco MJ, Kupesic S, et al. Assessment of placental vascularization by three-dimensional power Doppler "vascular biopsy" in normal pregnancies. Croat Med J. 2005;46:765-71.

26. Noguchi J, Hata K, Tanaka H, et al. Placental vascular sonobiopsy using three-dimensional power Doppler ultrasound in normal and growth restricted fetuses. Placenta. 2009;30:391-7.

27. Yu CH, Chang CH, Ko HC, et al. Assessment of placental fractional moving blood volume using quantitative three-dimensional power Doppler ultrasound. Ultrasound Med Biol. 2003;29:19-23.

28. De Pauls CF, Ruano R, Campsi JA, et al. Quantitative Analysis of Placental Vasculature by Three-dimensional Power Doppler Ultrasonography in Normal Pregnancies from 12 to 40 Weeks of Gestation. Placenta. 2008;30: 142-8.

29. Guoit C, Gaglioti P, Oberto M, et al. Is three-dimensional power Doppler ultrasound useful in the assessment of placental perfusion in normal and growth-restricted pregnancies? Ultrasound Obstet Gyecol. 2008;31:171-6.

30. Rizzo G, Capponi A, Pietrolucci ME, et al. Effects of maternal cigarette smoking on placental volume and vascularization measured by 3-dimensional power Doppler ultrasonography at 11+0 to 13+6 weeks of gestation. Am J Obstet Gynecol. 2009;200:415.e1-5.

31. Mercé LT, Barco MJ, Alcázar JL, et al. Intervillous and uteroplacental circulation in normal early pregnancy and early pregnancy loss assessed by 3-dimensional power Doppler angiography. Am J Obstet Gynecol. 2009;200:315. e1-8.

32. Odibo AO, Goetzinger KR, Huster KM, et al. Placental volume and vascular flow assessed by 3D power Doppler and adverse pregnancy outcomes. Placenta. 2011;32:230-4.

33. Brosens I, Pijnenborg R, Vercruysse L, et al. The "Great Obstetrical Syndromes" are associated with disorders of deep placentation. Am J Obstet Gynecol. 2011;204:193-201.

HDlive Flow Silhouette Mode for Fetal Heart

Toshiyuki Hata, Uiko Hanaoka, Kenji Kanenishi

INTRODUCTION

HDlive uses an adjustable light source, creating lighting, and shadowing effects, thereby increasing depth perception, to generate realistic images of the normal fetus and fetal anomalies.[1-17]

Using the HDlive silhouette mode, we can obtain novel information on normal fetal structures, congenital deformities, and placental abnormalities.[18-21] It can visualize outlines of structures of interest at the same time as visualizing the inner core, meaning that it is more effective for identifying normal anatomy and congenital deformities. The shadowing effect that enables the visualization of structures present behind the structure of interest makes it more effective than other advanced rendering modes that are available, such as three-dimensional (3D)/four-dimensional (4D) ultrasound and HDlive.

It allows more accurate assessments of the following: fetal heart and peripheral circulation, placental vasculature, and tumor vascularity in the presence of gynecologic disorders.[22-32] The use of HDlive to increase the resolution of 3D/4D color/power Doppler leads to a significant improvement on comparison with conventional 3D/4D color/power Doppler, facilitating clear visualization of: fetal heart with great vessels, peripheral vessels, placental blood flow, and tumor blood flow in the presence of gynecologic disorders.

As cutting-edge technology, the HDlive Flow silhouette mode provides vitreous-like clarity of fetal heart blood flow and gynecologic tumors.[33-38] The core is shown as semitransparent, while preserving the outline and borders of blood flow. Thus, it is possible to obtain holographic images of blood flow of the fetal heart and tumor vascularity, being its most unique feature.

In this chapter, the HDlive Flow silhouette mode features of the normal fetal heart and congenital heart anomalies with/without the HDlive silhouette mode are shown using various images.

HDLIVE FLOW AND HDLIVE FLOW SILHOUETTE MODE

HDlive Flow with Glass-body Rendering Mode

This has been suggested to improve the accuracy of diagnosing complex fetal cardiac anomalies, facilitating by its generation of images of outflow tracts and spatial relationships among cardiac structures (**Fig. 11.1**).[22,23]

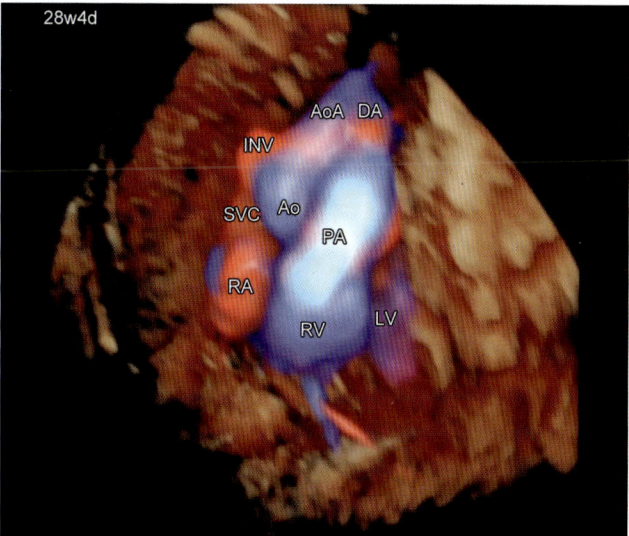

Fig. 11.1: HDlive Flow with glass-body rendering mode image of the normal fetal heart at 28 weeks and 4 days of gestation. (Ao: aorta; AoA: aortic arch; DA: ductus arteriosus; INV: innominate vein; LV: left ventricle; PA: pulmonary artery; RA: right atrium; RV: right ventricle; SVC: superior vena cava)

HDlive Flow with HDlive Silhouette Mode

When combining HDlive Flow with the HDlive silhouette mode, the spatial visualization of blood vessels in both the normal and abnormal fetal heart becomes possible **(Fig. 11.2)**, as well as that of peripheral blood vessels, placental abnormality, and gynecologic disorders, and so it is possible not only to spatially view these vessels, but also visualize landmarks of adjacent structures.[24-32]

HDlive Flow Silhouette Mode with Glass-body Rendering Mode

Use of HDlive Flow with the glass-body rendering mode enables a more accurate evaluation of the fetal heart and peripheral circulation.[24] The resolution of HDlive Flow is significantly more favorable than that of conventional 3D/4D color/power Doppler, and clear demonstration of the fetal heart with great vessels, small peripheral vessels, and blood flow in the placenta becomes possible **(Fig. 11.3)**.

HDlive Flow Silhouette Mode with HDlive Silhouette Mode

On combining the HDlive Flow silhouette mode and HDlive silhouette mode, we could clearly observe overlapping blood vessels, facilitating vitreous-like clarity of the fetal heart simultaneously with a transparent core.[33,36,37] The holography-like blood flow imaging of the fetal heart is the main merit of the system **(Figs. 11.4A to E)**. This technique clearly depicts the contour of cardiac chambers, and intracardiac-like flow can be identified.

NORMAL FETAL HEART

Frontal View

With this view, spatial relationships can be ascertained among the right atrium with superior vena cava and inferior vena cava, right ventricular outflow tract, ascending aorta, and descending aorta **(Figs. 11.5 and 11.6)**. The primary objective when adopting this view is to examine inflow of the right atrium (superior and inferior venae cavae to the right atrium).

Spatial Three-vessel View

With this view, we can ascertain the course of the outflow tracts (crisscross arrangements of pulmonary artery and aorta) and superior vena cava **(Figs. 11.7 to 11.11)**. This view is actually a superior or anterior view of the fetal heart, involving observation of the crisscross arrangements of the aorta, pulmonary artery, and superior vena cava, whose spatial relationships are easily identifiable.[33,37]

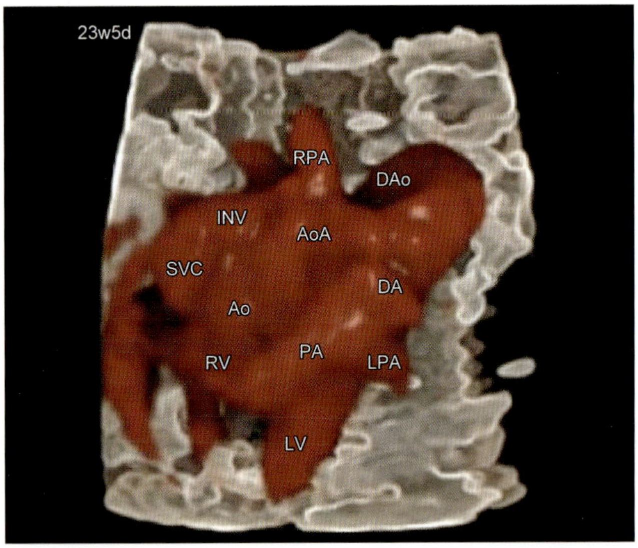

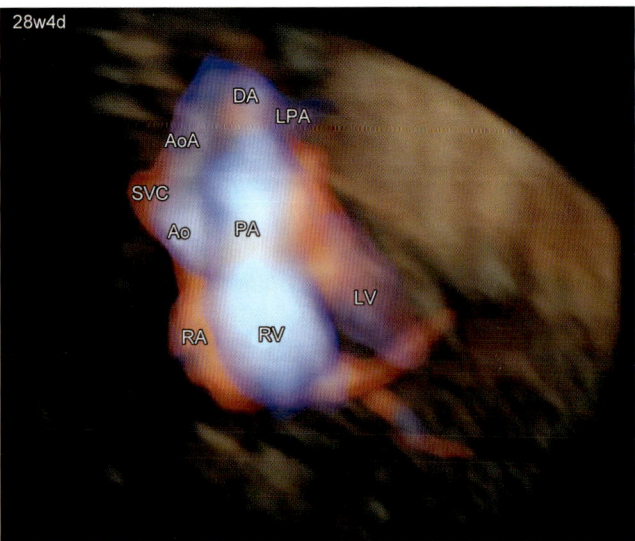

Fig. 11.2: HDlive Flow with HDlive silhouette mode image of the normal fetal heart at 23 weeks and 5 days of gestation. (Ao: aorta; AoA: aortic arch; DA: ductus arteriosus; DAo: descending aorta; INV: innominate vein; LPA: left pulmonary artery; LV: left ventricle; PA: pulmonary artery; RPA: right pulmonary artery; RV: right ventricle; SVC: superior vena cava)

Fig. 11.3: HDlive Flow silhouette mode with glass-body rendering mode image of the normal fetal heart at 28 weeks and 4 days of gestation. (Ao: aorta; AoA: aortic arch; DA: ductus arteriosus; LPA: left pulmonary artery; LV: left ventricle; PA: pulmonary artery; RA: right atrium; RV: right ventricle; SVC: superior vena cava)

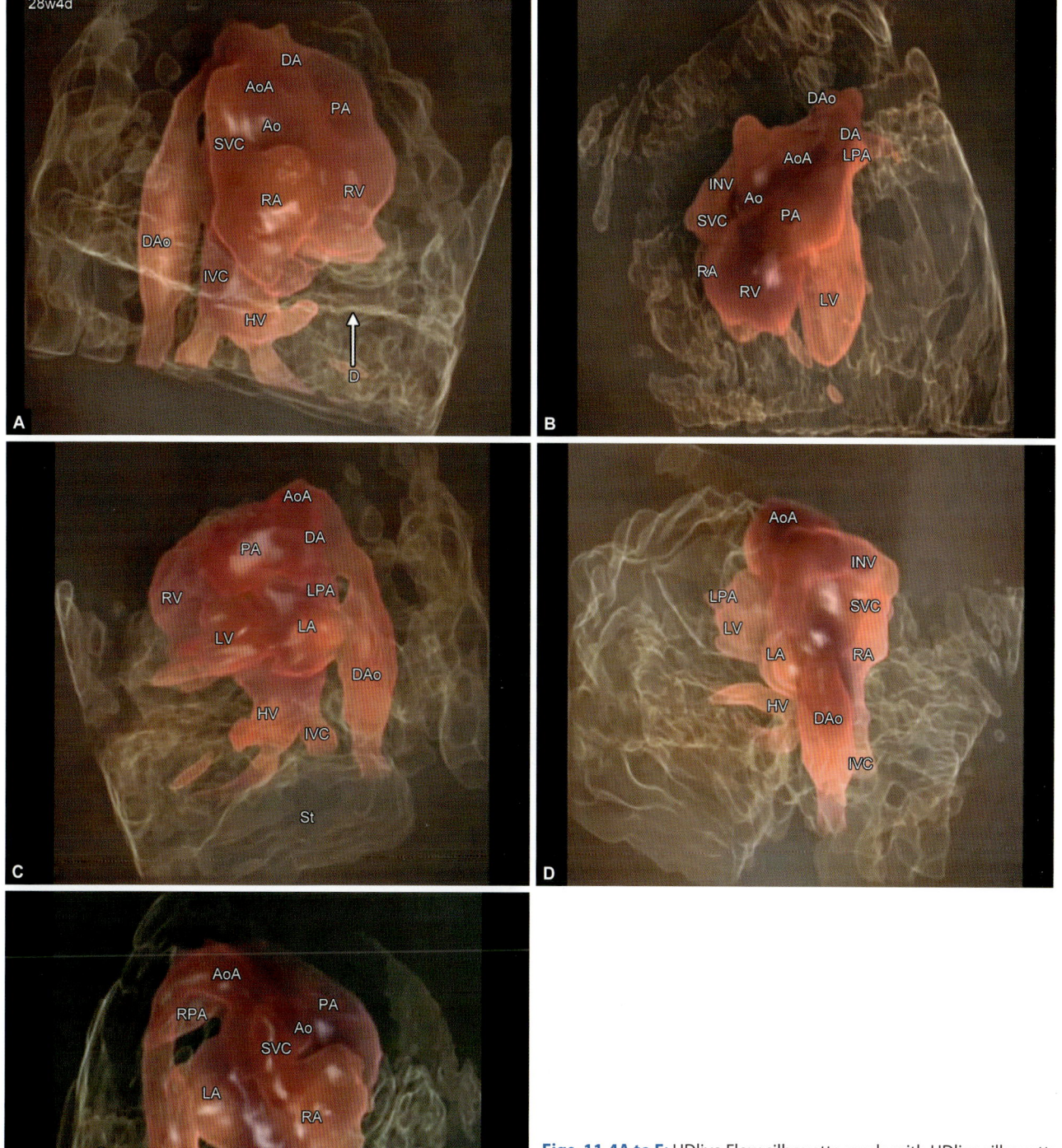

Figs. 11.4A to E: HDlive Flow silhouette mode with HDlive silhouette mode image of the normal fetal heart at 28 weeks and 4 days of gestation. (A) Frontal view; (B) Spatial three-vessel view; (C) Panoramic view; (D) Posterior view; (E) Right lateral view. (Ao: aorta; AoA: aortic arch; D: diaphragm; DA: ductus arteriosus; DAo: descending aorta; HV: hepatic vein; INV: innominate vein; IVC: inferior vena cava; LA: left atrium; LV: left ventricle; LPA: left pulmonary artery; PA: pulmonary artery; RA: right atrium; RPA: right pulmonary artery; RV: right ventricle; Sp: spine; St: stomach; SVC: superior vena cava)

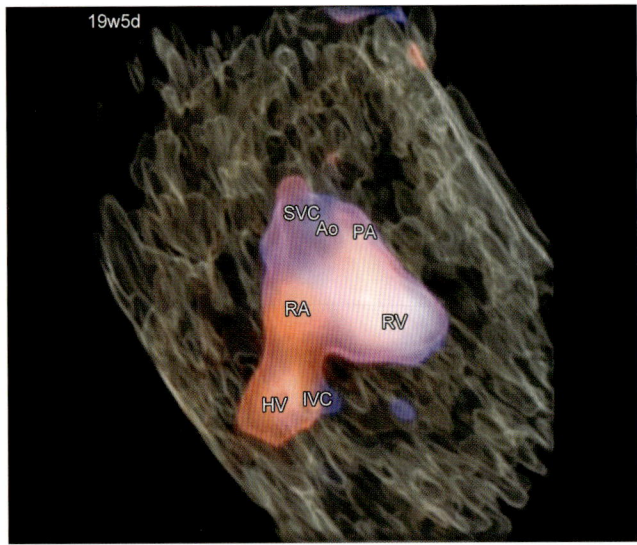

Fig. 11.5: Frontal view with HDlive Flow silhouette mode and HDlive silhouette mode of a normal fetal heart at 19 weeks and 5 days of gestation. (Ao: aorta; HV: hepatic vein; IVC: inferior vena cava; PA: pulmonary artery; RA: right atrium; RV: right ventricle; SVC: superior vena cava)

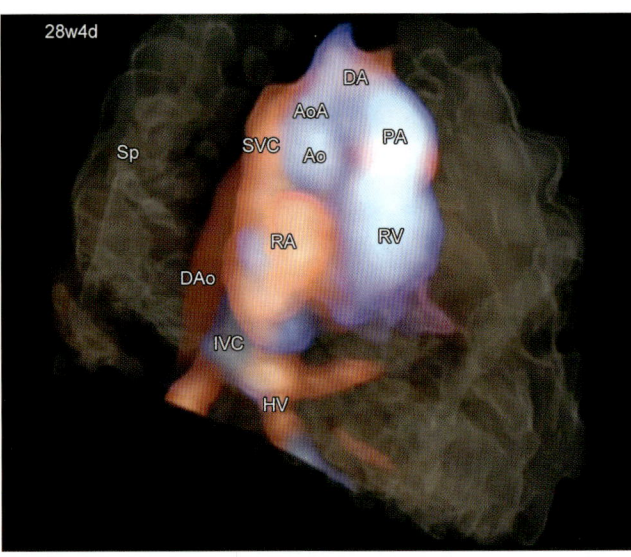

Fig. 11.6: Frontal view with HDlive Flow silhouette mode and HDlive silhouette mode of a normal fetal heart at 28 weeks and 4 days of gestation. (Ao: aorta; AoA: aortic arch; DAo: descending aorta; HV: hepatic vein; IVC: inferior vena cava; PA: pulmonary artery; RA: right atrium; RV: right ventricle; Sp: spine; SVC: superior vena cava)

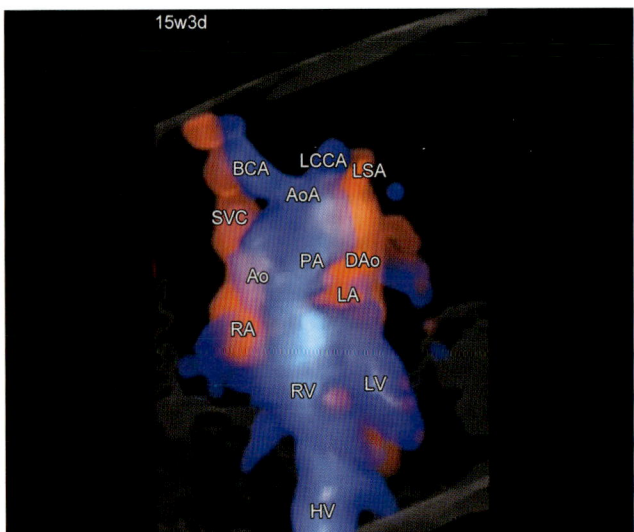

Fig. 11.7: Spatial three-vessel view with HDlive Flow silhouette mode and HDlive silhouette mode of a normal fetal heart at 15 weeks and 3 days of gestation. (Ao: aorta; AoA: aortic arch; BCA: brachiocephalic artery: DAo: descending aorta; HV: hepatic vein; LCCA: left common carotid artery; LSA: left subclavian artery; LV: left ventricle; PA: pulmonary artery; RA: right atrium; RV: right ventricle; SVC: superior vena cava)

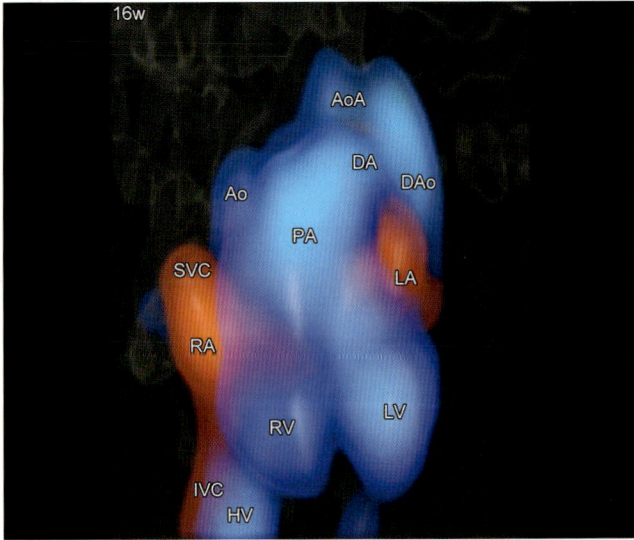

Fig. 11.8: Spatial three-vessel view with HDlive Flow silhouette mode and HDlive silhouette mode of a normal fetal heart at 16 weeks of gestation. (Ao: aorta; AoA: aortic arch; DA: ductus arteriosus; DAo: descending aorta; HV: hepatic vein; IVC: inferior vena cava; LA: left atrium; LV: left ventricle; PA: pulmonary artery; RA: right atrium; RV: right ventricle; SVC: superior vena cava)

Panoramic View

With this view, we can ascertain spatial relationships among cardiac chambers and vessels, allowing visualization of the out- and inflow tracts **(Figs. 11.12 to 11.16)**. This is actually a left, oblique, or lateral view, providing clear views of the two ventricles, two great arteries, and descending aorta.[33,37]

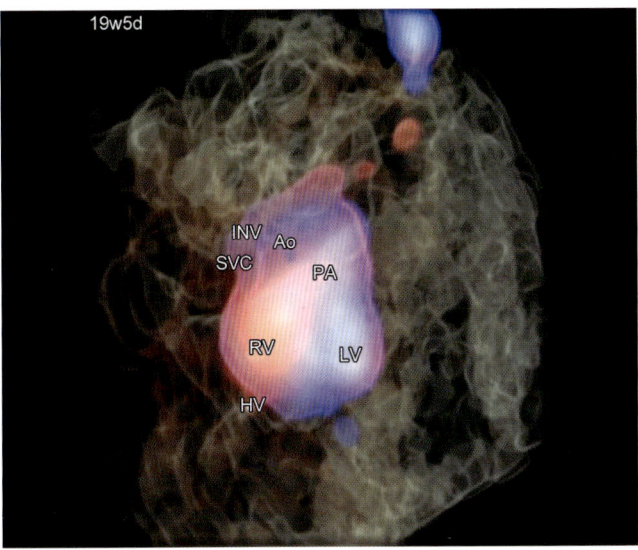

Fig. 11.9: Spatial three-vessel view with HDlive Flow silhouette mode and HDlive silhouette mode of a normal fetal heart at 19 weeks and 5 days of gestation. (Ao: aorta; HV: hepatic vein; INV: innominate vein; LV: left ventricle; PA: pulmonary artery; RV: right ventricle; SVC: superior vena cava)

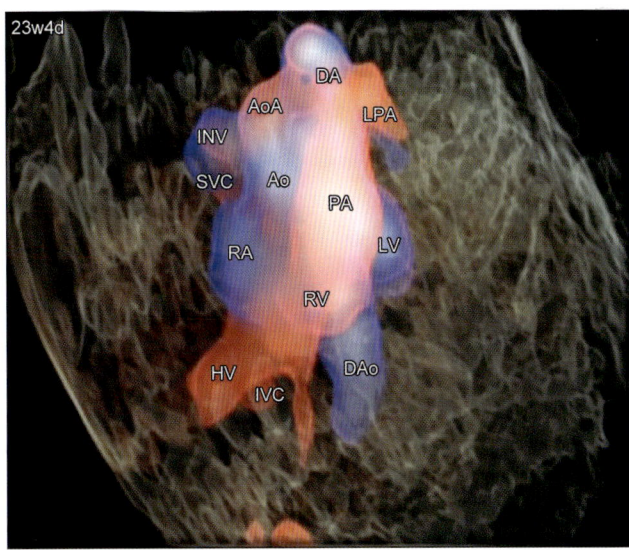

Fig. 11.10: Spatial three-vessel view with HDlive Flow silhouette mode and HDlive silhouette mode of a normal fetal heart at 23 weeks and 4 days of gestation. (Ao: aorta; AoA: aortic arch; DA: ductus arteriosus; DAo: descending aorta; HV: hepatic vein; INV: innominate vein; IVC: inferior vena cava; LPA: left pulmonary artery; LV: left ventricle; PA: pulmonary artery; RA: right atrium; RV: right ventricle; SVC: superior vena cava)

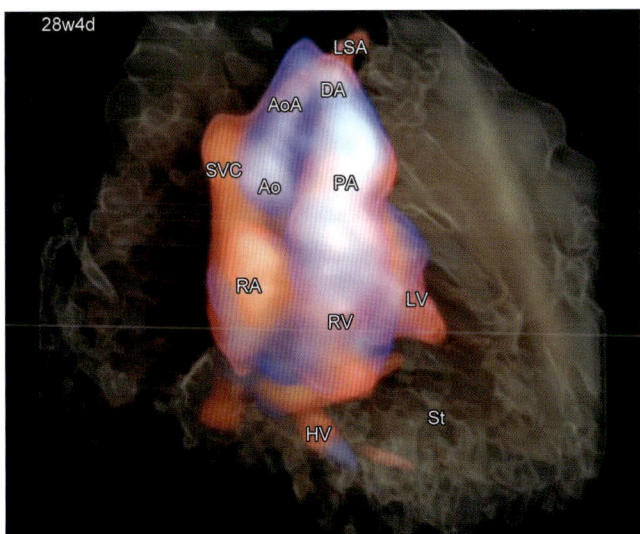

Fig. 11.11: Spatial three-vessel view with HDlive Flow silhouette mode and HDlive silhouette mode of a normal fetal heart at 28 weeks and 4 days of gestation. (Ao: aorta; AoA: aortic arch; DA: ductus arteriosus; HV: hepatic vein; LSA: left subclavian artery; LV: left ventricle; PA: pulmonary artery; RA: right atrium; RV: right ventricle; St: stomach; SVC: superior vena cava)

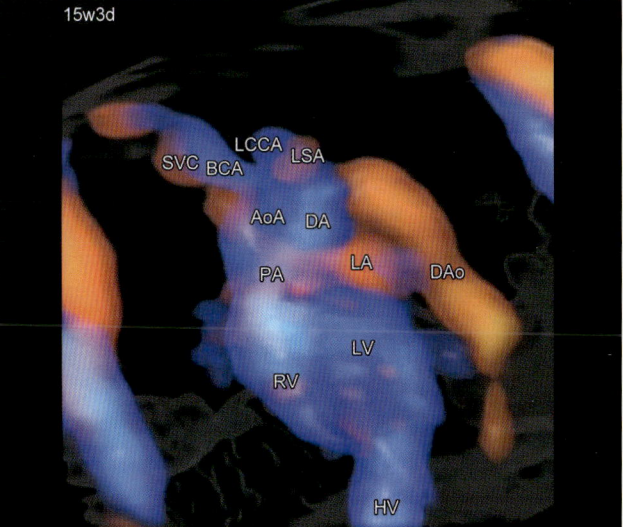

Fig. 11.12: Panoramic view with HDlive Flow silhouette mode and HDlive silhouette mode of a normal fetal heart at 15 weeks and 3 days of gestation. (AoA: aortic arch; BCA: brachiocephalic artery; DA: ductus arteriosus; DAo: descending aorta; HV: hepatic vein; LA: left atrium; LCCA: left common carotid artery; LSA: left subclavian artery; LV: left ventricle; PA: pulmonary artery; RV: right ventricle; SVC: superior vena cava)

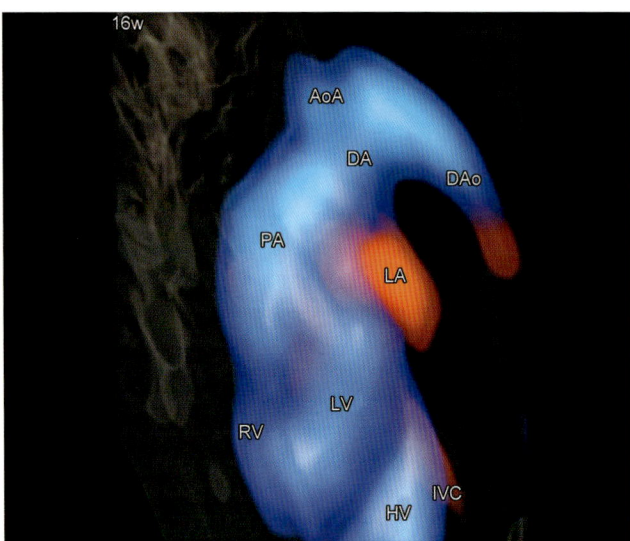

Fig. 11.13: Panoramic view with HDlive Flow silhouette mode and HDlive silhouette mode of a normal fetal heart at 16 weeks of gestation. (AoA: aortic arch; DA: ductus arteriosus; DAo: descending aorta; HV: hepatic vein; IVC: inferior vena cava; LA: left atrium; LV: left ventricle; PA: pulmonary artery; RV: right ventricle)

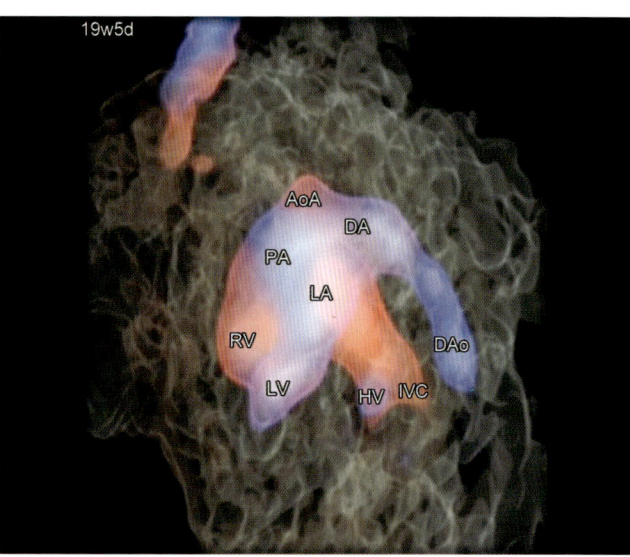

Fig. 11.14: Panoramic view with HDlive Flow silhouette mode and HDlive silhouette mode of a normal fetal heart at 19 weeks and 5 days of gestation. (AoA: aortic arch; DA: ductus arteriosus; DAo: descending aorta; HV: hepatic vein; IVC: inferior vena cava; LA: left atrium; LV: left ventricle; PA: pulmonary artery; RV: right ventricle)

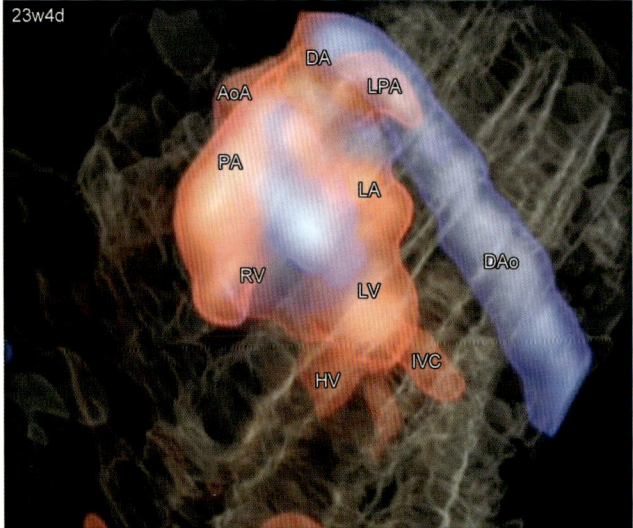

Fig. 11.15: Panoramic view with HDlive Flow silhouette mode and HDlive silhouette mode of a normal fetal heart at 23 weeks and 4 days of gestation. (AoA: aortic arch; DA: ductus arteriosus; DAo: descending aorta; HV: hepatic vein; IVC: inferior vena cava; LA: left atrium; LPA: left pulmonary artery; LV: left ventricle; PA: pulmonary artery; RV: right ventricle)

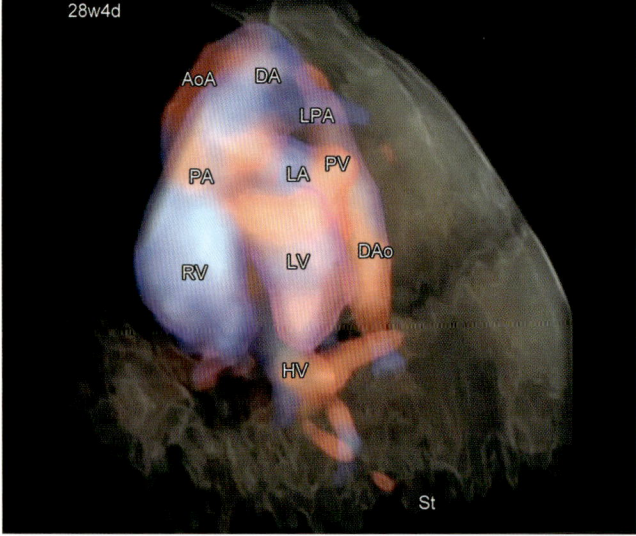

Fig. 11.16: Panoramic view with HDlive Flow silhouette mode and HDlive silhouette mode of a normal fetal heart at 28 weeks and 4 days of gestation. (AoA: aortic arch; DA: ductus arteriosus; DAo: descending aorta; HV: hepatic vein; LA: left atrium; LPA: left pulmonary artery; LV: left ventricle; PA: pulmonary artery; PV: pulmonary vein; RV: right ventricle; St: stomach)

Posterior View

With this view, we can observe the vertical descending aorta, left and right pulmonary arteries, left atrium with pulmonary veins, and right atrium with superior and inferior venae cavae **(Figs. 11.17 to 11.22)**. Conventional two-dimensional (2D) fetal echocardiography cannot provide this view, making it very unique.[37]

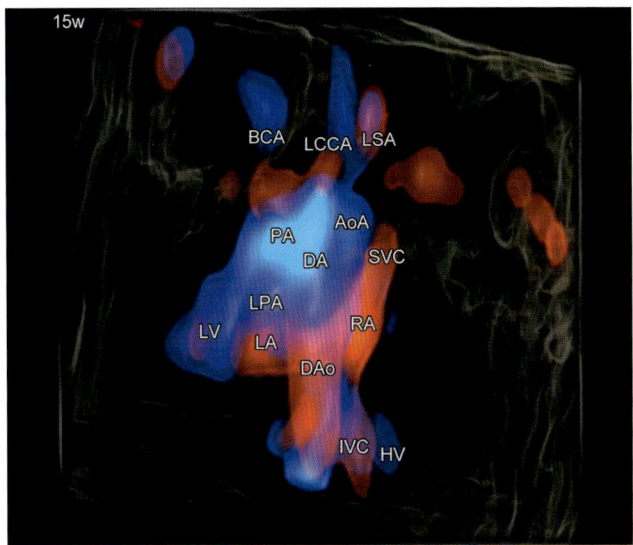

Fig. 11.17: Posterior view with HDlive Flow silhouette mode and HDlive silhouette mode of a normal fetal heart at 15 weeks of gestation. (AoA: aortic arch; BCA: brachiocephalic artery; DA: ductus arteriosus; DAo: descending aorta; HV: hepatic vein; IVC: inferior vena cava; LA: left atrium; LCCA: left common carotid artery; LPA: left pulmonary artery; LSA: left subclavian artery; LV: left ventricle; PA: pulmonary artery; RA: right atrium; RV: right ventricle)

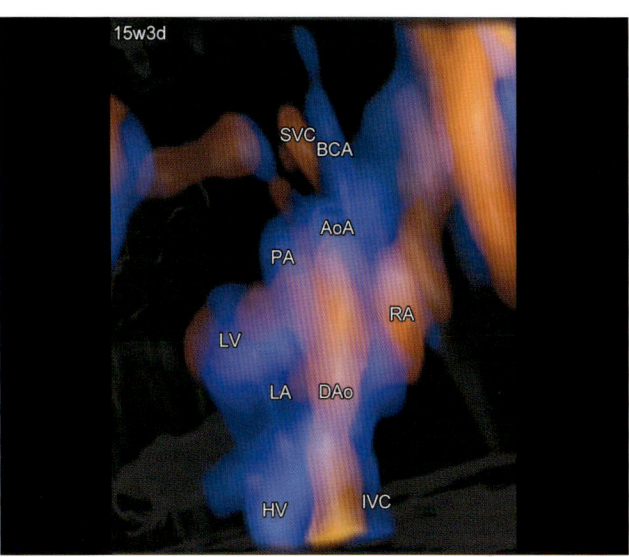

Fig. 11.18: Posterior view with HDlive Flow silhouette mode and HDlive silhouette mode of a normal fetal heart at 15 weeks and 3 days of gestation. (AoA: aortic arch; BCA: brachiocephalic artery; DAo: descending aorta; HV: hepatic vein; IVC: inferior vena cava; LA: left atrium; LV: left ventricle; PA: pulmonary artery; RA: right atrium; SVC: superior vena cava)

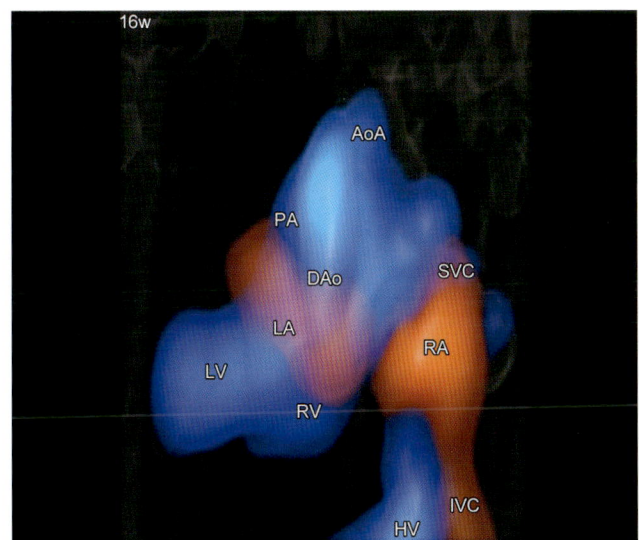

Fig. 11.19: Posterior view with HDlive Flow silhouette mode and HDlive silhouette mode of a normal fetal heart at 16 weeks of gestation. (AoA: aortic arch; DAo: descending aorta; HV: hepatic vein; IVC: inferior vena cava; LA: left atrium; LV: left ventricle; PA: pulmonary artery; RA: right atrium; RV: right ventricle; SVC: superior vena cava)

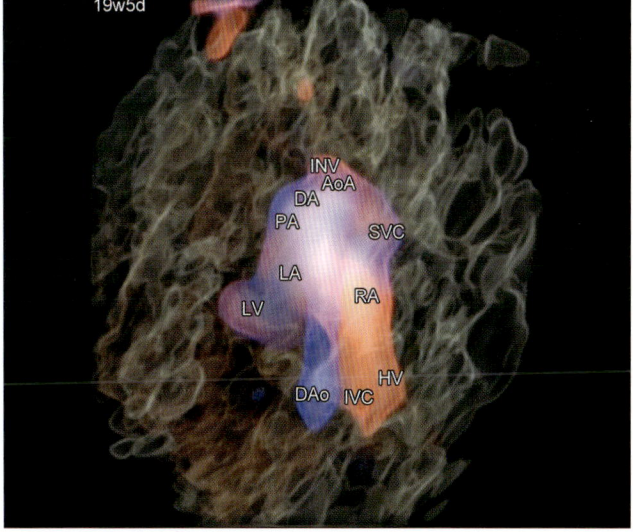

Fig. 11.20: Posterior view with HDlive Flow silhouette mode and HDlive silhouette mode of a normal fetal heart at 19 weeks and 5 days of gestation. (AoA: aortic arch; DA: ductus arteriosus; DAo: descending aorta; HV: hepatic vein; INV: innominate vein; IVC: inferior vena cava; LA: left atrium; LV: left ventricle; PA: pulmonary artery; RA: right atrium; SVC: superior vena cava)

Right Lateral View

With this view, we can identify the aortic arch and descending aorta, superior vena cava, and inferior vena cava **(Figs. 11.23 to 11.27).** In order to evaluate the aortic arch, this view is unique.[37]

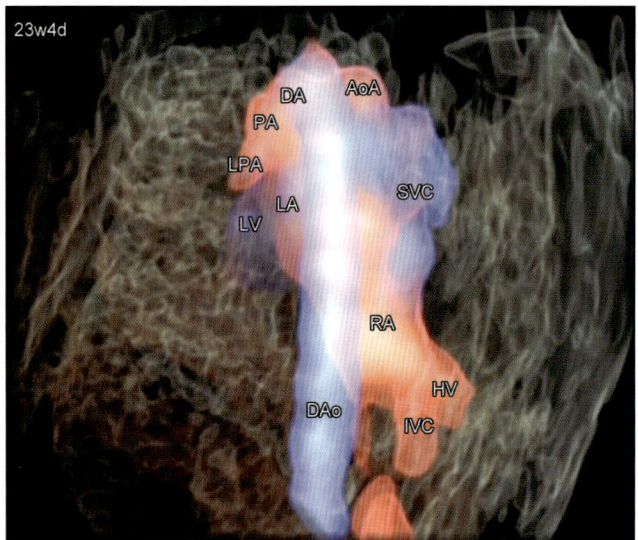

Fig. 11.21: Posterior view with HDlive Flow silhouette mode and HDlive silhouette mode of a normal fetal heart at 23 weeks and 4 days of gestation. (AoA: aortic arch; DA: ductus arteriosus; DAo: descending aorta; HV: hepatic vein; IVC: inferior vena cava; LA: left atrium; LPA: left pulmonary artery; LV: left ventricle; PA: pulmonary artery; RA: right atrium; SVC: superior vena cava)

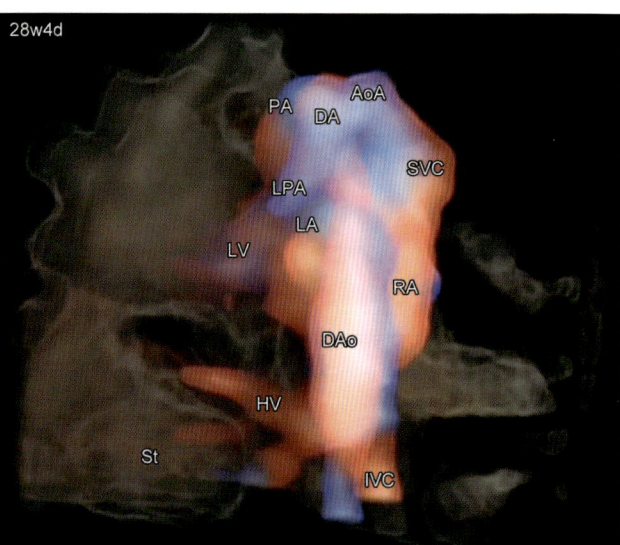

Fig. 11.22: Posterior view with HDlive Flow silhouette mode and HDlive silhouette mode of a normal fetal heart at 28 weeks and 4 days of gestation. (AoA: aortic arch; DA: ductus arteriosus; DAo: descending aorta; HV: hepatic vein; IVC: inferior vena cava; LA: left atrium; LPA: left pulmonary artery; LV: left ventricle; PA: pulmonary artery; RA: right atrium; St: stomach; SVC: superior vena cava)

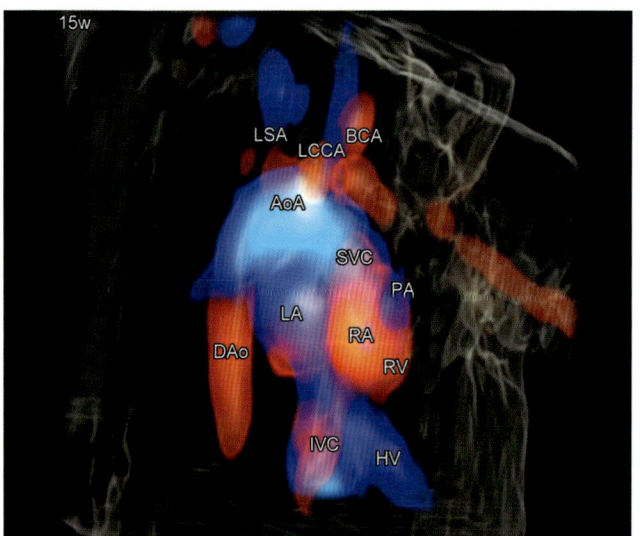

Fig. 11.23: Right lateral view with HDlive Flow silhouette mode and HDlive silhouette mode of a normal fetal heart at 15 weeks of gestation. (AoA: aortic arch; BCA: brachiocephalic artery; DAo: descending aorta; HV: hepatic vein; IVC: inferior vena cava; LA: left atrium; LCCA: left common carotid artery; LSA: left subclavian artery; PA: pulmonary artery; RA: right atrium; RV: right ventricle; SVC: superior vena cava)

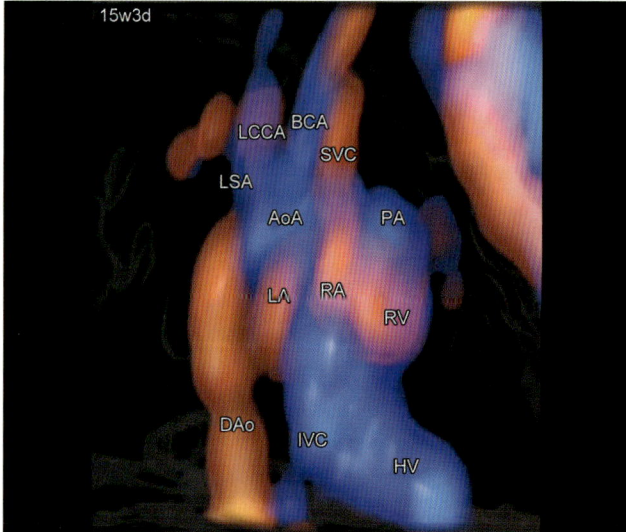

Fig. 11.24: Right lateral view with HDlive Flow silhouette mode and HDlive silhouette mode of a normal fetal heart at 15 weeks and 3 days of gestation. (AoA: aortic arch; BCA: brachiocephalic artery; DAo: descending aorta; HV: hepatic vein; IVC: inferior vena cava; LA: left atrium; LCCA: left common carotid artery; LSA: left subclavian artery; PA: pulmonary artery; RA: right atrium; RV: right ventricle; SVC: superior vena cava)

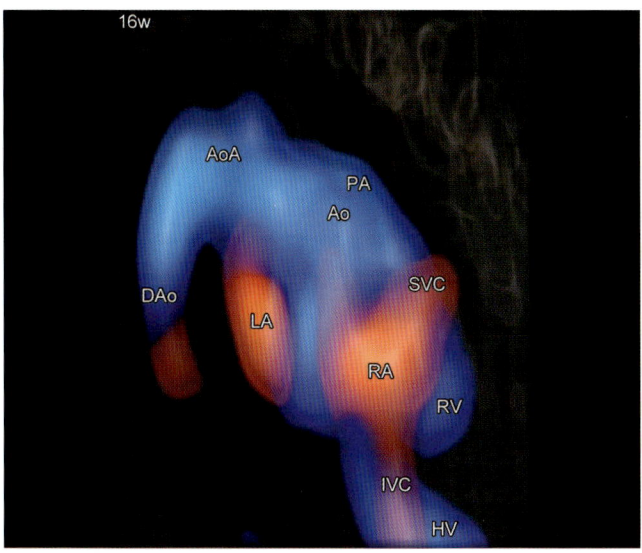

Fig. 11.25: Right lateral view with HDlive Flow silhouette mode and HDlive silhouette mode of a normal fetal heart at 16 weeks of gestation. (Ao: aorta; AoA: aortic arch; DAo: descending aorta; HV: hepatic vein; IVC: inferior vena cava; LA: left atrium; PA: pulmonary artery; RA: right atrium; RV: right ventricle; SVC: superior vena cava)

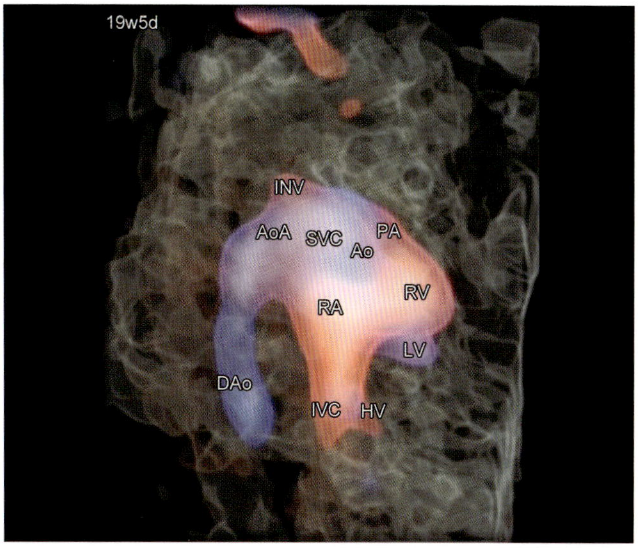

Fig. 11.26: Right lateral view with HDlive Flow silhouette mode and HDlive silhouette mode of a normal fetal heart at 19 weeks and 5 days of gestation. (Ao: aorta; AoA: aortic arch; DAo: descending aorta; HV: hepatic vein; INV: innominate vein; IVC: inferior vena cava; LV: left ventricle; PA: pulmonary artery; RA: right atrium; RV: right ventricle; SVC: superior vena cava)

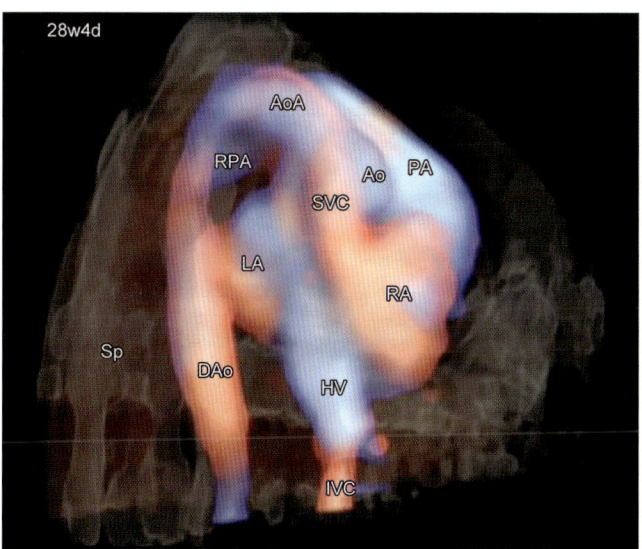

Fig. 11.27: Right lateral view with HDlive Flow silhouette mode and HDlive silhouette mode of a normal fetal heart at 28 weeks and 4 days of gestation. (Ao: aorta; AoA: aortic arch; DAo: descending aorta; HV: hepatic vein; IVC: inferior vena cava; LA: left atrium; PA: pulmonary artery; RA: right atrium; RPA: right pulmonary artery; Sp: spine; SVC: superior vena cava)

STRUCTURAL VARIANT OF THE FETAL HEART

Right Aortic Arch

In the presence of a right aortic arch (RAA) and an aberrant left subclavian artery in a fetus, the five views summarized provide clear visualization of the typical vascular ring of RAA **(Figs. 11.28A to E)**.[37] With a posterior view, the brachiocephalic and left common carotid arteries from

RAA, can be clearly demonstrated along with an aberrant left subclavian artery from the diverticulum of Kommerell **(Fig. 11.28D)**.

Persistent Left Superior Vena Cava

In a fetus with a persistent left superior vena cava (PLSVC), frontal, spatial three-vessel, and panoramic views clearly show the PLSVC on the left side of the pulmonary artery **(Figs. 11.29A to C)**.

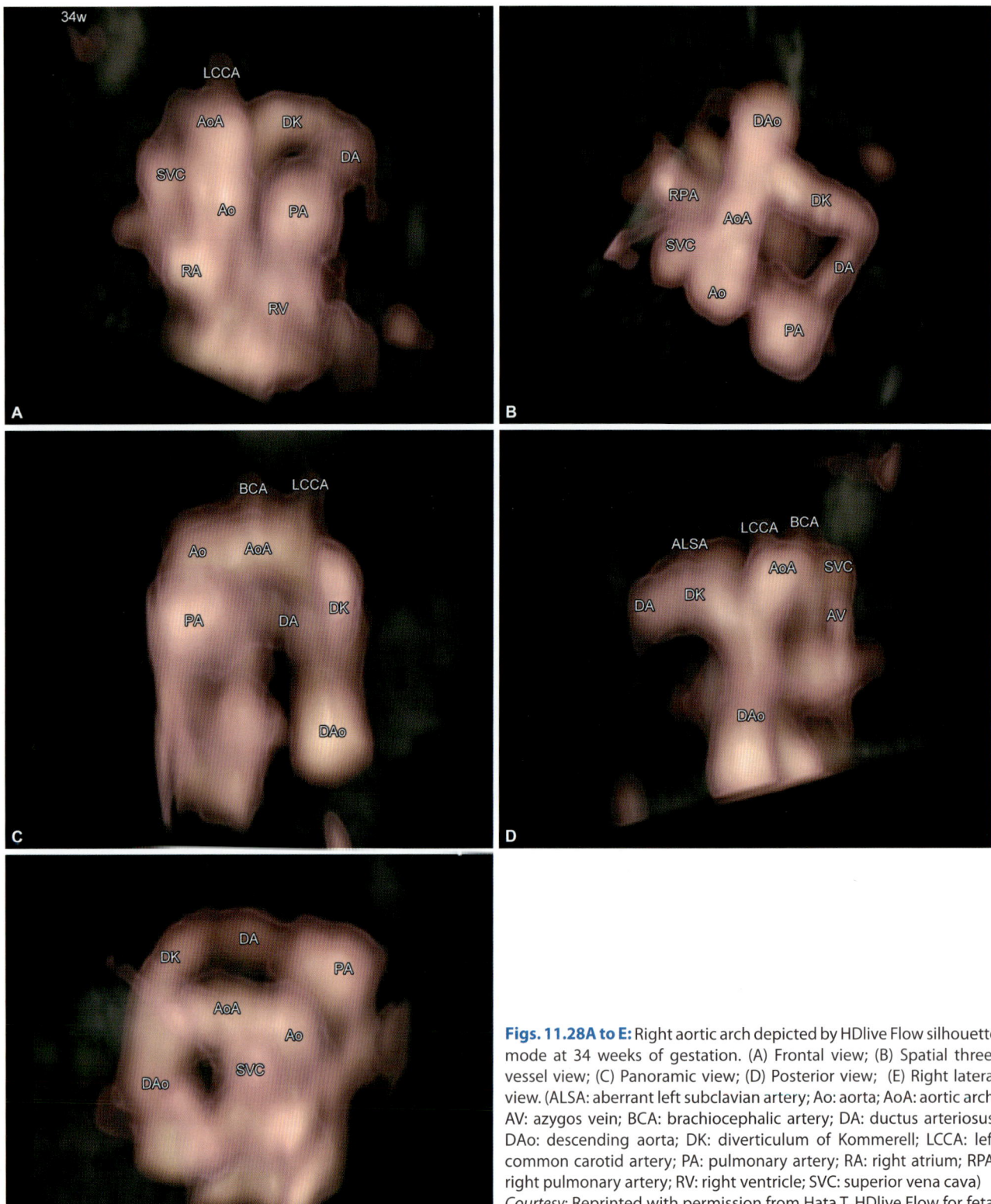

Figs. 11.28A to E: Right aortic arch depicted by HDlive Flow silhouette mode at 34 weeks of gestation. (A) Frontal view; (B) Spatial three-vessel view; (C) Panoramic view; (D) Posterior view; (E) Right lateral view. (ALSA: aberrant left subclavian artery; Ao: aorta; AoA: aortic arch; AV: azygos vein; BCA: brachiocephalic artery; DA: ductus arteriosus; DAo: descending aorta; DK: diverticulum of Kommerell; LCCA: left common carotid artery; PA: pulmonary artery; RA: right atrium; RPA: right pulmonary artery; RV: right ventricle; SVC: superior vena cava)
Courtesy: Reprinted with permission from Hata T. HDlive Flow for fetal heart. In: Sen C, Stanojevic M (Eds). Fetal Heart: Screening, Diagnosis and Intervention. New Delhi: Jaypee Brothers Medical Publishers (P) Ltd; 2018. pp. 200-16.

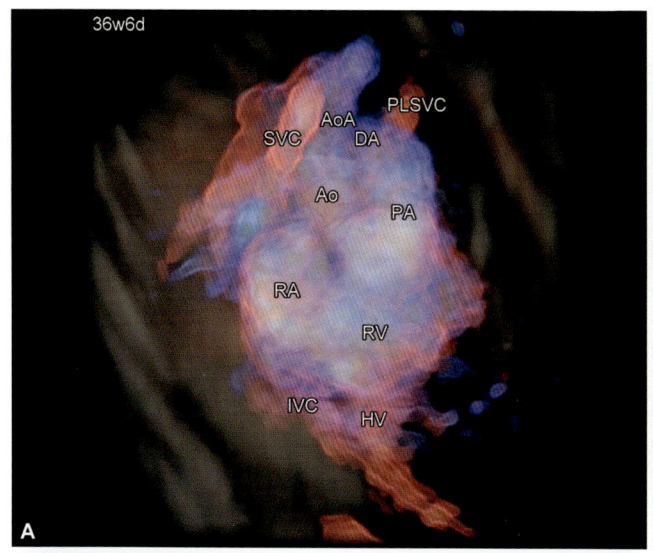

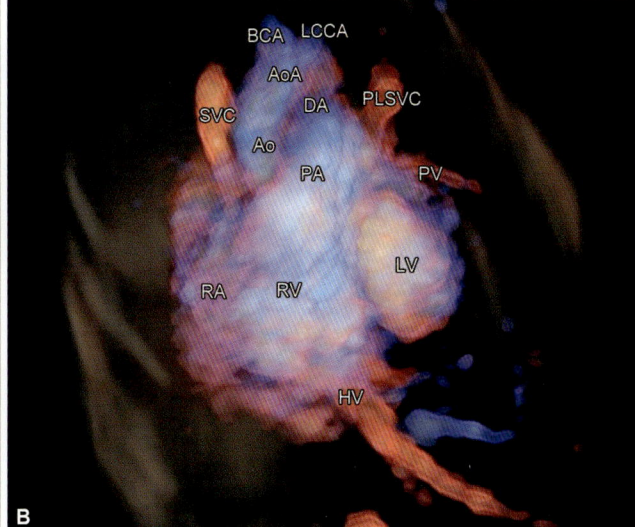

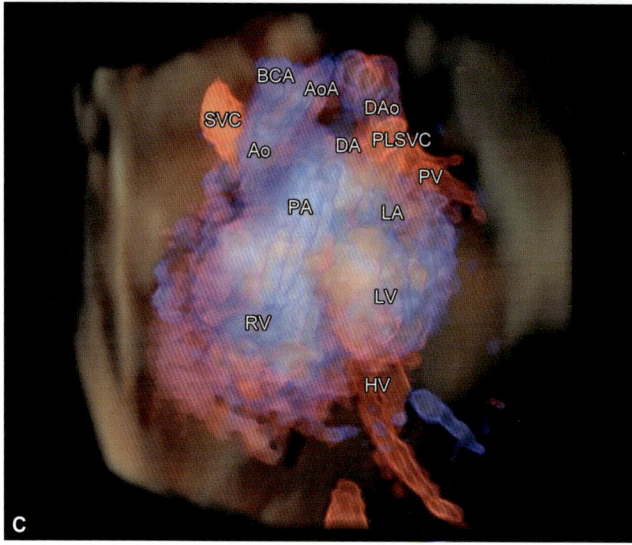

Figs. 11.29A to C: Persistent left superior vena cava (PLSVC) depicted by HDlive Flow silhouette mode with glass-body rendering mode at 36 weeks and 6 days of gestation. (A) Frontal view; (B) Spatial three-vessel view; (C) Panoramic view. (Ao: aorta; AoA: aortic arch; BCA: brachiocephalic artery; DAo: descending aorta; HV: hepatic vein; LA: left atrium; LV: left ventricle; LCCA: left common carotid artery; PA: pulmonary artery; PV: pulmonary vein; RA: right atrium; RV: right ventricle; SVC: superior vena cava)

CONGENITAL HEART ANOMALY

Transposition of the Great Arteries

In a fetus with transposition of the great arteries (TGA) at 32 weeks and 1 day of gestation, HDlive Flow clearly showed the spatial parallel arrangement of the aorta left from the right ventricle and pulmonary artery left from the left ventricle **(Fig. 11.30A)**.[33] Hidden vessels, such as pulmonary veins obscured by cardiac chambers could be observed using the HDlive Flow silhouette mode **(Figs. 11.30B and C)**.

Hypoplastic Left Heart Syndrome

In a fetus with hypoplastic left heart syndrome (HLHS) at 30 weeks and 1 day of gestation, a significant size difference could be noted on a spatial three-vessel view

between the pulmonary artery and aorta **(Figs. 11.31A and B)**.[33] With a panoramic view, a very small ascending aorta and teardrop-shaped heart could also be identified **(Figs. 11.31C and D)**. A difference in size between the aortic arch and descending aorta could also be noted. The mode allowed clear visualization of the contour of the right atrium, right ventricle, pulmonary artery, and small aorta **(Figs. 11.31B and D)**.

Pulmonary Valve Stenosis

In a fetus with pulmonary stenosis (PS) at 31 weeks and 5 days of gestation, HDlive Flow allowed the visualization of a large main pulmonary artery showing poststenotic dilatation **(Fig. 11.32A)**.[33] A holography-like image of the fetal heart with a dilated pulmonary artery and hidden vessels could be obtained with the HDlive Flow silhouette mode **(Fig. 11.32B)**.

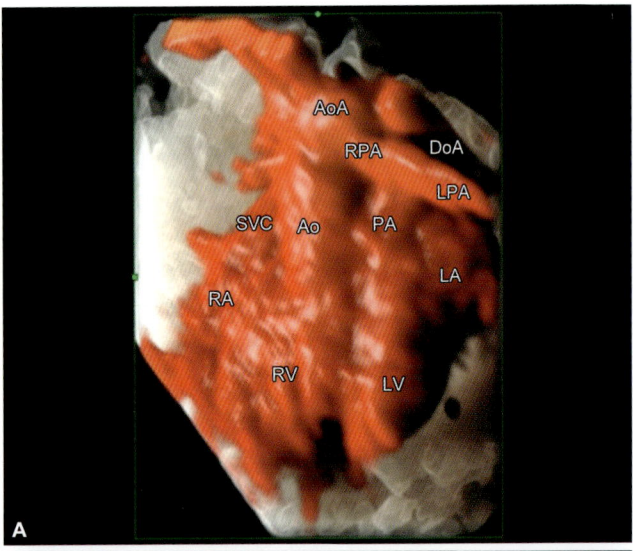

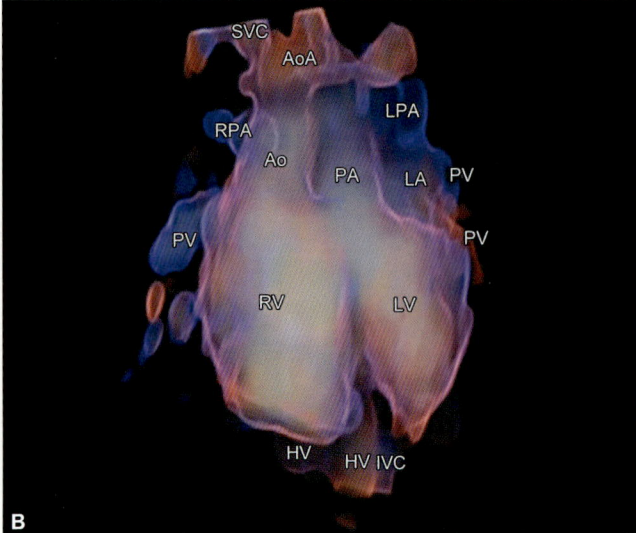

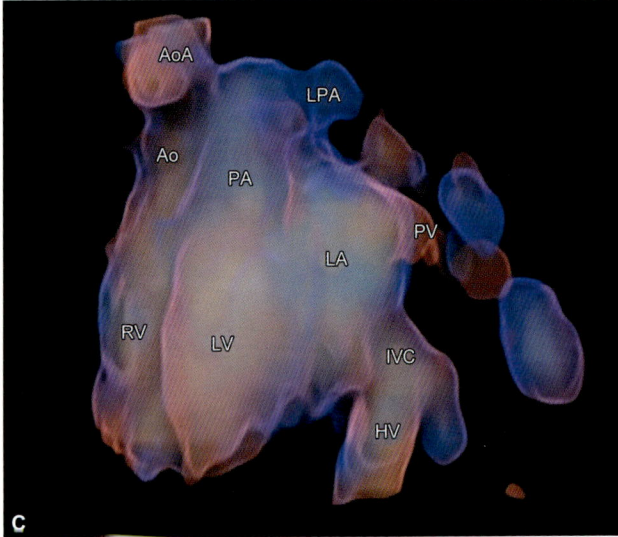

Figs. 11.30A to C: Transposition of great arteries depicted by HDlive Flow with HDlive silhouette mode (A) and HDlive Flow silhouette mode (B and C) at 32 weeks and 1 day of gestation. (A and B) Spatial three-vessel view; (C) Panoramic view. (Ao: aorta; AoA: aortic arch; DAo: descending aorta; HV: hepatic vein; IVC: inferior vena cava; LA: left atrium; LV: left ventricle; LPA: left pulmonary artery; PA: pulmonary artery; PV: pulmonary vein; RA: right atrium; RPA: right pulmonary artery; RV: right ventricle; SVC: superior vena cava)

Courtesy: Reprinted with permission from Ito M, AboEllail MA, Yamamoto K, et al. HDlive Flow silhouette mode and spatiotemporal image correlation for diagnosing congenital heart disease. Ultrasound Obstet Gynecol. 2017;50:411-5.

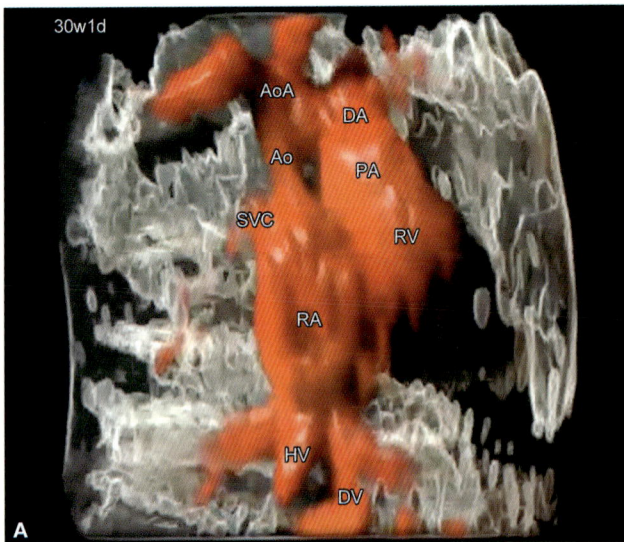

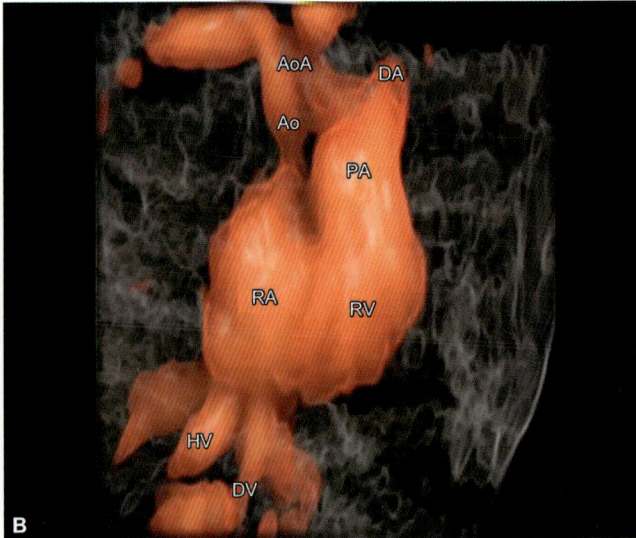

Figs. 11.31A and B

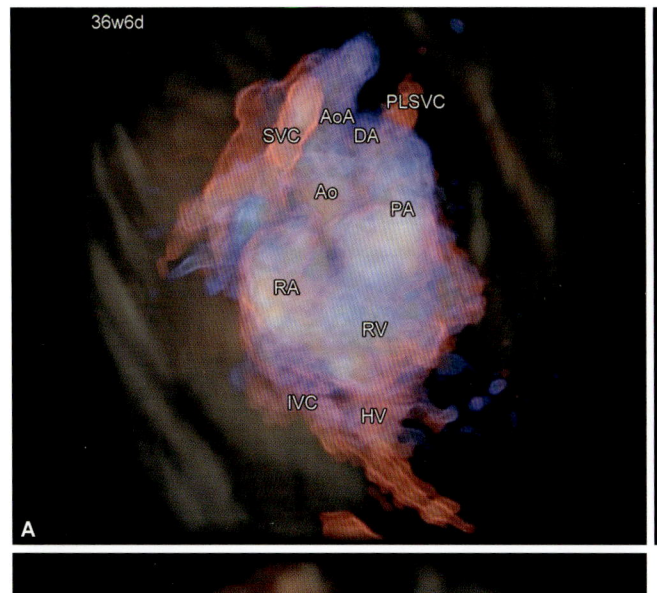

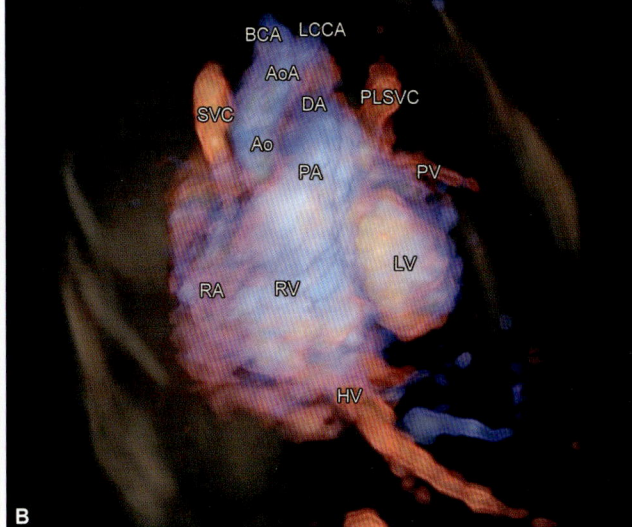

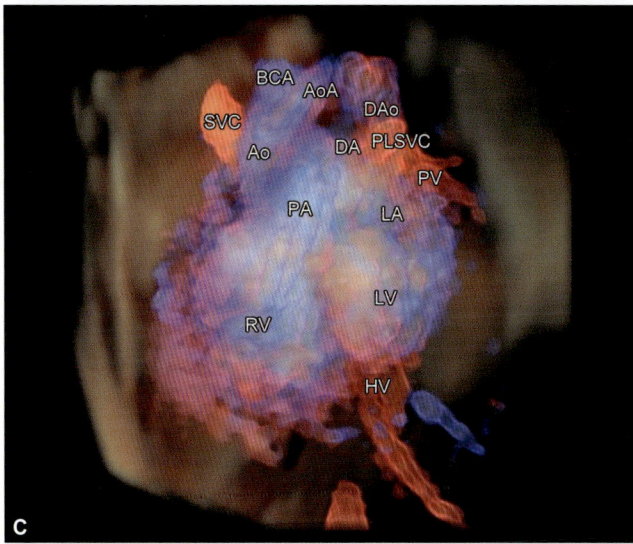

Figs. 11.29A to C: Persistent left superior vena cava (PLSVC) depicted by HDlive Flow silhouette mode with glass-body rendering mode at 36 weeks and 6 days of gestation. (A) Frontal view; (B) Spatial three-vessel view; (C) Panoramic view. (Ao: aorta; AoA: aortic arch; BCA: brachiocephalic artery; DAo: descending aorta; HV: hepatic vein; LA: left atrium; LV: left ventricle; LCCA: left common carotid artery; PA: pulmonary artery; PV: pulmonary vein; RA: right atrium; RV: right ventricle; SVC: superior vena cava)

CONGENITAL HEART ANOMALY

Transposition of the Great Arteries

In a fetus with transposition of the great arteries (TGA) at 32 weeks and 1 day of gestation, HDlive Flow clearly showed the spatial parallel arrangement of the aorta left from the right ventricle and pulmonary artery left from the left ventricle **(Fig. 11.30A)**.[33] Hidden vessels, such as pulmonary veins obscured by cardiac chambers could be observed using the HDlive Flow silhouette mode **(Figs. 11.30B and C)**.

Hypoplastic Left Heart Syndrome

In a fetus with hypoplastic left heart syndrome (HLHS) at 30 weeks and 1 day of gestation, a significant size difference could be noted on a spatial three-vessel view

between the pulmonary artery and aorta **(Figs. 11.31A and B)**.[33] With a panoramic view, a very small ascending aorta and teardrop-shaped heart could also be identified **(Figs. 11.31C and D)**. A difference in size between the aortic arch and descending aorta could also be noted. The mode allowed clear visualization of the contour of the right atrium, right ventricle, pulmonary artery, and small aorta **(Figs. 11.31B and D)**.

Pulmonary Valve Stenosis

In a fetus with pulmonary stenosis (PS) at 31 weeks and 5 days of gestation, HDlive Flow allowed the visualization of a large main pulmonary artery showing poststenotic dilatation **(Fig. 11.32A)**.[33] A holography-like image of the fetal heart with a dilated pulmonary artery and hidden vessels could be obtained with the HDlive Flow silhouette mode **(Fig. 11.32B)**.

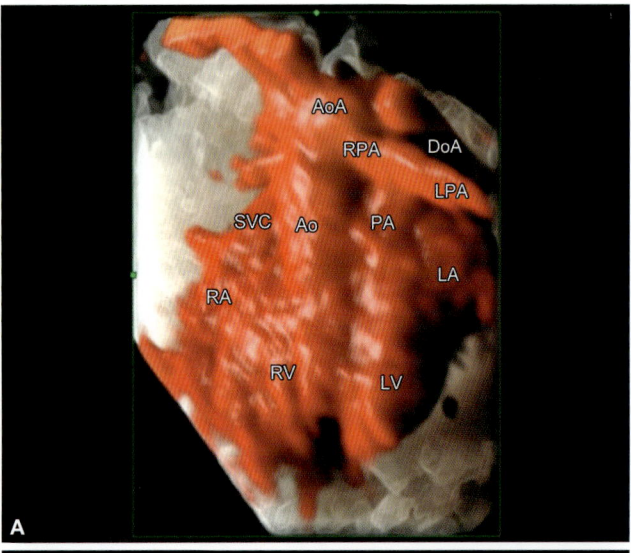

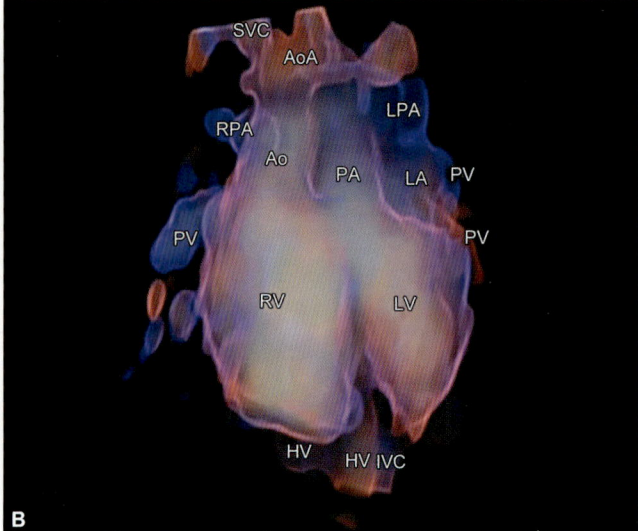

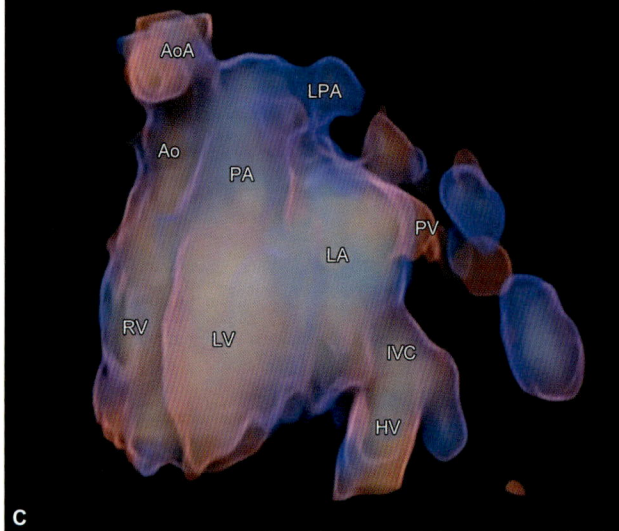

Figs. 11.30A to C: Transposition of great arteries depicted by HDlive Flow with HDlive silhouette mode (A) and HDlive Flow silhouette mode (B and C) at 32 weeks and 1 day of gestation. (A and B) Spatial three-vessel view; (C) Panoramic view. (Ao: aorta; AoA: aortic arch; DAo: descending aorta; HV: hepatic vein; IVC: inferior vena cava; LA: left atrium; LV: left ventricle; LPA: left pulmonary artery; PA: pulmonary artery; PV: pulmonary vein; RA: right atrium; RPA: right pulmonary artery; RV: right ventricle; SVC: superior vena cava)

Courtesy: Reprinted with permission from Ito M, AboEllail MA, Yamamoto K, et al. HDlive Flow silhouette mode and spatiotemporal image correlation for diagnosing congenital heart disease. Ultrasound Obstet Gynecol. 2017;50:411-5.

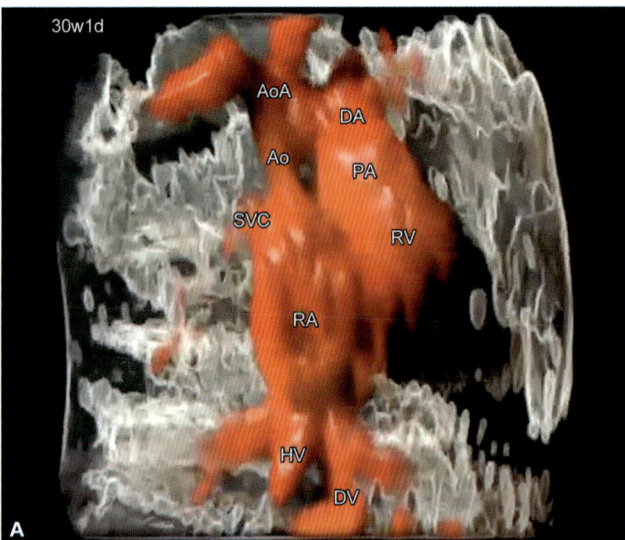

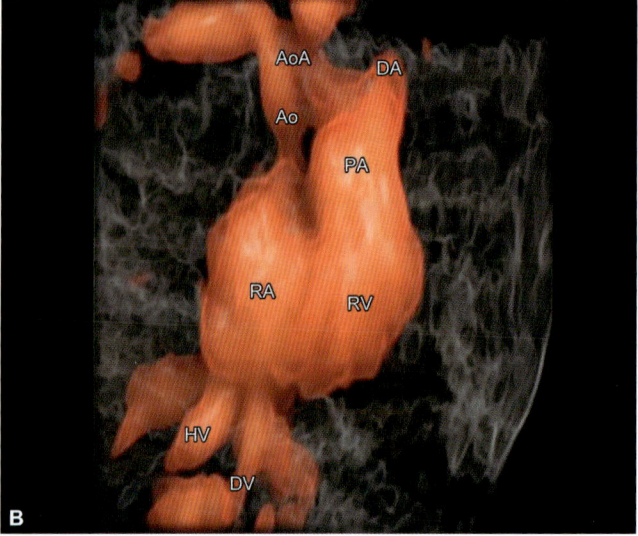

Figs. 11.31A and B

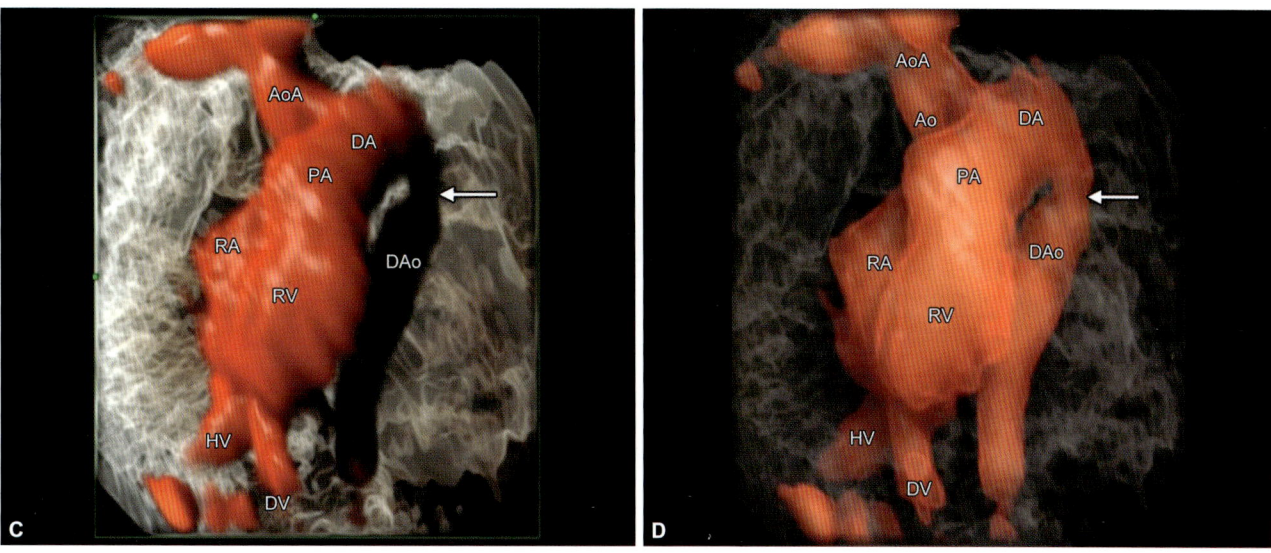

Figs. 11.31C and D

Figs. 11.31A to D: Hypoplastic left heart syndrome depicted by HDlive Flow with HDlive silhouette mode (A and C) and HDlive Flow silhouette mode with HDlive silhouette mode (B and D) at 30 weeks and 1 day of gestation. Arrow indicates isthmus (C and D). (A and B) Spatial three-vessel view; (C and D) Panoramic view. (Ao: aorta; AoA: aortic arch; DA: ductus arteriosus; DAo: descending aorta; DV: ductus venosus; HV: hepatic vein; PA: pulmonary artery; RA: right atrium; RV: right ventricle; SVC: superior vena cava)
Courtesy: Reprinted with permission from Ito M, AboEllail MA, Yamamoto K, et al. HDlive Flow silhouette mode and spatiotemporal image correlation for diagnosing congenital heart disease. Ultrasound Obstet Gynecol. 2017;50:411-5.

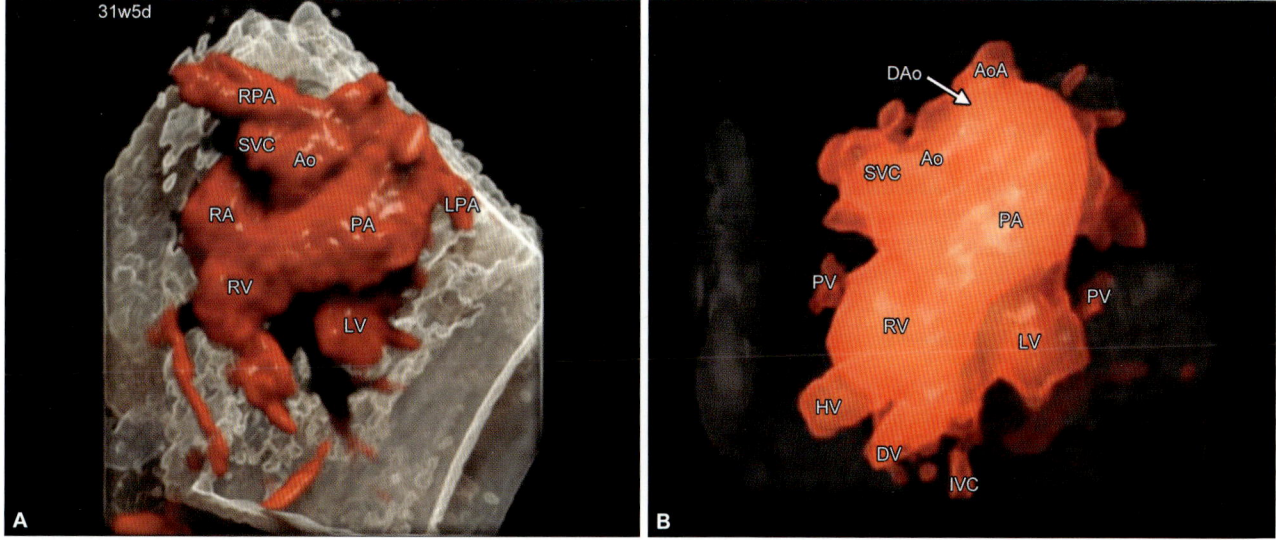

Figs. 11.32A and B: Pulmonary valve stenosis depicted by HDlive Flow with HDlive silhouette mode (A) and HDlive Flow silhouette mode (B) at 31 weeks and 5 days of gestation. (A and B) Spatial three-vessel view. (Ao: aorta; AoA: aortic arch; DAo: descending aorta; DV: ductus venosus; HV: hepatic vein; IVC: inferior vena cava; LV: left ventricle; LPA: left pulmonary artery; PA: pulmonary artery; PV: pulmonary vein; RA: right atrium; RPA: right pulmonary artery; RV: right ventricle; SVC: superior vena cava)
Courtesy: Reprinted with permission from Ito M, AboEllail MA, Yamamoto K, et al. HDlive Flow silhouette mode and spatiotemporal image correlation for diagnosing congenital heart disease. Ultrasound Obstet Gynecol. 2017;50:411-5.

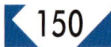
CONCLUSION

The HDlive Flow and HDlive Flow silhouette mode with spatiotemporal image correlation (STIC) may be more readily usable by inexperienced physicians to accurately diagnose normal fetal cardiac structures and congenital heart anomalies. This system's usefulness may also be evident when explaining abnormalities to doctors and students in the absence of patients. It is also straight-forward for parents and families to understand the conditions of fetuses in utero. HDlive Flow and the HDlive Flow silhouette mode provide families with important information, and their application as an adjunctive tool to conventional 2D fetal echocardiography to diagnose congenital heart anomalies may be possible. In clinical practice, to assess the normal fetal heart and congenital heart anomalies, HDlive Flow and the HDlive Flow silhouette mode may become significant.[37]

Conflict of interest: The authors have no conflict of interest.

REFERENCES

1. Hata T, Hanaoka U, Tenkumo C, et al. Three- and four-dimensional HDlive rendering images of normal and abnormal fetuses: pictorial essay. Arch Gynecol Obstet. 2012;286:1431-5.
2. Hata T, Mashima M, Ito M, et al. Three-dimensional HDlive rendering images of the fetal heart. Ultrasound Med Biol. 2013;39:1513-7.
3. Tanaka T, Ito M, Uketa E, et al. Antenatal three-dimensional sonographic features of multicystic dysplastic kidney. J Med Ultrasonics. 2012;40:181-3.
4. Hata T, Uketa E, Tenkumo C, et al. Three- and four-dimensional HDlive rendering image of fetal acrania/exencephaly in early pregnancy. J Med Ultrasonics. 2012;40:271-3.
5. Tenkumo C, Tanaka H, Ito M, et al. Three-dimensional HDlive rendering images of the TRAP sequence in the first trimester: Reverse end-diastolic umbilical artery velocity in a pump twin with an adverse pregnancy outcome. J Med Ultrasonics. 2012;40:293-6.
6. Hata T, Hanaoka U, Tenkumo C, et al. Three-dimensional HDlive rendering image of cystic hygroma. J Med Ultrasonics. 2012;40:297-9.
7. Hata T, Hanaoka U, Mashima M, et al. Four-dimensional HDlive rendering image of fetal facial expression: a pictorial essay. J Med Ultrasonics. 2013;40:437-41.
8. Hata T. HDlive rendering image at 6 weeks of gestation. J Med Ultrasonics. 2013;40:495-6.
9. Hata T, Hanaoka U, Mashima M. HDlive rendering image of cyclopia and a proboscis in a fetus with normal chromosomes at 32 weeks of gestation. J Med Ultrasonics. 2014;41:109-10.
10. Hanaoka U, Tanaka H, Koyano K, et al. HDlive imaging of the face of fetuses with autosomal trisomies. J Med Ultrasonics. 2014;41:339-42.
11. Nishizawa C, Mashima M, Mori N, et al. HDlive imaging of fetal enteric duplication cyst. J Med Ultrasonics. 2014;41:511-4.
12. Hata T, Kanenishi K, Hanaoka U, et al. HDlive of the fetal heart. Donald School J Ultrasound Obstet Gynecol. 2014;8:266-72.
13. Hata T, Hanaoka U, Uematsu R, et al. HDlive in the assessment of fetal facial abnormalities. Donald School J Ultrasound Obstet Gynecol. 2014;8:344-52.
14. Cajusay-Velasco S, Hata T. HDlive in the assessment of fetal intra-cranial, intra-thoracic, and intra-abdominal anomalies. Donald School J Ultrasound Obstet Gynecol. 2014;8:362-75.
15. AboEllail MA, Hanaoka U, Mashima M, et al. HDlive image of fetal endocardial cushion defect. Donald School J Ultrasound Obstet Gynecol. 2014;8:437-9.
16. AboEllail MA, Tanaka H, Mori N, et al. HDlive image of meconium peritonitis. Ultrasound Obstet Gynecol. 2015;45:494-6.
17. AboEllail MA, Hanaoka U, Numoto A, et al. HDlive image of giant fetal hemangioma. J Ultrasound Med. 2015;34:2315-8.
18. AboEllail MA, Kanenishi K, Mori N, et al. HDlive image of circumvallate placenta. Ultrasound Obstet Gynecol. 2015;46:513-4.
19. AboEllail MA, Kanenishi K, Marumo G, et al. Fetal HDlive silhouette mode in clinical practice. Donald School J Ultrasound Obstet Gynecol. 2015;9:413-9.
20. AboEllail MA, Tanaka H, Mori N, et al. HDlive silhouette mode in antenatal diagnosis of jejunal atresia. Ultrasound Obstet Gynecol. 2016;48:131-2.
21. Hata T, AboEllail MA, Sajapala S, et al. HDlive silhouette mode with spatiotemporal correlation for assessment of the fetal heart. J Ultrasound Med. 2016;35:1489-95.
22. Hata T, Kanenishi K, Mori N, et al. Four-dimensional color Doppler reconstruction of the fetal heart with glass-body rendering mode. Am J Cardiol. 2014;114:1603-6.
23. AboEllail MA, Kanenishi K, Tenkumo C, et al. Diagnosis of truncus arteriosus in first trimester of pregnancy using transvaginal four-dimensional color Doppler ultrasound. Ultrasound Obstet Gynecol. 2015;45:759-60.
24. Hata T, AboEllail MA, Sajapala S, et al. HDlive Flow in the assessment of fetal circulation. Donald School J Ultrasound Obstet Gynecol. 2015;9:462-70.
25. Yamamoto K, AboEllail MA, Ito M, et al. HDlive imaging in diagnosis of uterine artery pseudoaneurysm during pregnancy. Ultrasound Obstet Gynecol. 2016;48:125-8.
26. Sajapala S, AboEllail MA, Tanaka T, et al. Three-dimensional power Doppler with silhouette mode for diagnosis of malignant ovarian tumors. Ultrasound Obstet Gynecol. 2016;48:806-8.

27. AboEllail MA, Ishimura M, Sajapala S, et al. Three-dimensional color/power Doppler sonography and HDlive silhouette mode for diagnosis of molar pregnancy. J Ultrasound Med. 2016;35:2049-52.

28. Tanaka T, AboEllail MA, Ishimura M, et al. HDlive Flow with HDlive silhouette mode for diagnosis of malignant tumors of uterine cervix. Donald School J Ultrasound Obstet Gynecol. 2016;10:409-12.

29. Yang PY, Kanenishi K, Ishibashi M, et al. HDlive Flow with HDlive silhouette mode in antenatal diagnosis of bilobed placenta. Donald School J Ultrasound Obstet Gynecol. 2016;10:415-7.

30. Yang PY, Sajapala S, Yamamoto K, et al. Antenatal diagnosis of idiopathic dilatation of fetal pulmonary artery with 3D power Doppler imaging. J Clin Ultrasound. 2017;45:121-3.

31. Yamamoto K, AboEllail MA, Ishimura M, et al. HDlive silhouette inversion mode in diagnosis of complete hydatidiform mole. J Ultrasound Med. 2017;36:833-5.

32. Tenkumo C, Hanaoka U, AboEllail MA, et al. HDlive Flow with HDlive silhouette mode in diagnosis of fetal hepatic hemangioma. Ultrasound Obstet Gynecol. 2017;49:540-5.

33. Ito M, AboEllail MA, Yamamoto K, et al. HDlive Flow silhouette mode and spatiotemporal image correlation for diagnosing congenital heart disease. Ultrasound Obstet Gynecol. 2017;50:411-5.

34. Hata T, Kanenishi K, Tanaka T, et al. HDlive Flow silhouette mode for the diagnosis of uterine sarcoma. Donald School J Ultrasound Obstet Gynecol. 2017;11:259-60.

35. Tenkumo C, Kanenishi K, AboEllail MA, et al. HDlive Flow silhouette mode for the diagnosis of uterine enhanced myometrial vascularity/arteriovenous malformations. J Med Ultrasonics. 2018;45:349-52.

36. Hata T, Ito M, Nitta E, et al. HDlive Flow silhouette mode for diagnosis of ectopia cordis with a left ventricular diverticulum at 15 weeks' gestation. J Ultrasound Med. 2018;37:2465-7.

37. Hata T. HDlive Flow for fetal heart. In: Sen C, Stanojevic M (Eds). Fetal Heart: Screening, Diagnosis and Intervention. New Delhi: Jaypee Brothers Medical Publishers (P) Ltd; 2018. pp. 200-16.

38. Hata T, Kanenishi K, Nitta E, et al. HDlive Flow with HDlive silhouette mode in diagnosis of molar pregnancy. Ultrasound Obstet Gynecol. 2018;52:552-4.

Three-dimensional Ultrasound Imaging in the Diagnosis of Ectopic Pregnancy

Ulrich Honemeyer

INTRODUCTION

Ectopic pregnancy (EP) has remained a major cause of maternal morbidity and mortality. The incidence of EPs, denominated as the number of EPs per 1,000 pregnancies, it varies from 6.4 to 20.7.[1-3] EP is diagnosed in 6–16% of women seeking help in emergency departments with bleeding and/or pain in the first trimester.[4]

Reflecting the impact of socioeconomic factors on public healthcare, mortality rates of EP could be reduced by 50% in industrialized countries; while EP still remains a leading cause of maternal death in Africa and Asia.[5,6] In 2009, an EP mortality ratio of 0.48 per 100,000 live births (0.08% of 100 EP) was established for the USA,[3] compared with 1.4–2.79% in Nigeria and Ghana, probably resulting from delayed diagnosis and treatment.[7] The lack of research productivity concerning EP in low-income countries and their missing presence in international scientific working groups in the field[8] is another indirect sign that advances in diagnosis and management leading to earlier detection and better treatment of EP have reached developing countries only in urban areas. These advances include the serum beta-human chorionic gonadotropin (hCG) pregnancy test, transvaginal sonography (TVS) imaging, minimal invasive laparoscopic surgery, chemotherapy with methotrexate, and interventional radiology with uterine artery embolization (UAE).

To date, transvaginal sonography with high-resolution probes is an indispensable tool in any early pregnancy unit. One of its purposes there is to evaluate the spatial relationship of a suspicious mass—possibly representing an EP—to the inner genital organs, which is often difficult for nondynamic imaging such as computed tomography (CT) and magnetic resonance imaging (MRI). In contrast, TVS as a tool for "dynamic" investigation of structures within the pelvis can visualize whether the suspicious mass moves together or independently of ovary or uterus (sliding sign), by exerting gentle pressure with the tip of the ultrasound probe. Furthermore, with the tip of the TVS probe located in the topographic center of the pelvis/region of interest (ROI), image quality benefits from the ability to use close-range high frequencies with optimal resolution and image quality. Thirdly, TVS with color-, power-, and high-definition (HD) flow Doppler technology is able to show increased blood flow in the ROI and to detect typical trophoblast flow characterized by low resistance indices and low velocities, with peak systolic velocity (PSV) greater at and above 20 cm/s and pulsatility index (PI) lower than 1.[9]

With serum beta-hCG levels of 0–750 U/L at 1 week before the first missed period, and 200–7,000 U/L at 1 week after the first missed period, the threshold for sonographic visibility of the trophoblast is usually reached as early as 5 weeks after the last menstrual period (LMP).[10]

The term "visibility threshold" refers to visualization of an intrauterine trophoblast using TVS, which is achievable transvaginally already at a serum beta-hCG of 1,400 mIU/mL, versus 4,500 mIU/mL with transabdominal ultrasound (TUS) probes (**Fig. 12.1**).

Given all these improvements, modern TVS has led to a diagnostic paradigm change from "negative for intrauterine gestational sac (GS)" or "pregnancy of unknown location (PUL)", to a high percentage of positive identification of the site of the EP. High-resolution TVS is able to visualize 75% of all EPs during the first assessment, and even 87–99% of tubal EPs.[11] Last but not least, transvaginal three-dimensional (3D) ultrasound has created another diagnostic platform, with identification of new, equally efficient ways of diagnosing EP.

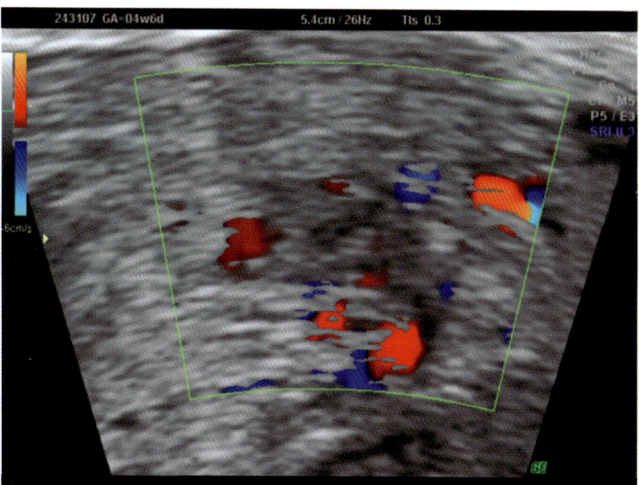

Fig. 12.1: B-mode color Doppler zoom of endometrium at 2 weeks postconception. Visualization of early intervillous trophoblast flow.

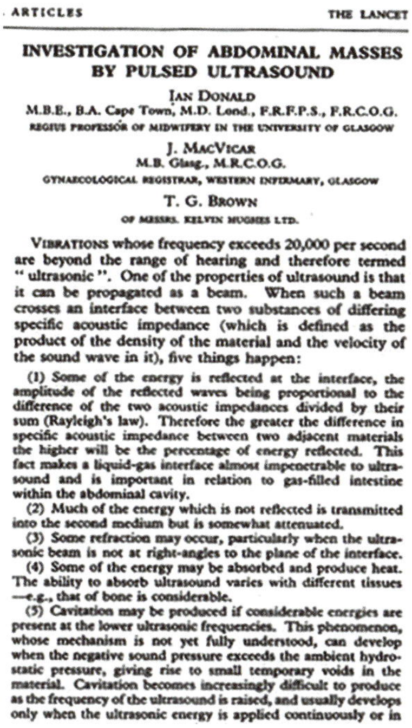

· ARTICLES   THE LANCET

INVESTIGATION OF ABDOMINAL MASSES BY PULSED ULTRASOUND

IAN DONALD
M.B.E., B.A. Cape Town, M.D. Lond., F.R.F.P.S., F.R.C.O.G.
REGIUS PROFESSOR OF MIDWIFERY IN THE UNIVERSITY OF GLASGOW

J. MacVICAR
M.B. Glasg., M.R.C.O.G.
GYNAECOLOGICAL REGISTRAR, WESTERN INFIRMARY, GLASGOW

T. G. BROWN
OF MESSRS. KELVIN HUGHES LTD.

VIBRATIONS whose frequency exceeds 20,000 per second are beyond the range of hearing and therefore termed "ultrasonic". One of the properties of ultrasound is that it can be propagated as a beam. When such a beam crosses an interface between two substances of differing specific acoustic impedance (which is defined as the product of the density of the material and the velocity of the sound wave in it), five things happen:

(1) Some of the energy is reflected at the interface, the amplitude of the reflected waves being proportional to the difference of the two acoustic impedances divided by their sum (Rayleigh's law). Therefore the greater the difference in specific acoustic impedance between two adjacent materials the higher will be the percentage of energy reflected. This fact makes a liquid-gas interface almost impenetrable to ultrasound and is important in relation to gas-filled intestine within the abdominal cavity.

(2) Much of the energy which is not reflected is transmitted into the second medium but is somewhat attenuated.

(3) Some refraction may occur, particularly when the ultrasonic beam is not at right-angles to the plane of the interface.

(4) Some of the energy may be absorbed and produce heat. The ability to absorb ultrasound varies with different tissues —e.g., that of bone is considerable.

(5) Cavitation may be produced if considerable energies are present at the lower ultrasonic frequencies. This phenomenon, whose mechanism is not yet fully understood, can develop when the negative sound pressure exceeds the ambient hydrostatic pressure, giving rise to small temporary voids in the material. Cavitation becomes increasingly difficult to produce as the frequency of the ultrasound is raised, and usually develops only when the ultrasonic energy is applied continuously or in

Fig. 12.2: First obstetrics and gynecology ultrasound publication in "The Lancet" by professor Ian Donald in 1958.

HISTORY

The first successful treatment of tubal pregnancy with salpingectomy was described in 1884 by Robert Lawson Tait (1845–1899).[12] As a result of improvements of surgical techniques, changing the approach from open salpingectomy to laparoscopy,[13,14] technological innovations in the field of ultrasonography **(Fig. 12.2)**[15-17] and biochemistry with the production of an antiserum highly specific to the P-subunit of hCG,[18] mortality rates could be reduced from 72%–90% in 1880 to 0.14% in 1990,[19,20] and this in spite of a sixfold increase of EP numbers for example in the US between 1970 and 1992.[21]

The increasing incidence of EP has to be attributed mainly to the following factors: more common pelvic inflammatory disease (PID) with tubal damage as a result of spreading chlamydia salpingitis,[22] ever-rising popularity of cesarean section,[23] and general availability and usage of assisted reproduction techniques.[24] Most tellingly, one of the first in vitro fertilization (IVF) attempts in history in 1976 resulted in an EP.[25]

ECTOPIC PREGNANCY LOCATIONS

The sites of EP can be divided into two groups—96% of EPs are found in the fallopian tubes, named after the 16th century Italian anatomist Gabriele Fallopio. The remaining 4% of EPs include uterine, ovarian, and abdominal locations.[26] It is this small group of nonfallopian EPs which is mainly responsible for morbidity and mortality— the mortality rate for interstitial pregnancy for example

was found to be 15 times higher than the mortality rate of tubal ectopic.[27]

TUBAL ECTOPIC PREGNANCY

The great majority of EPs (96%) implant within the fallopian tube. In 1,800 surgically treated cases, the distribution along the tube was found to be the following: 70% in the ampulla, 12% in the isthmus, and 11.1% fimbrial **(Fig. 12.3)**.[26] Other than the uterus, the fallopian tube has limitations of both vascularization and compliance, which explains that tubal ectopic pregnancies (TEPs) have a lower percentage of viable embryos and rupture earlier, at 6–8 weeks after the LMP, than uterine EPs (12–16 weeks). Under normal circumstances, the tube cannot be visualized by ultrasound. If, however, the tube is dilated by an ectopic trophoblast, this section of the tube becomes visible, and trophoblast flow can be demonstrated using color Doppler. In 70–85% of cases, corpus luteum and TEP are ipsilateral **(Figs. 12.4A to D)**.

The best approach to identification of the ectopic trophoblast is therefore visualization of the ovaries and determination of the site of the corpus luteum. The next step consists in careful exploration of the surroundings of the ovary containing the corpus luteum, looking for an adjacent inhomogeneous mass. Once this mass is seen, gentle pressure with the tip of the probe on the structures between ovary and the mass can provide knowledge whether or not the mass and the ovary are connected

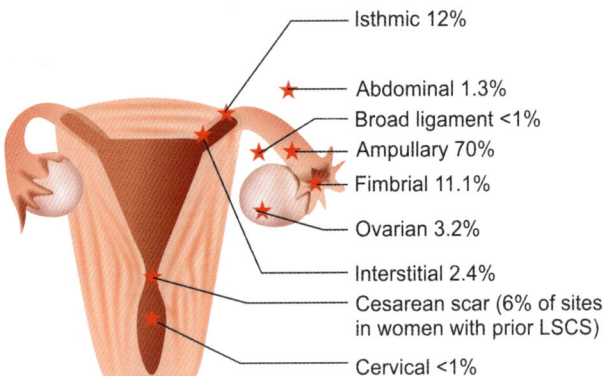

Fig. 12.3: Ectopic pregnancy sites and their distribution. The combination of quantitative assay for human chorionic gonadotropin (hCG) serum levels with findings of transvaginal high-resolution ultrasonography is the most common way to diagnose an ectopic pregnancy. However, abdominal or ovarian ectopic pregnancy may require transabdominal approach due to possible localization outside the small pelvis.

(sliding sign). Now color Doppler mode is activated and used to demonstrate corpus luteum neoangiogenesis in the ovary, the "ring of fire". The adjacent mass is interrogated in the same way to verify a similar vascular ring signal representing the trophoblast flow. Finally, 3D mode can give an idea of the spatial arrangement of ovary and mass and deliver additional proof that the mass, now identified as trophoblast, is not part of the ovary, but of the fallopian tube **(Figs. 12.5A and B)**.

OVARIAN ECTOPIC PREGNANCY

Ovarian ectopic pregnancy (OEP) results from the implantation of the trophoblast into the ovary, which happens in up to 3% of all EPs, or once in 7,000–15,000 pregnancies.[26] As per histological evidence, the implantation may occur as intra- or extrafollicular,[28] however this classification makes no difference for sonographic appearance and clinical manifestation. Like in other EPs, clinical symptoms may include vaginal bleeding and abdominal pain, with positive pregnancy test. Sonographic indicators for OEP are subtler than in other EPs. With a positive pregnancy test

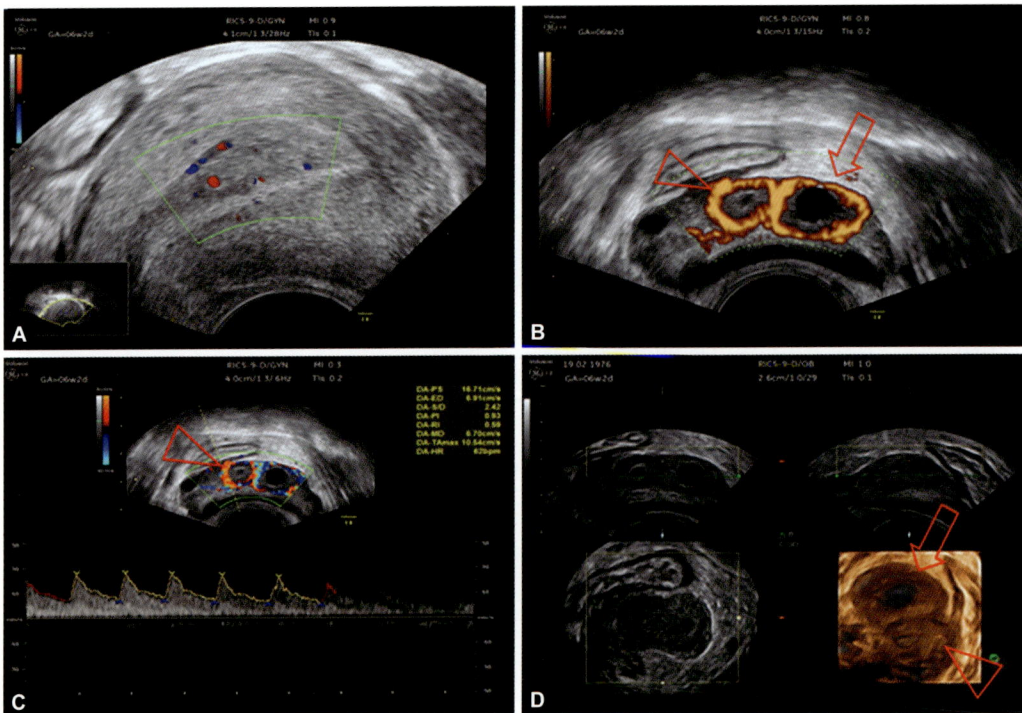

Figs. 12.4A to D: Ipsilateral tubal ectopic and corpus luteum. Follow-up transvaginal ultrasound (TVUS) at 44 days postmenstruation (PM). (A) B-mode color Doppler: Uterus shows thick endometrium without clear "comet sign" (trophoblastic flow); (B) Power Doppler: Double "ring of fire" around corpus luteum (arrow) and ectopic pregnancy (arrowhead); (C) Pulsed wave (PW) Doppler: Low-resistance-to-flow in ectopic pregnancy (neoangiogenesis and progesterone-induced vasodilatation); (D) 3D multiplanar: Clear "organ" boundaries of corpus luteum (arrow) and ectopic pregnancy (arrowhead).

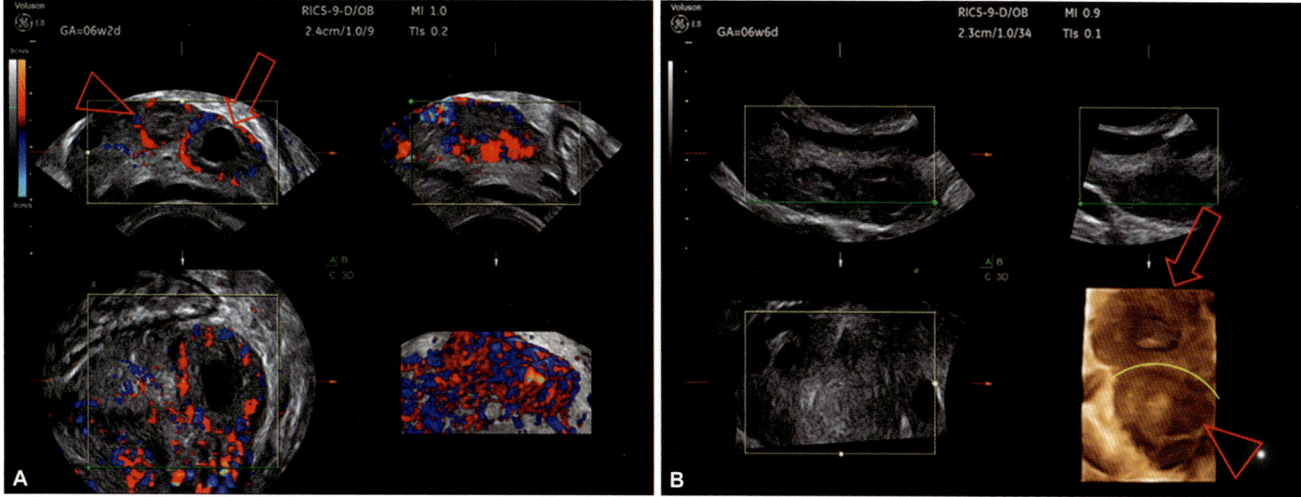

Figs. 12.5A and B: Tubal ectopic pregnancy, multiplanar, and surface rendered 3D ultrasound with high-definition (HD) flow Doppler. Follow-up transvaginal ultrasound (TVUS) at 48 days postmenstruation (PM) with suboptimal serial serum beta-human chorionic gonadotropin (hCG) levels. (A) 3D multiplanar HD flow demonstrates double "ring of fire" around corpus luteum (arrow) and tubal ectopic pregnancy (arrowhead); (B) Multiplanar surface rendering of the left adnexa. Note topographic discrimination of tube and ovary (yellow line) in 3D reconstructed image.

and the provisional diagnosis "PUL" overshadowing this clinical scenario, successful management depends on the cooperation between the main responsible obstetrician, sonographer, laparoscopic surgeon, and pathologist,[29] the first three often being the same person. OEP appearance in TVS can be misinterpreted as ovarian endometriosis or as corpus luteum; and even during laparoscopy, it usually presents as a hemorrhagic or ruptured corpus luteum cyst.[30] 3D ultrasound can demonstrate a small hypoechoic mass representing the GS, bulging from the ovarian cortex and being surrounded by a thick hyperechoic ring ("bagel sign").[31] The addition of color/power Doppler will highlight trophoblast flow within this hyperechoic ring and will eventually visualize a "ring of fire" of an adjacent corpus luteum graviditatis right next to it. Thus, 3D power Doppler ultrasound is able to establish OEP diagnosis by visualizing ectopic trophoblast and corpus luteum within the same ovarian volume.[31] The interested reader can find excellent images in the publication of Ghi T, Banfi A, Marconi R, Pilu G, et al. Three-dimensional sonographic diagnosis of ovarian pregnancy. Ultrasound Obstet Gynecol. 2005;26:102-4.[31]

UTERINE ECTOPIC PREGNANCY

All uterine EPs have higher beta-hCG levels and higher rates of embryonic viability in common, compared with tubal and OEPs, which is a limiting factor for the use of methotrexate in uterine EPs.

CORNUAL/INTERSTITIAL ECTOPIC PREGNANCY

The term "cornual" is often used as synonym for "interstitial" ectopic pregnancy (IEP). Strictly spoken, the cornual pregnancy (1% of all EPs), describes the location of an EP in the horn of a bicornuate or septate uterus, whereas an interstitial pregnancy (2–4% of all EPs) is defined as located in the interstitial or intramyometrial section of the fallopian tube **(Fig. 12.6)**.[32] In an emergency laparotomy situs, this differentiation may be rather difficult **(Figs. 12.7A and B)**. This intramural section of the tube may under ideal sonographic conditions and careful exploration of the 3D volume, for example by 3D tomographic ultrasound imaging (TUI), be visualized as a hyperechoic thin line in the cornual area. In IEP, the medial section of this line can be seen connecting the apex of the cornual endometrial angle with the medial aspect of the ectopic GS, as the "interstitial line" **(Fig. 12.8)**.[33]

Another sonographic marker for IEP is the "claw sign".[34] The myometrium, separating the central endometrium from the cornual mass in the lateral uterine fundus, forms a "claw" around this mass, with a remaining myometrial mantle of less than 5 mm thickness in the fundal area around the ectopic GS **(Fig. 12.8)**. Particularly because IEP occurs significantly more frequently after assisted reproduction, a delay of diagnosis and treatment is

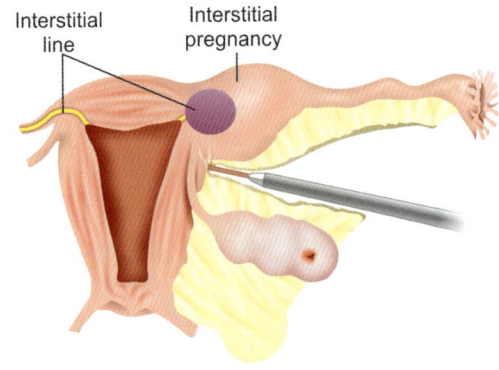

Fig. 12.6: Interstitial ectopic pregnancy.

unfortunately common and one of the reasons for a mortality rate 15 times higher (2–2.5%) than in TEP (0.14%) **(Figs. 12.7A and B)**.[27]

In analogy to the rather ominous naming of the arterioarterial anastomosis of obturator artery and inferior epigastric artery as "corona mortis", the severity of hemorrhage in IEP may be explained by the arterio-arterial anastomosis of the tubal branch of the ovarian artery and the uterine artery **(Figs. 12.9A and B)**.

Next to color Doppler mode for identification of cornual trophoblast flow **(Figs. 12.10A and B)**, 3D multi-planar **(Fig. 12.11)**, and 3D tomographic imaging are

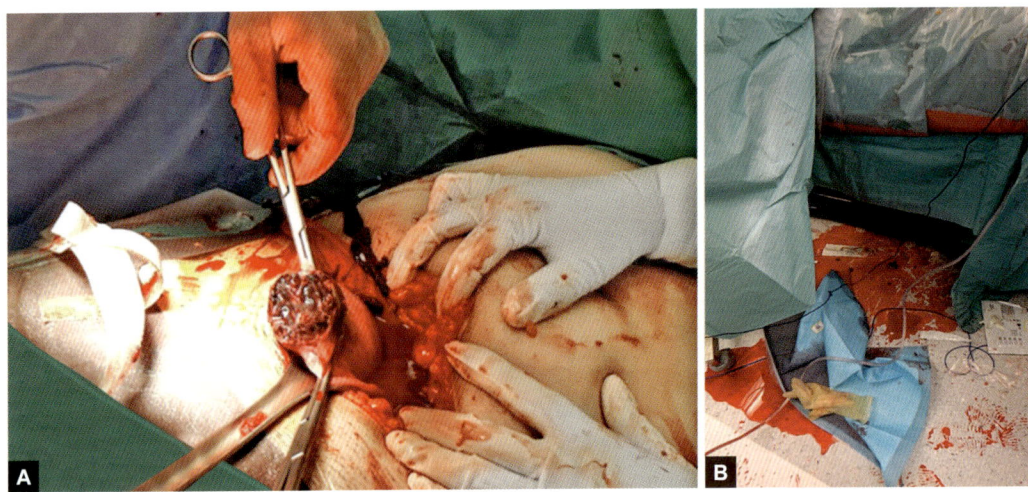

Figs. 12.7A and B: (A) Emergency laparotomy situs with ruptured cornual/interstitial ectopic pregnancy (EP); (B) Rupture of cornual/interstitial ectopic pregnancy is usually accompanied by massive blood loss.

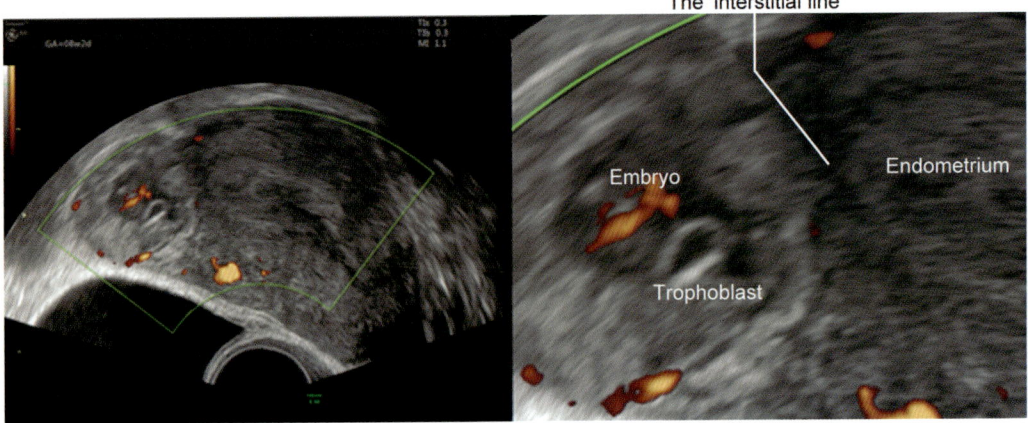

Fig. 12.8: Transvaginal sonography (TVS) visualization of the interstitial line.

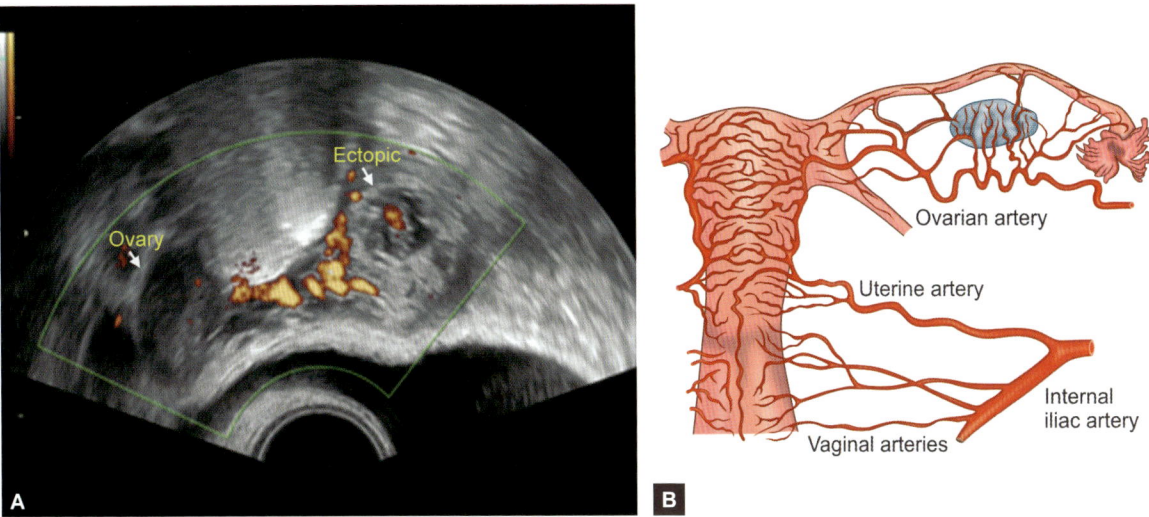

Figs. 12.9A and B: (A) Power Doppler image; (B) Vascular supply of interstitial ectopic pregnancy within the anastomosis of uterine and ovarian artery.

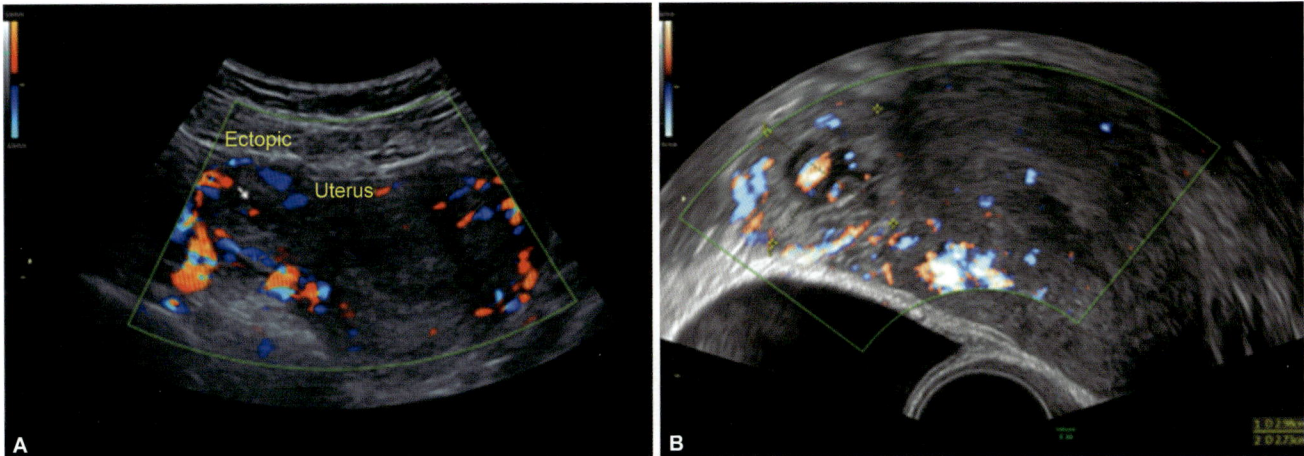

Figs. 12.10A and B: Cornual trophoblast flow.

excellent tools to deliver the decisive proof, that endometrium and trophoblast are separated by a layer of myometrium **(Fig. 12.12)**.

Various treatment options have been described in literature for cornual/interstitial pregnancy.[29] Of our three cases, one was ruptured and required emergency laparotomy with cornual resection. Of the other two, one was managed with laparoscopic cornual resection, the other with laparotomy and cornual resection **(Figs. 12.13 and 12.14)**.

CESAREAN SCAR ECTOPIC PREGNANCY

Cesarean scar ectopic pregnancy (CSEP) occurs in up to 0.05% of all pregnancies and is found in 0.15% of women who had a previous lower segment cesarean section (LSCS). In women after at least one LSCS, CSEP accounts for 6.1% of all EPs.[35] This rare form of uterine EP is defined by a trophoblast location in the niche of a lower segment cesarean scar, with the GS seen outside the endometrium and surrounded only by myometrium and scar tissue **(Figs. 12.15A to C)**.

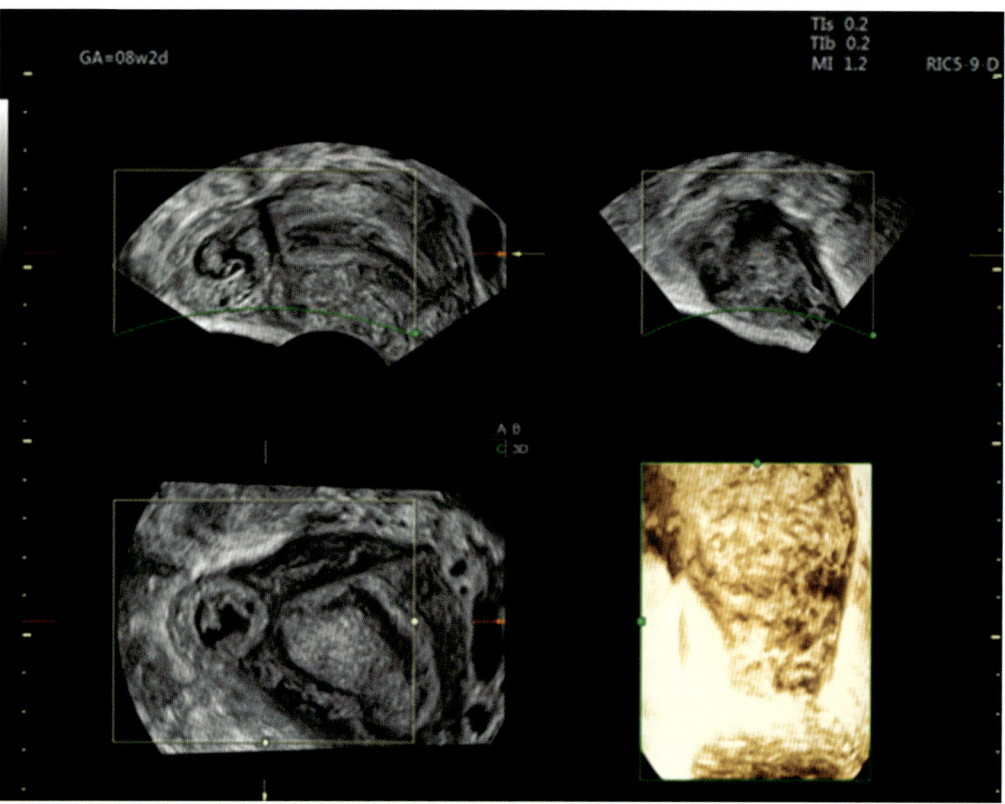

Fig. 12.11: 3D multiplanar imaging of interstitial ectopic pregnancy (EP). 3D tomographic imaging of interstitial ectopic pregnancy, with evidence of a myometrial layer which separates trophoblast and endometrium and forms a "claw" around the trophoblast (claw sign). Note the interposition of myometrium in between endometrium and trophoblast in the C-plane.

Clinical symptoms can occur already around 5 weeks postmenstruation in form of painless vaginal bleeding. CSEP might be mistaken for an isthmic intrauterine pregnancy or an incipient miscarriage of an initially regularly placed intrauterine pregnancy, though an inevitable spontaneous abortion is usually accompanied by lower abdominal cramps. In abortion, TVS presents images of a deformed or collapsed GS and vertical sliding movements of products of conception along the long axis of the lower uterine and cervical segment during uterine contractions (sliding sign) which can be provoked by gentle pressure on the myometrium. In contrast, the ultrasonographic evidence of an immobile trophoblast located atypically in the level of the cesarean scar and surrounded by rich blood flow in 3D power Doppler has to be taken as unmistakable sign of a viable CSEP.[36] Demonstration of embryonic heart action within the GS, rather common, given the excellent blood supply in vicinity of the uterine arteries, is additional proof. More differential diagnostic clues will be provided by 3D surface rendering of the uterus in the sagittal axis: the ballooning of the cervix, as typically seen in a cervical pregnancy (see section "cervical pregnancy"), is absent in CSEP. Since the CSEP expands within the cesarean scar niche, the main mass of the GS is not placed centrally in the uterocervical axis but anteriorly of it. Finally, the myometrial layer between GS and bladder is very thin or absent **(Figs. 12.16 to 12.18)**.

CERVICAL ECTOPIC PREGNANCY

Cervical ectopic pregnancy (CEP), defined as the implantation of a fertilized ovum in the endocervical canal below the inner cervical os, is a rare condition, with an incidence below 0.1% of all EPs **(Figs. 12.19A and B)**.[34] This ectopic implantation happens to be in the level where the uterine arteries reach the side of the uterus. Clinicians have to be cautioned that clinical and sonographic presentation of miscarriage and cervical pregnancy often have such features in common as early pregnancy vaginal bleeding,

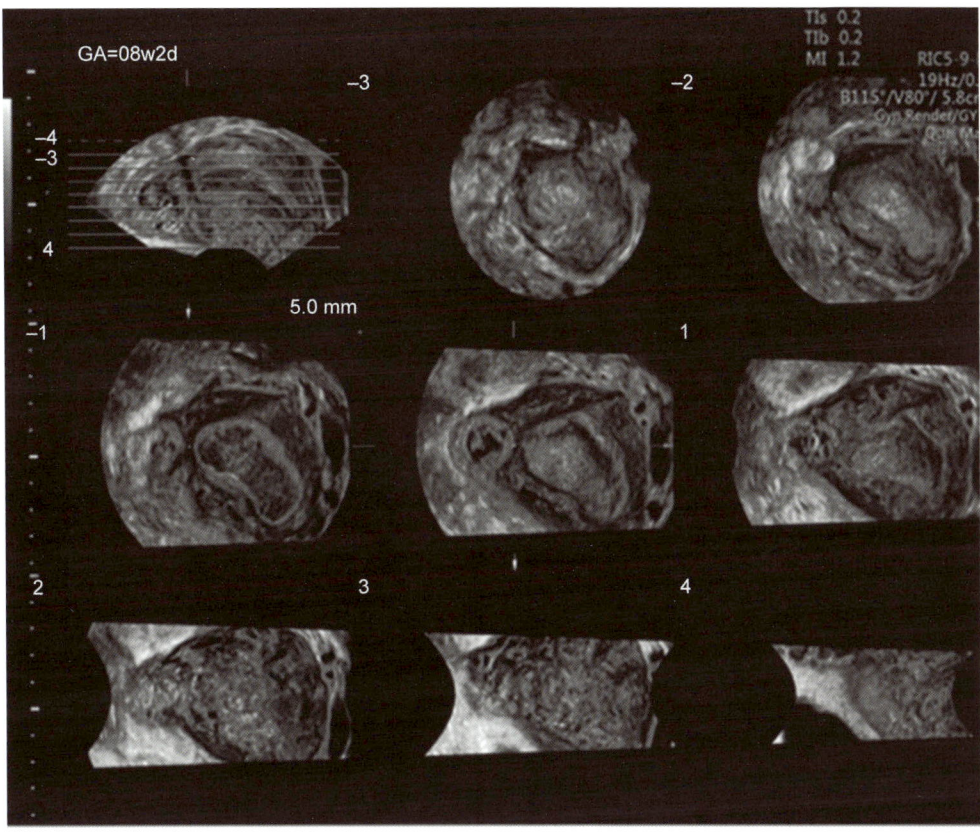

Fig. 12.12: 3D tomographic imaging.

speculum examination in both cases revealing an open external cervical os with a fleshy mass protruding,[29] a positive serum beta-hCG test, and TVS demonstration of a dilated cervical canal with heteroechogenic content. The response, however, to an attempt of evacuation of alleged "retained products of conception" could be deleterious in a CEP, disrupting placentation, and causing massive hemorrhage and even emergency hysterectomy. On the other hand, there is also need to differentiate between isthmic pregnancy with intraendometrial implantation just above the inner cervical os and cervical pregnancy because of opposite prognosis of the two. While a viable isthmic pregnancy is likely to have a normal outcome, cervical pregnancy—as uterine EP—has no chances of going to term and implies a high risk of maternal morbidity and mortality due to severe hemorrhage **(Figs. 12.20A and B)**.

3D vaginal sonography in combination with color Doppler has redefined the sonographic criteria of cervical pregnancy. 3D surface rendering with three orthogonal planes (sagittal, transversal, and coronal) shows an hourglass appearance of cervix, isthmus, and corpus uteri in the reconstructed image. The ballooned cervix contains the trophoblast, clearly located below a constricted isthmus.[36] With color/power Doppler mode added, atypically intense blood flow in the cervical area around the trophoblast can be demonstrated **(Figs. 12.21A and B)**.[37,38]

ABDOMINAL ECTOPIC PREGNANCY

Against the backdrop of a positive serum beta-hCG, the heteroechogenicity of a thickened endometrium, indicating a collection of debris and blood in the uterine cavity, resembles images of retained products of conception with a collapsed GS (pseudosac), in approximately 20% of all EPs.[39] It has therefore been argued that in the case of high and or increasing serum beta-hCG, a (diagnostic) curettage could provide histological clues—by demonstrating presence or absence of trophoblast villi within the endometrial tissue—to eventually abandon wrong assumptions of incomplete abortion, and in doing so, help to focus on the search for a PUL.[40,41] Depending on its location, an abdominal ectopic pregnancy (AEP)

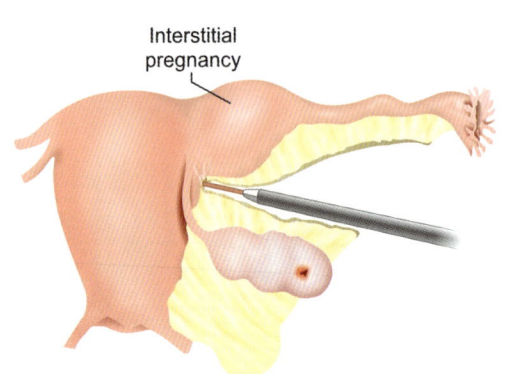

Interstitial pregnancy

A

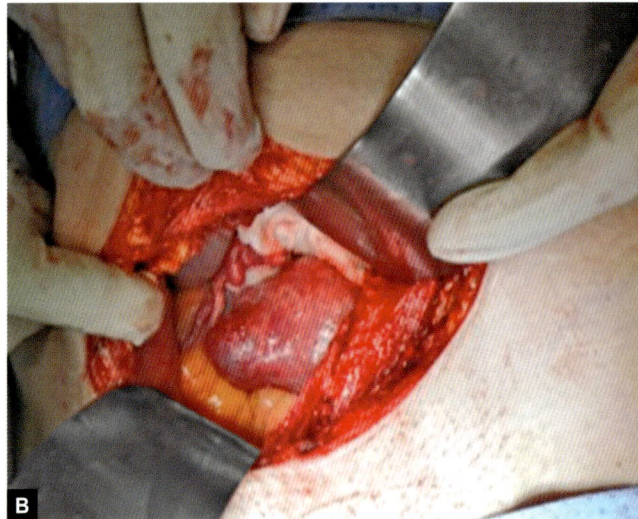

B

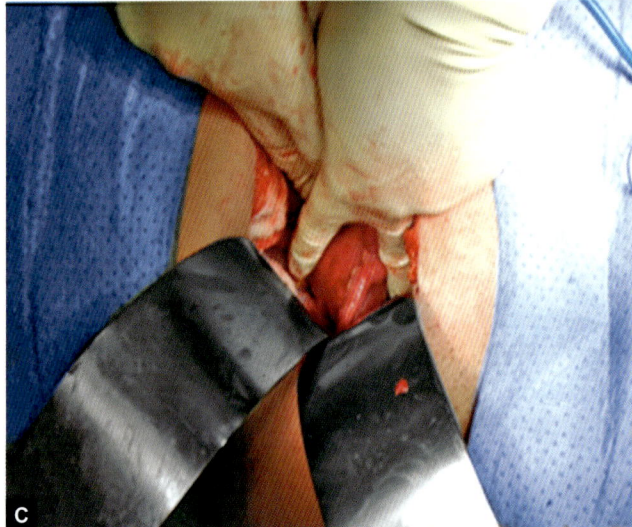

C

Figs. 12.13A to C: Cornual resection per laparotomy. Situs with distended horn of the uterus containing the ectopic pregnancy.

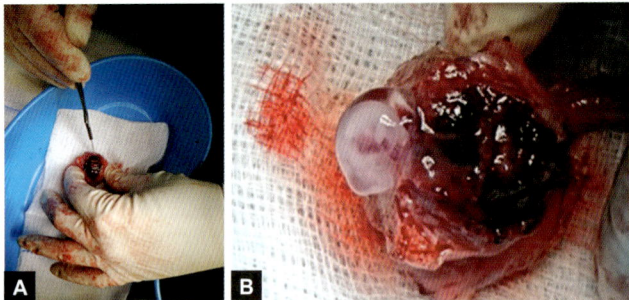

A

B

Figs. 12.14A and B: Cornual resection per laparotomy. Demonstration of the embryo within the resected horn.

can be accompanied by various symptoms, ranging from renal or gallbladder colic to symptoms of appendicitis. In clinically symptomatic PUL, careful transabdominal sonographic exploration of perihepatic and perisplenic spaces, and of the paracolic gutters, is always required to look for and to quantify free fluid, i.e. hemoperitoneum, but also to identify a possible AEP. Besides a good ultrasound equipment, sonographic skills and experience, a high degree of suspicion is needed in dealing with EPs. Abdominal pregnancy sites can be—in decreasing order of frequency—the pouch of Douglas (PoD), mesosalpinx, omentum, spleen, liver, and appendix.[42,43]

Abdominal ectopic pregnancy occurs as rarely as once in 8,000–10,000 pregnancies and makes up for 1–1.5% of all EPs.[44,45] Maternal mortality rates are high, which is explained by an often advanced gestational age at discovery, severe hemorrhage at any time in case of placenta separation, and predominance of occurrences

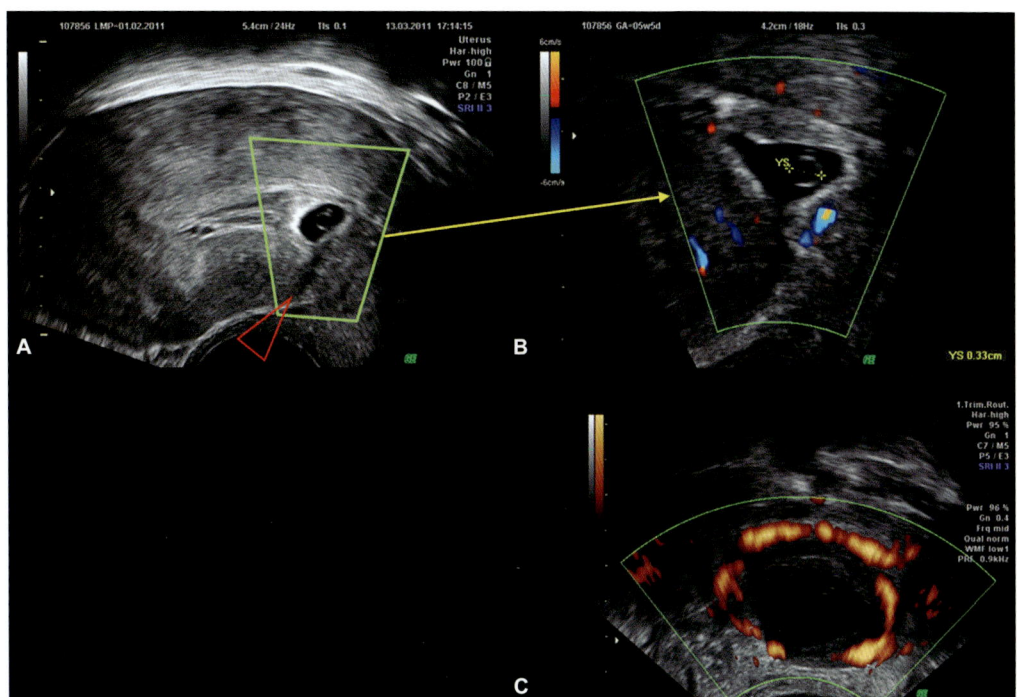

Figs. 12.15A to C: Diagnosis of cesarean scar ectopic pregnancy (CSEP) at 40 days postmenstruation (PM) with sonographic follow-up at 44 days PM. (A) Hysterotomy scar (arrowhead) with an adjacent gestational sac (GS); (B) Zoomed ROI: GS with yolk sac; (C) Power Doppler evidence of peritrophoblastic vasculature.

in developing countries with limitations of infrastructure and medical equipment. The following case presentation shall illustrate the specific challenges of an AEP.

Case presentation: Patient presented with vaginal bleeding and positive beta-hCG in the first trimester. TVS showed thickened endometrium with increased vascularization in color Doppler, interpreted as trophoblast flow in retained products of conception. She was admitted for daycare D&E. Five days later she was brought to ER with acute abdomen. Transabdominal ultrasound: large amount of free fluid in abdomen, empty uterus, fetus with cardiac activity under right liver lobe. Emergency laparotomy followed with removal of fetus and placenta, intraoperative blood loss 1500 mL. Patient was discharged 5 days later in good condition **(Figs. 12.22 to 12.25)**.

DIAGNOSTIC HINTS AND PITFALLS

Corpus Luteum

The corpus luteum, also called "the great imitator", can mimic not only ovarian malignancy, but also an EP. Its prominent vascularity (physiological benign neoangiogenesis) can be easily visualized by color/power/HD

flow Doppler as "ring of fire" using a low pulse repetition frequency (PRF). Likewise, the (ectopic) trophoblast, equally capable of neoangiogenesis, exhibits similar features in color Doppler imaging. It should be well noted that the majority of fallopian tube EPs are found on the same side as the corpus luteum.

Transabdominal Approach

Clinically symptomatic PUL with high and/or increasing serum beta-hCG suggest an abdominal pregnancy. TUS with high-resolution probes is the only way to detect such pregnancies, if they are not located within the small pelvis. TVS in cases of suspected EP should therefore always be complemented by transabdominal scan (TAS), not only for risk classification (free fluid), but also not to miss an AEP.

Pseudosac

As a response to pregnancy hormones produced by an EP, the endometrium proliferates and may bleed. The resulting arrangement of proliferated endometrium with fibrin and serum in between the endometrial layers can mimic a GS within the uterine cavity, termed "pseudosac". 3D TVS can give additional clues: while a normal

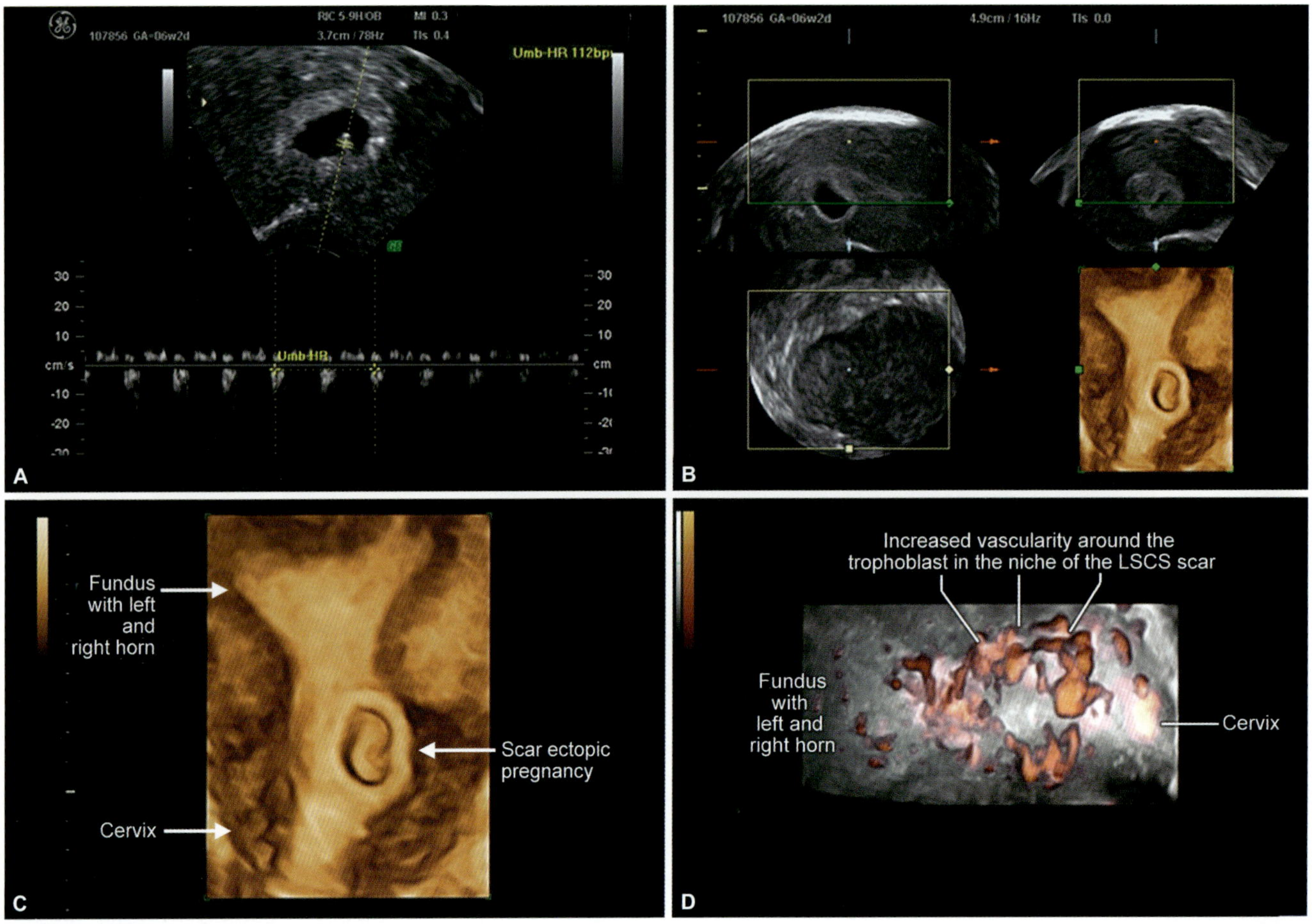

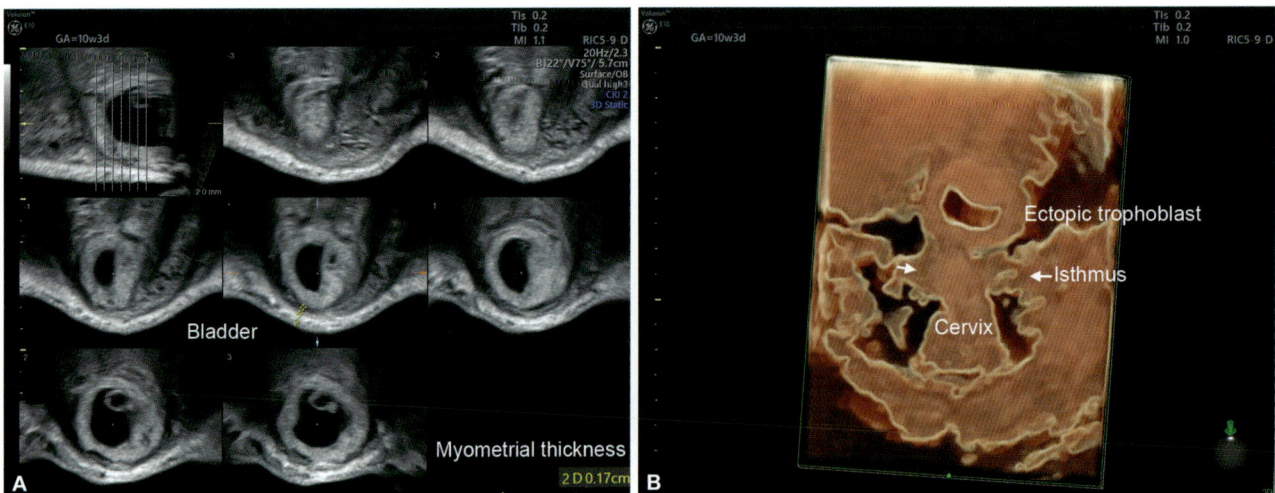

Figs. 12.16A to D: Follow-up at 44 days postmenstruation (PM). (A) Viable embryo with heart rate 112 bpm; (B and C) Multiplanar 3D surface rendered cervical glandular field and endometrium with cesarean scar ectopic pregnancy (CSEP); (D) Power Doppler glass body rendering: visualization of peritrophoblastic vasculature.

Figs. 12.17A and B: LSCS scar ectopic pregnancy, GA LMP 10 weeks 3 days, with viable embryo, CRL corresponding to 6 weeks 1 day. (A) Tomographic ultrasound imaging (TUI) of the transverse uterine plane shows best the minimal myometrial thickness between trophoblast and bladder mucosa; (B) HD skeleton mode of the coronal uterine plane demonstrates the spatial relationship between trophoblast and isthmus uteri, with uterine vasculature.

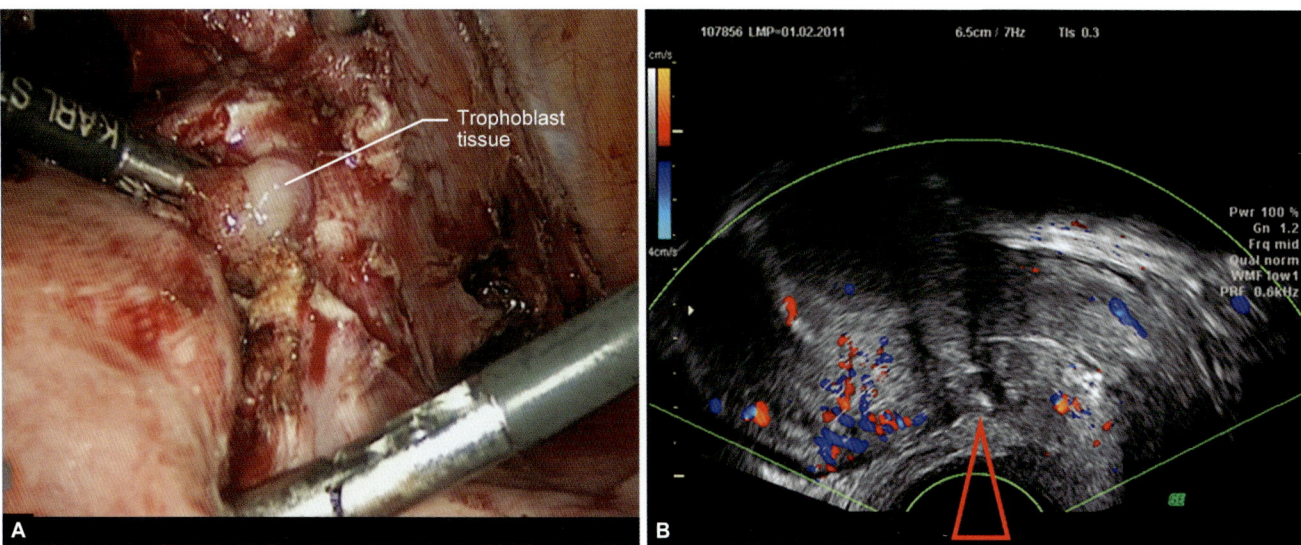

Figs. 12.18A and B: Cesarean scar ectopic pregnancy (CSEP), same patient as in Figure 16. (A) Laparoscopic incision of lower uterine segment and evacuation of the trophoblast; (B) Postoperative sagittal plane of the uterus, B-mode color Doppler: absence of abnormal vascularization in the area of the cesarean scar (arrowhead).

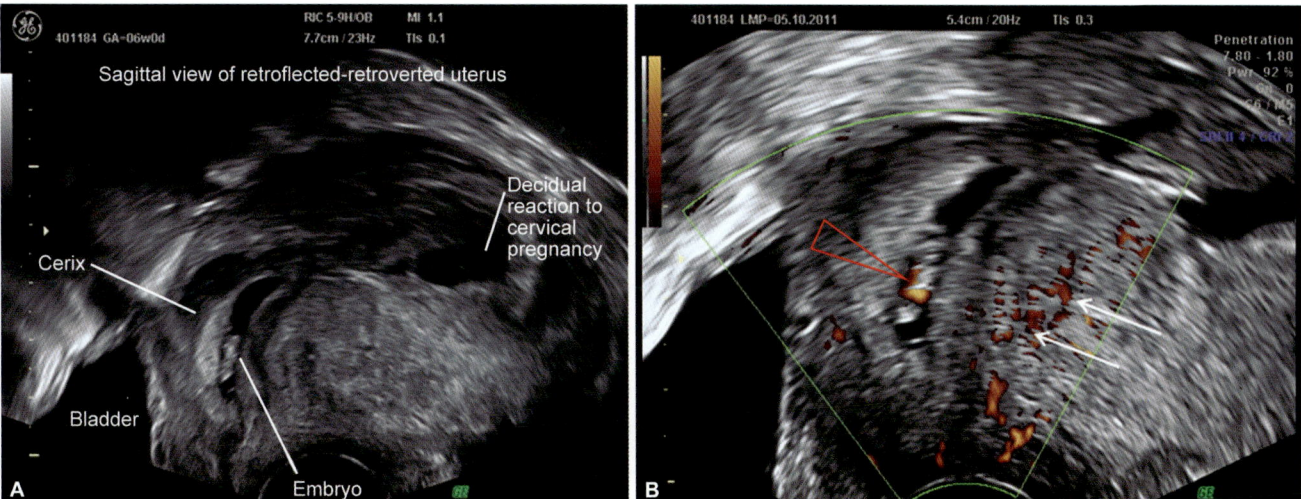

Figs. 12.19A and B: B-mode plus power Doppler, cervical ectopic pregnancy (CEP). (A) Sagittal B-mode view of retroflected uterus with CEP. *Note* marked decidual reaction; (B) Zoomed cervix, B-mode power Doppler with pericervical flow signals (arrows) and embryonic circulation (arrowhead).

implantation is eccentric within the endometrium of either the posterior or anterior face, a pseudosac is found centrally in between the two endometrial layers. With color Doppler applied, this pseudosac lacks surrounding peritrophoblast flow.

Unexplained Positive Pregnancy Test

When dealing with elevated serum beta-hCG levels above the "visibility threshold" in patients with "empty uterus" in TVS, a status after spontaneous abortion, and an EP are the most likely explanatory causes and can be confirmed by follow-up exams. Should these two have been ruled out, differential diagnosis should be widened to include other possible sources of beta-hCG production such as gestational trophoblastic neoplasia (GTN), ovarian germ cell tumors, tumors of the pituitary gland, and nontrophoblastic neoplasms of stomach, liver, pancreas, breast, as well as myeloma and melanoma.[48]

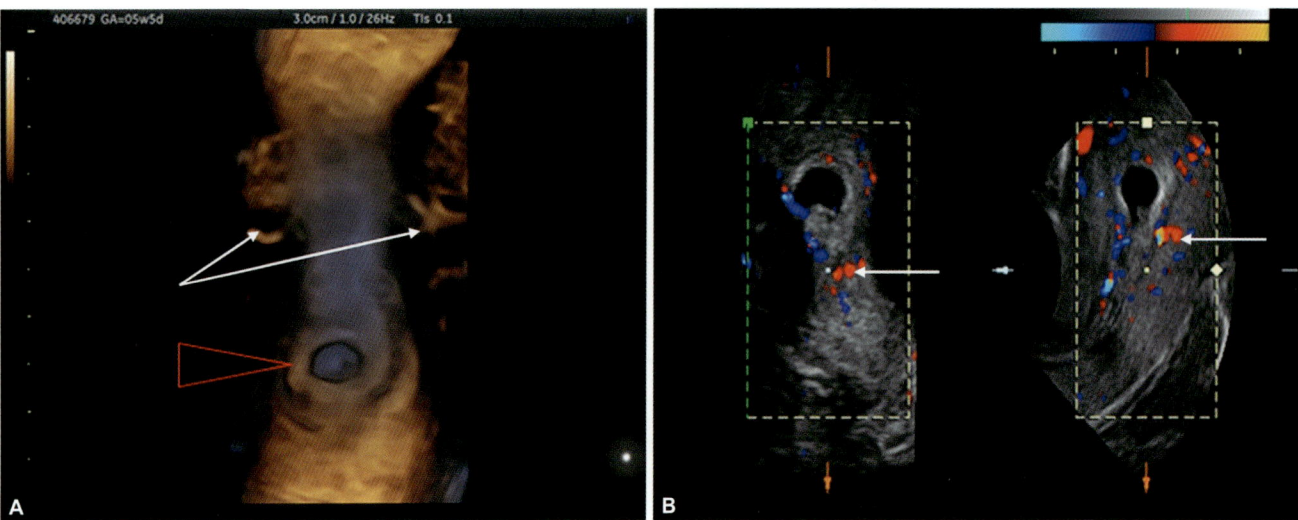

Figs. 12.20A and B: Sonographic differences between cervical ectopic and supraisthmic pregnancy. (A) Uterus with cervical ectopic pregnancy, 3D multiplanar surface rendered coronal view including cervix and lower uterine segment. *Note* paracervical structures of cardinal ligament and uterine artery, marking isthmus uteri (arrows). Gestational sac (arrowhead) clearly below isthmus uteri. (B) Multiplanar color Doppler image of the same region in a case of supraisthmic pregnancy which can go to term. *Note* color flow in level of uterine artery (arrows). Implantation low, however clearly above isthmus uteri.

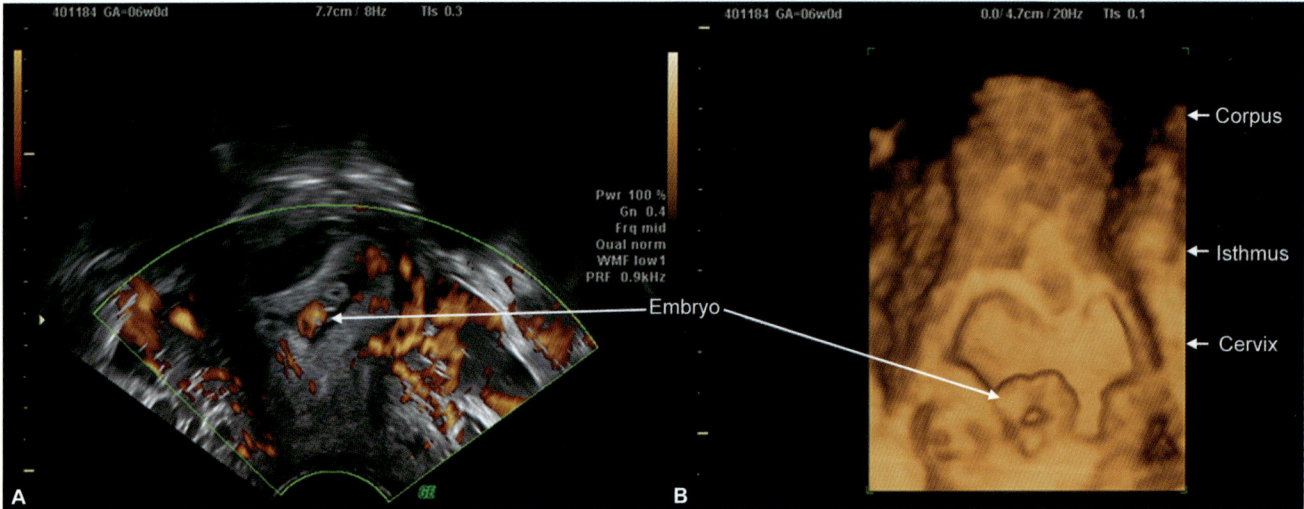

Figs. 12.21A and B: Cervical ectopic pregnancy (CEP) at 6 weeks. Power Doppler 2D and 3D visualization of cervical ectopic pregnancy. (A) Power Doppler, coronal view of the cervix with rich paracervical blood flow and embryonic cardiac activity; (B) 3D surface rendering, coronal view of the cervix and lower uterine segment. Clear visualization of the cervical ectopic pregnancy below the isthmus uteri.

SUMMARY

Transvaginal high-frequency 2D/3D ultrasound with color Doppler has emerged as the most important tool in diagnosing an EP. Applied in a dynamic real-time study of the pelvic organs, the TVS probe becomes the "seeing finger" of the examining clinician. The need of an experienced operator for the ultrasound machine in this encounter should not be conceived as disadvantage. If this operator is the gynecologist in-charge himself, he may find the answers to all his diagnostic questions, while interrogating the ROI methodically using all diagnostic

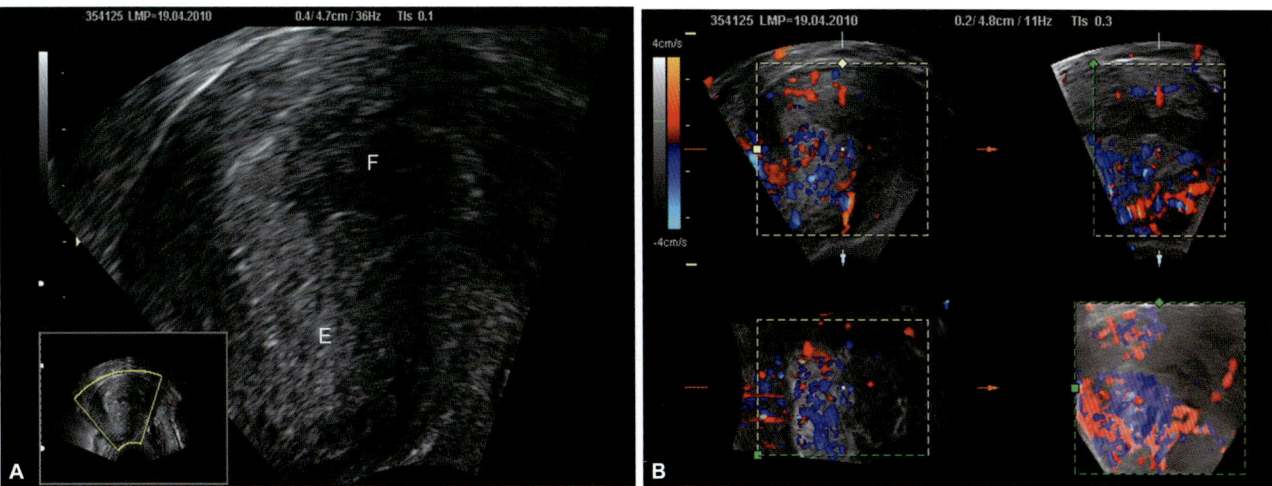

Figs. 12.22A and B: Abdominal ectopic pregnancy (AEP), case presentation of first visit of the patient. (A) B-mode, sagittal plane of corpus uteri. Thick endometrium (E) with low-echogenic fluid (F), interpreted as RPOC with blood; (B) Multiplanar color Doppler shows increased endometrial vascularization (decidual reaction). (RPOC: retained products of conception)

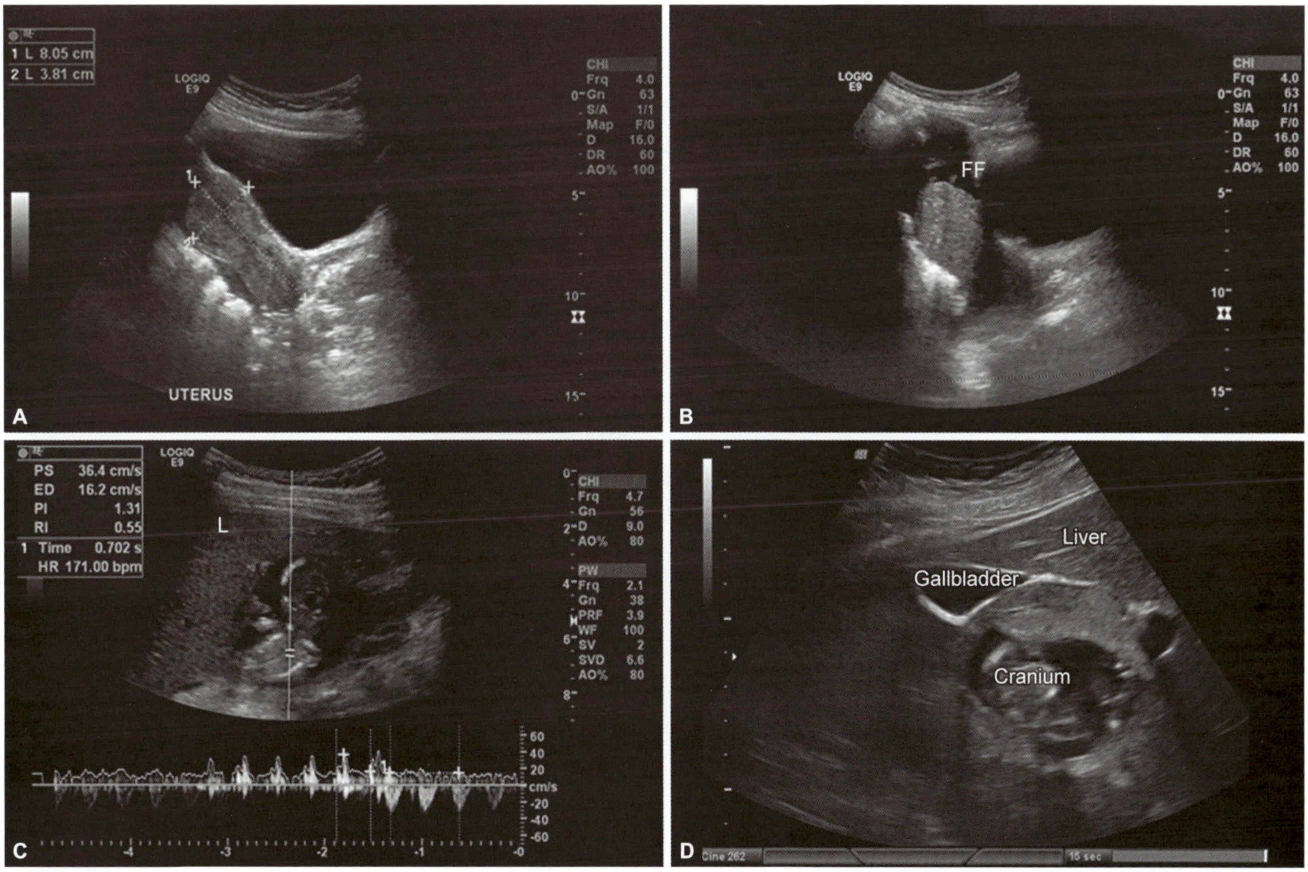

Figs. 12.23A to D: Abdominal ectopic pregnancy (case presentation continued). Ultrasound in emergency room 5 days later. (A) B-mode: Empty uterus, status post-dilation and evacuation (D&E); (B) B-mode: Free fluid in the abdomen (FF); (C) Pulsed wave (PW) Doppler: Viable fetus under the right liver lobe (L); (D) B-mode: Topographic arrangement of the abdominal ectopic pregnancy.

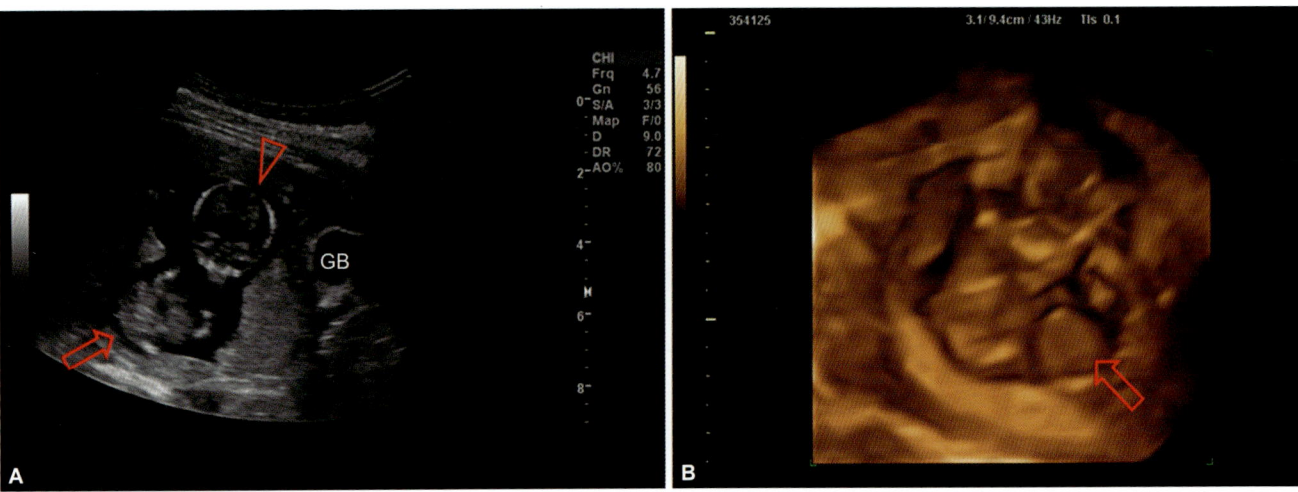

Figs. 12.24A and B: Abdominal pregnancy (case presentation continued). (A) B-mode image of a gestational sac with fetus, note head (arrowhead), omphalocele (arrow) and maternal gallbladder (GB); (B) Subhepatic ectopic pregnancy in 3D surface rendering, *note* the omphalocele (arrow) of this fetus.

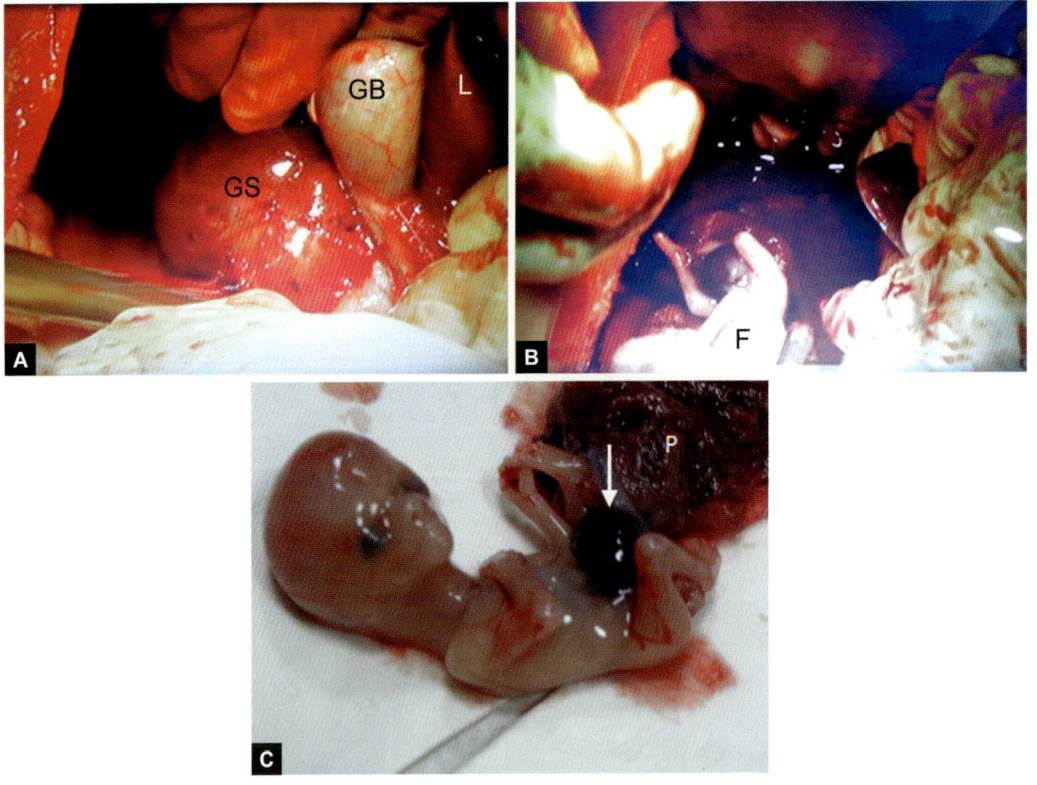

Figs. 12.25A to C: Abdominal ectopic pregnancy. Emergency laparotomy situs. (A) Situs with gestational sac (GS), gallbladder (GB), and liver (L); (B) GS ruptured, fetus (F), placenta is still in situ; (C) Aborted fetus with placenta (P). *Note* umbilical hernia (arrow).

modalities from 2D over color Doppler to 3D and 3D color Doppler. Tomographic imaging with postprocessing of volumes in different planes can be very useful as shown in section "interstitial ectopic pregnancy". Nevertheless, in analogy to CT and MRI, offline analysis of TVS-generated 3D datasets does not match the performance of 2D–3D real-time examination incorporating anamnestic data and clinical information during scanning.[46] Again the excellent diagnostic potential of TVS, with 3D mode added, is based on interactive dynamic real-time examination.[47]

REFERENCES

1. Van Den Eeden SK, Shan J, Bruce C, et al. Ectopic pregnancy rate and treatment utilization in a large managed care organization. Obstet Gynecol. 2005;105(5 Pt 1):1052-7.
2. Hoover KW, Tao G, Kent CK. Trends in the diagnosis and treatment of ectopic pregnancy in the United States. Obstet Gynecol. 2010;115(3):495-502.
3. Stulberg DB, Cain LR, Dahlquist I, et al. Ectopic pregnancy rates and racial disparities in the Medicaid population, 2004-2008. Fertil Steril. 2014;102(6):1671-6.
4. Murray H, Baakdah H, Bardell T, et al. Diagnosis and treatment of ectopic pregnancy. CMAJ. 2005;173(8): 905-12.
5. Creanga AA, Shapiro-Mendoza CK, Bish CL, et al. Trends in ectopic pregnancy mortality in the United States: 1980–2007. Obstet Gynecol. 2011;117:837-43.
6. Der EM, Moyer C, Gyasi RK, et al. Pregnancy-related causes of deaths in Ghana: a 5-year retrospective study. Ghana Med J. 2013;47:158-63.
7. Iklaki CU, Emechebe C. Njoku CO, et al. Review of Ectopic Pregnancy as a Cause of Maternal Morbidity and Mortality in a Developing Country. IOSR J Dent Med Sci. 2015;14(8):86-91.
8. Brüggmann D, Kollascheck J, Quarcoo D, et al. Ectopic pregnancy: exploration of its global research architecture using density-equalising mapping and socioeconomic benchmarks. BMJ Open. 2017;7:e018394.
9. Ouyang Y, Li X, Yi Y, et al. First-trimester diagnosis and management of cesarean scar pregnancies after in vitro fertilization embryo transfer: a retrospective clinical analysis of 12 cases. Reprod Biol Endocrinol. 2015;13: 126.
10. HealthDirect. (2017). hCG levels. [online] Available from https://www.healthdirect.gov.au/hcg-levels [Accessed December 2018].
11. Winder S, Reid S, Condous G. Ultrasound diagnosis of ectopic pregnancy. AJUM. 2011;14(2):29-33.
12. Tait RL. Five cases of extrauterine pregnancy operated upon at the time of rupture. Br Med J. 1884;1:1250-1.
13. Kalk H. Erfahrungen mit der Laparoskopie (zugleich mit Beschreibung eines neuen Instrumentes). Z Klin Med. 1929;111:303-48.
14. Hope RB. Differential diagnosis of ectopic gestation by peritonoscopy. Surg Gynecol Obstet. 1937;64:229-34.
15. Donald I, Macvikar MB, Brown TG. Investigation of abdominal masses by pulsed ultrasound. Lancet. 1958; 271(7032):1188-95.
16. Timor-Tritsch IE, Farine D, Rosen MG. A close look at early embryonic development with the high-frequency transvaginal transducer. Am J Obstet Gynecol. 1988;159: 676-81.
17. Kurjak A, Jurkovic D, Alfirevic Z, et al. Transvaginal color Doppler imaging. J Clin Ultrasound. 1990;18(4): 227-34.
18. Armstrong E, Ehrlich P, Birken S, et al. Use of a highly sensitive and specific immunoradiometric assay for detection of human chorionic gonadotropin in urine of normal, nonpregnant, and pregnant individuals. J Clin Endocrinol Metab. 1984;59:867-74.
19. Ben-Nagi J, Jurkovic D. Deaths in early pregnancy. The eighth report of the confidential enquiries into maternal deaths in the United Kingdom. BJOG. 2011;118(11): 1401-2.
20. Lurie S. The history of the diagnosis and treatment of ectopic pregnancy: a medical adventure. Eur J Obstet Gynecol Reprod Biol. 1992;43(1):1-7.
21. Institute of Obstetricians and Gynecologists, Royal College of Physicians in Ireland, Directorate of Clinical Strategies and Programmes, Health Service Executive. Clinical Practice Guideline: The Diagnosis and Management of Ectopic Pregnancy; 2014.
22. Centers for Disease Control and Prevention. Sexually Transmitted Disease Surveillance. Atlanta, GA: US Department of Health and Human Services; 2016.
23. Centers for Disease Control and Prevention. (2015). Births–Method of delivery. [online] Available from https://www.cdc.gov/nchs/fastats/delivery.htm [Accessed December 2018].
24. Li C, Zhao WH, Zhu Q, et al. Risk factors for ectopic pregnancy: a multi-center case-control study. BMC Pregnancy Childbirth. 2015;15:187.
25. Steptoe PC, Edwards RG. Reimplantation of the human embryo with subsequent tubal pregnancy. Lancet. 1976;1: 880-2.
26. Bouyer J, Coste J, Fernandez H, et al. Sites of ectopic pregnancy: a 10-year population-based study of 1800 cases. Hum Reprod. 2002;17:3224-30.
27. Tulandi T, Al-Jaroudi D. Interstitial pregnancy: results generated from the Society of Reproductive Surgeons registry. Obstet Gynecol. 2004;103:47-50.
28. Seo MR, Choi SC, Bae J, et al. Preoperative diagnostic clues to ovarian pregnancy: retrospective chart review of women with ovarian and tubal pregnancy. Obstet Gynecol Sci. 2017;60(5):462-8.
29. Fylstra DL. Ectopic pregnancy not within the (distal) fallopian tube: etiology, diagnosis, and treatment. Am J Obstet Gynecol. 2012;206(4):289-99.

30. Comstock C, Huston K, Lee W. The ultrasonographic appearance of ovarian ectopic pregnancies. Obstet Gynecol. 2005;105:42-5.

31. Ghi T, Banfi A, Marconi R, et al. Three-dimensional sonographic diagnosis of ovarian pregnancy. Ultrasound Obstet Gynecol. 2005;26:102-4.

32. Lau S, Tulandi T. Conservative medical and surgical management of interstitial ectopic pregnancy. Fertil Steril. 1999;72:207-15.

33. Yassin AS, Taha MS. Interstitial Ectopic Pregnancy, Diagnosis and Management: A Case Report and Literature Review. Ann Clin Case Rep. 2017;2:1352.

34. Kao LY, Scheinfeld MH, Chernyac V, et al. Beyond ultrasound: CT and MRI of ectopic pregnancy. AJR Am J Roentgenol. 2014;202(4):904-11.

35. Ash A, Smith A, Maxwell D. Caesarean scar pregnancy. BJOG. 2007;114:253-63.

36. Shih JC. Cesarean scar pregnancy: diagnosis with 3-dimensional (3D) ultrasound and 3D power Doppler. Ultrasound Obstet Gynecol. 2004;23:305-9.

37. Ruano R, Reya F, Picone O, et al. Three-dimensional ultrasonographic diagnosis of a cervical pregnancy. Clinics (Sao Paulo). 2006;61(4):355-8.

38. Lau WL, Cahn LL, Chan KS, et al. 3D ultrasound diagnosis of the cervical pregnancy. Hong Kong SAR, China: Department of Obstetrics and Gynaecology; 2011.

39. Ahmed AA, Brian DM, Calabrese P. Ectopic pregnancy and pseudo-sac. Fertil Steril. 2004;81(5):1225-8.

40. Rubal L, Chang K. Do you need to definitely diagnose the location of a pregnancy of unknown location? The case for "yes". Fertil Steril. 2012;98(5):1078-84.

41. Reid S, Condous G. Is there a need to definitely diagnose the location of a pregnancy of unknown location? The case for "no". Fertil Steril. 2012;98(5):1085-90.

42. Parekh VK, Bhatt S, Dogra VS. Abdominal pregnancy: An unusual presentation. J Ultrasound Med. 2008;27:679-81.

43. Abduljabbar N, Saquib S, Elhussein W. Successful management of abdominal pregnancy: two case reports. Oman Med J. 2018;33(2):171-5.

44. Gibbs RS. Danforth's Obstetrics and Gynecology, 10th edition. Philadelphia: Lippincott Williams & Wilkins; 2008. p. 84.

45. Atrash HK, Friede A, Hogue CJ. Abdominal pregnancy in the United States: frequency and maternal mortality. Obstet Gynecol. 1987;69(3 Pt 1):333-7.

46. Infante F, Espada Vaquero M, Bignardi T, et al. Prediction of tubal ectopic pregnancy using offline of 3-dimensional transvaginal ultrasonographic datasets: an interobserver and diagnostic accuracy study. J Ultrasound Med. 2018; 37(6):1467-72.

47. Testa AC, Van Holsbeke C, Mascilini F, et al. Dynamic and interactive gynecological ultrasound examination. Ultrasound Obstet Gynecol. 2009;34:225-9.

48. Braunstein GD, Vaitukaitis JL, Carbone PP, et al. Ectopic production of human chorionic gonadotropin by neoplasms. Ann Intern Med. 1973;78:39-45.

Recent Advances in 3D Assessment of Müllerian Anomalies

Ashok Khurana

INTRODUCTION AND BACKGROUND

Müllerian anomalies present with a variety of clinical manifestations,[1-6] including infertility (dysmorphic/T-shaped uterus), repeated first trimester spontaneous miscarriages (septate uterus), fetal growth restriction, fetal malposition, preterm labor, preterm delivery, obstructed or nonprogressive labor, and retained placenta. Paradoxically, a significant number of these anomalies are an incidental finding and this creates a dilemma with offering treatment options. An unambiguous label of the type of dysmorphology is central to the solution to this problem. Consequently, attempts are being made to define these better in order to optimize treatment offered.

Ever since Strassman[7] first described morphology and surgical management of common Müllerian anomalies and Jarcho[8] listed the gamut of uterine malformations, several classifications have emerged. The classification first proposed by Buttram and colleagues[9] was adopted by the American Fertility Society (AFS)[10] and has been in extensive use until recently. Oppelt and coworkers[11] have proposed a Vagina Cervix Uterus Adnex-associated Malformation (VCUAM) classification on the lines of a tumor nodes metastases (TNM) classification. This is exhaustive and systematic but not yet widely accepted, possibly because of its bulk. The efforts of Grimbizis et al.[12] and Acien and coworkers[13,14] have resulted in a new increasingly accepted classification now known as the ESHRE/ESGE (European Society of Human Reproduction and Embryology/European Society for Gynaecological Endoscopy) classification.[15] This classification connects embryology, anatomy, and the new array of treatment options that extend from expectant management to surgical correction. This classification is based on three-dimensional (3D) morphology and is currently undergoing external validation and will be presented in detail in this treatise.

This new ESHRE/ESGE classification was reached through a Delphi procedure, which involves an expert appraisal of a questionnaire system followed by a consensus. This new classification makes the clinical approach to Müllerian anomalies logical and clinically applicable, without making it too bulky or too brief.

Ninety-four observational studies were assessed with a total case tally of 89,861 women. The prevalence of Müllerian anomalies was 5.5% in the unselected population, 8.0% in infertile women, 13.3% in those with a history of miscarriage, and 24.5% in women with a history of miscarriage and infertility.[15] The classification arranges anomalies into increasingly severe subgroups and with increasing severity in each subgroup.

Over the years, several methods and techniques of imaging have been used to demonstrate the uterus and cervix. Hysterosalpingography (HSG) is good for delineation of the uterine cavity and for tubal patency, but is limited in the evaluation of developmental anomalies because it does not delineate the external contour of the uterus.[16-20] A similar limitation is encountered with sonohysterography and with hysteroscopy without a laparoscopy.[20-26] Ultrasound (US) is one imaging tool that is widely available, economical, lacks radiation, and can be achieved rapidly and is now the first step to diagnosis. Two-dimensional (2D) US, however, misses a large number of anomalies because it is often impossible to demonstrate a coronal plane. This plane is necessary to delineate the external uterine contour, which is central to labeling a Müllerian anomaly. Undoubtedly, a wide transverse diameter of the uterus or visualization of two cavities can be a clue on 2D US **(Figs. 13.1 to 13.3)**. However, these findings are shared by a septate and a bicorporeal

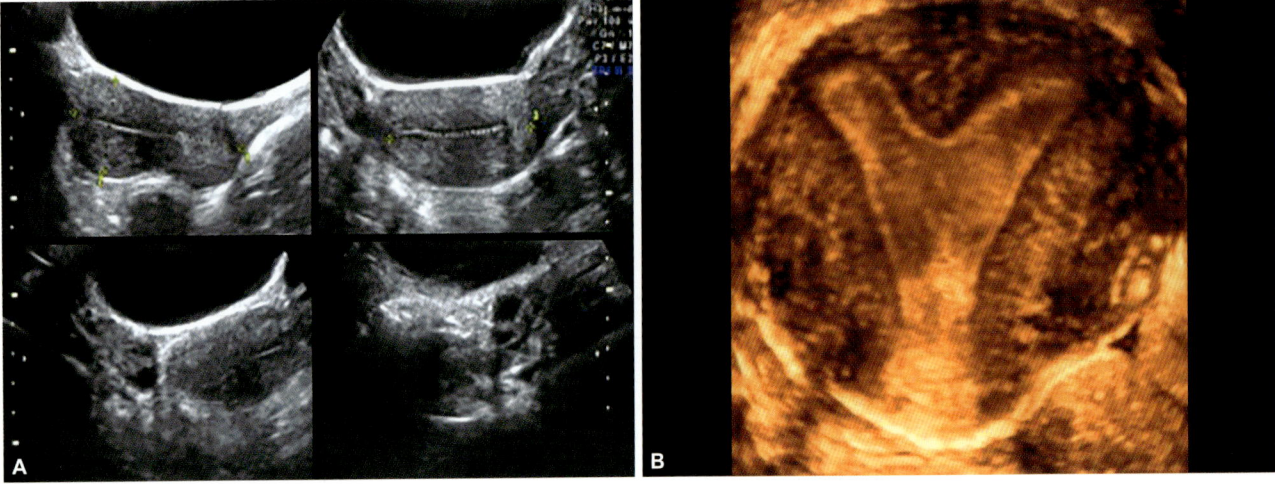

Figs. 13.1A and B: Increased transverse diameter.

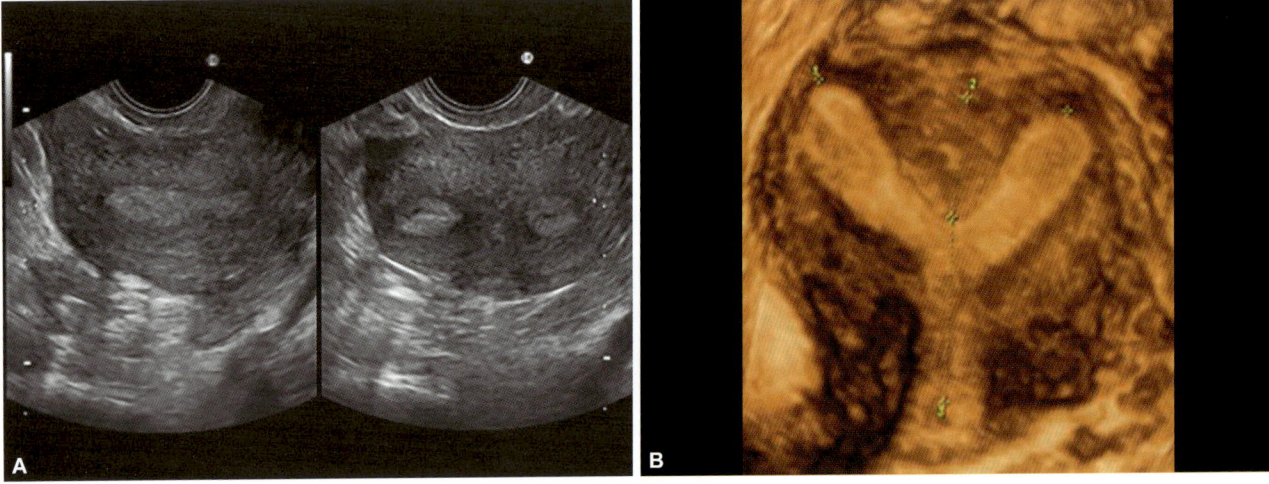

Figs. 13.2A and B: Two cavities septate.

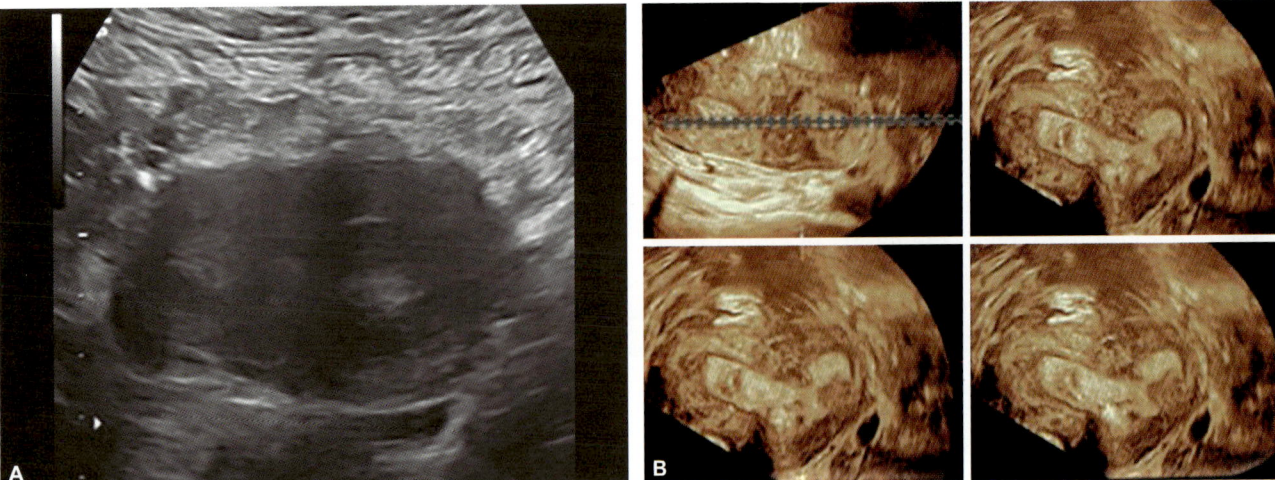

Figs. 13.3A and B: Two cavities bicorporeal uterus.

(bicornuate in the older classification) uterus. 3D US is a relatively new technique that is now widely practiced. This has been shown, to be far more accurate than 2D US and equal or better than magnetic resonance imaging (MRI) for assessing Müllerian anomalies.[27-36]

WHAT IS NEW AND DIFFERENT?

The new classification includes newer nomenclature and new mathematical calculations. The arcuate uterus is now mathematically defined and is either normal or septate as described later. The didelphys uterus is no longer a label. Bicornuate is now labeled as bicorporeal in keeping with embryological considerations. Bicorporeal septate is a new variant and is far more commonly encountered than expected, considering it has only recently been recognized. The T-shaped uterus is now labeled dysmorphic. Unicornuate uterus is now called a hemiuterus. "Not yet classified" is a new category. The vagina and cervix are now separately described. New measurements for an external cleft, wall thickness, and internal fundal indentation have been proposed to objectivize categorization.

Wall thickness is the distance between the interostial line and the highest point on the fundal contour **(Fig. 13.4)**. If this is not defined in the coronal view, then the anterior and posterior thickness of the myometrium is measured in the long axis and a mean is taken **(Fig. 13.5)**. The external cleft is measured from a line that connects the fundal aspect of the two humps of the externally indented uterus to the depth of indentation **(Figs. 13.6A to D)**. Internal fundal indentation is the depth of the indentation from the interostial line **(Figs. 13.7A to C)**. If the external cleft extends below the interostial line, then the depth is from the external aspect of the depressed fundus to the depth of the indentation **(Fig. 13.8)**.

THE ESHRE/ESGE CLASSIFICATION

Table 13.1 summarizes the various morphological Müllerian maldevelopment variants of the uterus, cervix, and vagina. These are illustrated in **Figure 13.9**. A comparison of the American Society for Reproductive Medicine (ASRM) classification and the ESHRE/ESGE classification is presented in **Table 13.2**.

Class U0 includes all normal uteri. The normal uterus has either a straight interostial line or a curved interostial line that has an internal indentation not exceeding 50% of the uterine wall thickness. The use of absolute numbers such as less than 5 mm indicating an arcuate uterus or more than 10 mm indicating a septate uterus has been avoided in definitions as uterine dimensions and wall thickness vary from one patient to another. It has, therefore, been decided to define the deformity as a fraction/percentage of wall thickness. Adding the normal uterus as an independent class permits defining isolated congenital malformations of the cervix and the vagina. This is illustrated in **Figures 13.10A to F**.

Class U1 or dysmorphic uterus includes those cases that have a normal outer uterine contour, but with an abnormal shape of the uterine cavity excluding septa. This is further subdivided into three categories. Class U1a or the T-shaped uterus consists of a long tubular vertical extent of the cavity, and a short-heighted horizontal extent **(Figs. 13.11A and B)**. The myometrium is thick.

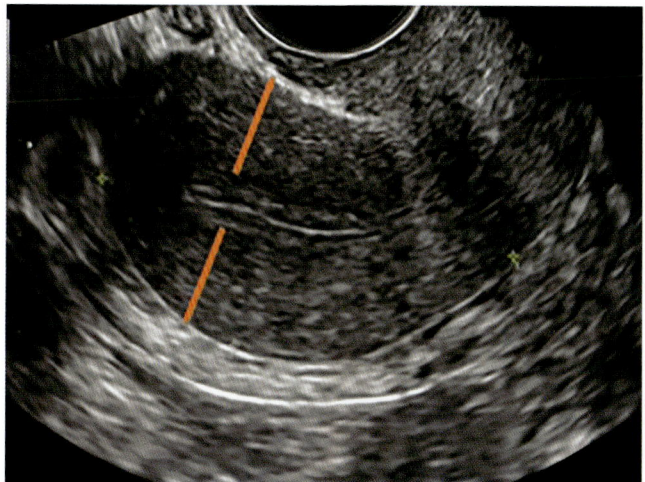

Fig. 13.4: Wall thickness—coronal.

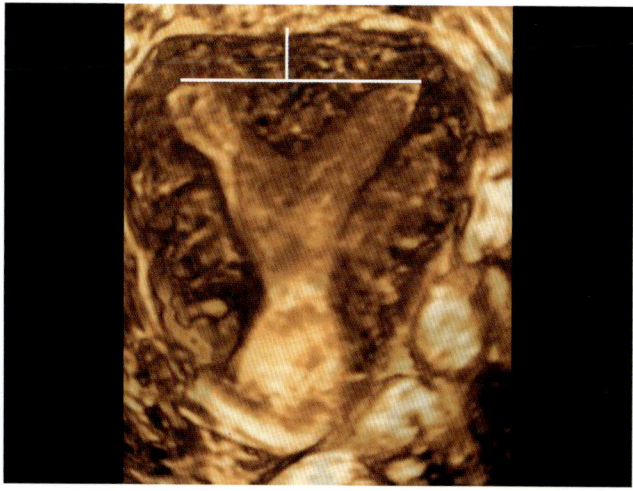

Fig. 13.5: Wall thickness—longitudinal.

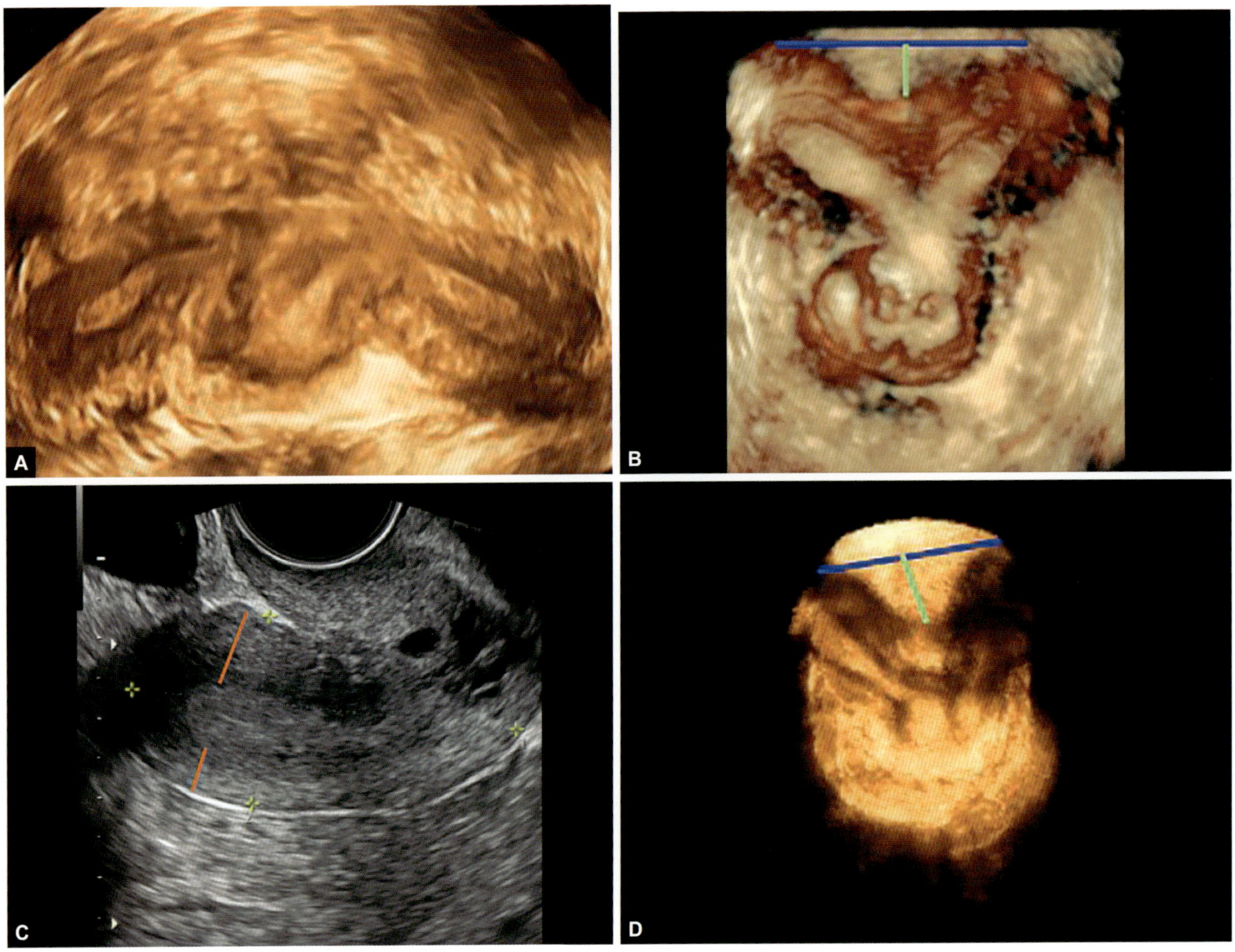

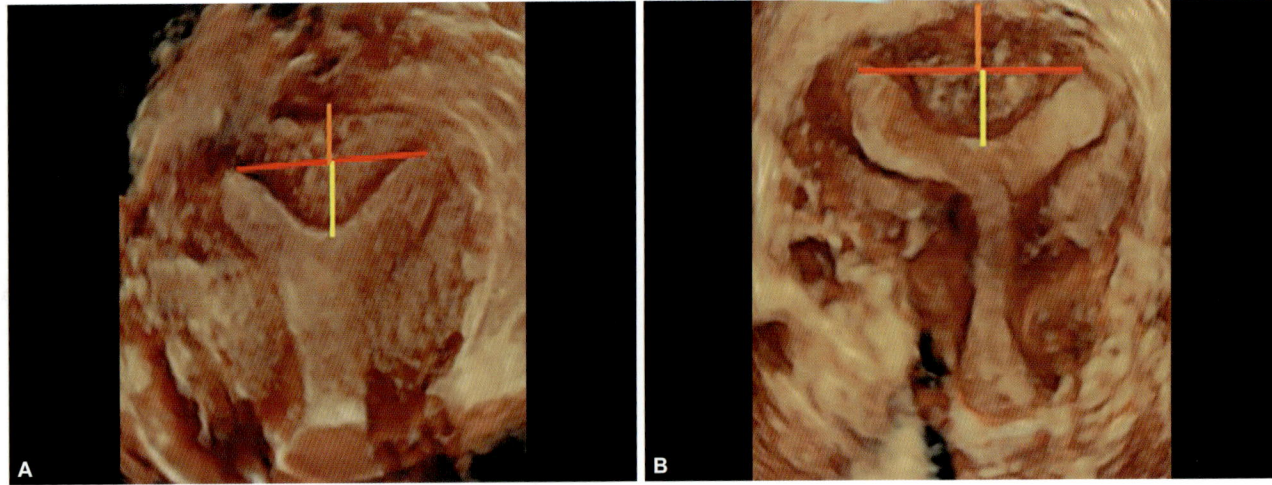

Figs. 13.6A to D: External cleft.

Figs. 13.7A and B

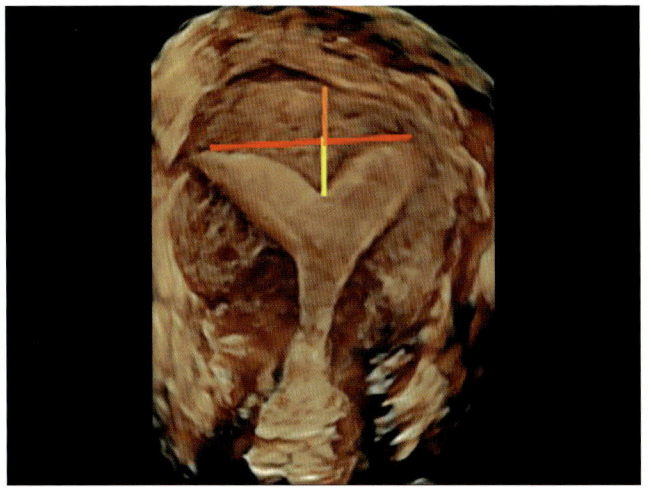

Fig. 13.7C

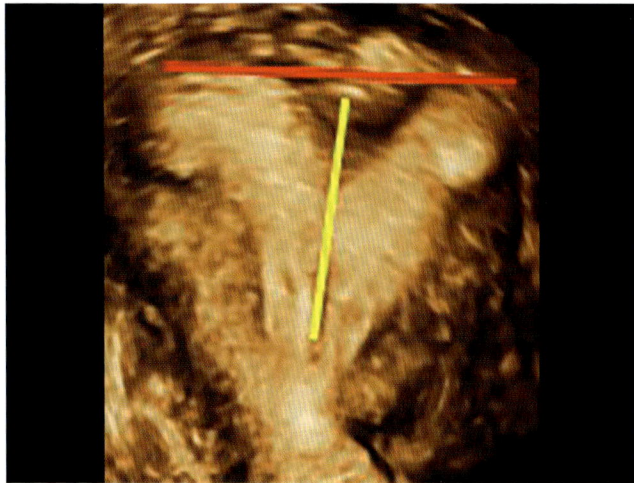

Fig. 13.8: Internal fundal indentation bicorporeal septate.

Figs. 13.7A to C: Internal fundal indentation septate.

Table 13.1: Morphological Müllerian maldevelopment variants of the uterus, cervix, and vagina.

Class	Uterine anomaly	Main subclass	Coexistent subclass cervical/vaginal anomaly
Class 0	Normal uterus		Cervix C0 normal
Class 1	Dysmorphic uterus	a. T-shaped b. Infantilis	C1 septate C2 double "normal"
Class 2	Septate uterus	a. Partial b. Complete	C3 unilateral aplasia/dysplasia C4 aplasia/dysplasia
Class 3	Dysfused uterus (including dysfused "septate"	a. Partial b. Complete	
Class 4	Unilaterally formed uterus	a. Rudimentary horn with cavity (communicating or not) b. Rudimentary horn without cavity/aplasia (no horn)	Vagina V0 normal vagina V1 longitudinal nonobstructing vaginal septum
Class 5	Aplastic/dysplastic	a. Rudimentary horn with cavity (bi- or unilateral) b. Rudimentary horn without cavity (bi- or unilateral)/aplasia	V2 longitudinal obstructing vaginal septum V3 transverse vaginal septum/imperforate hymen V4 vaginal aplasia
Class 6	Unclassified malformations		

Subjective evaluation reveals an adult type ratio of the uterine corpus to the cervix, two-thirds corpus to one-third cervix. Class U1b or uterus infantilis also shows a narrow uterine cavity, but without lateral wall thickening. There is an inverse proportion of one-third corpus and two-thirds cervix, on observing such a uterus **(Figs. 13.12A and B)**. Class U1c or "others" include all minor deformities of the uterine cavity including those with an inner indentation at the fundal midline level of less than 50% of the uterine wall thickness, formerly categorized as the arcuate uterus **(Figs. 13.13A and B)**.

Class U2 or septate uterus includes all cases with a normal fusion, but abnormal absorption of the midline septum. The septate uterus is characterized by a normal outline and a midline fundal internal indentation exceeding 50% of the uterine wall thickness. The septum may be partial (U2a) and end above the level of the cervix **(Figs. 13.14A to F)** or extend down to the cervix and completely divide the uterine cavity (U2b) **(Figs. 13.15A to D)**. It may extend into the cervix and/or into the vagina.

Class U3 is called the bicorporeal uterus. This was formerly called the bicornuate uterus. It includes all

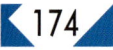

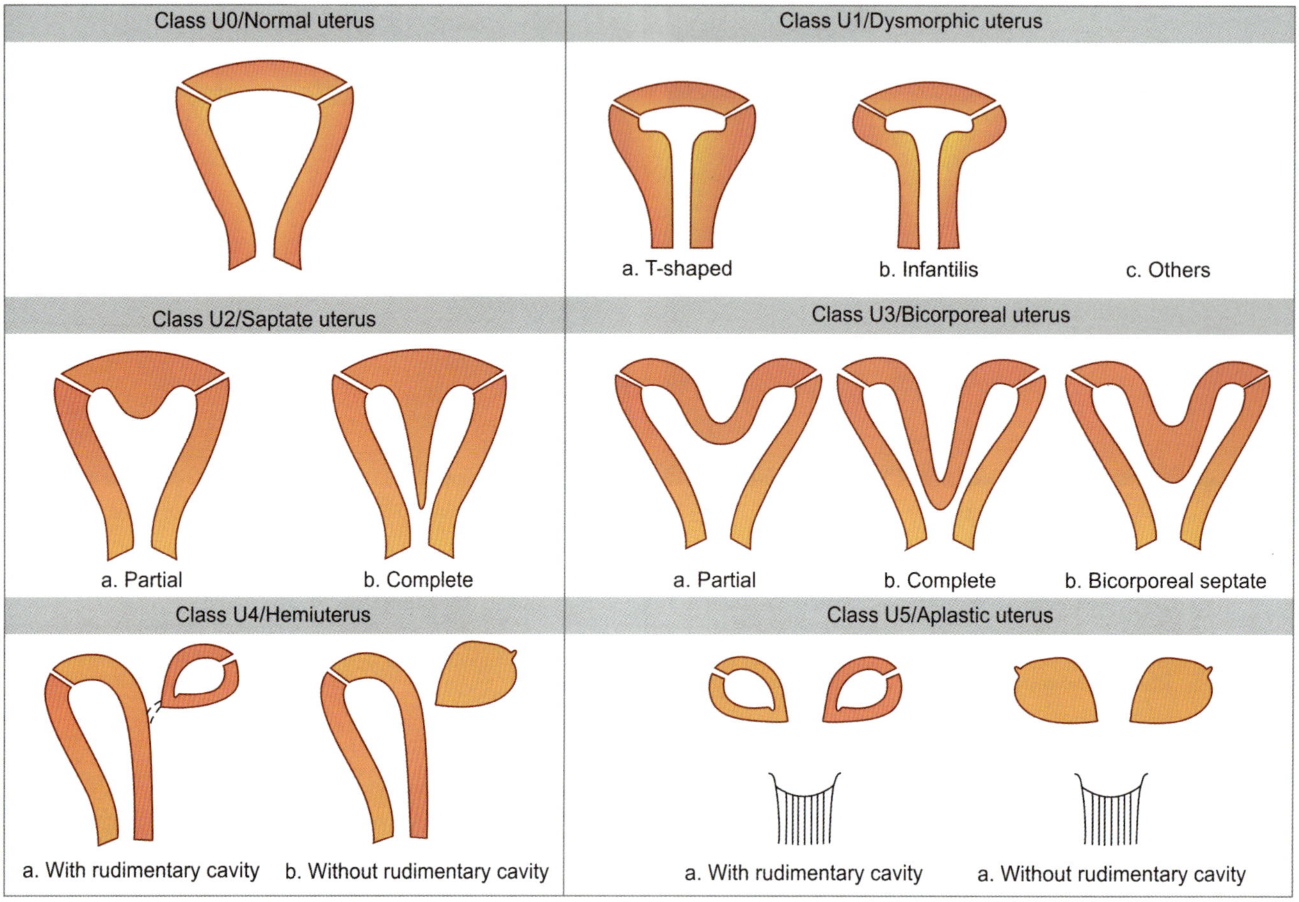

Class U0/Normal uterus	Class U1/Dysmorphic uterus
	a. T-shaped b. Infantilis c. Others
Class U2/Saptate uterus	Class U3/Bicorporeal uterus
a. Partial b. Complete	a. Partial b. Complete b. Bicorporeal septate
Class U4/Hemiuterus	Class U5/Aplastic uterus
a. With rudimentary cavity b. Without rudimentary cavity	a. With rudimentary cavity a. Without rudimentary cavity

Fig. 13.9: Graphic representation of the new uterus categories.

Table 13.2: Ultrasound criteria for the classification of congenital uterine anomalies by ASRM* and ESHRE/ESGE.

Classification	Uterine cavity shape	External contour	Differentiation
ASRM*			
Norm	Straight, convex fundal contour or internal indentation < 1 cm	Straight, convex or external cleft <1 cm	Subjective impression and measurements
Class I hypoplasia/ agenesis	a. vaginal, b. cervical, c. fundal, d. tubal, e. combined		Subjective impression
Class II uterus unicornuate	Single well-formed uterine cavity with a single interstitial portion of fallopian tube and concave fundal contour	Asymmetric ellipsoidal shape (banana-shaped) with or without smaller horn	Subjective impression
a. Communicating	Connected with smaller contralateral uterine cavity with or without interstitial portion of fallopian tube	External cleft > 1 cm dividing the two horns	a. Measurements
b. Noncommunicating	Unconnected with contralateral uterine cavity with or without interstitial portion of fallopian tube	External cleft > 1 cm dividing the two horn/variable if hemihematometra is present in rudimentary horn	b. Measurements/ subjective impression
c. No cavity	Without uterine cavity in rudimentary horn	External cleft > 1 cm dividing the two horns	c. Measurements
d. No horn		Rudimentary horn absent	d. Subjective impression

Contd…

Contd…

Classification	Uterine cavity shape	External contour	Differentiation
Class III uterus didelphys	Two separate unicornuate uterine cavities	Two corpus bodies with double cervix	Subjective impression
Class IV uterus bicornuate	Internal indentation ≥ 1.5 cm	External cleft ≥ 1 cm	Measurements
a. Complete		a. Division up to single normal cervix	a. Subjective impression
b. Partial		b. Division above the single normal cervix	b. Subjective impression
Class V septate uterus	Internal indentation ≥ 1.5 cm	External cleft < 1 cm	Measurements
a. Complete	Totally division of uterine cavity and cervical canal		a. Subjective impression
b. Partial	Partially or totally division of uterine cavity without or with partially septate cervix		b. Subjective impression
Class VI arcuate uterus	Internal indentation ≥ 1 cm; ≤ 1.5 cm	External cleft < 1 cm	Measurements
Class VII T-shaped uterus	T-shaped uterine cavity		Subjective impression
Anomaly without classification	Hybrid form, noncharacteristic conjunction of uterine, cervical and vaginal malformations		Subjective impression and measurements
ESHRE–ESGE			
Class U0: Normal uterus	Straight, curved interostial line or internal indentation < 50% myometrial thickness	Normal outline or external cleft <50% of uterine wall thickness	Subjective impression and measurements
Class U1: Dysmorphic uterus	Abnormal	Normal outline or external cleft <50% of uterine wall thickness	Subjective impression and measurements
a. T-shaped	Narrow cavity; thickened lateral walls; correlation of two-thirds uterine corpus and one-third cervix		
b. Infantilis	Narrow cavity without wall thickening; correlation of one-third uterine body and two-thirds cervix		
c. Others (?)	Internal indentation < 50% myometrial thickness (?)		
Class U2: Septate uterus	Internal indentation >50% myometrial thickness	Normal outline or external cleft <50% of uterine wall thickness	Measurements
a. Partial	a. Division above the internal cervical os		a. Subjective impression
b. Complete	b. Division up to the internal cervical os		b. Subjective impression
Class U3: Bicorporeal uterus		External cleft > 50% myometrial thickness	Measurements
a. Partial	Division above the internal cervical os	Division above the cervix	a. Subjective impression
b. Complete	Division up to the internal cervical os	Division up to the cervix	b. Subjective impression
c. Bicorporeal septate	Midline fundal indentation (myometrial thickness at the central point of the external cleft) >150% uterine wall thickness (average myometrial thickness)		c. Measurements
Class U4: Hemiuterus	Unilateral formed cavity	Unilateral formed corpus	Subjective impression
a. With a rudimentary (functional) cavity	With communicating or noncommunicating functional contralateral horn of cavity		

Contd…

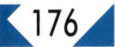

Contd…

Classification	Uterine cavity shape	External contour	Differentiation
b. Without rudimentary (functional) cavity	Without functional contralateral horn of cavity		
Class U5: Aplastic uterus			Subjective impression
a. With rudimentary (functional) cavity	Cavity remnant/s present	Uterine remnants present	
b. Without rudimentary (functional) cavity	Cavity remnants absent	Full uterine aplasia or uterine remnants present	
Class U6: Unclassified cases	Infrequent anomalies, subtle changes, or combined anomalies		Subjective impression and measurements

*Modified to include morphometric criteria.
(ASRM: American Society for Reproductive Medicine; ESHRE–ESGE: European Society of Human Reproduction and Embryology–European Society for Gynaecological Endoscopy)

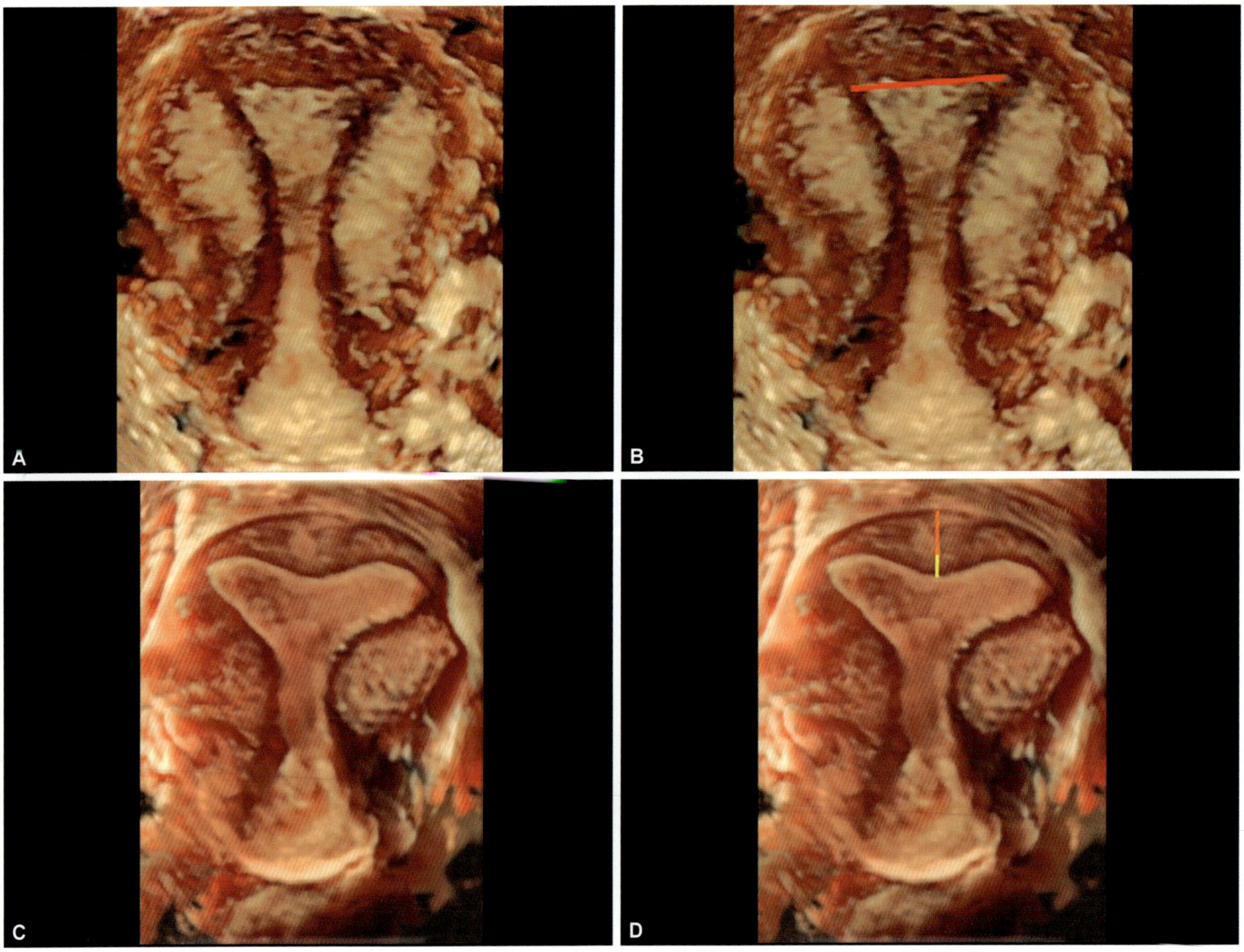

Figs. 13.10A to D

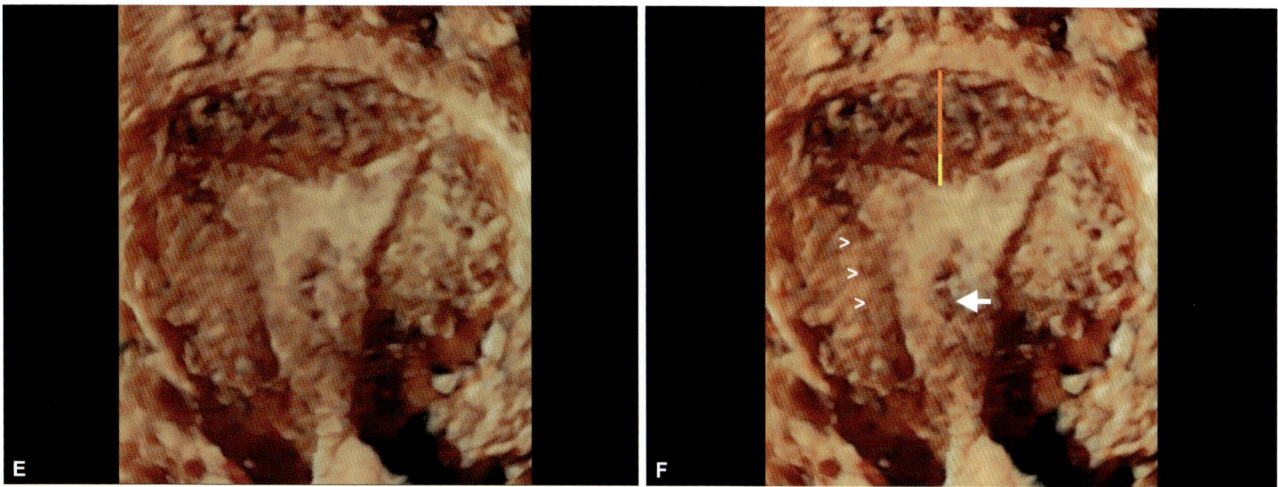

Figs. 13.10E and F

Figs. 13.10A to F: Normal and old arcuate uterus.

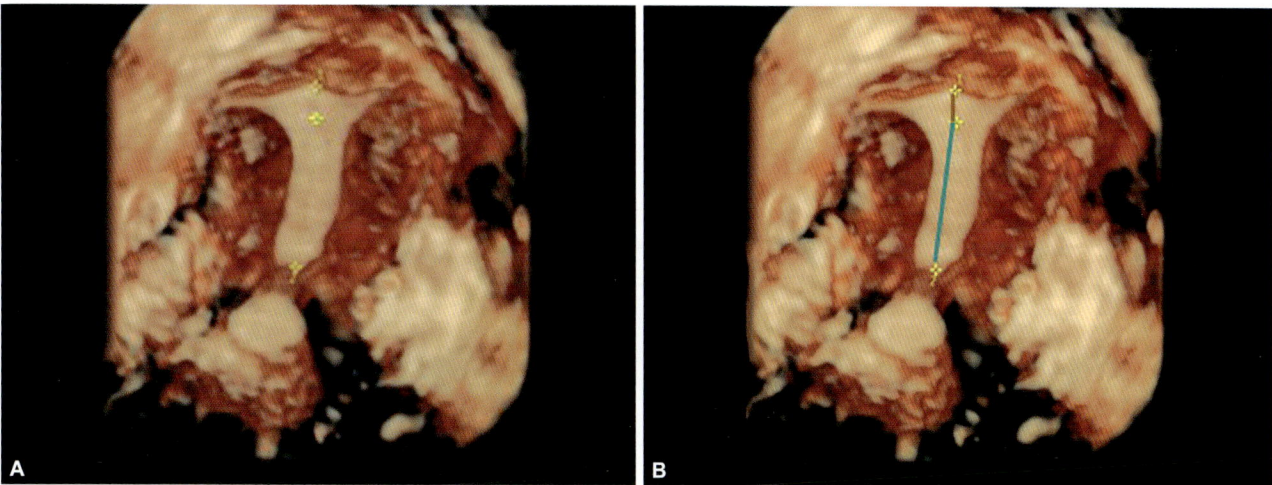

Figs. 13.11A and B: Dysmorphic old T-shape type.

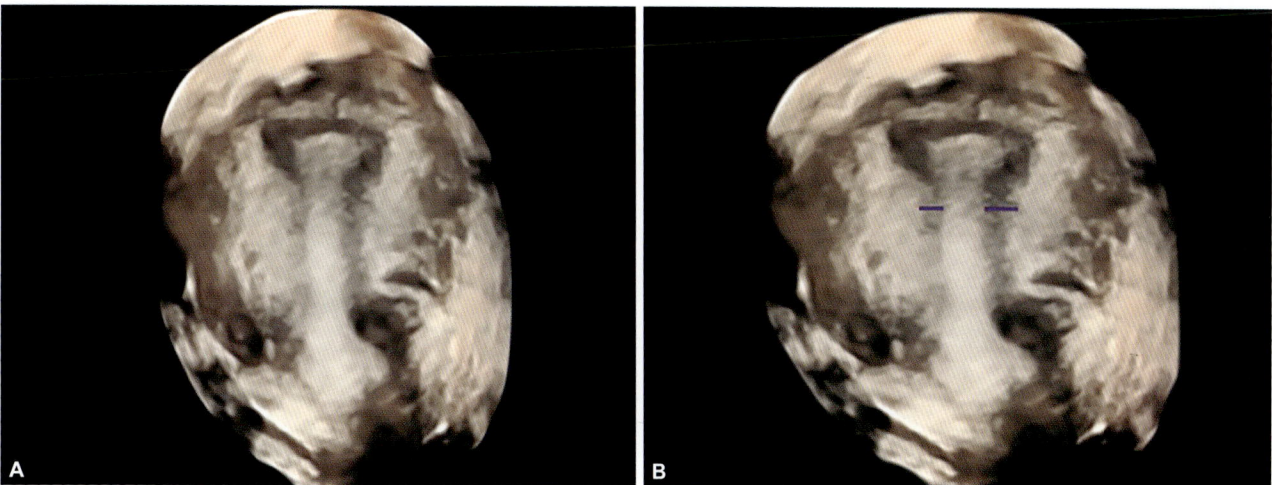

Figs. 13.12A and B: Dysmorphic infantile.

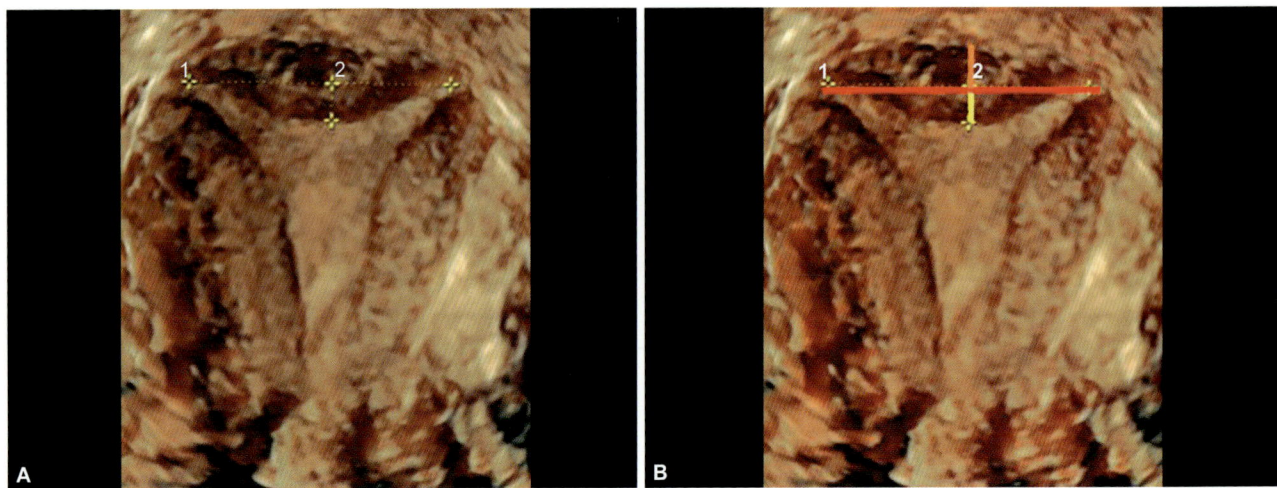

Figs. 13.13A and B: Arcuate uterus.

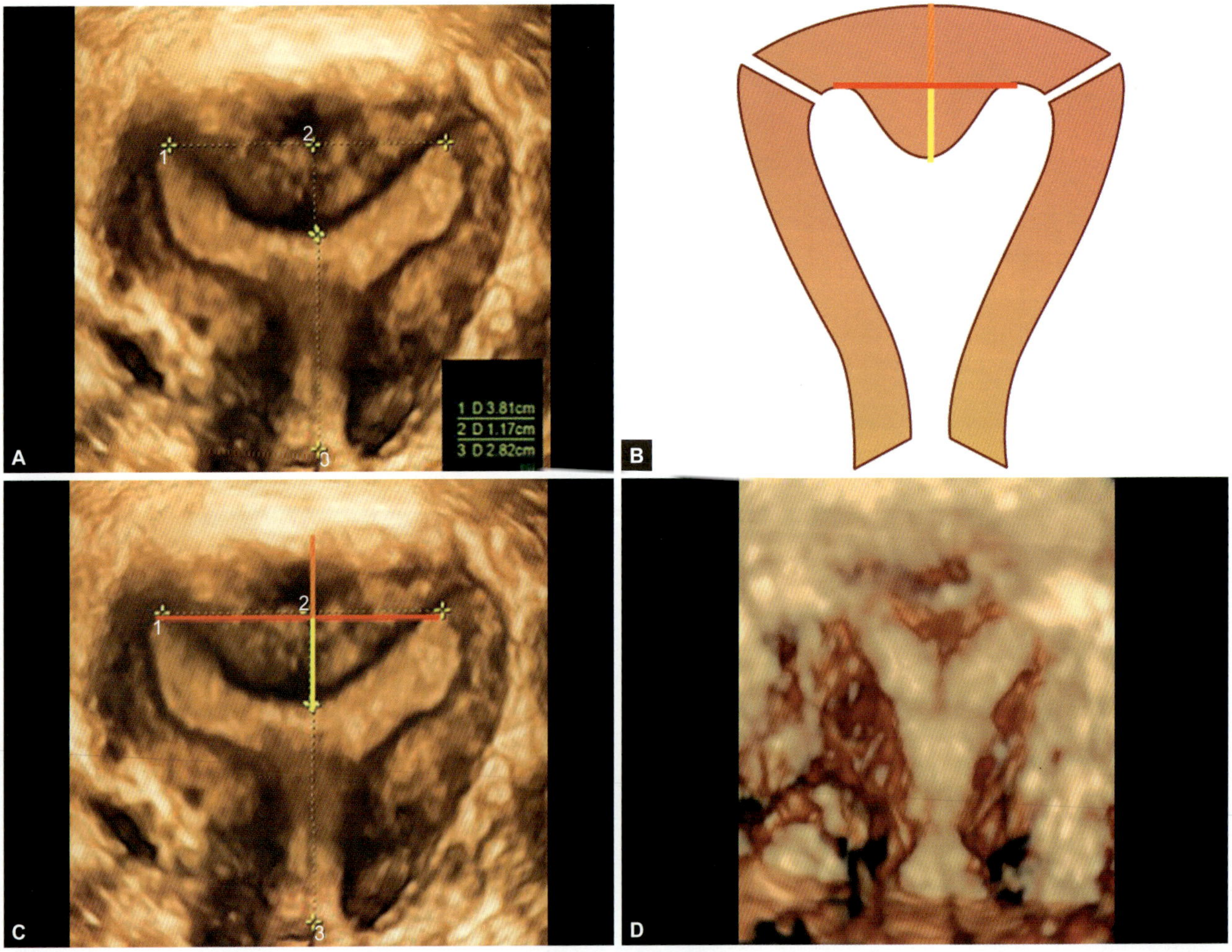

Figs. 13.14A to D

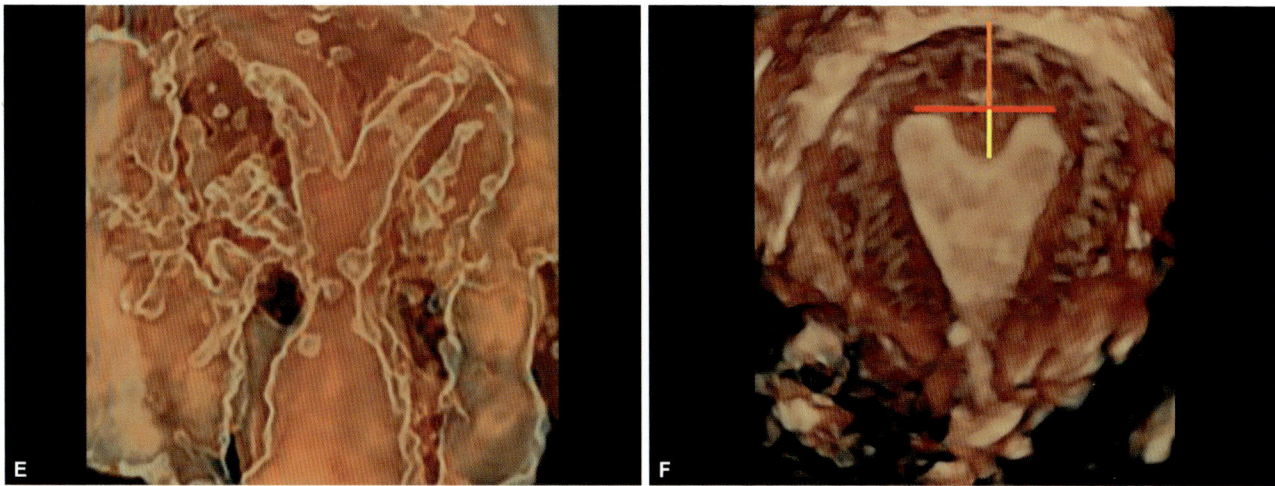

Figs. 13.14E and F

Figs. 13.14A to F: Incomplete septate.

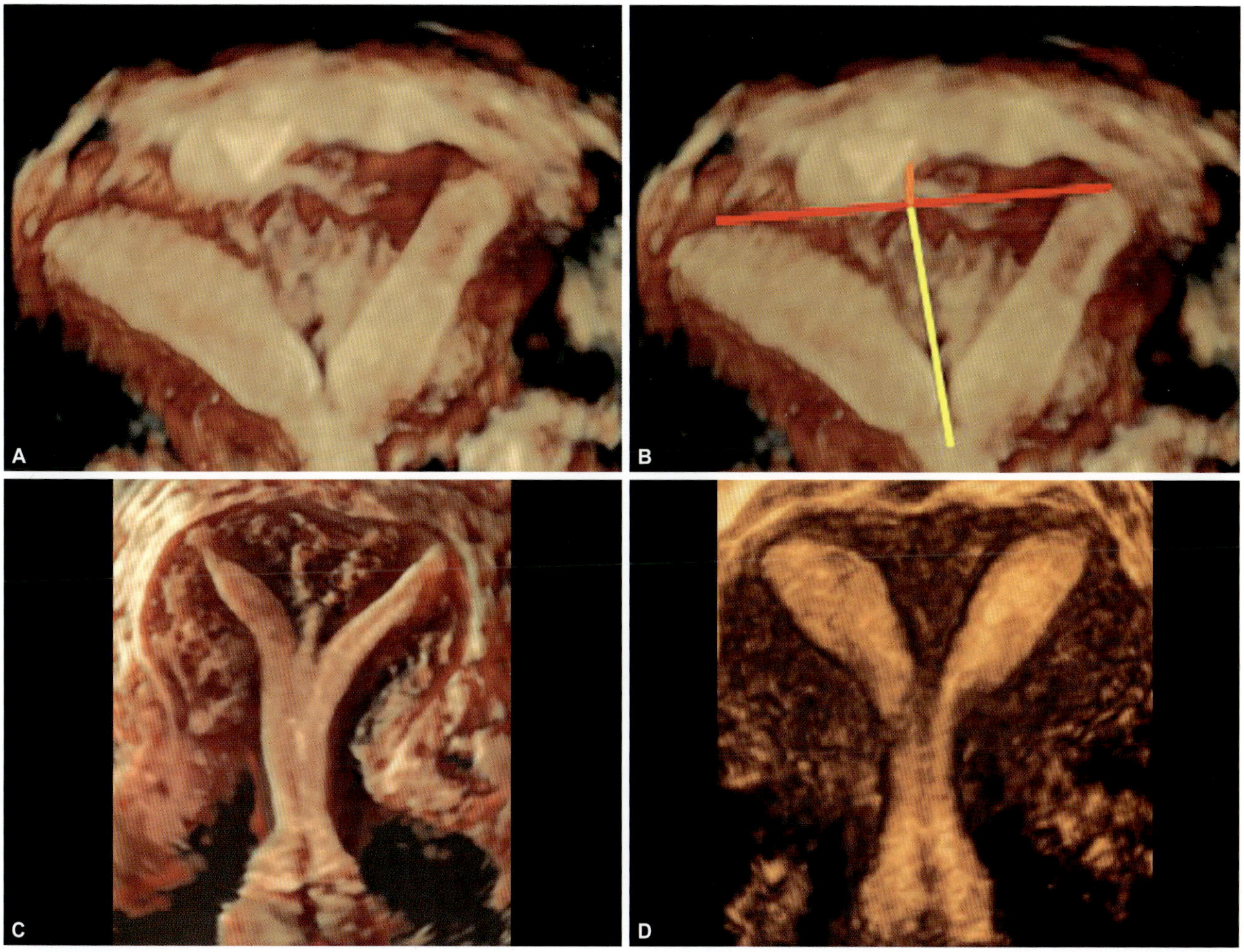

Figs. 13.15A to D: Complete septate and didelphys.

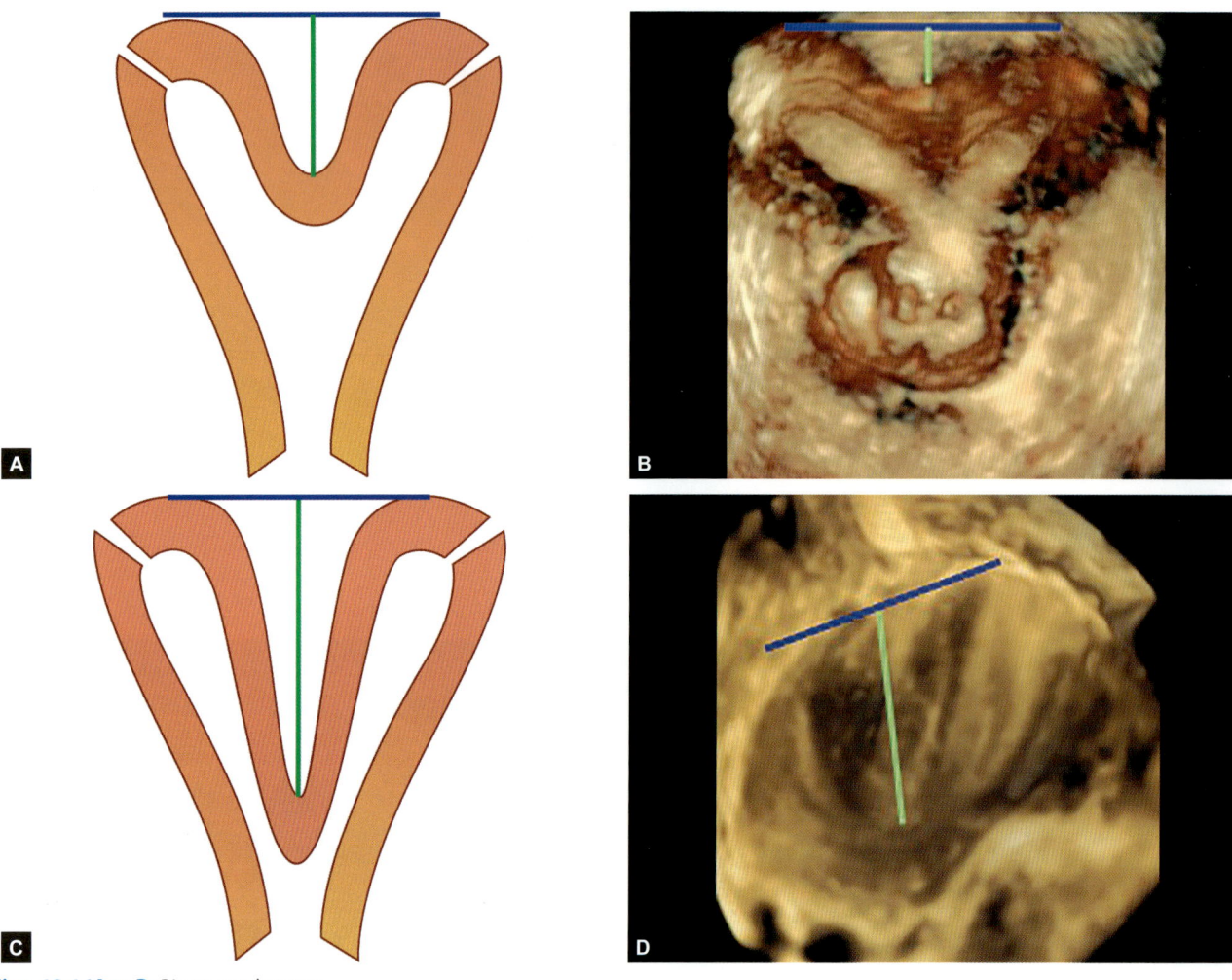

Figs. 13.16A to D: Bicorporeal uterus.

fusion defects and always has an abnormal fundal contour (**Figs. 13.16A to D**). The external indentation exceeds 50% of the uterine wall thickness. This indentation may divide the uterus partially (U3a) or completely (U3b). It may extend into the cervix and/or vagina. The bicorporeal uterus is always associated with an inner indentation at the midline level that divides the cavity as also happens in a septate uterus. Class U3c or bicorporeal septate uterus (**Figs. 13.17A and B**) is characterized by an absorption defect in addition to the main fusion defect. The width of the midline fundal indentation exceeds the uterine wall thickness by 50%. These patients may benefit from a hysteroscopic resection of the septate element of the defect.

Class U4 or hemiuterus is a formation defect that includes the unilateral formed uterus (**Fig. 13.18**), formerly known as the unicornuate uterus. The contralateral part may be incomplete or absent. Class U4a is a hemiuterus with a functional rudimentary cavity. This may be communicating or noncommunicating. A functional cavity in the contralateral part is the clinically important consideration for complications such as hematometra or ectopic pregnancy and laparoscopic removal is recommended even if the horn is communicating. Class U4b or hemiuterus is characterized either by the presence of a nonfunctional contralateral uterine horn or by aplasia of the contralateral part (**Figs. 13.19A to C**).

Class U5 includes all cases of uterine aplasia. It is a formation defect. In some cases, there could be unilateral or bilateral rudimentary horns with (U5a) or without (U5b) a functional cavity.

Class U6 has been created for hitherto unclassified cases. Consequent to technological advancements, newer rare anomalies, subtle variations or combinations may emerge.

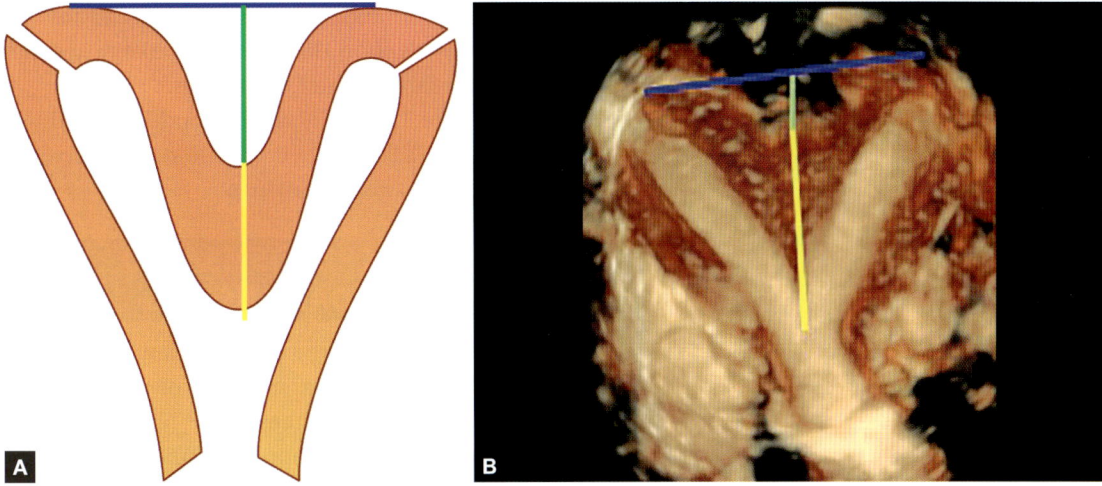

Figs. 13.17A and B: Bicorporeal septate.

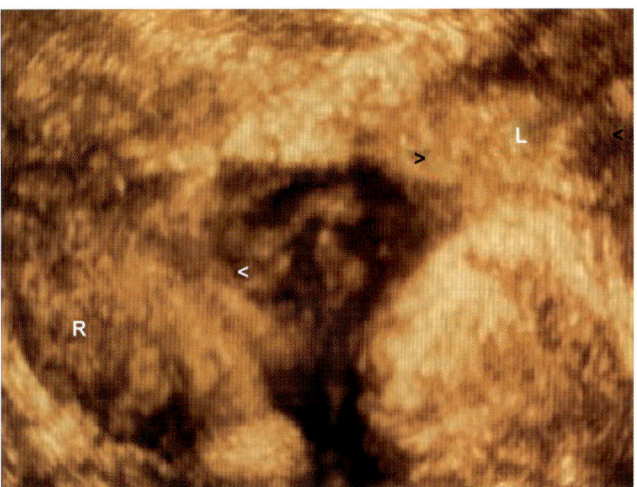

Fig. 13.18: Unicornuate with rudimentary horn.

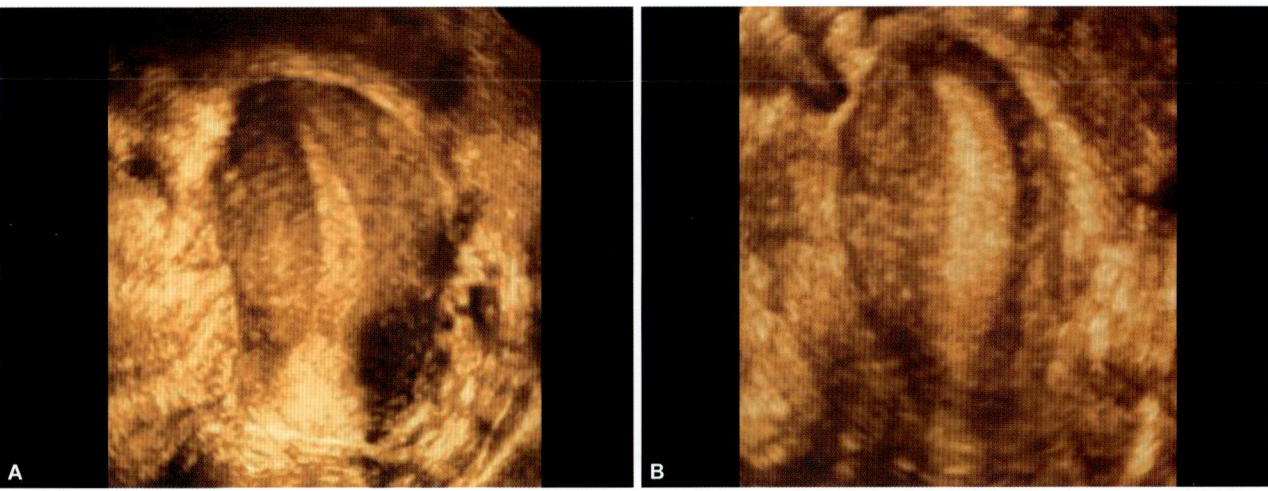

Figs. 13.19A and B

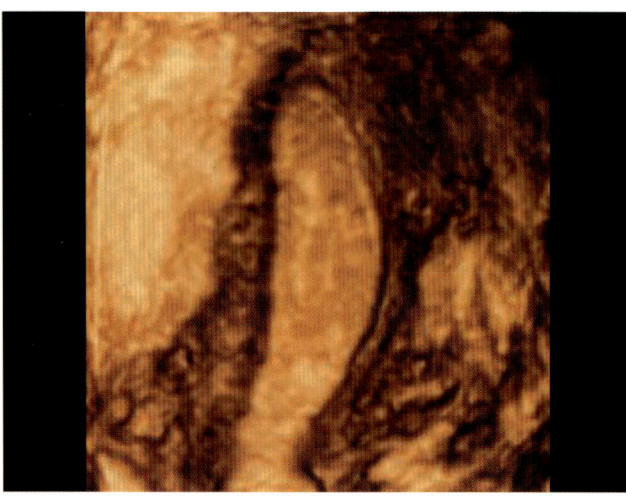

Fig. 13.19C

Figs. 13.19A to C: Unicornuate uterus.

Cervical and vaginal anomalies are not always clearly evident on US and a gynecological examination is indispensable in their evaluation.

Figure 13.20 is a recommended reporting form from ESHRE/ESGE and is a convenient summary including the possibility of hand drawings.

UPDATES, CRITICISMS, AND RECOMMENDATIONS

It has been suggested that the new classification significantly increases the number of septate uteruses and may result in overtreatment.[37-39] The original authors have published appropriate replies and rebuttals[40-42] and suggested a working algorithm. 3D US is recommended for the diagnosis of Müllerian anomalies in symptomatic patients belonging to high-risk groups and in any

ESHRE/ESGE classification				
Female genital tract anomalies				
Uterine anomaly			Cervical/vaginal anomaly	
Class	Main class	Subclass	Coexistent class	
U0	Normal uterus		C0 Normal cervix	
U1	Dysmorphic uterus	a. T-shaped b. Infantilis c. Others	C1 Septate cervix C2 Double "normal" cervix C3 Unilateral cervical aplasia	
U2	Septate uterus	a. Partial b. Complete	C4 Cervical aplasia	
U3	Bicorporeal uterus	a. Partial b. Complete c. Bicorporeal septate		
U4	Hemiuterus	a. With rudimentary cavity (communicating or not horn) b. Without rudimentary cavity (horn without cavity/no horn)	V0 Normal vagina V1 Longitudinal nonobstructing vaginal septum V2 Longitudinal obstructing vaginal septum	
U5	Aplastic	a. With rudimentary cavity (bi- or unilateral horn) b. Without rudimentary cavity (bi- or unilateral uterine remnants/aplasia)	V3 Transverse vaginal septum and/or imperforate hymen V4 Vaginal aplasia	
U6	Unclassified malformations			
U		C	V	

Associated anomalies of non-Müllerian origin:

Drawing of the anomaly

Fig. 13.20: Reporting format. (ESHRE/ESGE: European Society of Human Reproduction and Embryology/European Society for Gynaecological Endoscopy)

asymptomatic woman suspected to have an anomaly from routine evaluation. MRI and endoscopy should be carried out for patients with suspected complex malformations or in diagnostic dilemmas. Adolescents with symptoms should be thoroughly assessed with 2D and 3D US, MRI, and with endoscopy.

REFERENCES

1. Heinonen PK, Saarikoski S, Pystynen P. Reproductive performance of women with uterine anomalies: an evaluation of 182 cases. Acta Obstet Gynecol Scand. 1982;61:157-62.
2. Acien P. Reproductive performance of women with uterine malformations. Hum Reprod. 1993;8:122-6.
3. Rackow BW, Arici A. Reproductive performance of women with Müllerian anomalies. Curr Opin Obstet Gynecol. 2007;19:229-37.
4. Saravelos SH, Cocksedge KA, Li TC. Prevalence and diagnosis of congenital uterine anomalies in women with reproductive failure: a critical appraisal. Hum Reprod Update. 2008;14:415-9.
5. Chan YY, Jayaprakasan K, Zamora J, et al. The prevalence of congenital uterine anomalies in unselected and high-risk populations: a systematic review. Hum Reprod Update. 2011;17:761-71.
6. Brucker SY, Rall K, Campo R, et al. Treatment of congenital malformations. Semin Reprod Med. 2011;29:101-12.
7. Strassmann EO. Fertility and unification of double uterus. Fertil Steril. 1966;17:165-76.
8. Jarcho J. Malformations of the uterus. Am J Surg. 1946;71: 4106-66.
9. Buttram VC, Gibbons WE. Müllerian anomalies: a proposed classification (an analysis of 144 cases). Fertil Steril. 1979;32:40-6.
10. Buttram VC Jr, Gomel V, Siegler A, et al. The American Fertility Society classifications of adnexal adhesions, distal tubal occlusion, tubal occlusion secondary to tubal ligation, tubal pregnancies, Müllerian anomalies and intrauterine adhesions. Fertil Steril. 1988;49:944-55.
11. Oppelt P, Renner SP, Brucker S, et al. The VCUAM (Vagina Cervix Uterus Adnex-associated Malformation) classification: a new classification for genital malformations. Fertl Steril. 2005;91:1493-7.
12. Grimbizis GF, Camus M, Tarlatzis BC, et al. Clinical implications of uterine malformations and hysteroscopic treatment results. Hum Reprod Update. 2001;7:161-74.
13. Acién P, Acién MI, Sanchez-Ferrer M. Complex malformations of the female genital tract. New types and revision of classification. Hum Reprod. 2004;19:2377-84.
14. Acién P, Acién MI. The history of female genital tract malformation classifications and proposal of an updated system. Hum Reprod Update. 2011;17:693-705.
15. Grimbizis GF, Gordts S, Di Spiezio Sardo A, et al. The ESHRE/ESGE consensus on the classification of female genital tract congenital anomalies. Hum Reprod. 2013;28: 2032-44.
16. Braun P, Grau FV, Pons RM, et al. Is hysterosalpingography able to diagnose all uterine malformations correctly? A retrospective study. Eur J Radiol. 2005;53:274-9.
17. Roma Dalfo A, Ubeda B, Ubeda A, et al. Diagnostic value of hysterosalpingography in the detection of intrauterine abnormalities: a comparison with hysteroscopy. AJR Am J Roentgenol. 2004;183:1405-9.
18. Swart P, Mol BW, Veen F, et al. The accuracy of hysterosalpingography in the diagnosis of tubal pathology: a meta-analysis. Fertil Steril. 1995;64:486-91.
19. Guimarães Filho HA, Mattar R, Pires CR, et al. Comparison of hysterosalpingography, hysterosonography and hysteroscopy in evaluation of the uterine cavity in patients with recurrent pregnancy losses. Arch Gynecol Obstet. 2006;274: 284-8.
20. Dee Olpin J, Heilbrun M. Imaging of Müllerian duct anomalies. Clin Obstet Gynecol. 2009;52:40-56.
21. Kupesic S. Clinical implications of sonographic detection of uterine anomalies for reproductive outcome. Ultrasound Obstet Gynecol. 2001;18:387-400.
22. Lindheim SR, Adsuar N, Kushner DM, et al. Sonohysterography: a valuable tool in evaluating the female pelvis. Obstet Gynecol Surv. 2003;58:770-84.
23. Mazouni C, Girard G, Deter R, et al. Diagnosis of Müllerian anomalies in adults: evaluation of practice. Fertil Steril. 2008;89:219-22.
24. Cepni I, Ocal P, Erkan S, et al. Comparison of transvaginal sonography, saline infusion sonography and hysteroscopy in the evaluation of uterine cavity pathologies. ANZJ Obstet Gynecol. 2005;45:30-5.
25. Grimbizis GF, Tsolakidis D, Mikos T, et al. A prospective comparison of transvaginal ultrasound, saline infusion sonohysterography, and diagnostic hysteroscopy in the evaluation of endometrial pathology. Fertil Steril. 2010;94: 2720-5.
26. Guven MA, Bese T, Demirkiran F, et al. Hydrosonography in screening for intracavitary pathology in infertile women. Int J Gynecol Obstet. 2004;86:377-83.
27. Shokeir S, Abdelshaheed M. Sonohysterography as a first-line evaluation for uterine abnormalities in women with recurrent failed in vitro fertilization-embryo transfer. Fertil Steril. 2009;91(Suppl 4):1321-2.
28. Tur-Kaspa I, Gal M, Hartman M, et al. A prospective evaluation of uterine abnormalities by saline infusion sonohysterography in 1009 women with infertility or abnormal uterine bleeding. Fertil Steril. 2006;86:1731-5.
29. Valenzano MM, Mistrangelo E, Lijoi D, et al. Transvaginal sonohysterographic evaluation of uterine malformations. Eur J Obstet Gynecol Reprod Biol. 2006;124:246-9.
30. Jurkovic D, Geipel A, Gruboeck K, et al. Three-dimensional ultrasound for the assessment of uterine anatomy and detection of congenital anomalies: a comparison with hysterosalpingography and two-dimensional sonography. Ultrasound Obstet Gynecol. 1995;5:233-7.

31. Deutch TD, Abuhamad AZ. The role of 3-dimensional ultrasonography and magnetic resonance imaging in the diagnosis of Müllerian duct anomalies. J Ultrasound Med. 2008;27:413-23.

32. Raine-Fenning N, Fleischer AC. Clarifying the role of three-dimensional transvaginal sonography in reproductive medicine: an evidence-based appraisal. J Exper Clin Ass Reprod. 2005;2:10.

33. Salim R, Woelfer B, Backos M, et al. Reproducibility of three-dimensional ultrasound diagnosis of congenital uterine anomalies. Ultrasound Obstet Gynecol. 2003;21:578-82.

34. Minto CL, Hollings N, Hall-Craggs M, et al. Magnetic resonance imaging in the assessment of complex Müllerian anomalies. Br J Obstet Gynecol. 2001;108:791-7.

35. Scarsbrook AF, Moore NR. MRI appearances of Müllerian duct abnormalities. Clin Radiol. 2003;58:747-54.

36. Takagi H, Matsunami K, Noda K, et al. Magnetic resonance imaging in the evaluation double uterus and associated urinary tract anomalies: a report of five cases. J Obstet Gynaecol. 2003;23:525-7.

37. Marten K, Vosshenrich R, Funke M, et al. MRI in the evaluation of Müllerian duct anomalies. J Clin Imaging. 2003;27:346-50.

38. Pui MH. Imaging diagnosis of congenital uterine malformation. Comput Med Imag Graph. 2004;28:425-33.

39. Church DG, Vancil JM, Vasanawala SS. Magnetic resonance imaging for uterine and vaginal anomalies. Curr Opin Obstet Gynecol. 2009;21:379-89.

40. Ludwin A, Ludwin I. Comparison of the ESHRE–ESGE and ASRM classifications of Müllerian duct anomalies in everyday practice. Hum Reprod. 2015;30(3):569-80.

41. Knez J, Saridogan E, Van Den Bosch T, et al. ESHRE/ESGE female genital tract anomalies classification system—the potential impact of discarding arcuate uterus on clinical practice. Hum Reprod. 2018;33:600-6.

42. Ludwin A, Martins WP, Nastri CO, et al. Congenital Uterine Malformation by Experts (CUME): better criteria for distinguishing between normal/arcuate and septate uterus? Ultrasound Obstet Gynecol. 2018;51(1):101-9.

Fibroids and Infertility: The Added Value of Three-dimensional Ultrasound

Sanja Kupesic Plavsic

INTRODUCTION

Uterine fibroids, benign monoclonal tumors of the uterine smooth muscle cells, and fibrous connective tissue, are the most common tumors of the female pelvis, occurring in about 20–30% of women of reproductive age.[1] Other frequently used descriptive terms for uterine fibroids are myoma, leiomyoma, and fibromyoma. The cumulative rate of uterine fibroids increases with age, with a tendency of slower increase at older reproductive age. The rate of occurrence is markedly greater in African–Americans and patients with familial predisposition.[2] It is estimated that a woman whose mother or sister was diagnosed with fibroid uterus, has a 40% chance of developing a fibroid during her lifetime.[3]

Cytogenetic and molecular studies strongly suggest a genetic component in the etiology of uterine leiomyomas based on translocations found between chromosomes 12 and 14, 6 and 10, trisomy 12, and deletions of chromosomes 3 and 7.[3,4] The causes of leiomyomas are unknown; however, they typically arise after menarche and regress after menopause, implicating that estrogen (E), progesterone (P), and perimenopausal increase in luteinizing hormone (LH) act as promoters of their growth. Patients on tamoxifen treatment often experience an increase in leiomyoma growth, as well as patients with increasing body mass index (BMI).[5,6] It is estimated that the risk of fibroids increases 21% with each 10 kg increase in body weight. Increased risk of fibroids is also noted in patients with an earlier age of menarche, patients who consume alcohol and caffeinated drinks, and is proportional to the duration of alcohol/coffee consumption and a number of drinks per day.[4,6,7]

Fibroids may be of various sizes, single or multiple, and are described based on their relationship to the uterine cavity.[1,2] Those located within the myometrium are called intramural and are considered the most common, occurring in about 58–79% of all patients.[8-10] The submucous fibroids are located beneath the endometrium; they bulge into the uterine cavity, and eventually may become intracavitary. Subserous fibroids are at the serosal surface of the uterus, projecting into the peritoneal cavity. Imaging techniques used for the diagnosis of uterine fibroids include transabdominal and transvaginal two-dimensional (2D) and three-dimensional (3D) ultrasound, saline infusion sonography (SIS), and MRI.[11]

This chapter reviews the role of different ultrasound modalities, with emphasis on 3D ultrasound in the assessment of infertile patients with uterine fibroids.

UTERINE FIBROIDS AND INFERTILITY

Uterine fibroids are heterogeneous lesions, and their relationship with infertility is commonly explained by mechanical factors, such as distortion of the cervix and uterine cavity, impaired endometrial perfusion, increased and uncoordinated uterine contractility, and occlusion of the tubal ostia.[12] Numerous studies attempting to assess this relationship failed due to small sample size, insufficient study design, and lack of correction for important confounding variables.[13,14] While it is widely assumed that subserous fibroids do not affect fertility, patients with submucous fibroids show significantly lower pregnancy rates and their removal may enhance live-birth rates.[14] Currently, the most important unresolved issue is the assessment of the relationship between intramural fibroids and infertility, although it would appear logical that larger intramural fibroids interfere more with reproductive performance. Also, there is no clear evidence that myomectomy for intramural fibroids is beneficial to fertility.[14]

It has been reported that uterine contractility during the mid-luteal phase may play an important role in embryo implantation and pregnancy outcomes. Impaired uterine peristalsis noticed in some patients with intramural fibroids requires further evaluation. Yoshino et al.[15] used a cine-mode-display MRI to assess the frequency of uterine contractions in mid-luteal phase of 95 patients with regular menstrual cycles and evidence of intramural fibroids not distorting uterine cavity. After separating patients into the two groups: (1) patients exhibiting low-frequency peristalsis (<2 times in 3 minutes), and (2) patients with high-frequency peristalsis (≥2 times in 3 minutes), the authors found that none of the 22 patients with high-frequency peristalsis achieved pregnancy. Interestingly, the pregnancy rate in the group of 29 patients with low-frequency peristalsis was 34% (P <0.005).[15] These results indicate that the reproductive performance of patients with intramural fibroids may be compromised due to abnormal uterine contractility. Yan et al.[16] performed a retrospective study of 249 patients with intramural fibroids not distorting uterine cavity who underwent an in vitro fertilization (IVF)/intracytoplasmic sperm injection (ICSI) procedure. While no difference was detected in the IVF/ICSI outcomes between the patients with different sizes of the uterine fibroids, a significantly impaired live-birth rates (P <0.043) were reported for the patients whose intramural fibroid largest diameter exceeded 2.85 cm.[16]

According to the American Society for Reproductive Medicine (ASRM), uterine myomas are associated with infertility in 5–10% of cases and may be responsible for 2–3% of infertility cases.[17,18] All confounding variables are difficult to control when searching for the impact of fibroids on infertility, and the association between reproductive dysfunction, miscarriage, and fibroids is not clearly established. More studies are needed to determine the clinical importance of the size, location, morphology, and proximity to the endometrium of intramural fibroids regarding the reproductive potential and pregnancy complications rate.

Signs and Symptoms

The symptomatology of the uterine fibroids is determined by the size, location, and extension of the degenerative changes.[19] Many women with myomas remain asymptomatic.

Typically, submucous and intramural fibroids distorting the uterine cavity often result in abnormal uterine bleeding, clinically presenting as menorrhagia, dysmenorrhea, and intermenstrual spotting. Large uterine fibroids sometimes produce increasing abdominal girth associated with abdominal/pelvic discomfort or pain. An anterior leiomyoma often leads to urinary frequency and urgency, while posterior leiomyoma may be associated with lower back pain, rectal pressure, constipation, and rarely, leg discomfort and swelling.

Hormonal Pattern

Numerous studies have shown that E and P regulate most of the genes that encode growth factors which promote smooth muscle cells growth, while the use of gonadotropin-releasing hormone (GnRH) agonist (GnRHa) lead to a rapid decrease in the uterine fibroid size.[20-23] Bourlev et al.[24] compared the growth pattern of the uterine leiomyomas during proliferative and secretory phases of the menstrual cycle by assessing the expression of sex steroid receptors in their peripheral and central portions. Paired biopsy specimens confirm that during the secretory phase of the menstrual cycle, mitosis is significantly higher in the peripheral than in the central part of the uterine fibroids. During the proliferative phase, apoptosis shows the same pattern.[24] Wei et al.[25] compared the gene expression of selected genes in the uterine fibroids and normal myometrium. They confirmed that the expression of hypoxia-inducible factor-1 (HIF-1) is more pronounced in the peripheral portion of the fibroid compared to its central part. These observations illustrate that the fibroids typically grow from the periphery.[25-28] However, sex steroids are not the only regulators of the uterine leiomyoma growth. Numerous studies have demonstrated the presence of mesoderm-specific growth factors and their receptors in the myometrial and leiomyoma tissue.[29-34]

UTERINE FIBROIDS AND PREGNANCY

Fibroid growth in pregnancy may be affected by increase in E and P levels, human chorionic gonadotropin (hCG), and uterine blood flow. Several ultrasound and Doppler studies attempted to assess the effect of fibroid size, location, and number of pregnancies.[35-39] The conclusion of these studies is that the growth of fibroids during pregnancy cannot be predicted. Majority of the fibroids' growth occurred in the 1st trimester.[35,36] Fibroids measuring less than or equal to 5 cm in diameter were more likely to remain stable in size, while larger fibroids were more likely to grow. The mean increase in fibroid volume during pregnancy is on average 12%, and only a small proportion of the fibroids (22%) increased by more than 25%.[37-39]

Although majority of the patients with uterine fibroids do not report any complications, some authors reported slightly increased risk of complications, such as miscarriage, preterm labor, antepartum bleeding, placental abruption, malpresentation, and dysfunctional labor.[40-51] The available information is limited by inadequate methodology and study population selection, small sample size, different criteria used regarding the number, size, and location of the fibroids, limited number of adverse events, and inadequate adjustment of cofounding variables.[52-56] However, studies consistently report that uterine leiomyoma are associated with an increased risk of cesarean delivery.[57,58]

IMAGING

Diagnosis of the uterine fibroids is based on enlargement, distortion of the contour, and textural changes of the uterus.[59] Subserous and especially pedunculated fibroids can be mistaken for a number of conditions, including an ovarian neoplasm, bicornuate uterus, blind uterine horn, or even an ectopic pregnancy. Similarly, submucous and

intracavitary fibroids are often confused with endometrial polyps. The use of complementary imaging modalities, such as different forms of ultrasound (2D and 3D transabdominal and transvaginal ultrasound, 2D color Doppler, and 3D power Doppler ultrasound), contrast ultrasound studies (e.g. 2D and 3D-SIS), and MRI may be necessary to confirm the diagnosis.[60]

Two-dimensional Ultrasound and Color Doppler Features

Sonographic assessment of the uterine fibroids includes determination of their number, location, echotexture, and size, by measuring the three maximum diameters (length, width, and height). Serial examinations are necessary to document the interval growth and change in morphology.

Leiomyomas arise from the uterine myometrium and consist of the fascicles of smooth muscle cells and extracellular matrix.[61] Small fibroids typically appear as subtle changes in myometrial echogenicity. The increased amount of the extracellular matrix in an acellular area between the cells and a higher number of E and P receptors distinguishes the leiomyoma from the normal, surrounding myometrium. A well-delineated outline created by compressed muscle fibers forms a firm whorled surface, representing a pseudocapsule.[62,63] On transabdominal and transvaginal ultrasound, this area appears as an echogenic peripheral zone, while on color Doppler ultrasound, it is visualized as a "ring of fire" **(Figs. 14.1A and B)**.[64-66]

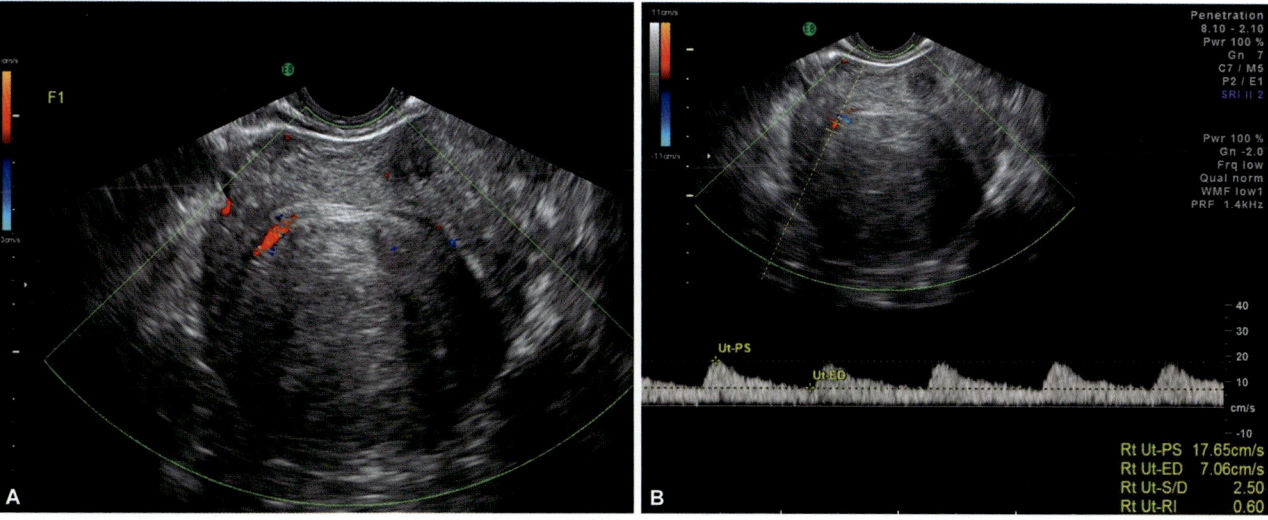

Figs. 14.1A and B: Transvaginal color Doppler image of a solitary intramural fibroid. (A) Note a well-delineated intramural fibroid with a regularly separated vessel within the pseudocapsule; (B) Pulsed Doppler waveform analysis reveals moderate vascular resistance signals [resistance index (RI) 0.60].

Submucous fibroids are visualized as round or elongated hypoechogenic, subendometrial lesions. Sometimes, they extend into the uterine cavity, may become intracavitary, pedunculated, and may even prolapse through the cervix.[63] They are differentiated from the endometrial polyps based on echogenicity and visualization in continuity with myometrium **(Figs. 14.2A and B)**. Color Doppler ultrasound typically reveals scattered vessels with moderate vascular impedance, although a wide range of vascularity signals may be obtained depending on the size, cellularity, and age of the fibroid. Degenerative submucous/intracavitary fibroids may display central low impedance blood flow signals.[65,66] After initial transvaginal ultrasound, SIS is recommended for improved visualization of the thickness of overlying myometrium and surgical planning.[67] Top differential diagnosis is an endometrial polyp, which is usually visualized as a hyperechogenic endometrial lesion with no continuity with the underlying myometrium. Contrary to leiomyoma scattered vascular pattern on color Doppler ultrasound, endometrial polyps show a single vascular pedicle.

Intramural fibroids are the most common fibroids, affecting about 40% of women after age 35 years.[3] If uncomplicated, they are visualized as homogeneous round, well-defined myometrial lesions. Majority of intramural fibroids are asymptomatic; however, 25–30% of the patients may present with menorrhagia, polymenorrhea, menometrorrhagia, bloating, pressure effects, dull ache, bloating, and/or pain.[3,64,65] Transabdominal ultrasound scan is necessary to obtain the overall size of the uterus, assess its contour, and leiomyoma locations, size, and echotexture changes.

Subserous fibroids are usually visualized as homogeneous, round, and well-defined masses protruding from the uterus with similar echogenicity as myometrium. Sometimes, pedunculated myomas cannot be detected by transvaginal ultrasound, but only with transabdominal approach. In this case, color Doppler ultrasound enables visualization of the vessels in the leiomyoma stalk. Identification of the vascular resistance of these vessels may assist in identification of the uterine origin of the tumor. Rarely, pedunculated fibroid may twists on its pedicle, infarct, and undergo necrosis. Eventually, they may detach and become infected.[65,66] In these cases, pulsed Doppler ultrasound reveals increased vascularity accompanied with low vascular impedance signals **(Figs. 14.3A and B)**.

Different types of degenerative changes are associated with alteration in fibroid's echotexture. With aging, the leiomyoma may undergo different types of degenerative changes. Hyaline degeneration is considered the most common, affecting about 60–70% of the uterine fibroids.[65,66] On ultrasound, it is recognized as loss of leiomyoma whorl appearance which occurs when the fibroid gradually outgrows its blood supply. When advanced, fibroids with hyaline degeneration may undergo fat degeneration, which is visualized as hyperechogenic well-delineated fatty deposits, with posterior attenuation **(Fig. 14.4)**. Calcific degeneration occurs when calcium binds to

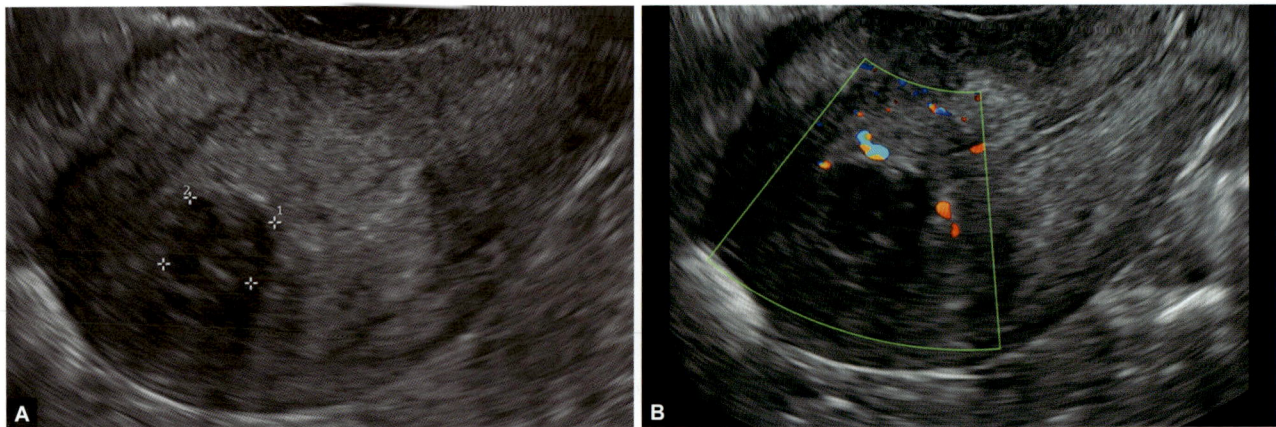

Figs. 14.2A and B: Transvaginal ultrasound of a hypoechoic fibroid in a patient with secondary infertility. (A) Hypoechoic fibroid measuring 1.3 × 1.5 cm is visualized in the fundal area, impinging upon a nearby endometrium; (B) Color Doppler displays discrete peripheral blood flow signals.

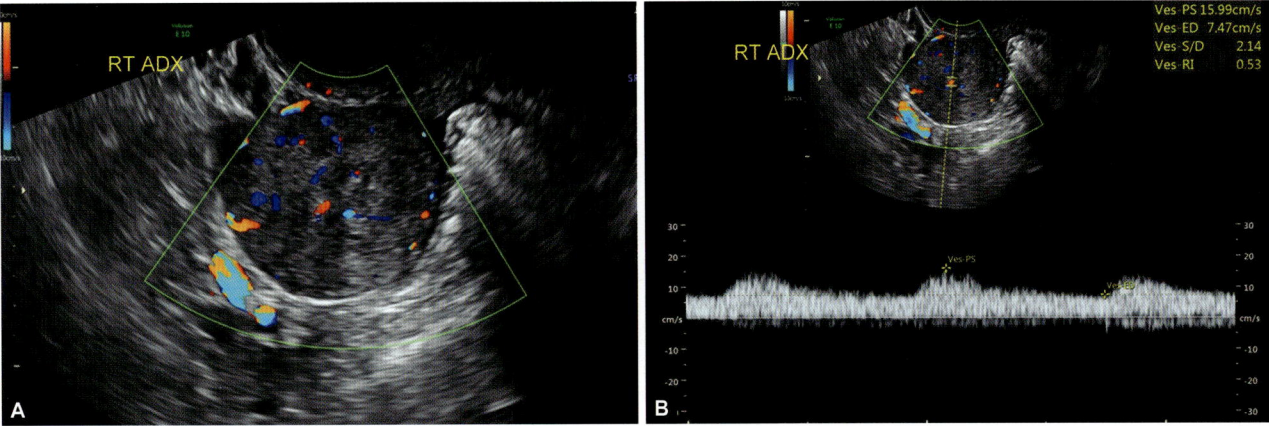

Figs. 14.3A and B: Transvaginal color Doppler image of a solid tumor in the right adnexal region in a primary infertile patient complaining of acute pelvic pain. (A) Solid mass is visualized in the right adnexal region. Transvaginal color Doppler image reveals scattered vascularity. The right ovary was visualized laterally from the lesion, and was within the normal sonographic limits; (B) Spectral Doppler analysis reveals moderate impedance blood flow signals [resistance index (RI) 0.53]. Comparison with transvaginal ultrasound which was performed 6 months earlier confirms prior diagnosis of a subserous fibroid. Laparoscopic surgery confirmed that the fibroid was twisted on its pedicle. Increased perfusion visualized within the pedunculated fibroid is consistent with necrosis which was confirmed by histology.

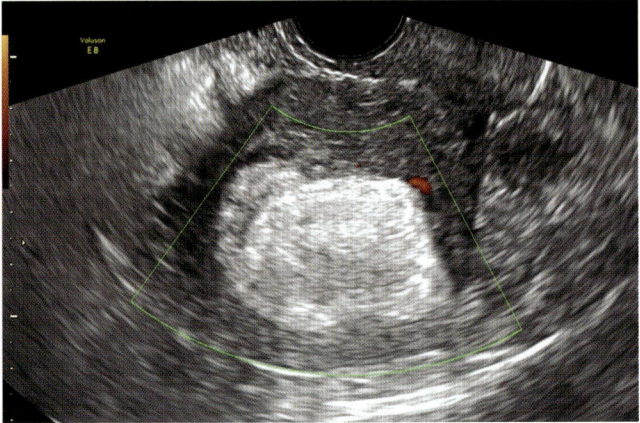

Fig. 14.4: Transvaginal color Doppler image of a fibroid with a well-delineated hyperechogenic area with posterior attenuation, suggestive of fat degeneration.

phospholipids within the membrane of the necrotic cells. These changes are recognized as bright reflectors with posterior shadowing, and may vary from focal areas to extensive calcifications, usually observed in older women **(Figs. 14.15A and B)**.[65] Cystic degeneration is recognized as the presence of hypoechoic areas within the leiomyoma. Cystic spaces appear as round and well-demarcated sonolucent areas **(Fig. 14.6)**.[66] Although the majority of degenerating fibroids are asymptomatic, sometimes they may present with acute pelvic pain, leukocytosis, nausea, and vomiting.

THE ADDED VALUE OF THREE-DIMENSIONAL ULTRASOUND

Ultrasound has evolved so quickly and now has it all: from real-time imaging, through functional Doppler assessment to volume rendering. By providing multiplanar imaging, 3D ultrasound not only gives an additional dimension to the uterine scan, but provides a similar quality and less expensive alternative to MRI. Automated volume acquisition minimizes the subjectivity of the ultrasound assessment and can be used for retrospective analysis (*re-evaluation at any time from any view and any orientation*).[64,65]

In patients with enlarged uterus and multiple fibroids, tomographic ultrasound imaging (TUI) is recommended for improved mapping of the uterine fibroids.[64] Simultaneous display of the coronal, sagittal, and transverse planes contributes to better localization and more accurate volume estimation of the uterine lesions. The volume display and OmniView improve the assessment of the continuity of the fibroids in different projections, leading to better concordance with intraoperative findings **(Figs. 14.7A and B)**.

Saline infusion sonography is a minimally invasive ultrasound technique that involves infusion of a small volume of sterile saline into the uterine cavity, followed by a pelvic ultrasound evaluation.[67] Saline acts as a negative contrast medium which clearly delineates hyperechogenic

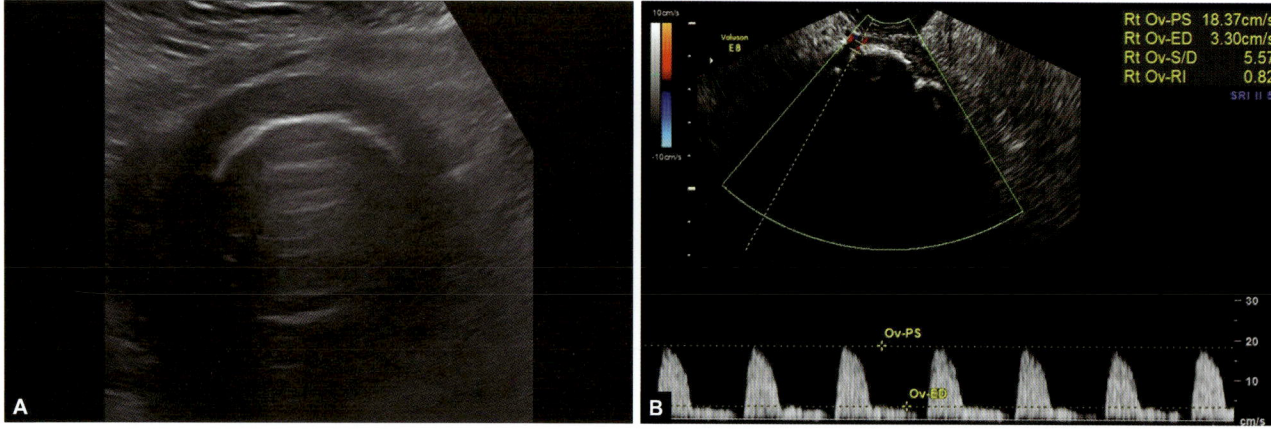

Figs. 14.5A and B: Transabdominal and transvaginal images of calcific degeneration. (A) Transabdominal ultrasound image of an intramural fibroid with calcific degeneration, recognized as ellipsoid-shaped bright signals; (B) Transvaginal color Doppler image of a fibroid with "popcorn-like" appearance of calcification. High impedance blood flow signals [resistance index (RI) 0.82] are obtained from the peripheral vessels.

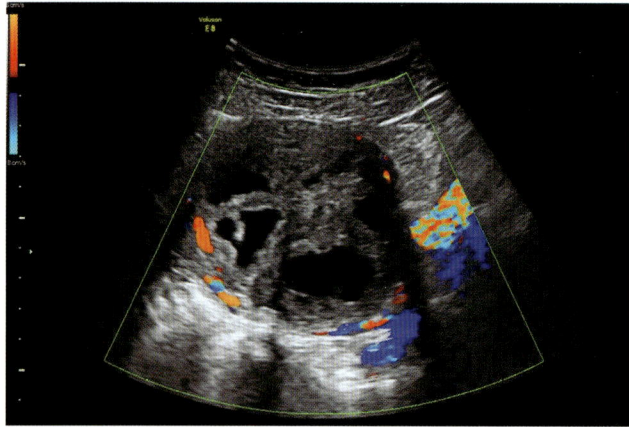

Fig. 14.6: Transabdominal color Doppler image illustrating cystic degeneration of a huge subserous fibroid. Color Doppler reveals regularly separated blood vessels at its periphery.

endometrial lining **(Fig. 14.8)**. The procedure can be performed under the guidance of 2D and 3D ultrasound. 3D SIS can precisely depict submucous and intracavitary fibroids, determine their size, and extent of protrusion, which is important for planning of a hysteroscopic resection **(Figs. 14.9A and B)**. When the entire fibroid is visualized arising from the pedicle, the lesion is classified as intracavitary **(Figs. 14.10A and B)**. 3D SIS is reported as superior to hysteroscopy for determining the depth of fibroid penetration to the endometrium and/or myometrium.[67]

It is well-known that malignant tumors are characterized with abundant and disorganized blood flow patterns, whereas benign lesions show regular, predominantly peripheral vessel distribution **(Figs. 14.11A and B)**.[68-70] Neovascularization represents a network of capillaries and larger vessels, whose wall are devoid of smooth muscle cells and elastic fibers, which on spectral Doppler analysis manifests as reduced vascular impedance. Vascular resistance measured by angle independent Doppler parameters, the resistance index (RI) and pulsatility index (PI), is largely dependent on the fraction of arterioles in the microcirculation.[71] Reported variations in blood flow in malignant tumors after radiotherapy suggest that the same technology has a potential to predict a response of a tumor to treatment.[72] 3D power Doppler angiography enables objective assessment of the vessels' density and quantification of the amount of blood within a volume of the tumor tissue, leading to a new concept of "virtual tumor biopsy".[73] The use of contrast agents is another possibility for enhancing the 3D power Doppler examination by increasing the detection rate of capillaries with small diameter.

Although uterine leiomyosarcoma is a rare tumor, accounting for only 1–3% of all genital tumors, it is characterized with poor prognosis due to early dissemination.[69,74-76] As gynecologists are more frequently choosing to use conservative treatment for uterine fibroids (e.g. pharmacologic treatment, uterine fibroid embolization, MR-guided focused ultrasound, and ultrasound-guided fibroid sclerosation), uterine leiomyosarcoma may become more common in the near future.[77] Clinically, this malignant tumor presents with atypical

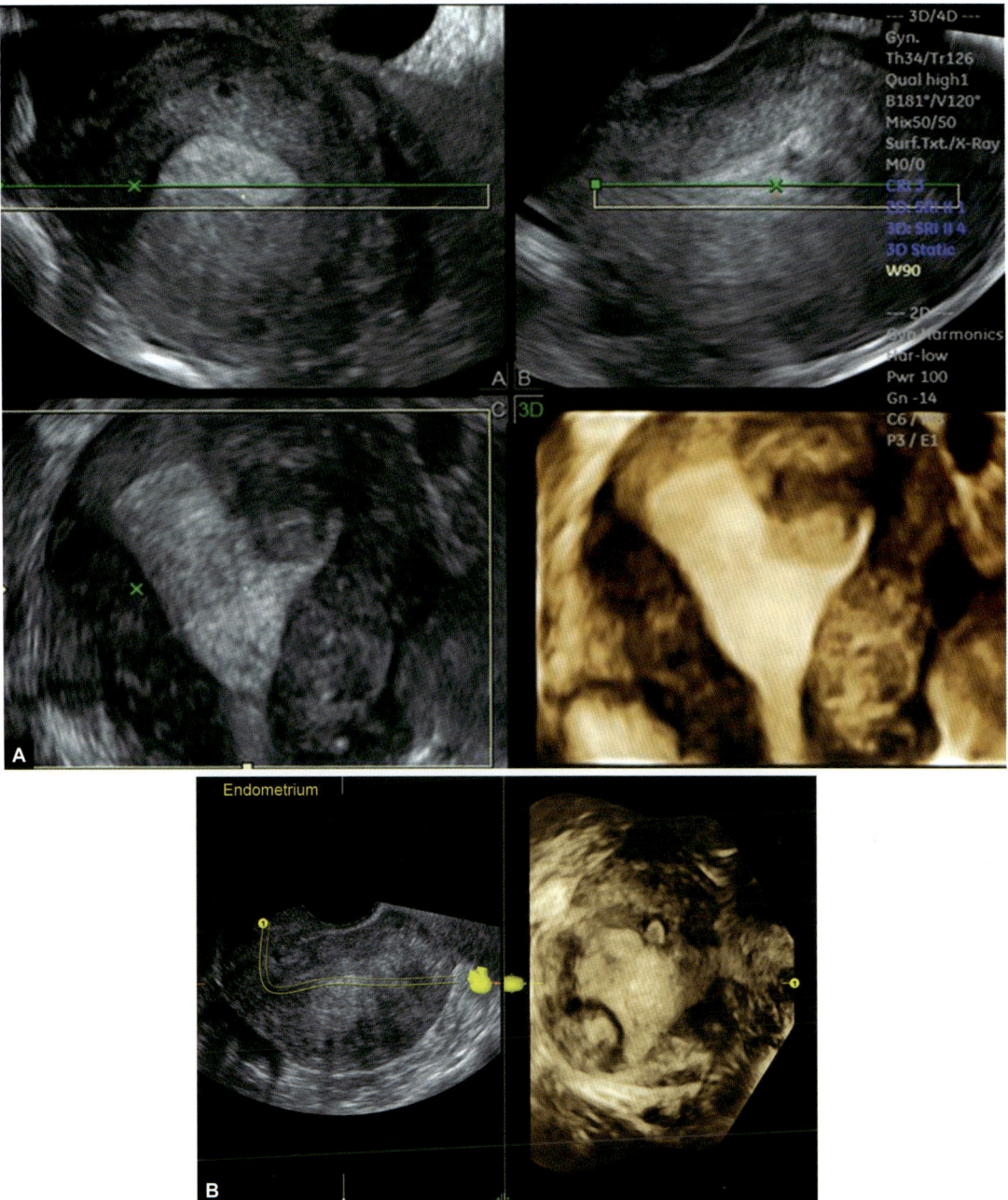

Figs. 14.7A and B: Transvaginal three-dimensional (3D) ultrasound of a submucous fibroid in an infertile patient. (A) Multiplanar view and surface rendering of a submucous fibroid impinging on the uterine cavity and blocking the intramural portion of the fallopian tube; (B) The same patient assessed by OmniView.

signs and symptoms, similar to the uterine leiomyoma such as abnormal uterine bleeding, palpable pelvic mass, lower abdominal pressure, and increase in size of the uterus after the onset of menopause.[64,78] On ultrasound, leiomyosarcoma is presented as solid or complex tumor. Color Doppler reveals irregular and randomly dispersed vessels with high velocity and low vascular impedance.[78] Demonstration of the irregular branching of the vessels with uneven diameter, microaneurysms and stenosis are typical 3D power Doppler angiography features of the leiomyosarcoma neovascularization **(Fig. 14.12)**.[79]

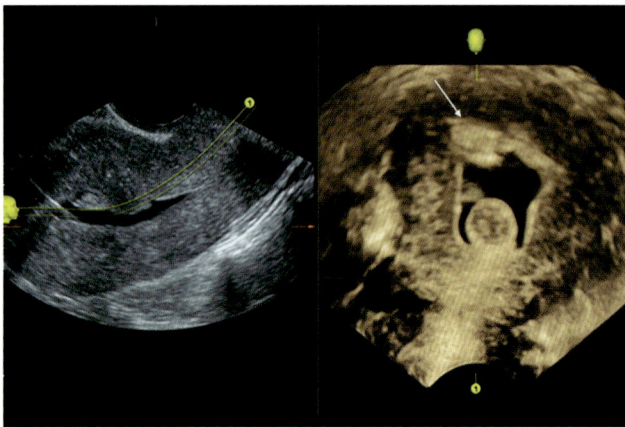

Fig. 14.8: Saline infusion sonography of a patient with a small intracavitary fibroid at the level of the internal cervical os. Hyperechogenic fundal polyp, shown by an arrow, is obstructing the opening of the right fallopian tube into the uterine cavity.

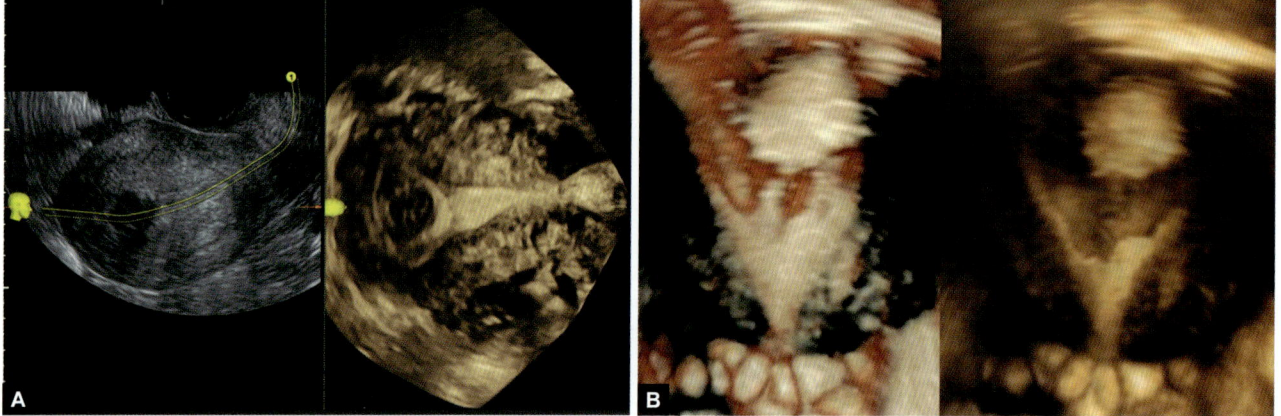

Figs. 14.9A and B: 3D imaging and 3D SIS of a submucous fibroid in a secondary infertile patient. (A) OmniView reveals a hypoechogenic intracavitary fibroid; (B) 3D SIS of the same patient. Sonographic finding of intracavitary fibroid was confirmed by hysteroscopy. (3D: three-dimensional; SIS: saline infusion sonography)

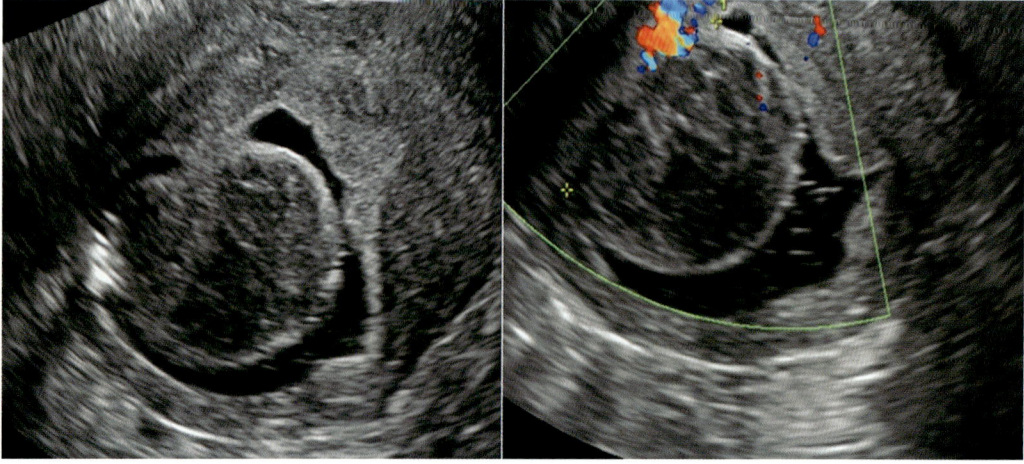

Fig. 14.10A

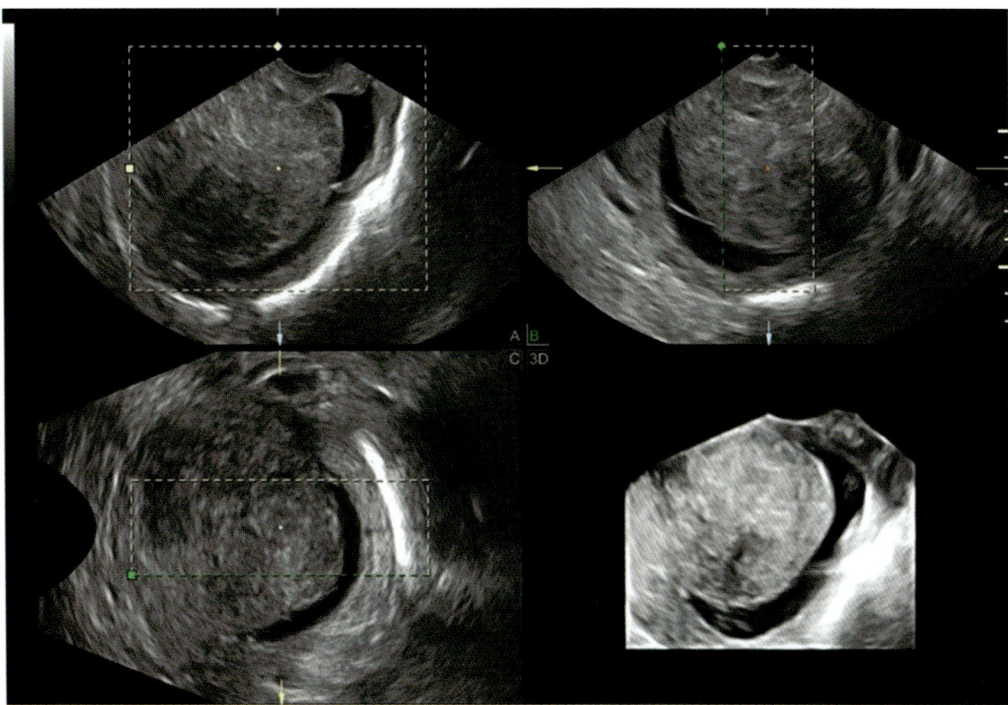

Fig. 14.10B

Figs. 14.10A and B: 2D and 3D SIS of an intracavitary fibroid in an infertile patient complaining of metrorrhagia. (A) 2D SIS of a huge intracavitary fibroid. Color Doppler reveals vascularized pedicle; (B) 3D SIS of another patient with a huge intracavitary fibroid. A protruding fibroid has a wide base, compared to a relatively thin connection pedicle of a fibroid displayed in Figure 10A. (2D: two-dimensional; SIS: saline infusion sonography)

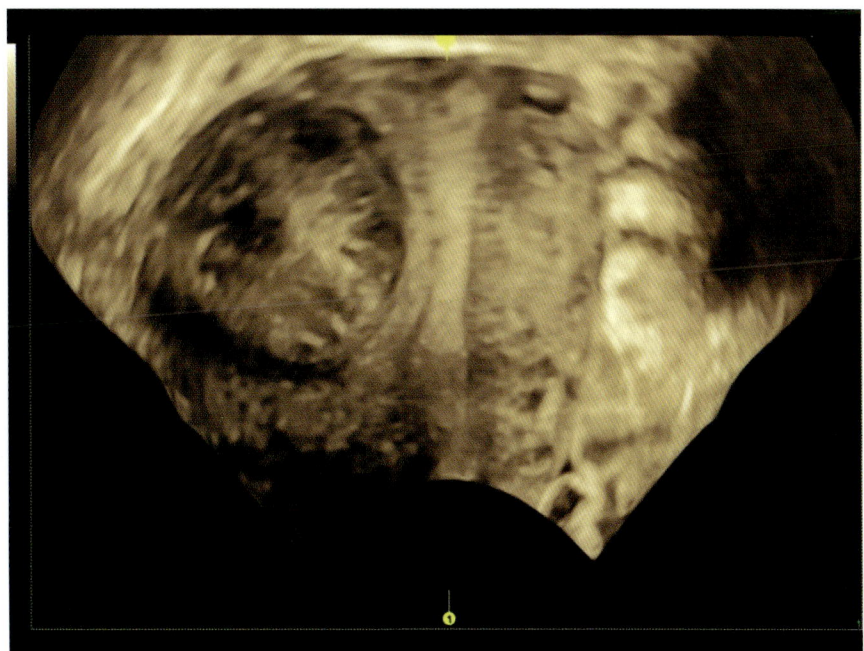

Fig. 14.11A

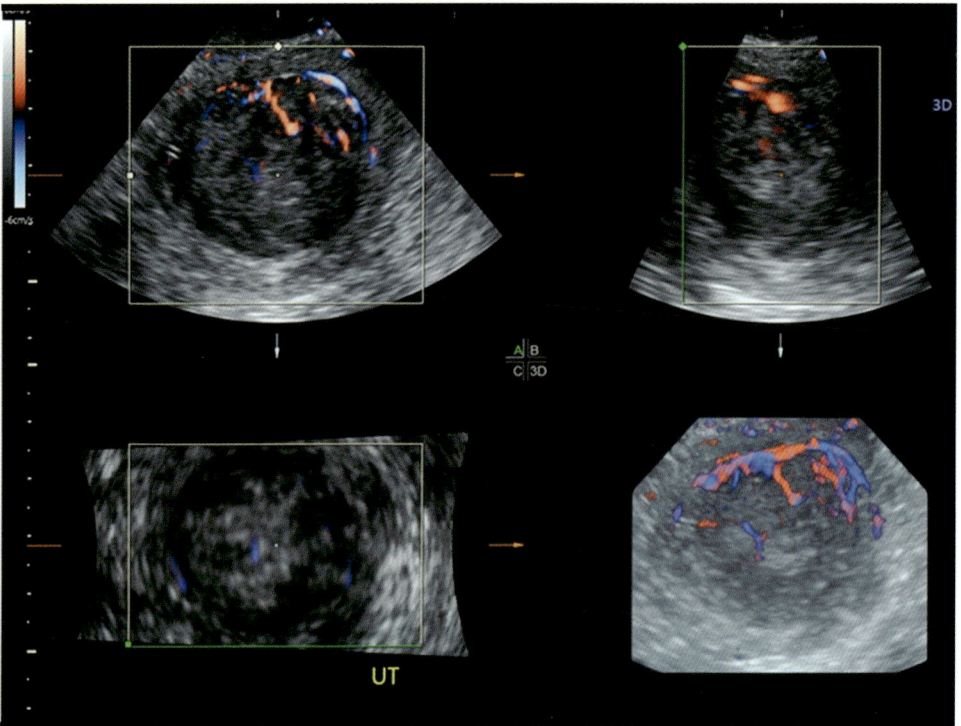

Fig. 14.11B

Figs. 14.11A and B: Three-dimensional (3D) ultrasound and 3D color Doppler image of an intramural fibroid. (A) 3D ultrasound image of an intramural fibroid; (B) 3D color/power Doppler angiography reveals regularly separated peripheral vessels, typical for a benign uterine growth.

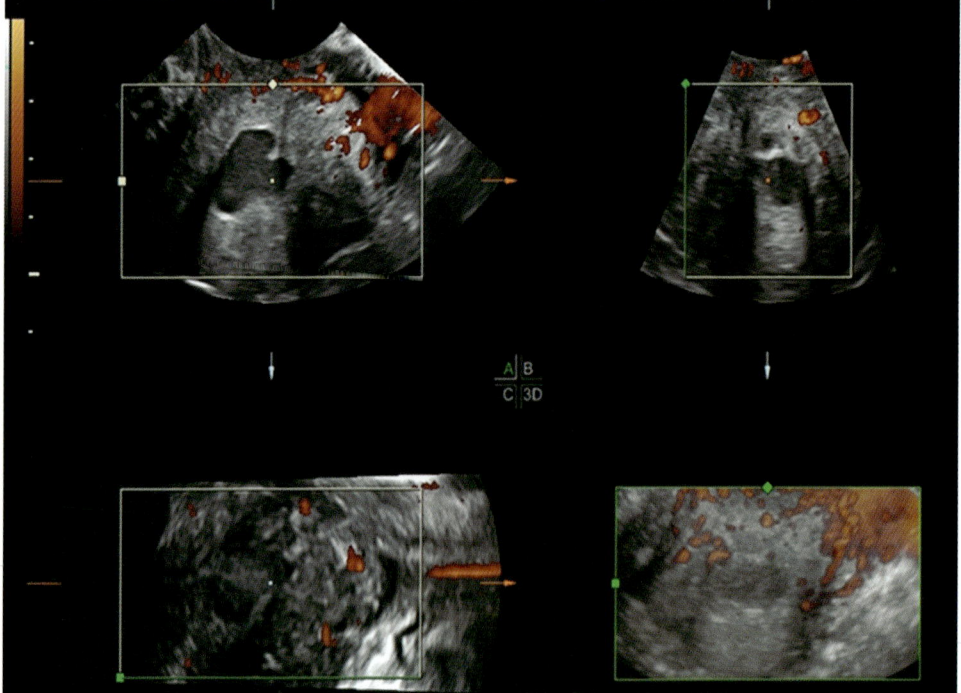

Fig. 14.12: Three-dimensional (3D) power Doppler image of a complex uterine mass in patient with increased size of the uterus in postmenopause. Irregular branching of the vessels with uneven diameter is suggestive of a malignant uterine lesion. Uterine leiomyosarcoma was confirmed by histology.

CONCLUSION

While there is a consensus that submucous uterine fibroids distorting the uterine cavity are associated with infertility and early pregnancy loss, the clinical relationship of intramural fibroids and infertility remains unclear. Because the effect of fibroids on implantation may not be reflected on the endometrium overlying the submucous or intramural fibroids, future studies should focus on the assessment of global effects, such as alteration of vasoconstriction factors, fibrinolytic and anticoagulant activity, and endometrial gene expression.[80]

Combining the advantages of multiple imaging modalities: ultrasound as a noninvasive, nonirradiation, and inexpensive method, and volume acquisition known from CT and MR imaging technologies, 3D ultrasound and 3D power Doppler angiography have become a valuable diagnostic tools for the assessment of uterine fibroids. Despite many advances in molecular and genetic linkage analysis, efficient diagnosis by high-resolution ultrasound imaging, introduction of minimally invasive techniques of leiomyoma embolization, uterine artery occlusion, and high-intensity focused ultrasound therapy, an integration of knowledge is required to assist in improved understanding of this most common gynecologic neoplasm of reproductive age women. Identification of the causes of the uterine fibroids is difficult because of their phenotypic complexity and variability. Therefore, combination of the basic science, genetic, clinical, and high-resolution multiplanar imaging studies is required for a better understanding of the etiopathogenesis and management of these common uterine tumors.

REFERENCES

1. Haney AF. Leiomyomata. In: Gibbs RS, Karlan BY, Haney AF, Nygaard IE (Eds). Danforth's Obstetrics and Gynecology, 10th edition. Philadelphia: Lippincott Williams & Wilkins; 2003.
2. Baird DD, Dunson DB, Hill MC, et al. High cumulative incidence of uterine leiomyoma in black and white women: Ultrasound evidence. Am J Obstet Gynecol. 2003;188(1):100-7.
3. Laughlin SK, Schroeder JC, Baird DD. New directions in the epidemiology of uterine fibroids. Semin Reprod Med. 2010;28(3):204-17.
4. Salem S, Wilson SR. Gynecologic ultrasound. In: Wilson SR (Ed). Diagnostic Ultrasound, 3rd edition. St. Louis: Elsevier; 2005.
5. Schwartz SM. Epidemiology of uterine leiomyomata. Clin Obstet Gynecol. 2001;44(2):316-26.
6. Wise LA, Palmer JR, Harlow BL, et al. Risk of uterine leiomyomata in relation to tobacco, alcohol and caffeine consumption in the Black Women's Health Study. Hum Reprod. 2004;19(8):1746-54.
7. Levine DJ, Berman JM, Harris M, et al. Sensitivity of myoma imaging using laparoscopic ultrasound compared with magnetic resonance imaging and transvaginal ultrasound. J Minim Invasive Gynecol. 2013;20(6):770-4.
8. Moshesh M, Peddada SD, Cooper T, et al. Intraobserver variability in fibroid size measurements. J Ultrasound Med. 2014;33(7):1217-24.
9. Mavrelos D, Ben-Nagi J, Holland T, et al. The natural history of fibroids. Ultrasound Obstet Gynecol. 2010;35(2):238-42.
10. Poder L. Ultrasound evaluation of the uterus. In: Callen P (Ed). Ultrasonography in Obstetrics and Gynecology, 5th edition. Philadelphia: Elsevier; 2008.
11. Parker WH. Etiology, symptomatology, and diagnosis of uterine myomas. Fertil Steril. 2007;87(4):725-36.
12. Cloke B, Brosens J, Brosens I. Leiomyomata and reproductive function. In: Brosens J (Ed). Uterine Leiomyomas: Pathogenesis and Management, 1st edition. London: Taylor & Francis; 2006. pp. 107-16.
13. Pritts EA. Fibroids and infertility: a systematic review of the evidence. Obstet Gynecol Surv. 2001;56(8):483-91.
14. Pritts EA, Parker WH, Ikuve DL. Fibroids and infertility: an updated systematic review of the evidence. Fertil Steril. 2009;91(4):1216-23.
15. Yoshino O, Hayashi T, Osuga Y, et al. Decreased pregnancy rate is linked to abnormal uterine peristalsis caused by intramural fibroids. Hum Reprod. 2010;25(10):2475-9.
16. Yan L, Ding L, Li C, et al. Effect of fibroids not distorting the endometrial cavity on the outcome of in vitro fertilization treatment: a retrospective cohort study. Fertil Steril. 2014; 101(3):716-21.
17. Practice Committee of the American Society for Reproductive Medicine. Myomas and reproductive function. Fertil Steril. 2004;82 (1):S111-6.
18. Buttram VC, Reiter RC. Uterine lciomyomata: Etiology, symptomatology, and management. Fertil Steril. 1981; 36(4):433-45.
19. Vander Werff BJ, Hagen-Ansert S. Pathology of the uterus. In: Callen P (Ed). Ultrasonography in Obstetrics and Gynecology, 5th edition. Philadelphia: Elsevier; 2008.
20. Ito F, Kawamura N, Ichimura T, et al. Ultrastructural comparison of uterine leiomyoma cells from the same myoma nodule before and after gonadotropin-releasing hormone agonist treatment. Fertil Steril. 2001;75(1):125-30.
21. Kurjak A, Kupesic S. Effetto degli analoghi del GnRH sul flusso ematico negli organi ginecologici. In: Nuovi aspetti clinici dei GnRH analoghi. Roma: CIC Edizioni Internazionali; 1994. pp. 45-85.
22. Kupesic S, Kurjak A. Blood flow in gynecological organs treated by GnRH agonists. Book of Abstracts. XIV FIGO World Congress, Montreal, Canada, September 25-30. IJGOAL. 1994;46 Suppl 2:60.
23. Garcia-Velasco JA, Kupesic S, Mrazek M, et al. Synchronization of the follicle cohort with the GnRH

antagonist Degarelix: A randomized assessor blind, placebo controlled trial. Fertil Steril. 2008;90(Suppl):S234.

24. Bourlev V, Pavlovitch S, Stygar D, et al. Different proliferative and apoptotic activity in peripheral versus central parts of human uterine leiomyomas. Gynecol Obstet Invest. 2003;55(4):199-204.

25. Wei JJ, Zhang XM, Chiriboga L, et al. Spatial differences in biologic activity of large uterine leiomyomata. Fertil Steril. 2006;85(1):179-87.

26. Dapunt O. Studies on the structure of the myoma capsule. Arch Gynecol. 1965;202(2):492-4.

27. Lindner V, Reidy MA. Proliferation of smooth muscle cells after vascular injury is inhibited by an antibody against basic fibroblast growth factor. Proc Natl Acad Sci USA. 1991;88(36):3739-43.

28. Stewart EA, Nowak RA. Leiomyoma-related bleeding: a classic hypothesis updated for the molecular era. Hum Reprod Update. 1996;2(4):295-306.

29. Olmos Gring AO, Lora V, Ferreira GD, et al. Protein expression of estrogen receptors α and β and aromatase in myometrium and uterine leiomyoma. Gynecol Obstet Invest. 2012;73(2):113-7.

30. Ishikawa H, Ishi V, AnnSerna V, et al. Progesterone is essential for maintenance and growth of uterine leiomyoma. Endocrinology. 2010;151(6):2433-42.

31. Barbarisi A, Petillo O, Di Lieto A, et al. 17-beta estradiol elicits an autocrine leiomyoma cell proliferation: evidence for a stimulation of protein kinase-dependent pathway. J Cell Physiol. 2001;186(3):414-24.

32. Park S, Ramachandran S, Kwon S, et al. Upregulation of ATP-sensitive potassium channels for estrogen-mediated cell proliferation in human uterine leiomyoma cells. Gynecol Endocrinol. 2008;24(5):250-6.

33. Rein MS, Barbieri RL, Friedman AJ. Progesterone: a critical role in the pathogenesis of uterine myomas. Am J Obstet Gynecol. 1995;172(3):14-8.

34. Andersen J. Growth factors and cytokines in uterine leiomyomas. Semin Reprod Endocrinol. 1996;14(3):269-82.

35. Kurjak A, Kupesic S, Miric D. Transvaginal color Doppler in the assessment of uterine blood flow changes during the pregnancy in patients with fibroids. J Perinat Med. 1991; 19(Suppl 2):81.

36. Kurjak A, Predanic M, Kupesic S, et al. Transvaginal color Doppler in the study of early pregnancies associated with fibroids. J Matern Fetal Invest. 1992;2(1):81-3.

37. Rosati P, Exacoustòs C, Mancuso S. Longitudinal evaluation of uterine myoma growth during pregnancy: a sonographic study. J Ultrasound Med. 1992;11(10):511.

38. Strobelt N, Ghidini A, Cavallone M, et al. Natural history of uterine leiomyomas in pregnancy. J Ultrasound Med. 1994;13(5):399-401.

39. Aharoni A, Reiter A, Golan D, et al. Patterns of growth of uterine leiomyomas during pregnancy. A prospective longitudinal study. Br J Obstet Gynaecol. 1988;95(5):510-3.

40. Klatsky PC, Tran ND, Caughey AB, et al. Fibroids and reproductive outcomes: a systematic literature review from conception to delivery. Am J Obstet Gynecol. 2008; 198(4):357-66.

41. Chen YH, Lin HC, Chen SF, et al. Increased risk of preterm births among women with uterine leiomyoma: a nation-wide population-based study. Hum Reprod. 2009;24(12): 3049-56.

42. Lam SJ, Best S, Kumar S. The impact of fibroid characteristics on pregnancy outcome. Am J Obstet Gynecol. 2014;211(4):395.e1-5.

43. Shavell VI, Thakur M, Sawant A, et al. Adverse obstetric outcomes associated with sonographically identified large uterine fibroids. Fertil Steril. 2012;97(1):107-10.

44. Roberts WE, Fulp KS, Morrison JC, et al. The impact of leiomyomas on pregnancy. Aust N Z J Obstet Gynaecol. 1999;39(1):43-7.

45. Davis JL, Ray-Mazumder S, Hobel CJ, et al. Uterine leiomyomas in pregnancy: a prospective study. Obstet Gynecol. 1990;75(1):41-4.

46. Vergani P, Ghidini A, Strobelt N, et al. Do uterine leiomyomas influence pregnancy outcome? Am J Perinatol. 1994;11(5):356-8.

47. Coronado GD, Marshall LM, Schwartz SM. Complications in pregnancy, labor, and delivery with uterine leiomyomas: a population-based study. Obstet Gynecol. 2000;95(5): 764-9.

48. Winer-Muram HT, Muram D, Gillieson MS. Uterine myomas in pregnancy. Can Med Assoc J. 1983;128(8): 949-50.

49. Forssman L. Distribution of blood flow in myomatous uteri as measured by locally injected 133Xenon. Acta Obstet Gynecol Scand. 1976;55(2):101-4.

50. Heinonen PK, Saarikoski S, Pystynen P. Reproductive performance of women with uterine anomalies. An evaluation of 182 cases. Acta Obstet Gynecol Scand. 1982;61(2):157-62.

51. Worthen NJ, Gonzalez F. Septate uterus: sonographic diagnosis and obstetric complications. Obstet Gynecol. 1984;64(3 Suppl):34S-8.

52. Phelan JP. Myomas and pregnancy. Obstet Gynecol Clin North Am. 1995;22(2):801-5.

53. Szamatowicz J, Laudanski T, Bulkszas B, et al. Fibromyomas and uterine contractions. Acta Obstet Gynecol Scand. 1997;76(10):973-6.

54. Hasan F, Arumugam K, Sivanesaratnam V. Uterine leiomyomata in pregnancy. Int J Gynaecol Obstet. 1991; 34(3):45-8.

55. Sheiner E, Biderman-Madar T, Katz M, et al. Higher rates of tachysystole among patients with clinically apparent uterine leiomyomas. Am J Obstet Gynecol. 2004;191(3): 945-8.

56. Koike T, Minakami H, Kosuge S, et al. Uterine leiomyoma in pregnancy: its influence on obstetric performance. J Obstet Gynaecol Res. 1999;25(5):309-13.

57. Vergani P, Locatelli A, Ghidini A, et al. Large uterine leiomyomata and risk of cesarean delivery. Obstet Gynecol. 2007;109(2 Pt 1):410-4.

58. Michels KA, Velez Edwards DR, Baird DD, et al. Uterine leiomyomata and cesarean birth risk: a prospective cohort with standardized imaging. Ann Epidemiol. 2014;24(2): 122-6.

59. Kupesic S, Plavsic BM. Sonography of uterine leiomyomata. In: Plavsic BM (Ed). Uterine Leiomyomata: Pathogenesis and Management, 1st edition. London: Taylor & Francis; 2006. pp. 139-51.

60. Stephenson SR. Benign diseases of female pelvis. In: Stephenson SR (Ed). Diagnostic Medical Sonography: Obstetrics and Gynecology, 3rd edition. Philadelphia: Lippincott Williams and Wilkins; 2012. pp. 175-211.

61. Stewart EA, Nowak RA. New concepts in the treatment of uterine leiomyomas. Obstet Gynecol. 1998;92(4 Pt 1): 624-7.

62. Vizza E, Motta PM. The skeleton fibrous and muscular of the uterus. In: Atti LXXVII Congresso SIGO. Rome: CIC Edizioni Internazionali; 2001. pp. 47-9.

63. Kupesic Plavsic S, Montgomery L, Tullius TG, et al. Uterine fibroids. In: Kupesic Plavsic S (Ed). Step by Step Case Studies in Obstetrics and Gynecology, 1st edition. New Delhi: Jaypee Brothers Medical Publishers (P) Ltd; 2014. pp. 183-99.

64. Kupesic S, Kurjak A, Baston K. Color Doppler and three-dimensional ultrasound of the uterine lesions. In: Kupesic S (Ed.) Color Doppler and Three-dimensional Ultrasound in Gynecology, Infertility and Obstetrics. New Delhi: Jaypee Brothers Medical Publishers (P) Ltd; 2011. pp. 22-33.

65. Kupesic Plavsic S, Honemeyer U, Kurjak A. Uterine lesions: advances in ultrasound diagnosis. In: Kurjak A, Chervenak F (Eds). Donald School Textbook of Ultrasound in Obstetrics and Gynecology. New Delhi: Jaypee Brothers Medical Publishers (P) Ltd; 2017. pp. 838-59.

66. Kupesic Plavsic S, Sparac V. Submucosal uterine fibroid. In: Reddy SY, Mendez M, Kupesic Plavsic S (Eds). Illustrated Problems in Obstetrics and Gynecology, 1st edition. New Delhi: Jaypee Brothers Medical Publishers (P) Ltd; 2018.

67. Padilla O, Arya S, Noble LS, et al. Saline infusion sonography: tips and tricks for improved visualization of the uterine cavity. Donald School J Ultrasound Obstet Gynecol. 2018;12(1):1-20.

68. Kurjak A, Kupesic S, Jukic S. Successful differentiation between fibroid and uterine sarcoma by TVCD. Fifth World Congress of Ultrasound in Obstetrics and Gynecology.

Book of abstracts. Ultrasound Obstet Gynecol. 1995; 6(Suppl 2):112.

69. Kupesic S, Kurjak A. Color Doppler assessment of uterine leiomyoma and sarcoma. In: Kurjak A, Kupesic S (Eds). An Atlas of Transvaginal Color Doppler. New York: Parthenon Publishing; 2000. p. 179.

70. Honemeyer U, Ross RJ, Barnard J, et al. Recurrent leiomyomatosis disseminata: sonographic and laparo-scopic correlation. Donald School J Ultrasound Obstet Gynecol. 2012;6(3):327-32.

71. Kidron D, Berheim J, Aviram R, et al. Resistance to blood flow in ovarian tumors: correlation between resistance index and histological pattern of vascularization. Ultrasound Obstet Gynecol. 1999;13(6):425-30.

72. Prompuntagorn C, Saldivar JS, Kupesic Plavsic S. Ultrasound assessment of ovarian function following radiation therapy. Donald School J Ultrasound Obstet Gynecol. 2014;8(3):288-92.

73. Kupesic S, Kurjak A, Bjelos D. The assessment of uterine lesions. In: Kurjak A, Kupesic S (Ed). Clinical Application of 3D Sonography. New York: Parthenon Publishing; 2000. pp. 55-67.

74. Kurjak A, Kupesic S, Shalan H, et al. Uterine sarcoma: a report of 10 cases studied by transvaginal color and pulsed Doppler sonography. Gynecol Oncol. 1995;59(3):342-6.

75. Kupesic S, Kurjak A. Uterine sarcoma. In: Kurjak A, Fleischer A (Eds). Doppler Ultrasound in Gynecology. New York: Parthenon Publishing; 1998. pp. 125-32.

76. Ortiz C, Mendez MD, Padilla O, et al. Leiomyosarcoma. In: Reddy SY, Mendez M, Kupesic Plavsic S. (Eds). Illustrated Problems in Obstetrics and Gynecology, 1st edition. New Delhi: Jaypee Brothers Medical Publishers (P) Ltd; 2018.

77. Ljubic A, Bozanovic T. Uterine fibroid. In: Kurjak A, Chervenak F (Eds). Donald School Textbook of Ultrasound in Obstetrics and Gynecology. New Delhi: Jaypee Brothers Medical Publishers (P) Ltd; 2017. pp. 859-74.

78. Exacoustos C, Romanini ME, Amadio A, et al. Can gray-scale and color Doppler sonography differentiate between uterine leiomyosarcoma and leiomyoma? J Clin Ultrasound. 2007;35(8):449-57.

79. Aragon L, Terreros D, Ho H, et al. Ultrasound imaging of ovarian angiosarcoma. J Clin Ultrasound. 2011;39(6):351-5.

80. Rackow BW, Taylor HS. Submucous uterine leiomyomas have a global effect on molecular determinants of endometrial receptivity. Fertil Steril. 2010;93(6):2027-34.

Four-dimensional Ultrasound in Functional Studies of the Fetus

Asim Kurjak, Panagiotis (Panos) Antsaklis

INTRODUCTION

Assessing the fetal neurobehavior has been a great challenge since the first steps of fetal medicine. The introduction of three-dimensional (3D) and four-dimensional (4D) ultrasound (US) technology offered the opportunity to not only examine the fetus anatomically with explicit detail, but also to observe directly the fetus and examine its behavior in real time, as one would examine a neonate.[1-3] The development of the fetal central nervous system (CNS) follows a very structured path and these developmental steps are reflected by the behavior of the fetus in utero for each corresponding week or trimester. Which fetal movements develop during each month and which fetal behavioral patterns are normal or abnormal have been identified. In the same way that a neonatologist can understand by its motoric function if a neonate is premature or not, similarly we can now understand which fetal movements–behavioral pattern correspond to each trimester of pregnancy.[4] On the other hand, pregnancy is a long period and there is always a possibility that different factors or incidents can affect this very sensitive and delicate course of fetal brain development. And if this incidence causes an anatomical abnormality to the fetal CNS, which can be detected prenatally by ultrasound, then a neurological impairment may be suspected; but if an anatomical abnormality is not seen, then a neurological impairment of the fetus will not be suspected and, of course, will be only diagnosed sometime after birth, and possibly wrongly attributed to intrapartum or even postpartum events. What is more is a delayed diagnosis of a neurological problem will make the possibility of treating it rather impossible. So, what is needed for such cases is a timely diagnosis which will also offer the chance of

early treatment intervention which would aim to a better outcome of these fetuses. It is clear that the assessment of fetal neurological status is of utmost importance, and should be practiced not only as a screening test for low-risk pregnancies, but also for cases where there is suspicion of neurological impairment prenatally.[4-6] The most complete method so far for the assessment of fetal neurobehavior, that relays on real-time observation of the fetal behavior with 4D ultrasound and its efficacy has been tested through many multicentric studies, is Kurjak's Antenatal Neurodevelopmental Test (KANET). KANET has been introduced in everyday clinical practice and aims to assess the fetal behavior in a similar way that a neonate is assessed postnatally, through 4D ultrasound technology.

ASSESSMENT OF FETAL BEHAVIOR OVER THE YEARS

When two-dimensional (2D) ultrasound was introduced into clinical practice, the fetal movements were observed in order to draw conclusions regarding the fetal well-being and the fetal behavior.[7-10] Of course, this method is very subjective and inadequate to assess the fetal behavior as a whole. The method that offered a complete and real-time assessment of the fetus and not just information on isolated limb movements was 4D ultrasonography.[11-14] 4D gives the opportunity to examine not only gross fetal movements but also small details such as finger movements, facial expressions, eye blinking, etc. details that are not visible by applying 2D ultrasound.[15-17]

Kurjak's Antenatal Neurodevelopmental Test used the advantages of 4D technology and succeeded to assess the fetus in the same way that neonates are assessed neurologically after birth by neonatologists.[18-21] Apart from the classical fetal movements, KANET through 4D ultrasound, introduced all the markers that are used for postnatal neurological assessment according to the Amiel–Tison Neurological Assessment at Term (ATNAT) test.[19,22] So, it also includes the cranial sutures, head circumference and finger movements, detection of neurological thumb (adducted thumb in the clenched feast), and more specifically it includes: isolated head ante-flexion, overlapping cranial sutures, head circumference, isolated eye blinking, facial alterations, mouth opening (yawning or mouthing), isolated hand and leg movements and thumb position, and gestalt perception of general movements (overall perception of the body and limb movements with their qualitative assessment) **(Figs. 15.1 to 15.3)**. KANET consists of eight parameters and its aim is to evaluate fetal motoric activity and through that to assess the development and integrity of the fetal nervous system **(Table 15.1)**. The maturation of fetal CNS and the transition from fetal to neonatal behavior are a very smooth process, with all movements that are present in postnatal life have been documented with 4D ultrasound in fetal life (with the exception of Moro's reflex, which is not present in fetuses) and that is exactly what KANET has managed to demonstrate and succeed.[23]

Kurjak's antenatal neurodevelopmental test is already a standardized method, with good reproducibility as proved by many multicentric studies. Training modules on KANET have been formed and the training centers show that the learning curve is very reasonable for physicians and medical staff with good ultrasound background.[24] Regarding the gestational age at which KANET should be performed, it has been decided that the best period is the 3rd trimester of pregnancy, and particularly after 28 weeks. The duration of KANET should be around 15–20 minutes, and should be preferably performed at periods that the fetus is awake. If this is not possible, as it is not always easy to predict when a fetus will be active awake, and the fetus is quite for a prolonged period of time, KANET should be repeated within 30 minutes or the following day, at a minimum interval of 14–16 hours.

When KANET is abnormal or the score is borderline, it is proposed that test is repeated every 2 weeks until delivery. Very important features are facial movements and eye blinking—"the face is the mirror of the brain". The overall number of movements must be documented in all cases.[22,25]

Examiners who apply KANET should have proper training, and adequate experience in low- and high-risk pregnancies. Interobserver and intraobserver variability has to be documented. The suggestion regarding the ultra-sonographic machines used is to have a frame rate of at least 24 volumes/s. The results of KANET are divided in three groups: (1) abnormal, when the score is 0–5, (2) borderline for a score from 6 to 13, and finally (3) normal for a score 14–20 **(Table 15.2)**. A 2-year follow-up should be available and documented for all fetuses that KANET has been applied, in order to draw safe conclusions.

Kurjak's antenatal neurodevelopmental test has been introduced in training and has been calculated that the number of KANET needed to be performed by experienced ultrasound specialist in order to be familiar to assess a fetus with 4D US in 20 minutes is 80. The success rate of the test ranges from 91% to 95% and further study of each parameter revealed a success rate for the assessment of particular signs of 88% for isolated eye blinking and 100% for mouth opening and isolated leg movement. KANET has almost 100% negative predictive value, interobserver variability was satisfactory with lowest being for the facial expression (K = 0.68) and highest for the finger movements (K = 0.84).

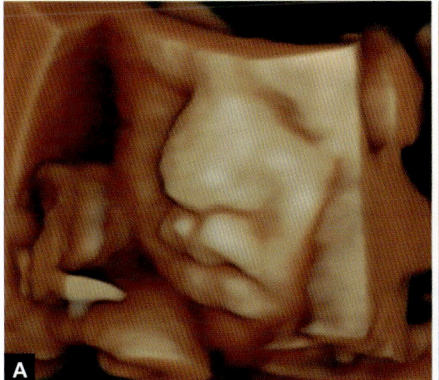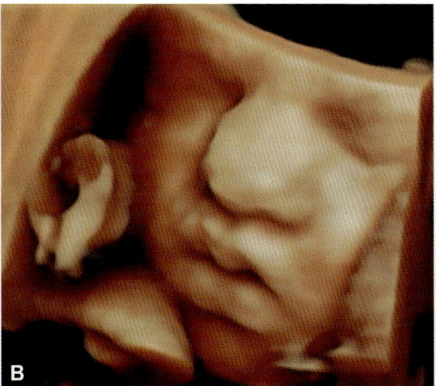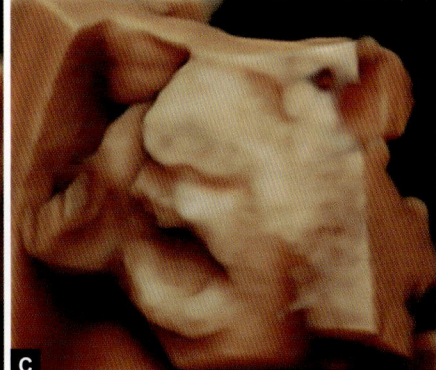

Figs. 15.1A to C: Mouthing as part of the assessment of fetal neurobehavior.

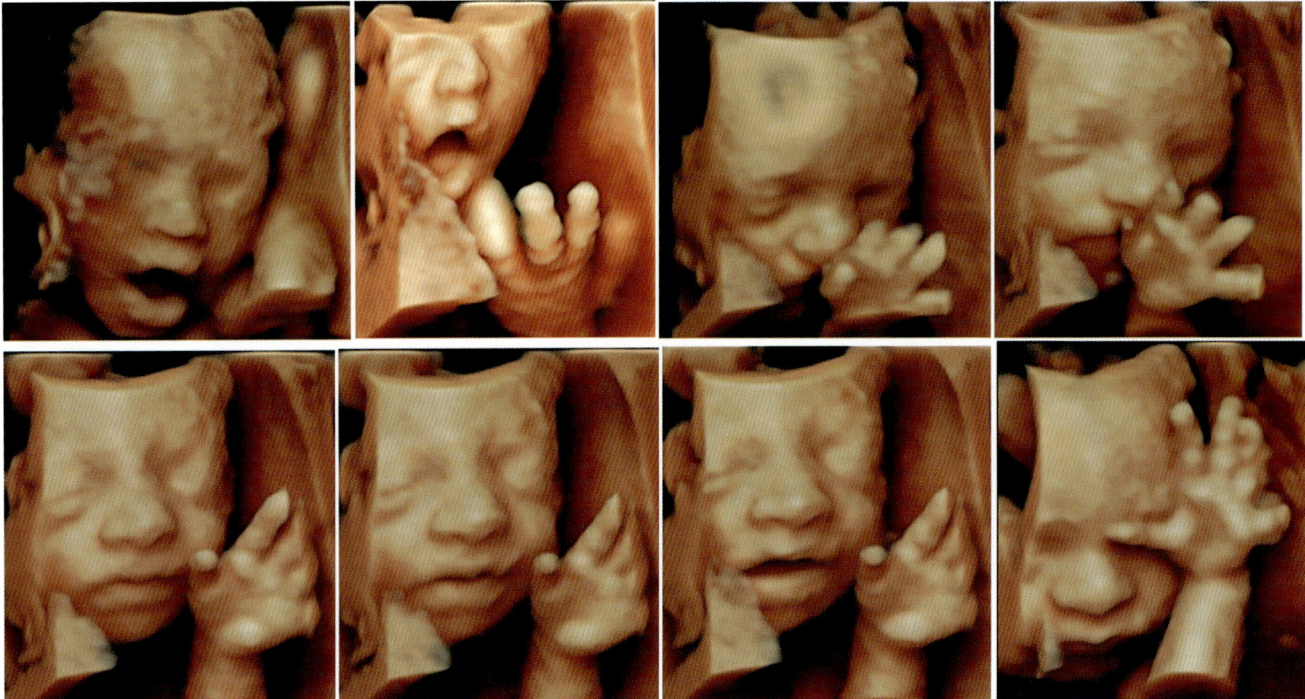

Fig. 15.2: Parameters of Kurjak's antenatal neurodevelopmental test (KANET) test: mouthing, yawning, and hand movements.

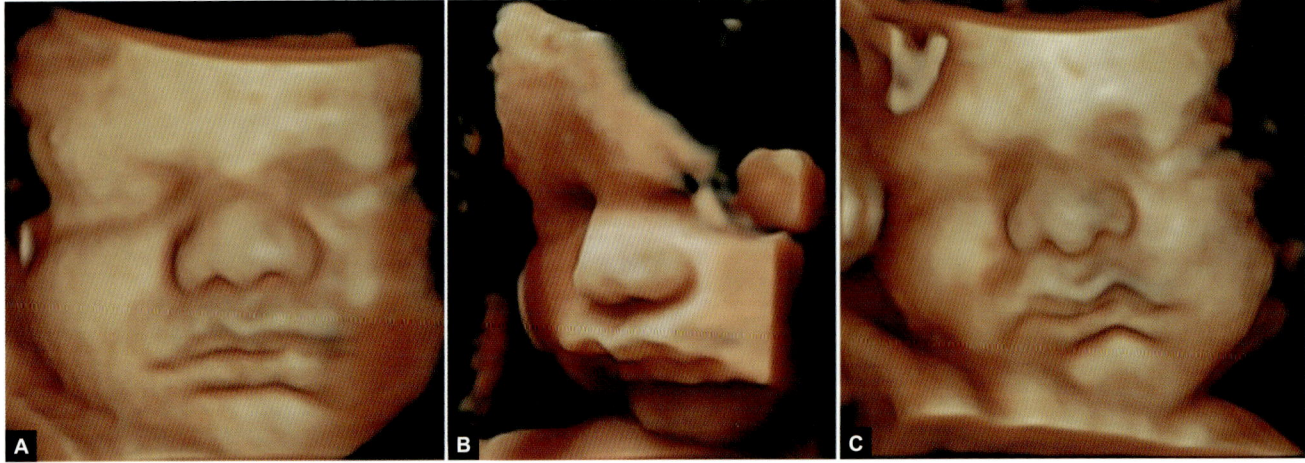

Figs. 15.3A to C: Facial alterations and grimacing.

CLINICAL RESULTS OF KURJAK'S ANTENATAL NEURODEVELOPMENTAL TEST (TABLE 15.3)

The first application of KANET was on growth-restricted fetuses,[26] where mainly facial expressions and body movements were studied and what was noticed was a decreased behavioral activity in the intrauterine growth restriction (IUGR) fetuses compared with normal growth cases. The study that followed was the first with complete neurologic postnatal assessment for all studied fetuses and according to the criteria, they used neonates that were divided into three groups: (1) normal, (2) mildly or moderately abnormal, and (3) abnormal. According to these groups,

Table 15.1: The parameters of standardized Kurjak's antenatal neurodevelopmental test (KANET).[24]

Sign	Score			Sign score
	0	1	2	
Isolated head anteflexion	Abrupt	Small range (0–3 times of movement	Variable in full range, many alternations (>3 times of movements)	
Cranial sutures and head circumference	Overlapping of cranial sutures	Normal cranial sutures with measurement of HC below or above the normal limit (–2 SD) according to GA	Normal cranial sutures with normal measurement of HC according to GA	
Isolated eye blinking	Not present	Not fluent (1–5 times of blinking)	Fluency (>5 times of blinking)	
Facial alterations (grimace or tongue expulsion)				
Or Mouth opening (yawning or mouthing)	Not present	Not fluent (1–5 times of alteration)	Fluency (>5 times of alteration)	

Contd…

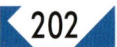

Contd...

	Score			Sign score
Sign	**0**	**1**	**2**	
Isolated leg movement	Cramped	Poor repertoire or small in range (0–5 times of movement)	Variable in full range, many alternations (>5 times of movements)	
Isolated hand movement	Cramped or abrupt	Poor repertoire or small in range (0–5 times of movement)	Variable in full range, many alternations (>5 times of movements)	
Or Hand to face movements				
Fingers movements	Unilateral or bilateral clenched fist (neurological thumb)	Cramped invariable finger movements	Smooth and complex, variable finger movements	
Gestalt perception of GMs	Definitely abnormal	Borderline	Normal Total score	

Contd...

Authors	Year	Study	Study design	Study population	Indication	No.	GA (weeks)	Time (minutes)	Result	Summary
Hata et al.[47]	2016	Cohort	Prospective	Mixed (male vs female)	Multiple	112	3rd trimester	20	NO	No difference in fetal behavior between male and female fetuses in the 3rd trimester of pregnancy. These results suggest that 4D ultrasound study examining fetal behavior does not need to consider the factor of fetal sex
Antsaklis et al.[40]	2017	Cohort	Prospective	High & low risk (diabetic vs nondiabetic)	Multiple	80	3rd trimester	20	Positive	Differences in the fetal behavior between diabetic and nondiabetic fetuses were shown, and also the specific parameters—movements that were different between the two groups were identified

(ATNAT: Amiel–Tison neurological assessment at term; GDM: gestational diabetes mellitus; IUGR: intrauterine growth restriction; KANET: Kurjak's antenatal neurodevelopmental test; MCA: middle cerebral artery; No.: number of patients; PTD: preterm delivery; PPROM: preterm premature rupture of membrane; PET: preeclampsia)

identified seven cases with abnormal score and 25 with a borderline KANET score. There were also 11 cases which either died in utero or had a termination of pregnancy and all of these cases had an abnormal KANET score. The seven remaining neonates with abnormal KANET were followed up postnatally at 10 weeks of neonatal life and three had confirmed pathological ATNAT score. These three cases included a neonate with arthrogryposis, a neonate with cerebellar vermis complete aplasia, and one case with a history of cerebral palsy in a previous pregnancy. Out of the parameters that KANET uses, facial expressions appeared to be most pathological—the fetal faces were characterized as "masks" by the authors, due to lack of expressions on 4D ultrasound. The remaining four pathological KANET cases had normal postnatal assessment. These four cases, however, had complications of pregnancy: one case with ventriculomegaly, one case with preeclampsia, one case with maternal thrombophilia, and one case with oligohydramnios. From the 25 cases diagnosed with borderline KANET result, 22 neonates showed a borderline ATNAT score and were followed up, while the three remaining cases showed normal ATNAT result. An interesting paper was the one that studied a case of a fetus with prenatally diagnosed acrania. The authors studied the fetal behavior and managed to document how it altered from 20 weeks of gestation onward. It was noticed that as pregnancy progressed and the control center of motoric activity shifted from the lower to the upper part, KANET score was decreasing,

respectively suggesting that neurological damage in later pregnancy is possible.[28]

A study with[29] 226 cases, including different study populations, identified three cases with pathological KANET score. All three cases had chromosomal abnormalities and all three of them postnatally also had an abnormal ATNAT score. Scores from antenatal KANET and postnatal ATNAT were compared between low and high-risk groups, and showed differences between them, for eight out of the 10 parameters—these included: head anteflexion, eye blinking, facial expressions—grimacing, tongue expulsion, mouth movement such as yawning, jawing, swallowing—isolated hand movements, hand to face movements, fist and finger movements, and general movements.

The comparison of the two tests revealed correlation between them, proving that the neonatal examination (ATNAT) was a satisfactory confirmation of the prenatal ultrasound examination (KANET), stating that KANET could offer useful information about the neurological status of the fetus and can be applied in clinical practice.

One of the largest studies regarding KANET,[30] including 620 cases, of both low and high-risk populations (100 low-risk and 520 high-risk cases) showed differences in the scores between the two groups. What was interesting in this study was that most abnormal cases were noted from pregnancies with a previous history of CP (23.8%) and that most borderline scores were noted in cases with possible chorioamnionitis (56.4%). The parameters of

KANET that were more notably different between the two groups were: overlapping cranial sutures, head circumference, isolated eye blinking, facial expressions, mouth movements, isolated hand movements, isolated leg movements, hand to face movements, finger movements, and general movements. This study confirmed the relationship of pathological KANET with increased risk of perinatal mortality and neurological impairment and showed that the results can be confirmed and are reproducible postnatally.

A recent study with a complete follow-up[31] postnatally up to 3 months of life, with complete postnatal documentation in all cases and showed that a normal KANET score is very reassuring of a good neonatal outcome, confirming the consistency of prenatal and postnatal assessments. Understanding the evolution of fetal movements by 4D ultrasound throughout pregnancy, and how these movements reflect the development and integrity of fetal nervous system were a great challenge. What was shown was that during the 1st weeks of pregnancy, the development of the frequency and the complexity of fetal movements are more important, while during the 2nd trimester, the variation of fetal movements develops, with more detailed movements (facial expressions and eye blinking) appearing at the end of this trimester. Finally, at the end of 3rd trimester, the number of fetal movements decline as a result of the increase of fetal rest periods, due to fetal cerebral maturation, and this is something that most pregnant women notice nearterm.[12-14] A very interesting study which tried to shed some light on the clinical dilemmas caused by the prenatal diagnosis of ventriculomegaly, compared fetuses with ventriculomegaly[32] with apparently low-risk fetuses (normal CNS appearance on ultrasound examination). A significant difference was noted between the two groups, with the KANET score decreasing as the degree of ventriculomegaly was increasing. For isolated cases of mild or moderate ventriculomegaly, no pathological KANET scores were noted and postnatal evaluation confirmed the prenatal KANET, offering valuable information for the more complete assessment of these fetuses and better counseling regarding their prognosis.

Abo-Yaqoub et al.[33] aimed to study how practical is to apply 4D ultrasonography for the assessment of fetal neurobehavior and also how useful it is for the prediction of neurological impairment. Their results showed agreement of prenatal scores with postnatal assessment. The parameters that were significantly different between the two groups were: isolated head anteflexion, isolated eye blinking, facial expressions, mouth movements, isolated hand movements, hand-to-face movements, finger movements, and general movements. Regarding isolated leg movements and cranial sutures, the difference was not statistically significant.

Vladareanu et al.[34] noted that the majority of normal KANET scores derived from low-risk populations that they studied, while the majority of cases with borderline or pathological KANET scores derived from the high-risk groups and in some cases were related to abnormal values of Doppler studies in IUGR fetuses. The authors concluded that KANET can be useful for the detection of neurological impairment which could become obvious during the antenatal or postnatal period.

The average KANET score was introduced for fetuses who had more than one assessments in order to have a more complete picture of the behavior of these fetuses. The average KANET score derived from the mean calculation of KANET scores for each fetus throughout pregnancy, since these fetuses had more than one KANET assessments. What was new from this study was the association of KANET score with fetal diurnal rhythm. For the high-risk group, 89% of the borderline scores were recorded at times that the mothers characterized them as active periods, compared with 33.3%, respectively in the low-risk pregnancies.[35]

Other studies[36,37] confirmed the feasibility of neurodevelopment assessment by 4D ultrasound and showed further evidence that KANET test is useful in early identification of fetuses prone to neurological impairment.

What was also important was to compare all parameters of KANET between high and low-risk pregnancies and observe differences in fetal behavior between them. For pathological KANET score, five out of eight parameters were significant different: isolated head anteflexion, cranial sutures and head circumference, isolated hand movement or hand to face movements, isolated leg movement, and fingers movements.[38] Further results showed that only high-risk patients had abnormal scores (8.5%), while comparing high and low-risk groups, it was noticed that 80.6% of high-risk patients had borderline results while 85.3% of low-risk patients were normal, both being statistically significant. For abnormal KANET results (score between 0 and 5), some were related to pregnancy complications (preeclampsia, threatened preterm labor, and drug abuse) and some were related to fetal conditions (trisomy 13, 18 and 21, and IUGR).

When comparing Caucasian to Asian populations in order to check for ethnic differences, the total KANET score was normal in both populations, but there was a difference noted in total KANET scores between these two populations. When individual KANET parameters were compared, significant differences were observed in four fetal movements (isolated head anteflexion, isolated eye blinking, facial alteration or mouth opening, and isolated leg movement). No significant differences were noted in the four other parameters (cranial suture and head circumference, isolated hand movement or hand to face movements, fingers movements, and gestalt of general movements), showing that ethnicity is a parameter that should be considered when evaluating fetal behavior, especially during assessment of fetal facial expressions. The authors concluded that although there was a difference in the total KANET score between Asian and Caucasian populations, all the scores in both groups were within normal range proving that ethnical differences in fetal behavior do not affect the total KANET score, but close follow-up should be continued in some borderline cases.[39]

Unpublished data from Greece, from 655 singleton pregnancies, showed that KANET is a method which is feasible in everyday clinical practice, with a success rate of 95% and a very low negative predictive value. For the cases that KANET could not be completed, the reason was severe oligohydramnios, fibroid uterus (difficult imaging), very increased body mass index (BMI), and a case that due to vasovagal reaction—supine hypotensive syndrome, ultrasound examination could not be completed. From the 655 cases, 1,712 KANET were performed from only two operators and the interobserver variability was calculated showing adequate results for all parameters, with the lowest being for facial alterations (k-value = 0.68) and the highest for finger movements (k-value = 0.84). This study was primarily designed to compare the neurological status of pregnancies complicated by diabetes, compared with low-risk pregnancies and it did show that there was a difference between the fetal neurobehavior of these two groups, with the diabetic pregnancies having lower scores.[40]

DISCUSSION

One of the greatest challenges in perinatal medicine is the assessment of fetal neurobehavior and detection of fetal neurological impairment in utero. KANET is the first method that applied 4D ultrasound for the assessment of the fetus in the same way that a neonate is assessed neurologically after birth by neonatologists and it appears to be a strong diagnostic method for the detection of neurological impairment and for the assessment of fetal neurobehavior, conditions that were inaccessible with the traditional prenatal diagnostic methods used so far.[23] Studies have proved the validity of this method,[13,41,42] its applicability in everyday clinical practice, especially for high-risk cases, how and by whom it should be performed and what is the value of the result of KANET, and how it should be managed. Diagnosis of neurological impairment prenatally is very difficult and usually all these diagnoses are made postnatally, even months or years after delivery. What is more, neurological conditions, such as cerebral palsy are not adequately understood and falsely attributed to incidents during labor, although it has been proven that the majority of CP cases originate sometime during in utero life and are not related to intrapartum events. All these things lead to delayed diagnoses of neurological conditions. The later a neurological impairment is diagnosed, the less is the possibility of an effective intervention. It would be extremely challenging to have a timely diagnosis of such conditions, even during in utero life, in order to increase the possibility of an effective intervention or even treatment. KANET offers the possibility of prenatal detection of fetuses at risk for neurological problems, offering the possibility of even an in utero intervention or at least an early postpartum intervention.[43] The earliest physiotherapy is commenced and intervention programs are applied in neonates that are born prematurely or with neurological problems—the better the neurodevelopmental outcome of these neonates, with the cognitive benefits persisting into preschool age. KANET appears to be able to offer this advantage of early identification of these fetuses with neurological problems, so that they could be put under treatment as early as possible, aiming to a better outcome.[36,44]

What is more the explicitly detailed pictures obtained by the new ultrasound machines but also the advanced techniques of molecular genetics, many times brings us as ultrasound specialists, across findings (anatomical and chromosomal) of uncertain clinical significance and prognosis, especially regarding the neurological integrity of the fetus.[45-47] A method like KANET offers a more comprehensive diagnostic approach to such dilemmas and hopefully in the near future with more data we could

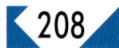

form a complete neurobehavioral assessment of the fetus and a more complete counseling of these couples.[48]

Kurjak's antenatal neurodevelopmental test has currently been introduced in everyday clinical practice by many centers for the assessment of fetal neurobehavior of not only high-risk cases, but also low-risk pregnancies. Studies show that the sensitivity and specificity of the test are satisfactory, as are the positive and negative predictive values and the inter- and intraobserver variability of this method. The KANET has been introduced into systematical training and already ultrasound specialists have been certified to perform this examination. Hopefully, application of KANET on larger populations, both high and low risk, will give more knowledge regarding early detection of fetuses at risk for neurological impairment, in order to allow accurate diagnosis prenatally, and as a consequence prompt intervention that could possibly improve the outcome of some of these neonates.

REFERENCES

1. Yigiter AB, Kavak ZN. Normal standards of fetal behavior assessed by four-dimensional sonography. J Matern Fetal Neonatal Med. 2006;19:707-21.
2. Rees S, Harding R. Brain development during fetal life: influences of the intrauterine environment. Neurosci Lett. 2004;361:111-4.
3. Joseph R. Fetal brain and cognitive development. Dev Rev. 1999;20:81-98.
4. Kurjak A, Carrera JM, Stanojevic M, et al. The role of 4D sonography in the neurological assessment of early human development. Ultrasound Rev Obstet Gynecol. 2004;4:148-59.
5. Stanojevic M, Zaputovic S, Bosnjak AP. Continuity between fetal and neonatal neurobehavior. Semin Fetal Neonatal Med. 2012;17:324-9.
6. Haak P, Lenski M, Hidecker MJ, et al. Cerebral palsy and aging. Dev Med Child Neurol. 2009;51:16-23.
7. Precht HF. Qualitative changes of spontaneous movements in fetus and preterm infant are a marker of neurological dysfunction. Early Hum Dev. 1990;23:151-8.
8. de Vries JI, Visser GH, Prechtl HF. The emergence of fetal behaviour. II. Quantitative aspects. Early Hum Dev. 1985;12:99-120.
9. de Vries JI, Visser GH, Prechtl HF. The emergence of fetal behaviour. III. Individual differences and consistencies. Early Hum Dev. 1988;16:85-103.
10. de Vries JI, Visser GH, Prechtl HF. The emergence of fetal behaviour. I. Qualitative aspects. Early Hum Dev. 1982;7:301-22.
11. Kurjak A, Luetic AT. Fetal neurobehavior assessed by three-dimensional/four-dimensional sonography. Zdrav Vestn. 2010;79:790-9.
12. Salihagic-Kadic A, Medic M, Kurjak A, et al. 4D sonography in the assessment of fetal functional neurodevelopment and behavioural patterns. Ultrasound Rev Obstet Gynecol. 2005;5:1-15.
13. Kurjak A, Pooh R, Tikvica A, et al. Assessment of fetal neurobehavior by 3D/4D ultrasound. Fetal Neurol. 2009;2:222-50.
14. Lebit DF, Vladareanu PD. The role of 4D ultrasound in the assessment of fetal behaviour. Maedica (Buchar). 2011;6:120-7.
15. Merz E, Abramowicz JS. 3D/4D ultrasound in prenatal diagnosis: Is it time for routine use? Clin Obstet Gynecol. 2012;55:336-51.
16. Kurjak A, Vecek N, Hafner T, et al. Prenatal diagnosis: what does four-dimensional ultrasound add? J Perinat Med. 2002;30:57-62.
17. Kurjak A, Vecek N, Kupesic S, et al. Four-dimensional ultrasound: how much does it improve perinatal practice? In: Carrera JM, Chervenak FA, Kurjak A (Eds). Controversies in Perinatal Medicine, Studies on the Fetus as a Patient. New York: Parthenon Publishing; 2003. p. 222.
18. Kurjak A, Miskovic B, Stanojevic M, et al. New scoring system for fetal neurobehavior assessed by three- and four-dimensional sonography. J Perinat Med. 2008;36:73-81.
19. Gosselin J, Gahagan S, Amiel-Tison C. The Amiel-Tison Neurological Assessment at Term: conceptual and methodological continuity in the course of follow-up. Ment Retard Dev Disabil Res Rev. 2005;11:34-51.
20. Amiel-Tison C, Gosselin J, Kurjak A. Neurosonography in the second half of fetal life: a neonatologist's point of view. J Perinat Med. 2006;34:437-46.
21. Tomasovic S, Predojevic M. 4D Ultrasound—Medical Devices for Recent Advances on the Etiology of Cerebral Palsy. Acta Inform Med. 2011;19:228-34.
22. Kurjak A, Stanojevic M, Andonotopo W, et al. Fetal behavior assessed in all three trimesters of normal pregnancy by four-dimensional ultrasonography. Croat Med J. 2005;46:772-80.
23. Stanojevic M, Kurjak A, Salihagic-Kadic A, et al. Neurobehavioral continuity from fetus to neonate. J Perinat Med. 2011;39:171-7.
24. Stanojevic M, Talic A, Miskovic B, et al. An attempt to standardize Kurjak's antenatal neurodevelopmental test: Osaka Consensus Statement. Donald School J Ultrasound Obstet Gynecol. 2011;5:317-29.
25. Kurjak A, Andonotopo W, Hafner T, et al. Normal standards for fetal neurobehavioral developments—longitudinal quantification by four-dimensional sonography. J Perinat Med. 2006;34:56-65.
26. Andonotopo W, Kurjak A. The assessment of fetal behavior of growth-restricted fetuses by 4D sonography. J Perinat Med. 2006;34:471-8.
27. Kurjak A, Carrera J, Medic M, et al. The antenatal development of fetal behavioral patterns assessed by four-dimensional sonography. J Matern Fetal Neonatal Med. 2005;17:401-16.

28. Kurjak A, Abo-Yaqoub S, Stanojevic M, et al. The potential of 4D sonography in the assessment of fetal neurobehavior—multicentric study in high-risk pregnancies. J Perinat Med. 2010;38:77-82.

29. Miskovic B, Vasilj O, Stanojevic M, et al. The comparison of fetal behavior in high-risk and normal pregnancies assessed by four-dimensional ultrasound. J Matern Fetal Neonatal Med. 2010;23:1461-7.

30. Talic A, Kurjak A, Ahmed B, et al. The potential of 4D sonography in the assessment of fetal behavior in high-risk pregnancies. J Matern Fetal Neonatal Med. 2011;24:948-54.

31. Honemeyer U, Kurjak A. The use of KANET test to assess fetal CNS function. First 100 cases. 10th World Congress of Perinatal Medicine 8-11 November 2011. Uruguay. 2011;3:p209.

32. Talic A, Kurjak A, Stanojevic M, et al. The assessment of fetal brain function in fetuses with ventriculomegaly: the role of the KANET test. J Matern Fetal Neonatal Med. 2012;25:1267-72.

33. Abo-Yaqoub S, Kurjak A, Mohammed AB, et al. The role of 4D ultrasonography in prenatal assessment of fetal neurobehaviour and prediction of neurological outcome. J Matern Fetal Neonatal Med. 2012;25:231-6.

34. Vladareanu R, Lebit D, Constantinescu S. Ultrasound assessment of fetal neurobehaviour in high-risk pregnancies. Donald School J Ultrasound Obstet Gynecol. 2012;6:132-47.

35. Honemeyer U, Talic A, Therwat A, et al. The clinical value of KANET in studying fetal neurobehavior in normal and at-risk pregnancies. J Perinat Med. 2013;41:187-97.

36. Kurjak A, Talic A, Honemeyer U, et al. Comparison between antenatal neurodevelopmental test and fetal Doppler in the assessment of fetal well being. J Perinat Med. 2013;41:107-14.

37. Athanasiadis AP, Mikos T, Tambakoudis GP, et al. Neuro-developmental fetal assessment using KANET scoring system in low- and high-risk pregnancies. J Matern Fetal Neonatal Med. 2013;26:363-8.

38. Neto RM. KANET in Brazil: First Experience. Donald School J Ultrasound Obstet Gynecol. 2015;9:1-5.

39. Hanaoka U, Hata T, Kananishi K, et al. Does ethnicity have an effect on fetal behavior? A comparison of Asian and Caucasian populations. J Perinat Med. 2016;44:217-21.

40. Antsaklis P, Porovic S, Daskalakis G, et al. 4D assessment of fetal brain function in diabetic patients. J Perinat Med. 2017;45:711-5.

41. Kurjak A, Stanojevic M, Andonotopo W, et al. Behavioral pattern continuity from prenatal to postnatal life—a study by four-dimensional (4D) ultrasonography. J Perinat Med. 2004;32:346-53.

42. Andonotopo W, Kurjak A, Kosuta MI. Behavior of an anencephalic fetus studied by 4D sonography. J Matern Fetal Neonatal Med. 2005;17:165-8.

43. Kurjak A, Predojevic M, Salihagic-Kadic A. Fetal brain function: lessons learned and future challenges of 4D sonography. Donald School J Ultrasound Obstet Gynecol. 2010;2:85-92.

44. Stanojevic M, Antsaklis P, Salihadic-Kadic A, et al. Is Kurjak Antenatal Neurodevelopmental Test Ready for Routine Clinical Application? Bucharest Consensus Statement. Donald School J Ultrasound Obstet Gynecol. 2015;3:260-5.

45. Spencer-Smith MM, Spittle AJ, Doyle LW, et al. Long-term benefits of home-based preventive care for preterm infants: a randomized trial. Pediatrics. 2012;130:1094-101.

46. Predojević M, Talić A, Stanojević M, et al. Assessment of motoric and hemodynamic parameters in growth restricted fetuses—case study. J Matern Fetal Neonatal Med. 2014;27:247-51.

47. Hata T, Hanaoka U, Mostafa AboEllail MA, et al. Is there a sex difference in fetal behavior? A comparison of the KANET test between male and female fetuses. J Perinat Med. 2016;44:585-8.

48. Kurjak A, Antsaklis P, Stanojevic M, et al. Multicentric studies of the fetal neurobehavior by KANET test. J Perinat Med. 2017;45:717-27.

Anomalies of the Fetal Face

Eberhard Merz, Sonila Pashaj

INTRODUCTION

Visualization of the fetal face with three-dimensional/four-dimensional (3D/4D) ultrasound is a unique experience for both, the parents-to-be and the operator. While the future parents are primarily interested in seeing the surface of the fetal face and facial movements, the operator uses the different display modes for a precise fetal malformation check.[1] The multiplanar mode with a simultaneous display of the three perpendicular planes allows an accurate demonstration of a normal or an abnormal fetal profile. Even if an image of the fetal face is acquired in an oblique position, the stored volume can be rotated by the rotational controls in all three directions, until the face is seen precisely in the median plane. The different surface modes enable the operator to detect abnormal protuberant structures or surface defects, while the transparent mode (maximum mode) reveals ossification defects.

During a targeted ultrasound examination of the fetal face, five different regions have to be assessed: (1) the forehead, (2) orbits and eyes, (3) nose, (4) mouth, and (5) chin.

ANOMALIES INCLUDING THE FOREHEAD

Anencephaly

Anencephaly is the most common and severe anomaly of the central nervous system with an incidence rate of 1:1,000 births. The surface demonstration of the fetal head shows an absent superior vault, the missing cerebrum, and large bulging eyes ("frog eyes") **(Fig. 16.1)**. The respective ultrasound appearance of the face has also been described as "Mickey Mouse face".[2] Anencephaly can be detected as early as 9–10 weeks gestation.[3,4]

Protuberant Forehead

The term frontal bossing refers to the development of an unusually pronounced forehead caused by an enlargement of the frontal bone. In several cases it has been observed in conjunction with an abnormal enlargement of other facial bones. A protuberant forehead may be observed in different fetal abnormalities, such as achondroplasia, Crouzon syndrome, Fragile X syndrome, Hurler syndrome, Marfan syndrome, Pfeiffer syndrome, Rubinstein–Taybi syndrome, and Russell–Silver syndrome. Moderate frontal bossing may also be seen in some normal fetuses.

Sonographically, frontal bossing is best seen in a side view **(Fig. 16.2)**, but it can also be unambiguously demonstrated in a frontal surface view.

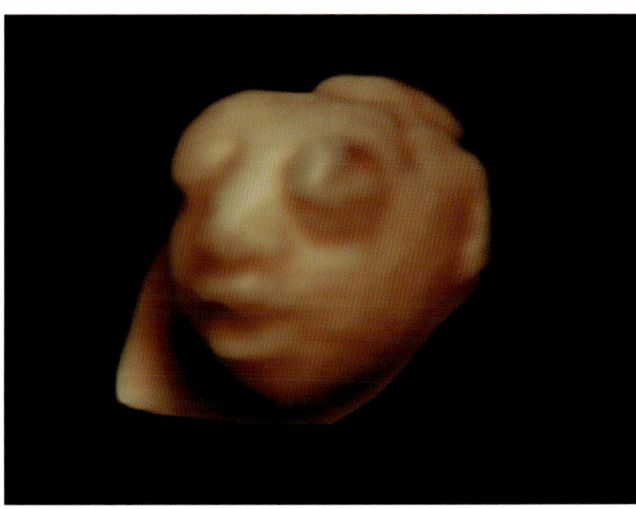

Fig. 16.1: Surface view (HDlive) of an anencephalus at 30 weeks gestation.

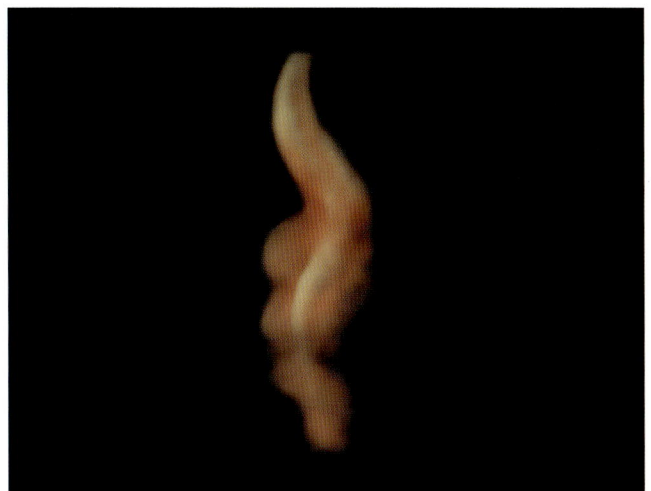

Fig. 16.2: Achondroplasia (37 weeks gestation). The profile (lateral surface view) of the fetal face shows pronounced frontal bossing.

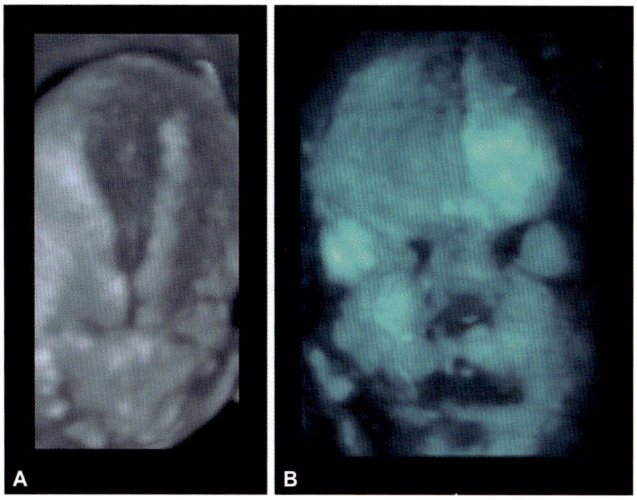

Figs. 16.3A and B: Transparent demonstration of the skull from a front view. (A) Wide V-shaped metopic suture in a fetus with trisomy 22 (20 weeks gestation); (B) Premature closure of the metopic suture in Apert syndrome (37 weeks gestation).

Abnormal Metopic Suture

The metopic suture can be clearly demonstrated in the transparent mode from a front view **(Figs. 16.3A and B)**.

Wide Metopic Suture

Wide V-, Y-, and U-shaped metopic sutures have been observed in fetuses with facial defects involving the orbits, nasal bones, lip, the palate, and mandible, as well as in fetuses with cerebellar abnormalities.[5] A wide V-shaped metopic suture can also be observed in fetuses with chromosomal defects **(Fig. 16.3A)** or in those with osteogenesis imperfecta type II.

Narrow Metopic Suture

Premature closure of the suture (craniosynostosis) or the presence of an additional bone between the frontal bones may be a sign for holoprosencephaly and abnormalities of the corpus callosum.[5] Premature closure of the metopic suture is also found in Apert syndrome **(Fig. 16.3B)**. Fetal neurosonography is mandatory in all fetuses with craniosynostosis.

Frontal Encephalocele/Meningocele

Frontoethmoidal encephalocele represents a frontal skull defect with herniated brain substance. This is in contrast to frontal meningocele where the herniation contains only leptomeninges with cerebrospinal fluid. The incidence

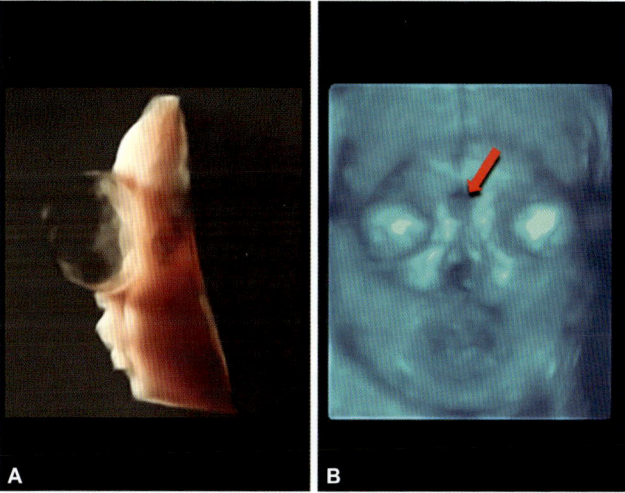

Figs. 16.4A and B: Frontal meningocele at 34 weeks gestation. (A) Surface side view (HDlive Studio), showing cystic mass in front of the orbits. Only liquid but no brain tissue is seen inside the herniated sac; (B) Transparent view of the fetal face, demonstrating the bony defect between the orbits (arrow).

of frontoethmoidal encephalocele is 1:40,000 live births.[6] The presence of a frontal lesion has been observed in 15% of all encephaloceles.[7]

A frontoethmoidal encephalocele is identified sonographically as a cystic solid mass between the orbits. In the presence of a frontal meningocele only a hernial sac filled with liquid is be observed between the orbits **(Fig. 16.4A)**. In both findings a skull defect is visualized behind the protrusion **[Fig. 16.4B (arrow)]**.

ANOMALIES OF THE ORBITS AND THE EYES

Orbital Hypoplasia/Microphthalmia

In orbital hypoplasia the orbital size ranges below the 5th percentile and the eye may be abnormally small (**Fig. 16.5**).[8] The most extreme situation is encountered in *anophthalmia* where the eye is completely missing from the orbit. Microphthalmia may occur as an isolated abnormality, but is also seen in chromosomal defects (trisomy 13 and triploidy), holoprosencephaly and various other syndromes (Aicardi and Treacher Collins).[9]

Hypertelorism

Hypertelorism is defined as an abnormally increased interorbital distance (inner and outer orbital distances) above the 95th percentile.[8] A number of different fetal anomalies associated with hypertelorism have been described: chromosome anomalies, various syndromes (e.g. Apert syndrome and Crouzon syndrome), ethmoidal encephalocele, and facial hemangioma.[9]

Ultrasonic measurements of the inner and the outer orbital distances can be performed in both the coronal (**Fig. 16.6A**) and axial demonstration of the orbits.

The high risk for associated malformations requires both, a targeted ultrasound examination and karyotyping.

Hypotelorism

Hypotelorism is defined as a decreased interorbital distance below the 5th percentile.[8] There is a high risk for associated malformations (chromosome anomalies, holoprosencephaly, microcephaly, and Meckel syndrome.[9] As in hypertelorism, measurements of the inner and the outer orbital distances can be performed in the coronal (**Fig. 16.6B**) or axial demonstration of the orbits.

Cataract

A cataract is an opacification of the crystalline lens in the eye. Cataracts represent a rare fetal condition that may be caused by intrauterine infections (cytomegaly, rubella, and varicella), and chromosome abnormalities (trisomy 13, 18, and 21), or it may form a part of a syndrome (Walker–Warburg, Smith–Lemli–Opitz, and cerebro-ocular muscle dystrophy).[10-15]

A beginning cataract appears sonographically as a hyperechoic dot in the fetal lens, a complete cataract is visualized as a solid hyperechoic disk in the lens (**Fig. 16.7**).

Nasolacrimal Cyst/Dacryocystocele

The nasolacrimal duct cyst is a unilateral or bilateral benign cyst of the nasolacrimal duct. Embryogenesis is attributed to the failure of the valve of Hasner at the distal

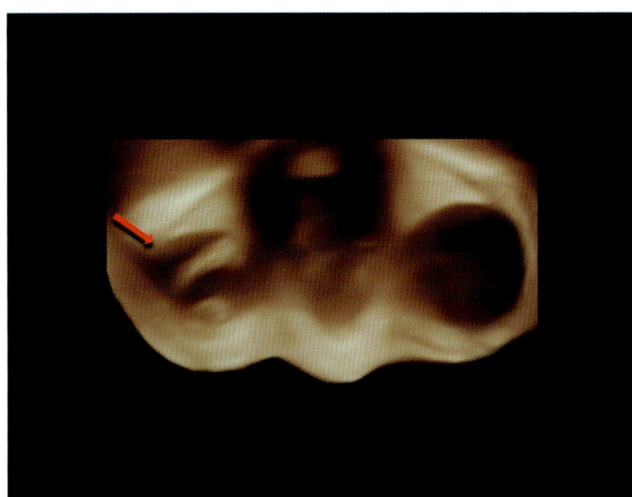

Fig. 16.5: Orbital hypoplasia with detachment of the retina right (arrow). Axial surface view, showing small orbital size (right) in comparison to normal orbita (left). 33 weeks gestation.

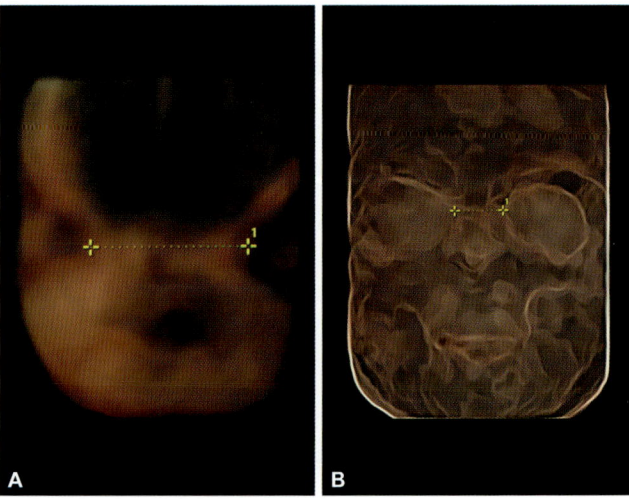

Figs. 16.6A and B: (A) Enlarged interorbital distance (34 mm) revealing hypertelorism (transparent mode, 32 weeks gestation); (B) Reduced interorbital distance (8 mm) showing hypotelorism (silhouette mode, 28 weeks gestation).

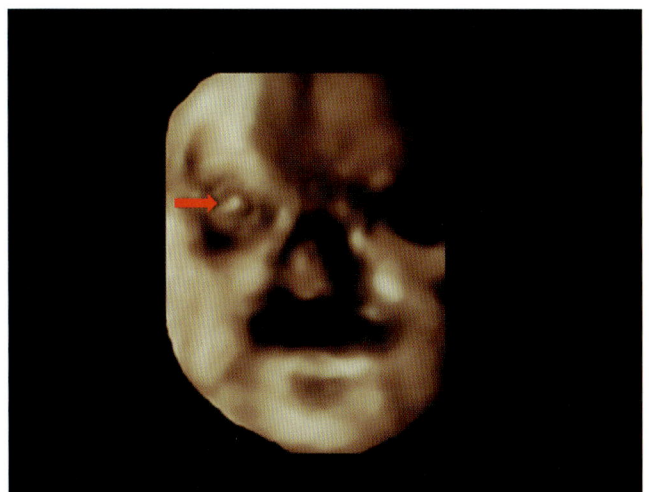

Fig. 16.7: Cataract (hyperechoic disk) in the right lens (arrow). Surface rendered image. 33 weeks gestation.

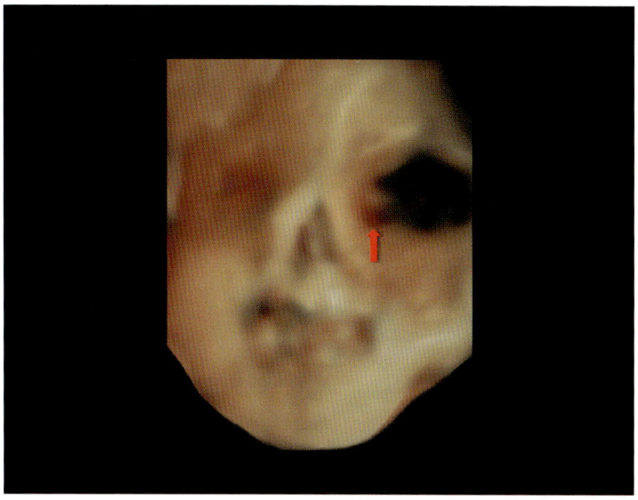

Fig. 16.8: Dacryocystocele in the inferomedial canthus left (arrow). Surface/transparent view of the face. 31 weeks gestation.

end of the nasolacrimal duct. In dacryocystocele there is an obstruction of the lacrimal drainage system both above (Rosenmuller valve) and below the sac (valve of Hasner).[16,17]

A lacrimal cyst/dacryocystocele appears sonographically as a cystic mass in the inferomedial canthus **(Fig. 16.8)**. Dacryocystoceles are typically not identifiable until 30 weeks gestation.[18] In view of the fact that they may be a part of various syndromes, the investigator should carefully examine the fetus for other associated anomalies.[19]

Cyclopia/Proboscis

Cyclopia is a rare facial abnormality characterized by the failure of the embryonic prosencephalon to properly divide the orbits of one eye into two cavities. Instead of the nose a proboscis is usually present, i.e. a trunk like appendage in the midline of the face originating above the eye level. Cyclopia and proboscis occur in association with holoprosencephaly.[20,21]

Ultrasound of the fetal face reveals a single orbit that is best demonstrated in the coronal or axial transparent view **(Fig. 16.9A)**. The proboscis is best seen in a lateral surface view **(Fig. 16.9B)**.

NOSE ABNORMALITIES

Flat Nose (Flat Profile)

A flat profile is a known marker for a chromosomal abnormality (trisomy 21) in the second trimester.[22-25]

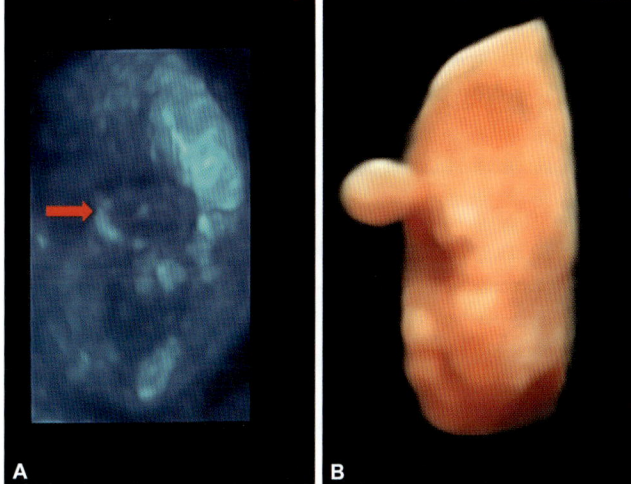

Figs. 16.9A and B: Cyclopia with proboscis (24 weeks gestation). (A) Transparent view of the face, showing one central orbit (arrow); (B) Lateral surface view of cyclopia with proboscis (HDlive).

One of the main advantages of 3D ultrasound technology is the ability to provide the operator with a true median plane of the face, using the multiplanar mode.[1] After identification of the precise profile in the multiplanar mode, several fetal measurements can be performed to confirm a flat profile.[24-26] A frontal fetal facial angle of more than 145° identified in the second trimester should raise suspicion for trisomy 21.[24]

A flat face can also be demonstrated with the surface mode from a lateral view **(Fig. 16.10)**.

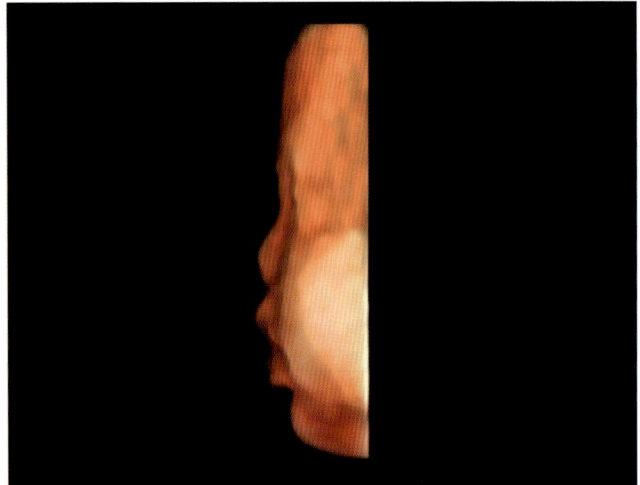

Fig. 16.10: Surface view of a fetus with trisomy 21, showing a flat profile (34 weeks gestation).

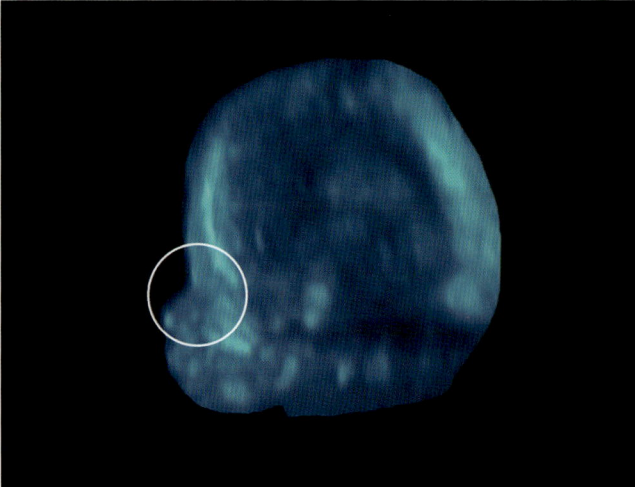

Fig. 16.11: Absent nasal bone in trisomy 21 (O). Transparent side view. 16 weeks gestation.

Every flat profile requires a targeted ultrasound examination with a diligent search for additional anomalies, and fetal karyotyping should be performed.

Absent Nasal Bone

Missing ossification of the two bilateral nasal bones is a further marker for trisomy 21.[27,28]

3D ultrasound allows the identification of an absent nasal bone in both the multiplanar and the transparent mode **(Fig. 16.11)**.

ABNORMALITIES OF THE MOUTH

Cleft Lip/Cleft Palate

Orofacial clefts are one of the most common congenital anomalies. The group of orofacial anomalies is heterogeneous. It comprises "typical" orofacial clefts [cleft lip (CL), cleft lip and cleft palate (CLP), and cleft palate only (CPO)], as well as "atypical" clefts (median, transversal, oblique, and other Tessier facial clefts).[29]

Both typical and atypical clefts can occur as an isolated anomaly, as part of a sequence of the primary defect, or as a multiple congenital anomaly.[29] More than 300 syndromes are associated with facial clefting. The most common chromosomal aberrations with orofacial clefts are trisomy 13, trisomy 18, and trisomy 21.[29,30] CLP can be unilateral, bilateral or median.

The ultrasound demonstration of different CLs is most successful in the surface mode **(Figs. 16.12A to C)**.[31]

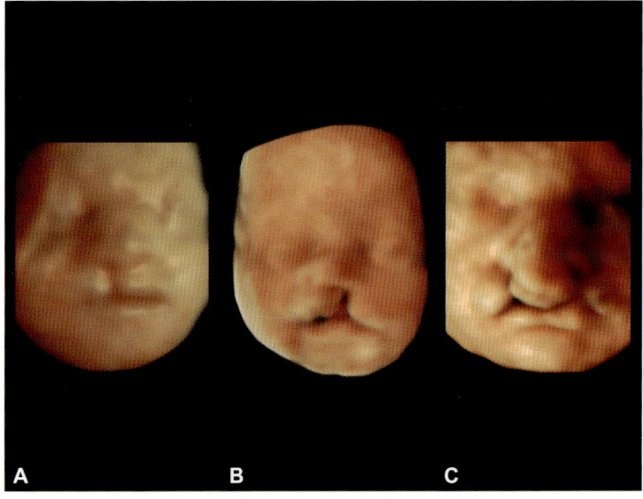

Figs. 16.12A to C: Surface views (HDlive) of different cleft lip. (A). Cleft lip right (30 weeks gestation); (B) Cleft lip left left (29 weeks gestation); (C) Bilateral cleft lip (25 weeks gestation).

The detection of cleft palate is more difficult, particularly in the presence of an isolated cleft palate. Several 3D techniques have been described for the detection of cleft palate.[1,32-35] The defect can be demonstrated in different modes: the multiplanar mode, tomographic mode, surface mode, and Omniview/volume contrast imaging (VCI) mode. The defect is most readily demonstrated when the fetus is yawning and the oral cavity is filled with amniotic fluid **(Fig. 16.13)**.

Fetal karyotyping is recommended with a view to the risk for a chromosomal abnormality.

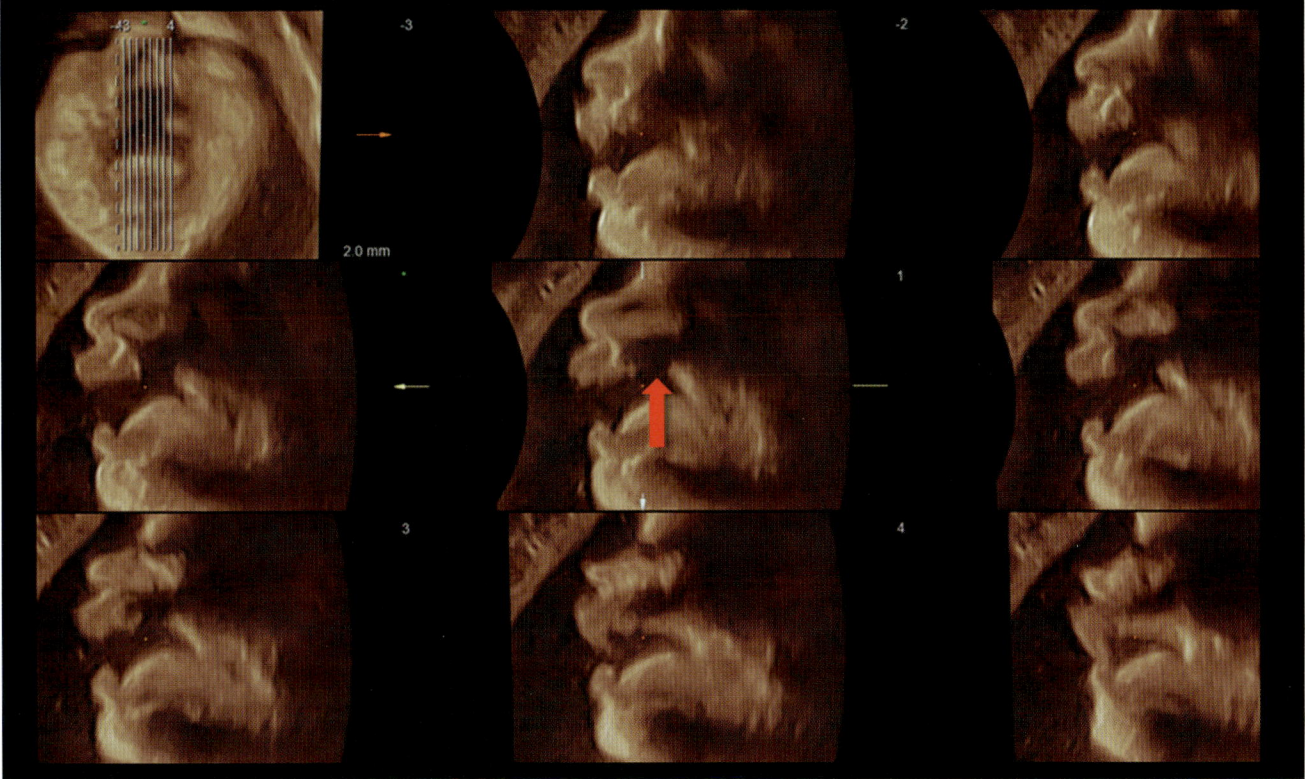

Fig. 16.13: Tomographic demonstration of yawning fetus with cleft palate (34 weeks gestation). The parallel sagittal planes of the face reveal a central defect of the palate (arrow).

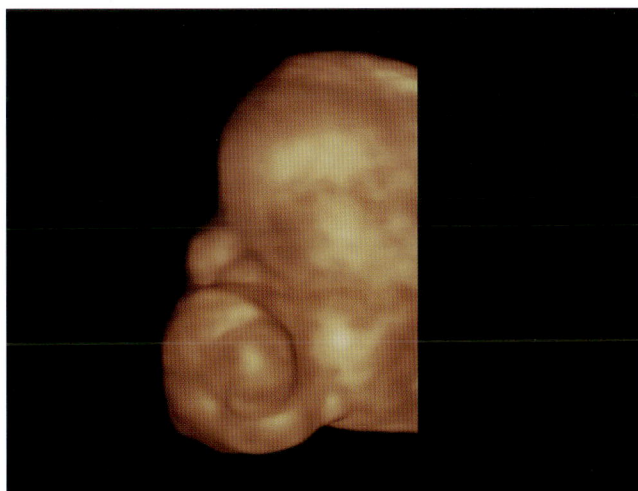

Fig. 16.14: Surface view of an epignathus arising as a solid mass from the oral cavity (22 weeks gestation).

Epignathus

Epignathus is a rare type of teratoma arising in the oral cavity. In most cases it is a benign tumor. However, it is associated with high mortality and morbidity rates because of severe airway obstruction and other malformations.[36] Rare malignant cases have also been described in the literature.[37]

The 3D surface mode shows a solid tumor in front of the fetal mouth **(Fig. 16.14)**.

Macroglossia

Macroglossia is a disorder characterized by an abnormal enlargement of the tongue. It may occur as an isolated and sporadic trait, as a familial trait, or in association with Beckwith–Wiedemann syndrome[38] or Down syndrome.[39]

Ultrasound demonstration of macroglossia is best achieved in the surface mode and demonstrates an enlarged tongue in the open mouth **(Fig. 16.15)**.

CHIN ANOMALY

Micrognathia/Retrognathia

Both micrognathia and retrognathia involve an abnormal, arrested development of the mandible **(Fig. 16.16)**. Micrognathia refers to the size of the mandible whereas retrognathia refers to its position in relation to the maxilla.[40]

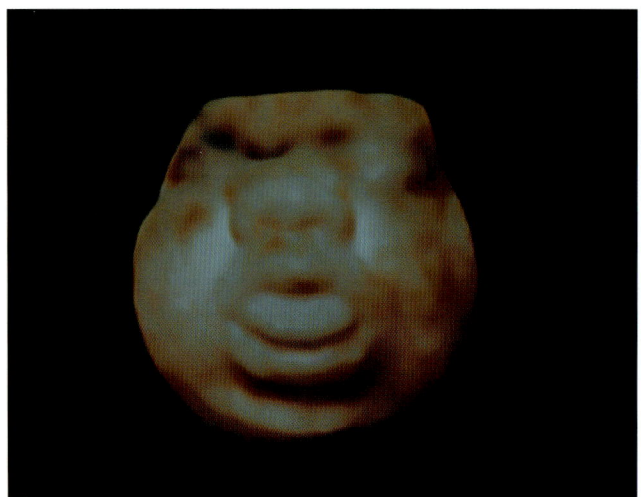

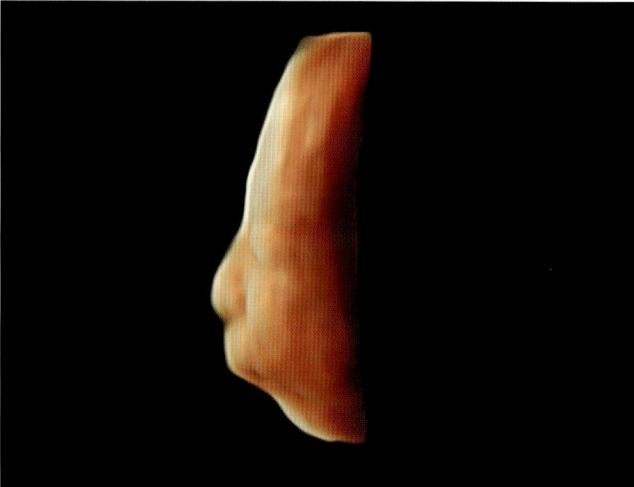

Fig. 16.15: Macroglossia in a fetus with trisomy 21 (27 weeks gestation). The surface rendered image shows permanently open mouth with protruding enlarged tongue.

Fig. 16.16: Micro-retrognathia at 24 weeks gestation. The lateral surface representation shows small mandible.

Micrognathia is frequently associated with a number of different syndromes, skeletal, and neuromuscular diseases, as well as with chromosome anomalies (primarily trisomy 18).[39-41]

The sonographic diagnosis can be made on a subjective or an objective basis. The subjective diagnosis is carried out by evaluating the midsagittal view of the facial profile and by assessing the geometric relationship between the mandible and the rest of the profile. For an objective diagnosis both the inferior facial angle (IFA)[42] and the jaw index[43] are used.

When micro-/retrognathia is detected, a detailed search for additional fetal abnormalities and fetal karyotyping is required.

CONCLUSION

3D ultrasonography allows a comprehensive evaluation of the fetal face with the different display modes. In contrast to 2D ultrasound, 3D ultrasound enables a detailed demonstration of the soft tissue of the fetal face and thus contributes to a better understanding of the malformation by both the physician and the future parents.[31]

REFERENCES

1. Merz E, Abramovicz J, Baba K, et al. 3D imaging of the fetal face—recommendations from the International 3D Focus Group. Ultraschall Med. 2012;33:175-82.
2. Chatzipapas IK, Whitlow BJ, Economides DL. The 'Mickey Mouse' sign and diagnosis of anencephaly in early pregnancy. Ultrasound Obstet Gynecol. 1999;13:196-9.
3. Becker R, Mende B, Stiemer B, et al. Sonographic markers of exencephaly at 9 + 3 weeks of gestation. Ultrasound Obstet Gynecol. 2000;16(6):582-4.
4. Sepulveda W, Sebire NJ, Fung TY, et al. Crown chin length in normal and anencephalic fetuses at 10-14 weeks' gestation. Am J Obstet Gynecol. 1997;176:852-5.
5. Chaoui R, Levaillant JM, Benoit B, et al. Three-dimensional sonographic description of abnormal metopic suture in second- and third-trimester fetuses. Ultrasound Obstet Gynecol. 2005;26:761-4.
6. Donnenfeld AE, Hughes H, Weiner S. Prenatal diagnosis and perinatal management of frontoethmoidal meningo-encephalocele. Am J Perinat. 1988;5:51-3.
7. Weichert J, Hoellen F, Krapp M, et al. Fetal cephaloceles: prenatal diagnosis and course of pregnancy in 65 consecutive cases. Arch Gynecol Obstet. 2017;296:455-63.
8. Merz E, Wellek S, Püttmann S, et al. Orbital diameter, interorbital and binocular diameters—a growth model for fetal orbital parameters. Ultraschall in Med. 1995;16:12-7.
9. Merz E. Ultrasound in Obstetrics and Gynecology. Stuttgart: Thieme; 2005.
10. Francois J. Genetics of cataract. Ophthalmologica. 1982;184;61-71.
11. Francis PJ, Bery V, Bhattacharya SS, et al. The genetics of childhood cataract. J Med Genet. 2000;37:481.
12. Lambert S, Drack A. Infantile cataracts. Surv Ophthalmol. 1996;40:427-58.
13. Rahi JS, Dezateux C. Congenital and infantile cataract in the United Kingdom: underlying or associated factors. Invest Ophthalmol Vis Sci. 2000;41:2108-14.

14. Brasseur-Daudruy M, Vivier PH, Ickowicz V, et al. Walker-Warburg syndrome diagnosed by findings of typical ocular abnormalities on prenatal ultrasound. Pediatr Radiol. 2012;42:488-90.

15. Drought A, Wimalasundera R, Holder S. Ultrasound diagnosis of bilateral cataracts in a fetus with possible cerebro-ocular congenital muscular dystrophy during the routine second trimester anomaly scan. Ultrasound. 2015;23:181-5.

16. Cavazza S, Laffi GL, Lodi L, et al. Congenital dacryocystocele: diagnosis and treatment. Acta Otorhinolaryngol Italica. 2008;28:298-301.

17. Barham HP, Wudel JM, Enzenauer RW, et al. Congenital nasolacrimal duct cyst/dacryocystocele: An argument for a genetic basis. Allergy Rhinol (Providence). 2012;3(1):e46-9.

18. Sherer D, Eisenberg C, Hammerman R, et al. Prenatal sonographic diagnosis of dacryocystocele: a case and review of the literature. Amer J Perinatol. 1997;14(8):479-81.

19. Sharon R, Raz J, Aviram R, et al. Prenatal diagnosis of dacryocystocele: a possible marker for syndromes. Ultrasound Obstet Gynecol. 1999;14:71-3.

20. Olejek A, Bodzek P, Skutil M, et al. Cyclopia—literature review and a case report. Ginekol Pol. 2011;82:221-5.

21. Mălutan AM, Dudea M, Ciortea R, et al. Cyclopia and proboscis—the extreme end of holoprosencephaly. Rom J Morphol Embryol. 2017;58:1555-9.

22. Sonek J, Borenstein M, Downing C, et al. Frontomaxillary facial angles in screening for trisomy 21 at 14–23 weeks' gestation. Am J Obstet Gynecol. 2007;197:160.e1-5.

23. Vos FI, de Jong-Pleij EA, Bakker M, et al. Fetal facial profile markers of Down syndrome in the second and third trimesters of pregnancy. Ultrasound Obstet Gynecol. 2015;46:168-73.

24. Merz E, Pashaj S. The frontal fetal facial (FFF) angle in the second trimester measured by 3D ultrasound in normal fetuses and fetuses with trisomy 21. Ultrasound Obstet Gynecol. 2015;46 (Suppl 1):88.

25. Vos FI, Bakker M, de Jong-Pleij EA, et al. Is 3D technique superior to 2D in Down syndrome screening? Evaluation of six second and third trimester fetal profile markers. Prenat Diagn. 2015;35:207-13.

26. Vos FI, De Jong-Pleij EA, Ribbert LS, et al. Three-dimensional ultrasound imaging and measurement of nasal bone length, prenasal thickness and frontomaxillary facial angle in normal second- and third-trimester fetuses. Ultrasound Obstet Gynecol. 2012;39:636-41.

27. Agathokleous M, Chaveeva P, Poon LC, et al. Meta-analysis of second-trimester markers for trisomy 21. Ultrasound Obstet Gynecol. 2013;41(3):247-61.

28. Du Y, Ren Y, Yan Y, et al. Absent fetal nasal bone in the second trimester and risk of abnormal karyotype in a prescreened population of Chinese women. Acta Obstet Gynecol Scand. 2018;97:180-6.

29. Tolarová MM, Cervenka J. Classification and birth prevalence of orofacial clefts. Am J Med Genet. 1998;75:126-37.

30. Doray B, Badila-Timbolschi D, Schaefer E, et al. Epidemiology of orofacial clefts (1995-2006) in France (Congenital Malformations of Alsace Registry). Arch Pediatr. 2012;19:1021-9.

31. Merz E, Pashaj S. Prenatal detection of orofacial clefts. Ultraschall in Med. 2016;37:137-9.

32. Campbell S, Lees C, Moscoso G, et al. Ultrasound antenatal diagnosis of cleft palate by a new technique: the 3D "reverse face" view. Ultrasound Obstet Gynecol. 2005;25:12-8.

33. Platt LD, Devore GR, Pretorius DH. Improving cleft palate/cleft lip antenatal diagnosis by 3-dimensional sonography: the "flipped face" view. J Ultrasound Med. 2006;25:1423-30.

34. Pilu G, Segata M. A novel technique for visualization of the normal and cleft secondary palate: angled insonation and three-dimensional ultrasound. Ultrasound Obstet Gynecol. 2007;29:166-9.

35. Merz E, Pashaj S. Advantages of 3D ultrasound in the assessment of fetal abnormalities. J Perinat Med. 2017;45:643-50.

36. Moon NR, Min JY, Kim YH, et al. Prenatal diagnosis of epignathus with multiple malformations in one fetus of a twin pregnancy using three-dimensional ultrasonography and magnetic resonance imaging. Obstet Gynecol Sci. 2015;58:65-8.

37. Too SC, Sarji SA, Yik YI, et al. Malignant epignathus teratoma. Biomed Imaging Interv J. 2008;4:e18.

38. Reish O, Lerer I, Amiel A, et al. Wiedemann-Beckwith syndrome: further prenatal characterization of the condition. Am J Med Genet. 2002;107:209-13.

39. Nicolaides KH, Salvesen DR, Snijders RJM, et al. Fetal facial defects: associated malformations and chromosomal abnormalities. Fetal Diagn Ther. 1993;8:1-9.

40. Paladini D. Fetal micrognathia: almost an ominous finding. Ultrasound Obstet Gynecol. 2010;35:377-84.

41. Luedders DW, Bohlmann MK, Germer U, et al. Fetal micrognathia: objective assessment and associated anomalies on prenatal sonogram. Prenat Diagn. 2011;31:146-51.

42. Rotten D, Levaillant JM, Martinez H, et al. The fetal mandible: a 2D and 3D sonographic approach to the diagnosis of retrognathia and micrognathia. Ultrasound Obstet Gynecol. 2002;19:122-30.

43. Paladini D, Morra T, Teodoro A, et al. Objective diagnosis of micrognathia in the fetus: the Jaw Index. Obstet Gynecol. 1999;93:382-6.

Artifacts and Pitfalls in 3D Ultrasound

Danka Miric Tesanic, Eberhard Merz

INTRODUCTION

Three-dimensional (3D) ultrasound in prenatal diagnosis and its different visualization modes give the operator the possibility to examine the fetus more precisely than with two-dimensional (2D) sonography. Multiplanar mode and tomographic ultrasound imaging (TUI) enable detailed examinations of the fetal structures in three perpendicular respectively parallel planes while 3D surface view shows the surface of the fetus and the surface of cut planes in a photorealistic demonstration. Volume contrast imaging (VCI) and maximum mode enable the visualization of the fetal skeleton and bony structures. Volume postprocessing allows the operator to rotate the acquired volume on the screen and to examine fetal structures from different viewing angles. Therefore, combining all possibilities offered by 3D technology, a well-trained sonographer can be even more self-confident in establishing the final diagnosis. Furthermore, for the parents-to-be 3D technology represents a unique visual experience giving them the opportunity to see their fetus comparable to a photograph.[1-7] By introducing four-dimensional (4D) sonography in obstetrics as a real-time surface demonstration, the operator is able to visualize not only general fetal movements but also facial movements and facial expressions.

Although 3D ultrasound may produce excellent 3D images, the 3D technique in daily obstetrical sonographic practice is quite demanding. To perform a detailed diagnostic examination with high-quality 3D surface images takes time and requires operator's knowledge and skill. Furthermore, using 3D ultrasound, the operator should always be aware of potential artifacts and pitfalls that

Box 17.1: Different types of artifacts that can occur during three-dimensional (3D) sonographic examination.

3D artifacts caused by:
- Fetal movements
- Acoustic shadowing
- Amputation of objects by the volume box
- Unfavorable threshold adjustment
- Electronic scalpel
- Superimposed objects

may occur during volume acquisition and volume post-processing. Artifacts are a common problem in sonography in general. Sonographic artifacts have already been reported in conventional 2D ultrasound and in color Doppler. They may also be part of any 3D sonographic examination and can disturb a routine diagnostic procedure.[5,7-17] They can arise during volume acquisition, volume rendering or image postprocessing.[15] The artifacts present in everyday practical work may occur due to fetal movements, acoustic shadowing, and superimposed structures. Further, artifacts can be caused by improper use of the electronic scalpel and the threshold. If properly recognized during the sonographic examination, the risk of misinterpretation of the sonographic findings can be reduced.

The basic artifacts are listed in **Box 17.1** according to the origin of their appearance.

MOTION ARTIFACTS

Motion artifacts are the most common artifacts in 3D volume acquisition and visualization. They are the result of fetal movements during 3D volume acquisition. Fetal

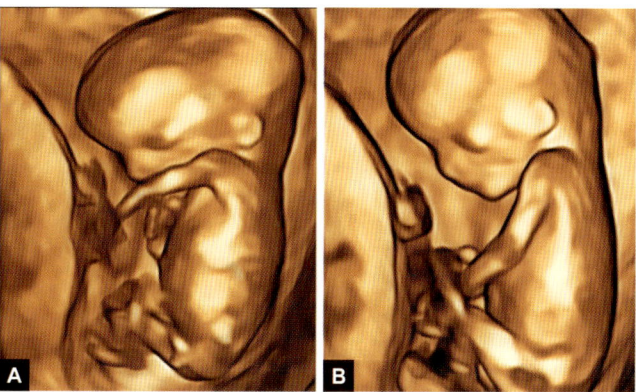

Figs. 17.1A and B: (A) A horizontal fetal movement during volume acquisition providing horizontal widening/deformity of the fetal head (12 weeks gestation). (B) The rescanned volume reveals a completely normal fetal anatomy.

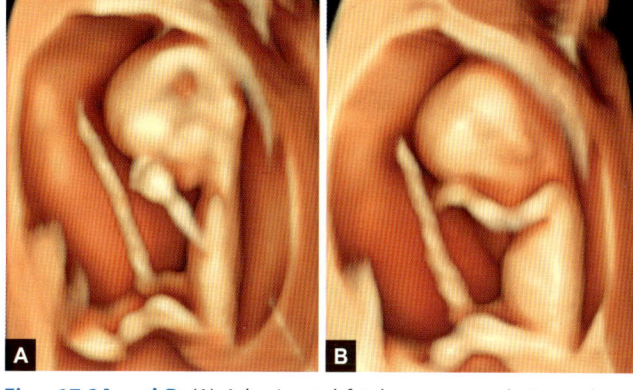

Figs. 17.2A and B: (A) A horizontal fetal movement during volume acquisition providing narrow body (12 weeks gestation). (B) The rescanned volume reveals a completely normal fetal anatomy.

movement can be slight or strong. Slight fetal movement can provide only mild unevenness on the fetal surface, whereas strong fetal movement can result in severe deformities of the fetal structures. Fetal movement artifacts are always visible in the 3D surface image. In multiplanar view, a motion artifact can only be recognized in planes B and C, while it is not visible in plane A. Due to the direction of the fetal movement, motion artifacts can be divided into horizontal and vertical artifacts. Horizontal fetal movements during acquisition provide horizontal deformities of the fetal structures such as widening **(Figs. 17.1A and B)** or narrowing of anatomical structures **(Figs. 17.2A and B)**. Strong horizontal movements of the fetal head provide severe facial deformities, e.g. hypertelorism. Slight horizontal head movements can even mimic fetal anomaly, e.g. horizontal cleft lip. Vertical fetal movements during acquisition can cause vertical deformities of the fetal structures and can feign cleft lip or spina bifida. Images with motion artifacts, especially those with suspected fetal anomalies have to be viewed with caution and the acquisition process has to be repeated in order to get an image with an adequate quality to avoid a false diagnosis.

ACOUSTIC SHADOWING

Shadow artifacts are the result of hyperechoic and bony structures like the fetal spine or the limb bones. Shadows affected by the vertebrae prevent the evaluation of the underlying fetal thoracic and abdominal organs in the 3D surface image and also in the multiplanar view.

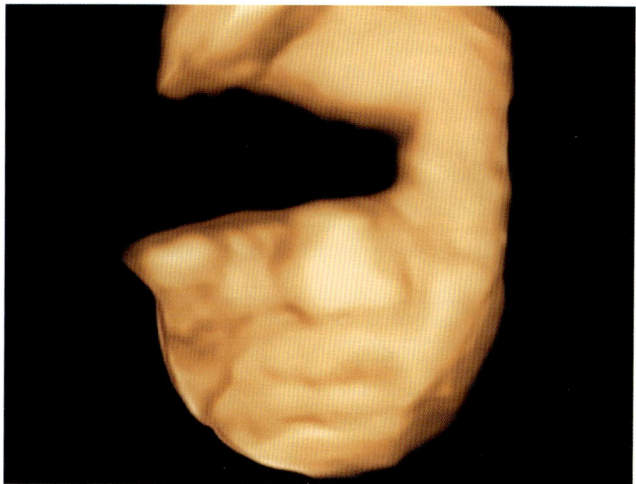

Fig. 17.3: Acoustic shadow artifact caused by a superimposed limb bone (fetal ulna) in front of the fetal face (29 weeks gestation).

Limb bones in front of the fetal face can provide cut-like shadows across the region of interest or hole-like artifacts in the middle of the face **(Fig. 17.3)**. In case of large shadows, the underlying structures are only partially visible on the screen or sometimes even completely invisible. Sometimes shadow artifacts can feign fetal anomaly, e.g. cleft lip **(Figs. 17.4A to C)**. In such cases volume acquisition has to be repeated at a different scanning angle. If this is not possible, the operator can try to provoke a movement of the fetus by slightly pressing the mother's abdomen with the hand and repeat the scanning procedure in order to get an image with sufficient quality for further diagnostic evaluation.

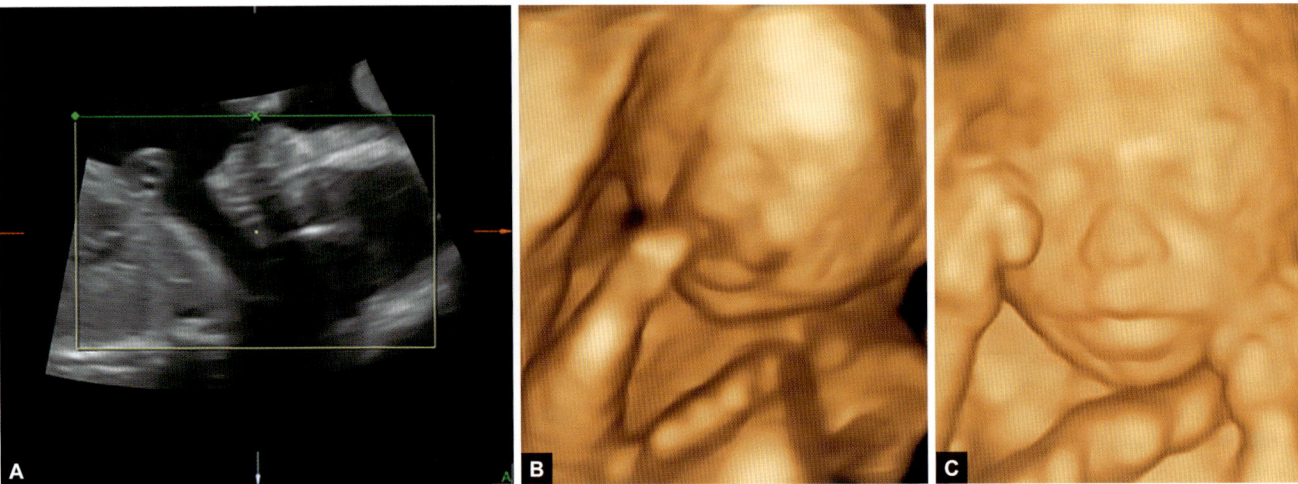

Figs. 17.4A to C: Acoustic shadow artifact feigning cleft lip (21 weeks gestation). This artifact is caused by the fetal hand lying in front of the fetal face. In the multiplanar mode (A) the superimposed fetal hand is visible lying partially outside the volume box and therefore is not completely presented in the 3D surface image. (B) Hyperechoic bony structures of the fetal hand are causing shadow artifact that looks like a cleft lip. (C) Normal fetal face after repeated volume acquisition.

AMPUTATION OF OBJECTS BY THE VOLUME BOX

Amputation artifacts are caused by the size and position of the volume box. Structures of the fetus which are not within the volume box during volume acquisition are not visible on the screen after the scanning procedure. As a result, it may look like a limb amputation, fetal head or face defect (**Figs. 17.5A and B**), or even like a spinal or eye anomaly in the rendered image. In such cases, it is always important to explain the image presented on the screen to the parents, and it is also necessary to rescan the volume in order to visualize the apparently missing fetal structures on the screen.

UNFAVORABLE THRESHOLD ADJUSTMENT

The threshold is a useful filter to remove small floating particles from the amniotic fluid electronically. Optimal threshold adjustment is necessary in order to get a high-quality image.[1] If the threshold is set too low, the small echoes in front of the region of interest do not allow a proper visualization of the fetal structures, resulting in a poor image quality. By setting the threshold too high, the sonographer can cause artifacts mimicking fetal defects (**Figs. 17.6A to C**).

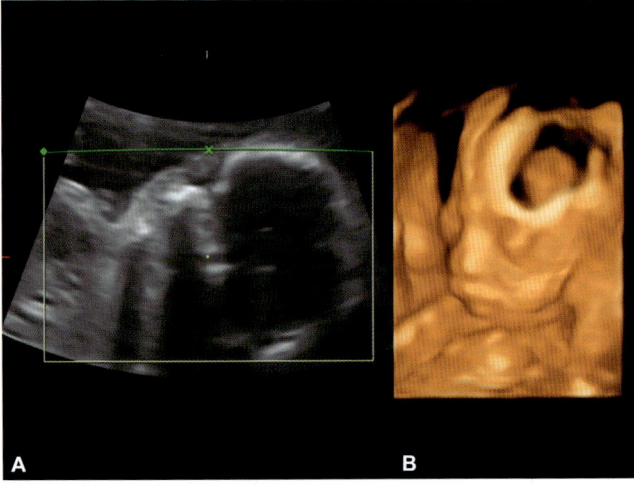

Figs. 17.5A and B: Amputation artifact of the fetal forehead left due to a too small volume box (20 weeks gestation). (A) In the 2D image, it can be seen clearly that the fetal forehead is partially outside the volume box. (B) The amputation defect can be observed in the surface-rendered image.

DEFECTS CAUSED BY THE ELECTRONIC SCALPEL

Usually the electronic scalpel is used to improve the image quality by removing superimposed structures that obstruct the view to the region of interest.[3] Sometimes the operator can cause the artifacts by improper use

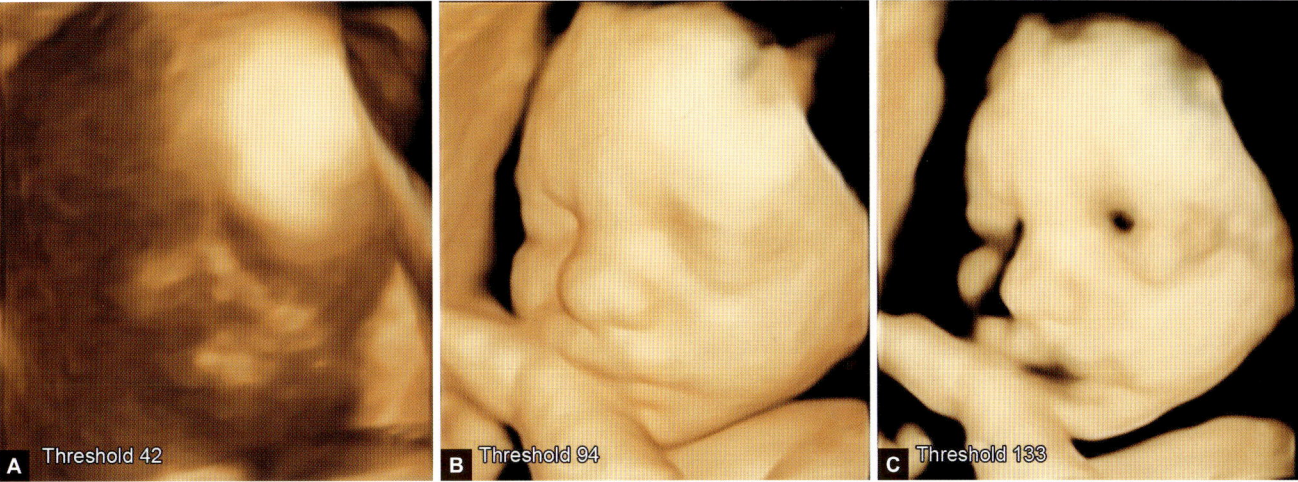

Figs. 17.6A to C: Threshold artifacts (31 weeks gestation). (A) If the threshold is set to low, the small echoes in the amniotic fluid in front of the region of interest avoid the demonstration of the fetal surface. (B) If the threshold is set properly, it improves the image quality. (C) By setting the threshold to a high, the sonographer can partially delete normal fetal face structures causing iatrogenic artifacts.

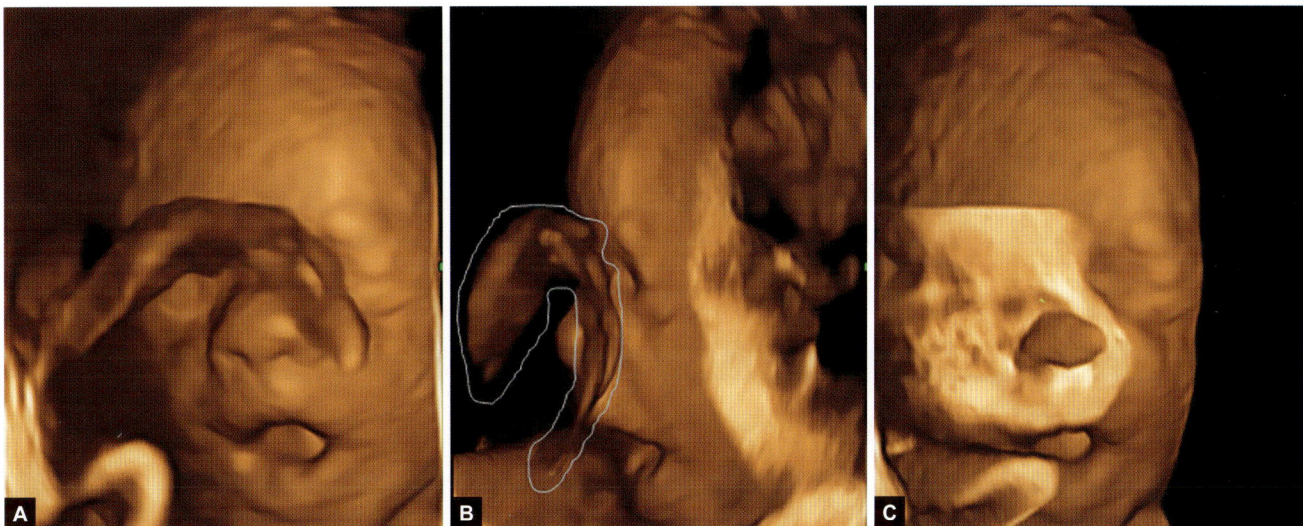

Figs. 17.7A to C: Defects caused by the electronic scalpel. Structures positioned in front of the fetal face [e.g. umbilical cord] (A) which prevent viewing of the region of interest, can be removed with the electronic scalpel (B). If the cutting process is performed to intense the structures in front of the face, e.g. the right eye and cheek, can be removed as well (C) (28 weeks gestation).

of the electronic scalpel. If the cutting process is too intense, normal structures are also accidentally removed providing a defect of the fetal surface, e.g. missing tip of the nose or missing chin **(Figs. 17.7A to C)**. In such cases, it is necessary to use the redo button and to perform the cutting process once again with more precision. Sometimes, such cutting defects may even simulate an anomaly like spina bifida. To exclude such a defect it is necessary to perform a multiplanar or tomographic analysis in order to avoid a misinterpretation of the finding. In some other

situations, it is necessary to repeat the volume acquisition from a different scanning angle in order to clarify whether it is an anomaly or artifact, before establishing the final diagnosis.

ARTIFACTS DUE TO SUPERIMPOSED OBJECTS

Superimposed structures can provide funny images in 3D rendered images. This can result in a Pinocchio nose,

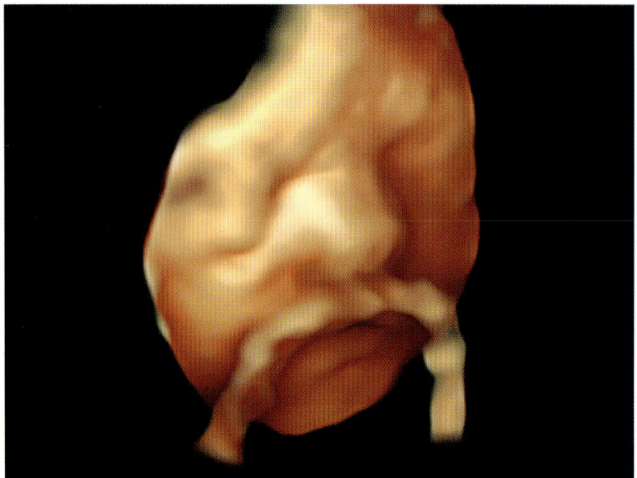

Fig. 17.8: Fetus with "moustache". Superimposed structures, e.g. the umbilical cord may sometimes provide funny images in 3D surface view (30 weeks gestation)—3D HDlive surface image.

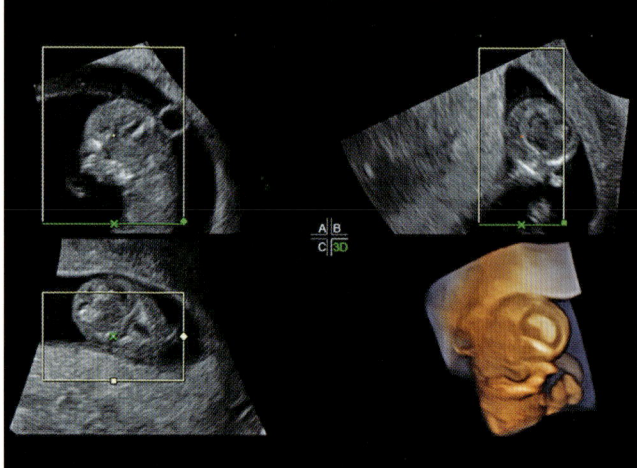

Fig. 17.9: Overlapping structures next to the head can simulate fetal anomaly. In this case, the yolk sac can be misinterpreted as a meningocele (11 weeks gestation). The evaluation of the region of interest in the multiplanar mode can exclude possible diagnostic vagueness.

vampire teeth or a fetus with a mustache **(Fig. 17.8)**. In other cases the overlapping structures in front of the region of interest can also simulate a fetal anomaly, e.g. a yolk sac can simulate a meningocele **(Fig. 17.9)**. In cases like this, the superimposed structure can be removed with the electronic scalpel, or the volume has to be acquired once again using a different acquisition angle.

SONOGRAPHIC PITFALLS

In daily routine, a sonographer has to deal with pitfalls that could lead to an incorrect diagnosis. An unfavorable viewing angle, as presented in **Figure 17.10A**, allows only demonstration of four fingers on the screen. By rotating the obtained volume around the y-axis, all fingers can be seen on the screen **(Fig. 17.10B)**.

Looking at the umbilical cord in **Figure 17.11A**, the diagnosis of a true umbilical knot can be falsely assumed. After rotating the obtained volume and looking at the umbilical cord from different viewing angles, the operator can see that the umbilical cord is twisted and overlapped, but there is no true knot **(Figs. 17.11B and C)**. In such situations, it is always important to rotate the acquired volume on the screen to see the structures from different viewing angles and to get the correct diagnosis.

Another doubtful situation may be seen in **Figure 17.12A**. A postaxial adnexa visible on the fetal hand may be misinterpreted as a superimposed structure

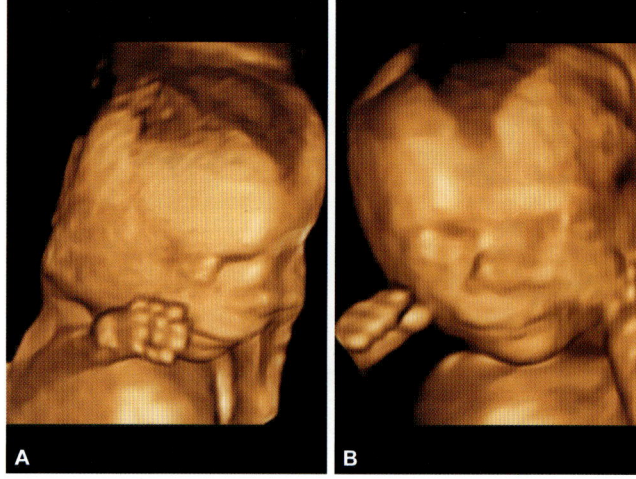

Figs. 17.10A and B: Sonographic pitfall. (A) Due to an unfavorable viewing angle, only four fingers are visible on the screen (20 weeks gestation). (B) By rotating the acquired volume and examining the fetal hand from an optimal viewing angle, all five fingers are visible.

and be removed with the electronic scalpel **(Fig. 17.12B)**. Only if the fetal hand is controlled with a different viewing angle, a hexadactyly can be precisely demonstrated in the multiplanar **(Fig. 17.12C)** and in the surface view.

To avoid such pitfalls in daily work, it is always necessary to see the object of interest from different angles and in different rendering modes to find the correct diagnosis.

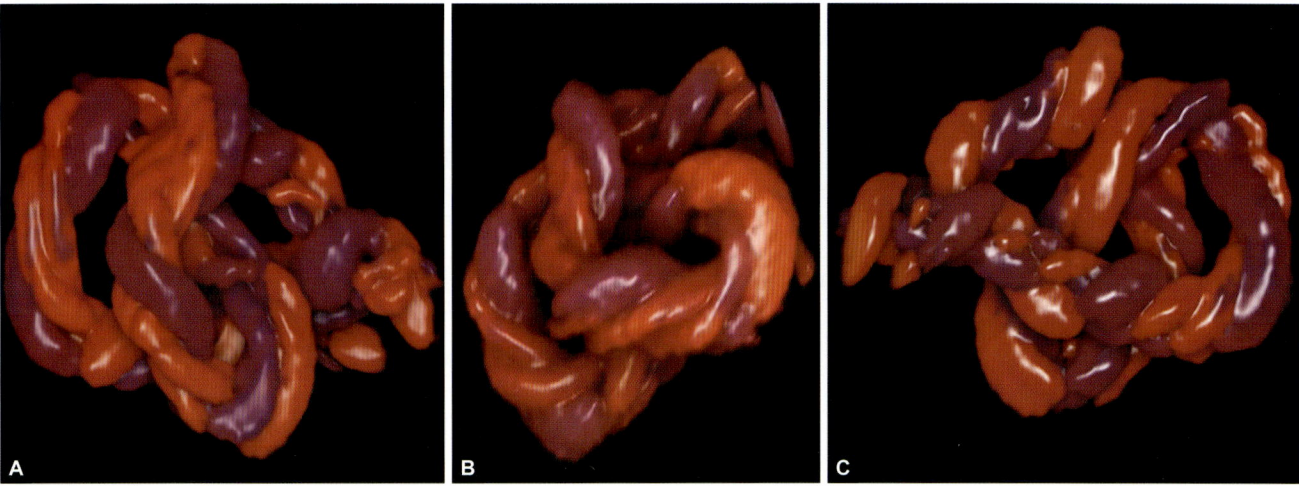

Figs. 17.11A to C: Sonographic pitfall. (A) Due to an unfavorable viewing angle, the umbilical cord is seen like a true knot on screen. (B and C) By rotating the acquired volume and examining the umbilical cord from different viewing angles, it is obvious that the umbilical cord is only twisted and without true umbilical knot.

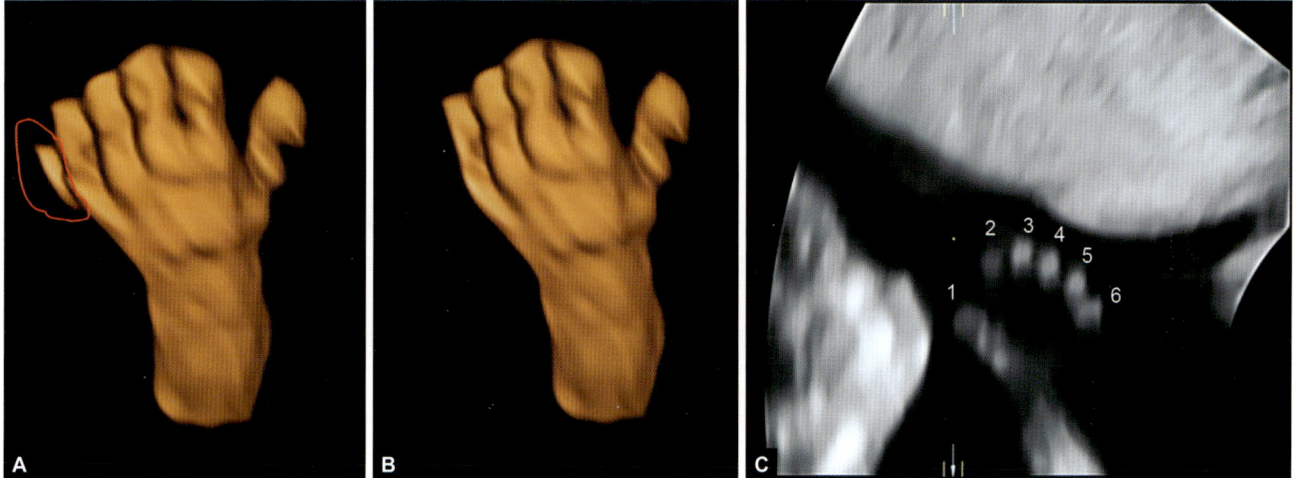

Figs. 17.12A to C: Sonographic pitfall. A small postaxial adnexa visible on the left fetal hand can be interpreted as an artifact instead of an anomaly (13 weeks gestation). With the use of the electronical scalpel, this small superimposed structure can be easily removed (A) resulting in a completely normal looking hand (B). However, reexamination of the obtained volume and rotating the volume reveals the correct diagnosis of postaxial hexadactyly in the multiplanar mode (C).

CONCLUSION

Three-dimensional ultrasound is based on 2D ultrasound. Therefore, it is always necessary to start the examination always with the best possible 2D sonographic image quality.

In prenatal 3D sonography, artifacts can arise during volume acquisition, volume rendering or volume postprocessing. Some artifacts can be avoided by optimizing the size and position of the volume box or by using a different scanning angle. Other artifacts can be minimized by the proper use of the threshold and the precise use of the electronic scalpel during the postprocessing of the image.

In all doubtful 3D findings, it is always necessary to rescan the region of interest and to assess the fetal structures in the multiplanar mode once again before making a final diagnosis.

REFERENCES

1. Merz E, Bahlmann F, Weber G, et al. Application of transvaginal and transabdominal 3D-ultrasound for detection or exclusion of fetal malformations of the fetal face. Ultrasound Obstet Gynecol. 1997;9:237-43.

2. Merz E, Pashaj S. Advantages of 3D ultrasound in the assessment of fetal abnormalities. J Perinat Med. 2017; 45(6):643-50.

3. Merz E, Miric-Tesanic D, Welter C. Value of the electronic scalpel (cut mode) in the evaluation of the fetal face. Ultrasound Obstet Gynecol. 2000;16:564-8.

4. Merz E. 3D-Sonographie in der Pränatalen Diagnostik. In: E Merz (Ed). Sonographische Diagnostik in Gynäkologie und Geburtshilfe. Stuttgart: Thieme Verlag; 2002. pp. 517-30.

5. Merz E, Bahlmann F, Weber G, et al. Fetal malformations: assessment by three-dimensional ultrasound in the surface mode. In: Merz E (Ed). 3-D Ultrasound in Obstetrics and Gynecology. Philadelphia, New York: Lippincott Williams & Wilkins; 1998. pp. 109-19.

6. Merz E. 3D/4D-Ultrasound in Obstetrics—Baby TV without Diagnostics? Ultraschall Med. 2008;29:156-8.

7. Kratochwil A. Importance and possibilities of multiplanar examination in three-dimensional sonography. In: Merz E (Ed). 3-D Ultrasonography in Obstetrics and Gynecology. Philadelphia: Lippincott Williams & Wilkins; 1998. pp. 105-8.

8. Ahn H, Hernández-Andrade E, Romero R, et al. Mirror artifacts in obstetric ultrasound; case presentation of a ghost twin during the second trimester ultrasound scan. Fetal Diagn Ther. 2013;34:248-52.

9. Zalud I. Artifacts, pitfalls and normal variants. In: Kurjak A, Chervenak FA (Eds). Donald School Textbook of Ultrasound in Obstetrics and Gynecology. New Delhi: Jaypee Brothers Medical Publishers (P) Ltd.; 2008. pp. 26-34.

10. Zalud I, Rocha F. Pitfalls and normal variants. In: Kurjak A, Chervenak FA. (Eds.): Donald School Textbook of Ultrasound in Obstetrics and Gynecology. New Delhi: Jaypee Brothers Medical Publishers (P) Ltd.; 2011. pp. 85-93.

11. Zalud I, Rocha F. Artifacts, pitfalls and normal variants. Donald. School J Ultrasound Obstet Gynecol. 2012;6(1): 1-8.

12. Lim BH, Amos M, Fairhead AC. The mirror image artifacts in early pregnancy. Ultrasound Obstet Gynecol. 2003;21:518-20.

13. Benacerraf BR, Benson C, Abuhamad AZ, et al. Three- and 4-dimensional ultrasound in obstetrics and gynecology: proceedings of the American Institute of Ultrasound in Medicine Consensus Conference. J Ultrasound Med. 2005; 24:1587-97.

14. Shapiro I, Degani S, Ohel G. Pitfalls and artifacts in 3D ultrasound. Ultrasound Obstet Gynecol. 2004;24:232.

15. Nelson TR, Pretorius DH, Hull A, et al. Sources and impacts of artifacts on clinical three-dimensional ultrasound images. Ultrasound Obstet Gynecol. 2000;16:374-83.

16. Leung KY, Ngai CSW, Tang MHY. Facial cleft or shadowing artifact? Ultrasound Obstet Gynecol. 2006;27: 231-2.

17. Merz E, Abramovicz J, Baba K, et al. 3D imaging of the fetal face—recommendations from the International 3D Focus Group. Ultraschall Med. 2012;33:175-82.

Three-dimensional Ultrasound in Infertility and Ectopic Pregnancy

Sonal Panchal

INTRODUCTION

Three-dimensional (3D) ultrasound (US) is now a well-developed technology, and it has proved its superiority over the B mode US in several applications. In the patients with infertility or gynecological complaints, some abnormalities are suspected in the uterus, tubes, or ovaries in the female, but the male factor is also equally important in infertility. For the assessment of the female, transvaginal scan is the scanning method of choice and the first-line investigation. Adding dynamic examination, Doppler and 3D US markedly increase the information available. 3D US can be used for the assessment of uterine congenital anomalies, intrauterine pathologies, adnexal lesions, tubal patency assessment, polycystic ovaries, ovarian follicular monitoring, and endometrial receptivity assessment. In the infertile male, 3D US has a role in the assessment of the seminal vesicles and ejaculatory ducts, especially with transrectal US. This means it may help differentiate between the obstructive and nonobstructive azoospermia. Though in this article, we shall discuss the role of 3D US in female infertility.

3D ULTRASOUND FOR ABNORMALITIES OF THE UTERUS

Amongst the *uterine abnormalities*, Müllerian abnormalities and fibroids have been discussed elsewhere in this book. So, in this article, we shall discuss the other abnormalities of the uterus that affect fertility. These include endometritis, polyps, adenomyosis, chiefly. Though endometritis is a B mode and Doppler diagnosis, polyps and adenomyosis have a definite role of 3D US.

ENDOMETRIAL POLYP

Polyp is a soft tissue solid projection from the endometrial wall into the endometrial cavity. This may have a pedicle or may be sessile. Polyps may be of variable sizes and may involve the endometrial cavity and may also arise in the cervical canal. Polyps are fairly easy to diagnose during the periovulatory phase of the menstrual cycle **(Fig. 18.1)** but are obscured in the secretory phase due to the hyperechoic endometrium. In such cases, localized area of subtly increased echogenicity **(Fig. 18.2)**, with Doppler showing a single feeding vessel, may be diagnostic. Single feeding vessel has high sensitivity and specificity for the diagnosis of polyps[1] **(Fig. 18.3)**.

In early proliferative phase when the endometrium is thin, smaller polyps can be easily missed **(Figs. 18.4A and B)** but the larger ones may show bulbous irregularity

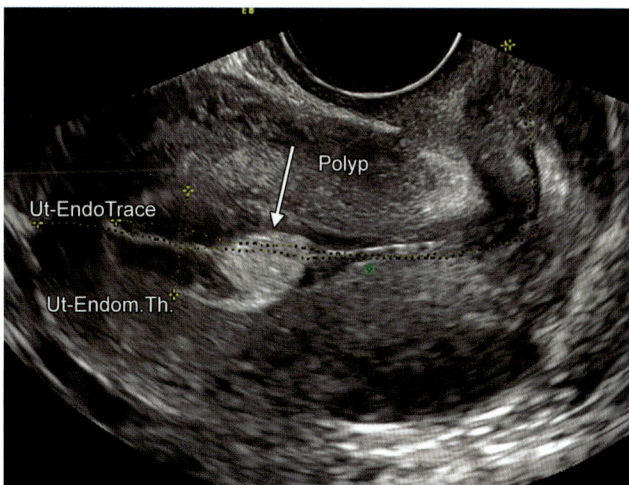

Fig. 18.1: B mode ultrasound image showing endometrial polyp in preovulatory phase.

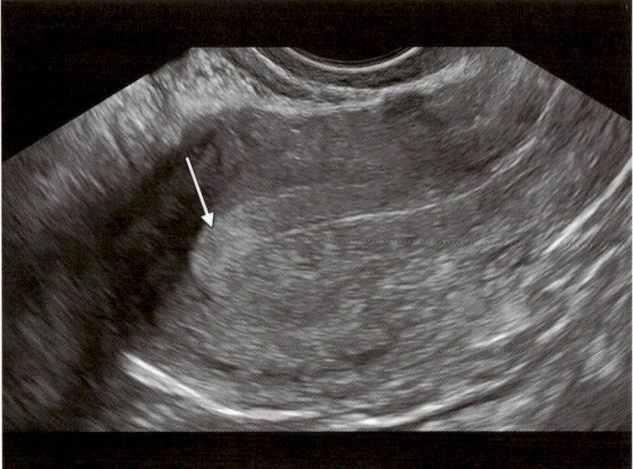

Fig. 18.2: B mode ultrasound image showing endometrial polyp in secretory phase.

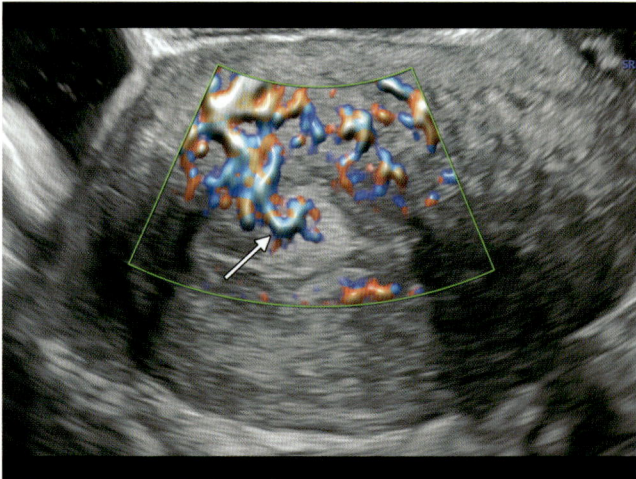

Fig. 18.3: High definition flow showing single feeding vessel in the polyp.

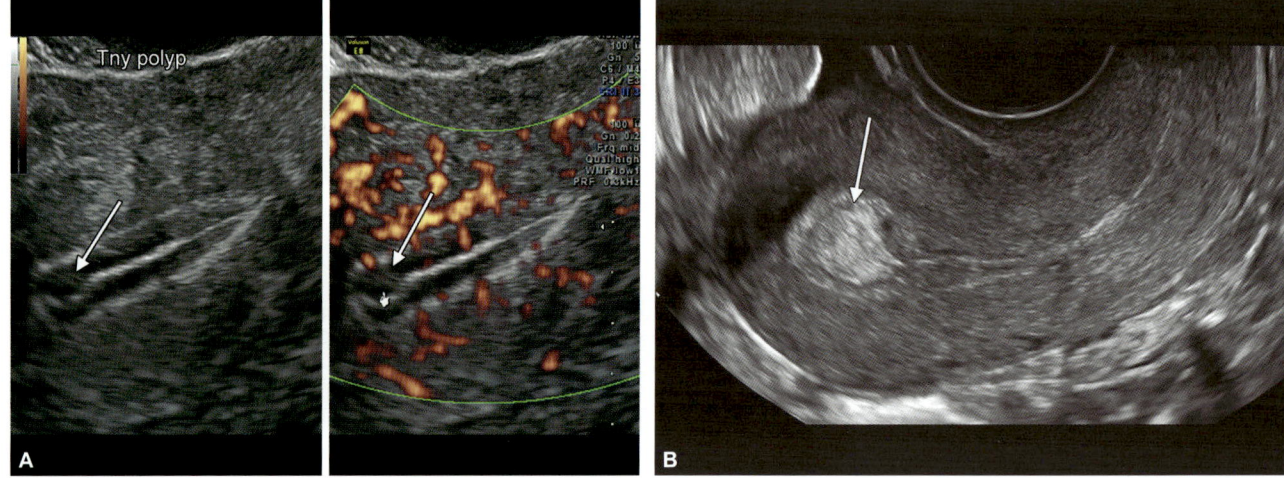

Figs. 18.4A and B: (A) B mode and power Doppler image showing a small polyp; (B) B mode ultrasound image of a polyp filling the fundal endometrium.

of the endometrium. 3D US helps differentiate large polyps with sessile base from hyperplasia. Whatever the phase of the cycle, saline infusion sonohysterography is the investigation that will allow the lesion to be clearly visualized **(Fig. 18.5)**. But 3D US with sonohysterography is the most reliable investigation for the diagnosis of polyp.

SONOHYSTEROGRAPHY TECHNIQUE

A 6-Fg Foley's catheter with external diameter of 1.6 mm and internal diameter of 1.1 mm is introduced through the cervix and is so placed that the bulb remains in the cervix. Distend the balloon by 1.5–2 mL of distilled water. Slowly inject 5–10 mL of normal saline with 20 mL syringe.

Introduce the probe into the vagina after removing the speculum and tenaculum, but with catheter in situ. While filling the syringe and injecting the fluid, take care not to introduce any air, which will cause artifacts. Take a 3D sweep of the uterus and reconstruct in coronal view. Two-dimensional (2D) US may also be used with fluid in situ for identifying the endometrial pathologies. Lately; gel has been used instead of saline and has been found to be more convenient with equivalent results. Normal saline gives negative contrast better for intracavitary lesions. Instillagel and Endosgel are the commonly available preparations. These contain lidocaine hydrochloride, 20 mg/g, chlorhexidine digluconate, methyl hydro-xybenzoate, propyl hydroxybenzoate, sodium lactate,

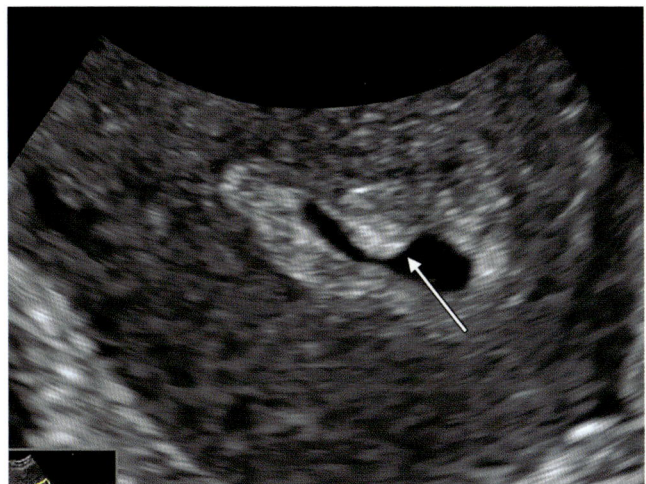

Fig. 18.5: B mode ultrasound image of a small polyp on sonohysterography.

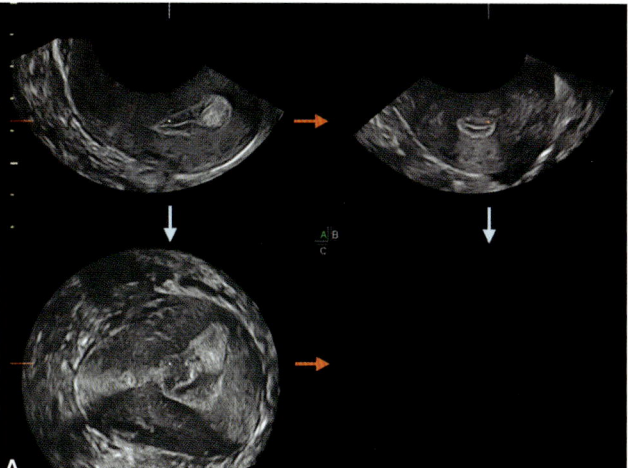

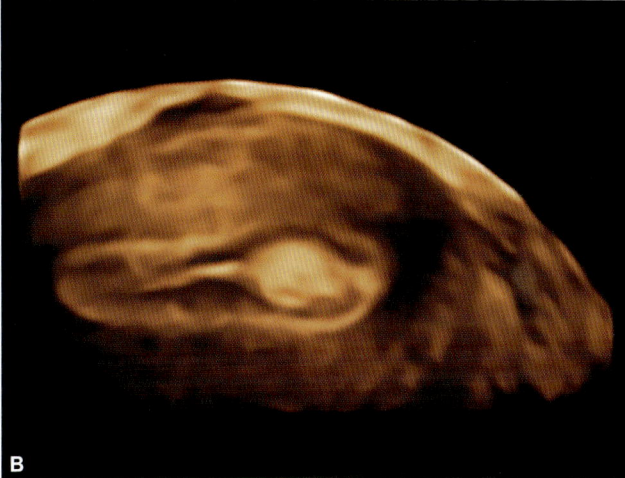

Figs. 18.6A and B: (A) 3D ultrasound multiplanar image of the endometrial polyp; (B) Polyp seen with clear margins and high contrast on 4D ultrasound volume contrast imaging (A).

hydroxyethylcellulose, and purified water. It does not flow out the uterus very quickly because of its viscosity.

Three-dimensional ultrasound techniques used for diagnosis and demonstration of polyp are as follows:

Volume contrast imaging (VCI) A: This is a thick slice imaging and therefore increases the contrast of the subtle lesions. This significantly improves the visualization of small polyps. Depending on the size of the polyp, the slice thickness of the VCI is selected **(Figs. 18.6A and B)**. VCI can also be used to see the coronal plane, and this is called VCI C. This gives rendered like images **(Fig. 18.7)**.

Three-dimensional rendering: 3D volume acquired with or without sonohysterography and rendering will demonstrate the polyp. Rendering also can demonstrate the exact location of the polyp in the endometrial cavity, the pedicle location and the thickness of the pedicle that can be of help to plan the surgery **(Fig. 18.8)**.

ENDOMETRIAL HYPERPLASIA

Overgrowth of endometrial epithelium—endometrial hyperplasia leads to partial or generalized thickening of the endometrium with a broad base on the endometrium unlike the polyp. On 3D, it is seen as a thickening of one or both lips, complete or incomplete. The endometriomyometrial junction (hypoechoic halo) is well preserved **(Fig. 18.9)**. Doppler shows multiple vessels symmetrically arranged, supplying this thickening, that are regularly placed and can be better confirmed on 3D-power Doppler **(Figs. 18.10A to C)**.

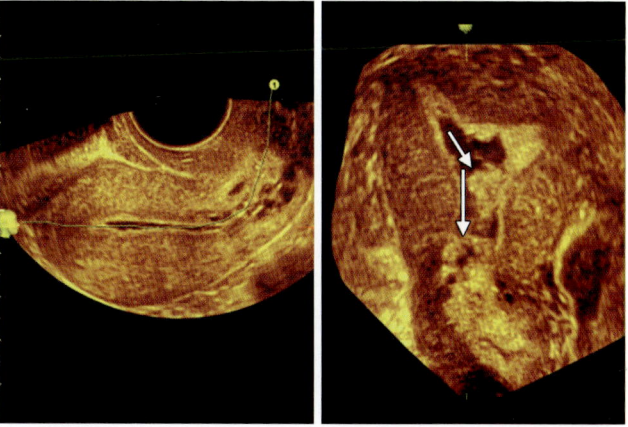

Fig. 18.7: 3D ultrasound, VCI C image of the uterus showing multiple polyps in coronal section.

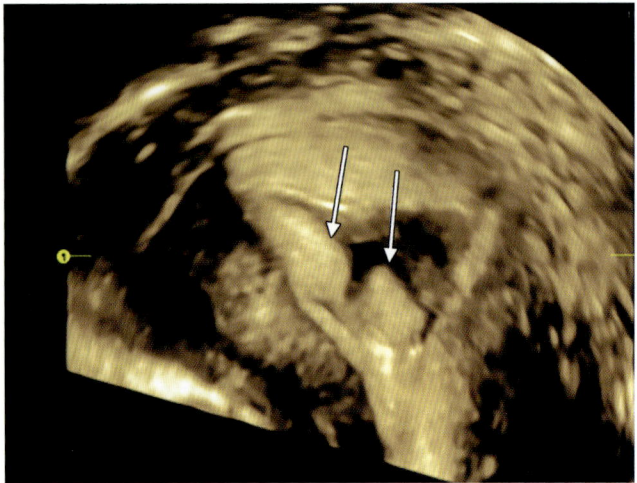

Fig. 18.8: 3D ultrasound rendered image of sonohysterography showing two polyps.

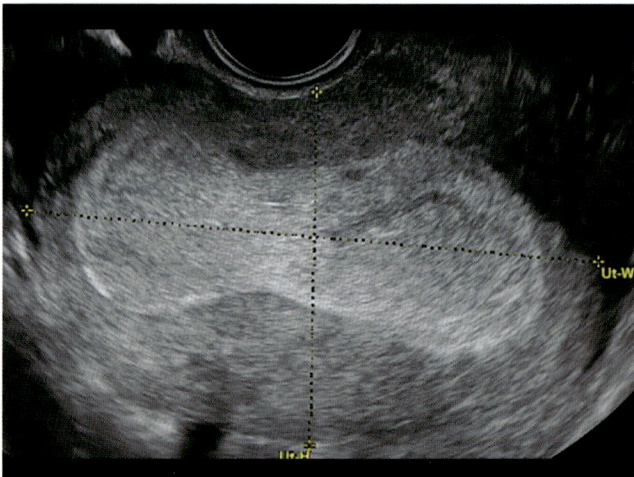

Fig. 18.9: B mode ultrasound image of the uterus showing endometrial hyperplasia.

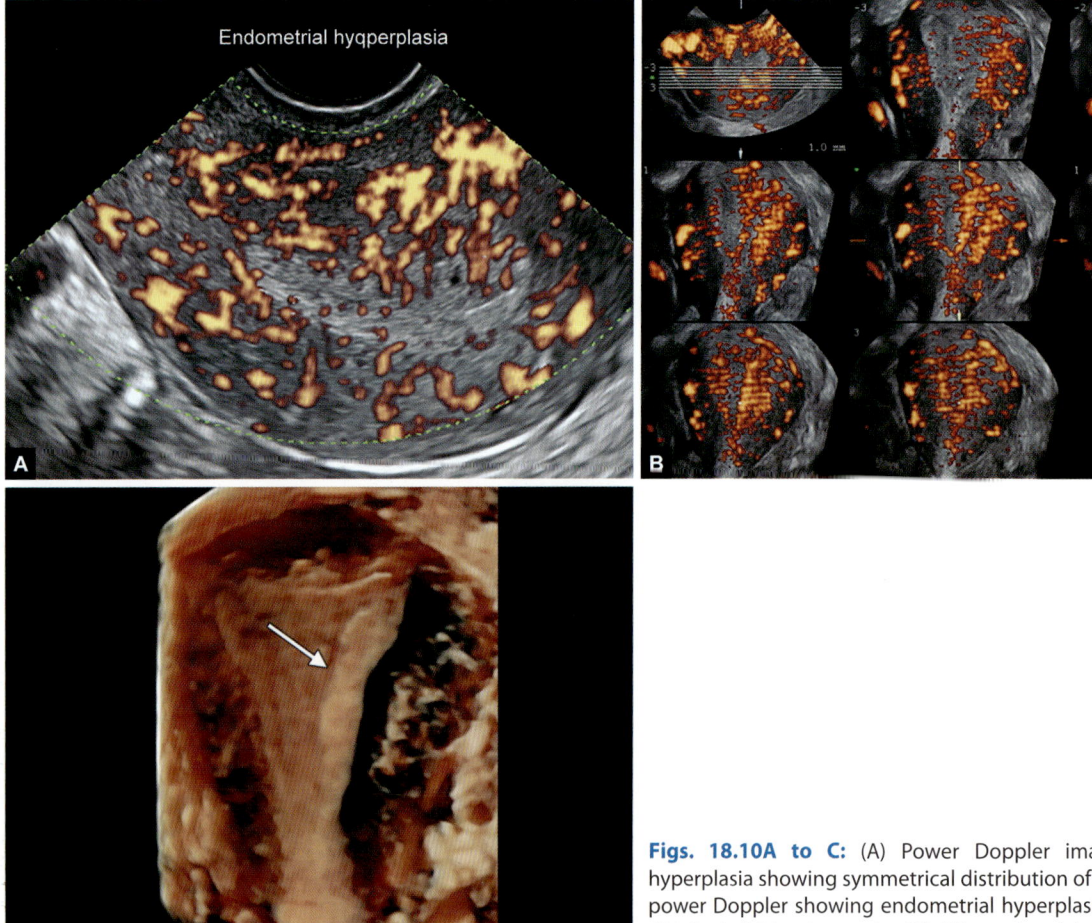

Figs. 18.10A to C: (A) Power Doppler image of endometrial hyperplasia showing symmetrical distribution of blood vessels; (B) 3D power Doppler showing endometrial hyperplasia and symmetrically distributed blood vessels; (C) 3D rendered image of endometrial hyperplasia.

INTRAUTERINE DEVICE PLACEMENT

Intrauterine device (IUD) is known to be properly placed if distance between the fundus and the tip of the IUD is less than 5 mm on rendered coronal image or distance from tip of IUCD to outer wall of uterine fundus is less than or equal to (anterior wall + posterior wall)/2 × 1.33. For displaced IUD, US is the choice of investigation. It not only demonstrates the exact location of IUD but also determines the route of removal whether abdominal or hysteroscopic. 3D US is the modality of choice to assess the displacement of IUD **(Figs. 18.11A and B)**.

ADENOMYOSIS

Adenomyosis is a dichotomous disease characterized primarily by disruption of the inner myometrial architecture and function, with secondary infiltration of endometrial elements into the myometrium. Patients present with dysmenorrhea, menorrhagia, dyspareunia, infertility, and recurrent abortions. Adenomyosis leads to derangement of normal myometrial peristalsis and blood supply and also leads to immunological reaction leading to these symptoms. Prevalence of adenomyosis in infertile population is as high as 50%.[2]

On US, this typically shows as thickening of the myometrium. This may be of one or both walls of the myometrium. The myometrium shows heterogeneous echogenicity with hyperechoic dots and lines. It also shows small anechoic myometrial cysts. The hyperechoic and anechoic areas together lead to a "salt and pepper" appearance **(Fig. 18.12)**. The endometrial cavity typically may show an abnormal curvature in the fundal area, and this is described as "ear sign" or question mark sign **(Fig. 18.13)**. The Doppler typically shows translesional vessels. The vessel diameter is more than that of normal spiral vessels **(Fig. 18.14)**. The endometrio–myometrial junction becomes irregular thick at places and is obliterated in other areas due to extension of the endometrial strands into myometrium. This irregularity of the junctional zone is not well appreciated on B mode US. Therefore magnetic resonance imaging (MRI) was considered a superior modality for the diagnosis of adenomyosis.

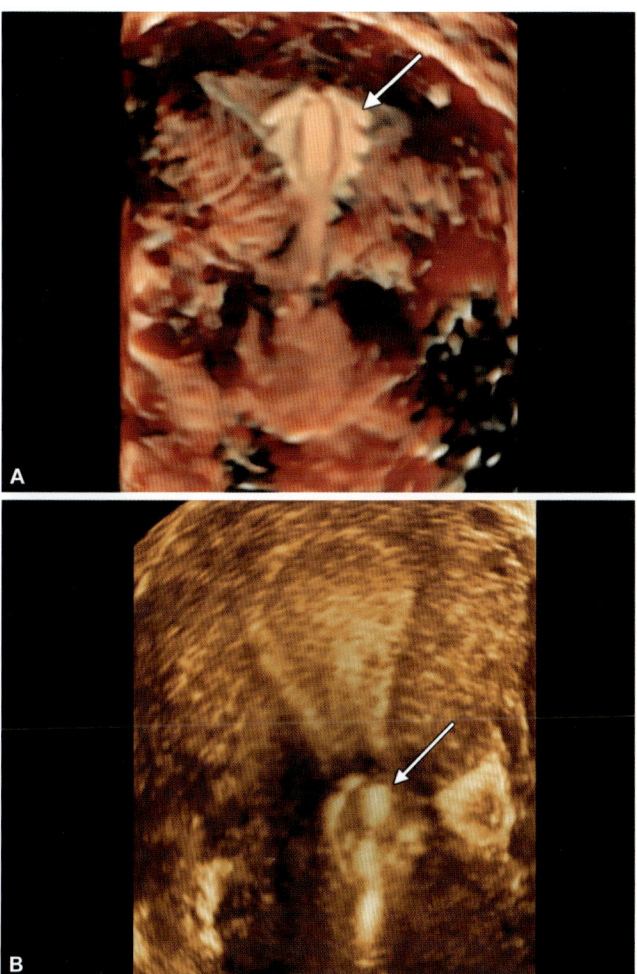

Figs. 18.11A and B: (A) 3D rendered ultrasound image showing normally positioned intrauterine device; (B) 3D ultrasound image showing displaced intrauterine device in the cervix.

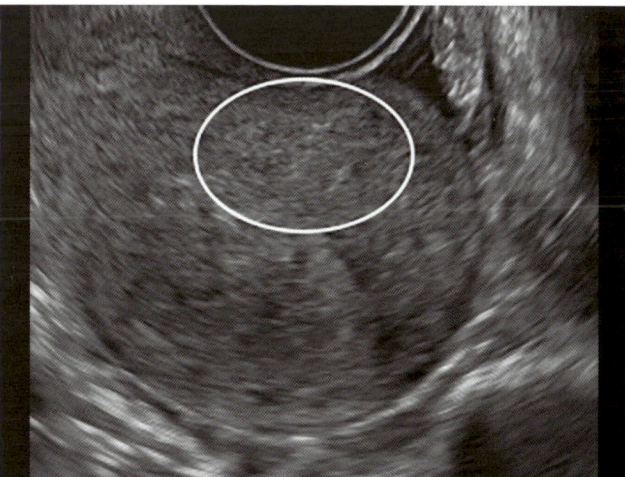

Fig. 18.12: B mode ultrasound image of uterus with adenomyosis (salt and pepper appearance).

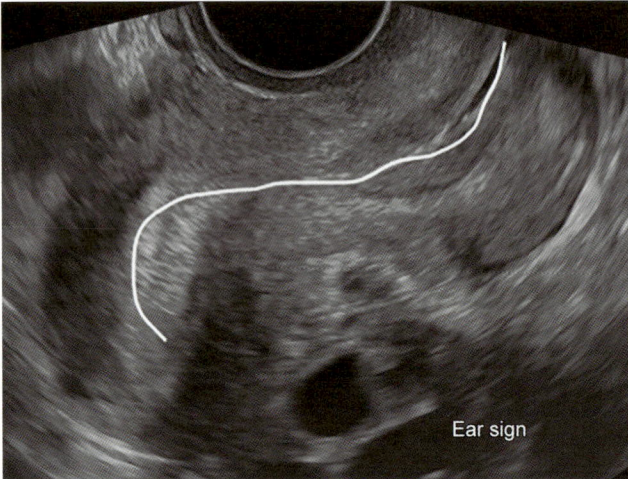

Fig. 18.13: B mode ultrasound image of adenomyotic uterus, demonstrating question mark sign of endometrium.

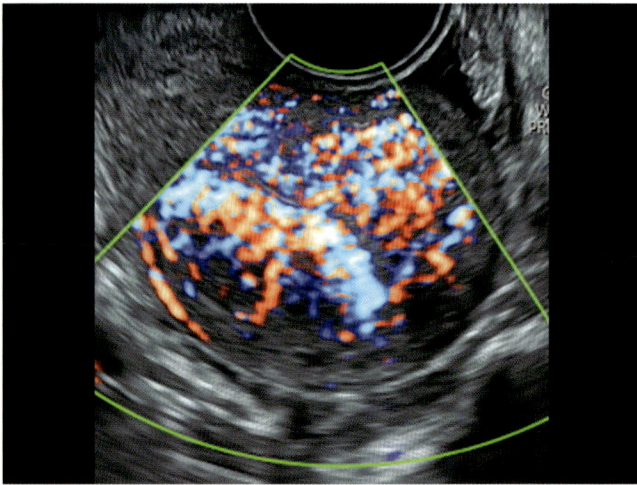

Fig. 18.14: High definition flow in an adenomyotic uterus, showing dilated and translesional vascularity.

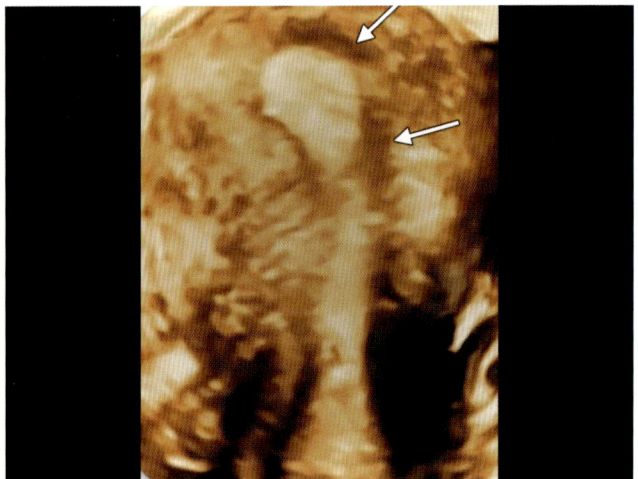

Fig. 18.15: 3D ultrasound rendered image of adenomyotic uterus showing irregular junctional zone.

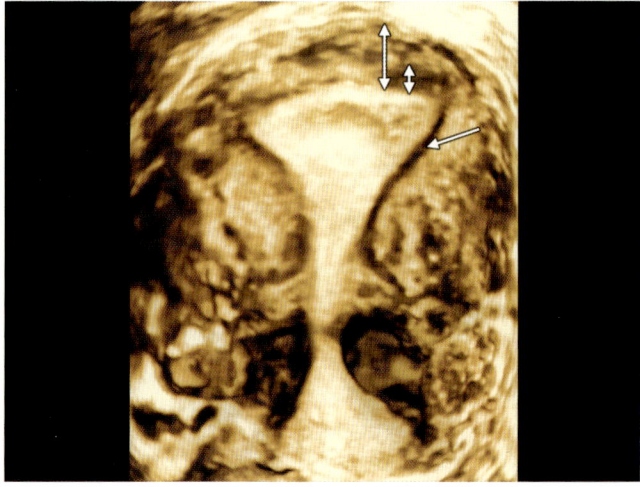

Fig. 18.16: 3D ultrasound rendered image of the uterus showing irregularity of the junctional zone. The double-headed arrows demonstrate the myometrial thickness and thickness of the irregular junctional zone. Single-headed arrow shows the thickness of the normal junctional zone.

But 3D US allows clear visualization of the junctional zone and also allows assessment of its thickness at different places in the uterus **(Figs. 18.15 and 18.16)**. It is for this reason that all the parameters that were used for the diagnosis of adenomyosis on MRI can also be used for 3D US also. Thickening of the transition zone thickness of 12 mm or greater has been shown to be associated with adenomyosis. Difference in the junctional zone thickness of more than 4 mm (JZdiff >4 mm), JZ infiltration and distortion are also diagnostic criteria for adenomyosis. These have 88% sensitivity and 85% and 82% accuracy, respectively.[3] Junctional zone can be measured on 3D US.

Severity of irregularity is measured as thickness of the thickest part of the junctional zone and thickness of the entire myometrial thickness. Magnitude of a JZ irregularity is expressed as the difference between the maximum and minimum JZ thickness: (JZdif) = JZmax – Jzmin.[4]

Polypoid adenomyosis is seen as polyps with heterogeneous echogenicity, well appreciated on 3D US. Its feeding vessel shows abundant branching inside the polyp and is most impressively demonstrated on 3D-power Doppler **(Figs. 18.17A and B)**.

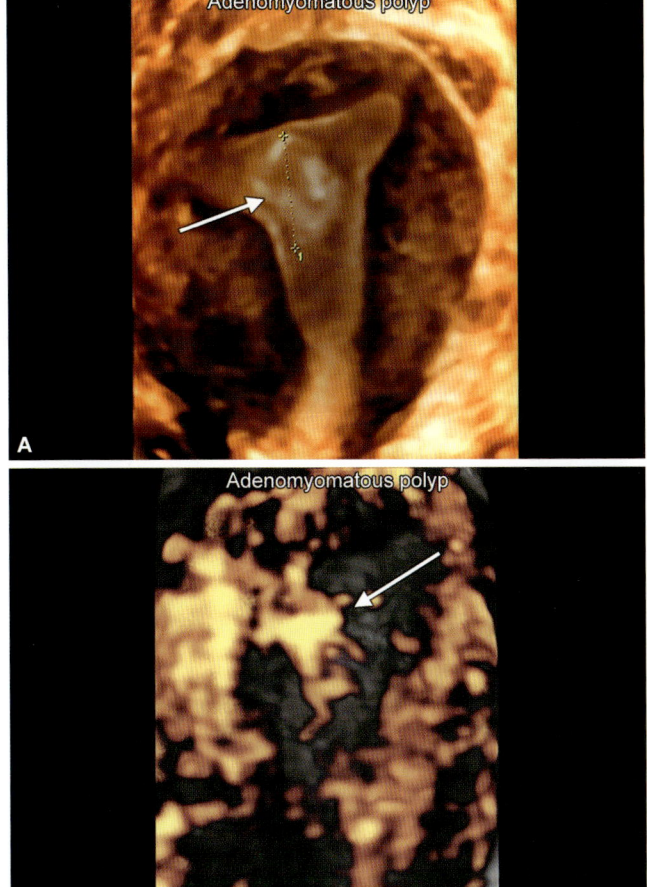

Figs. 18.17A and B: (A) 3D ultrasound rendered image of the uterus showing adenomyomatous polyp; (B) 3D power Doppler angio-rendered image of adenomyomatous polyp showing feeding vessel with abundant vascularity.

FIBROIDS

Fibroids are benign tumors made of fibrous and muscular tissue. As these are benign overgrowths, these displace the surrounding myometrial fibers and create a pseudo-capsule. Therefore fibroids are usually seen as well defined, roundish, and hypoechoic lesions. These are diagnosed on 2D US and may be subserosal, intramural, or submucosal. It is the later type in which 3D US has a role for diagnosis. Submucous fibroids are divided as T0, T1, and T2 depending on whether entire fibroid is inside the endometrial cavity, more than 50% is in the endometrial cavity or less than 50% is inside the endometrial cavity. This distortion or invasion depends on location and size of the fibroids. Moreover, a large fibroid in submucous

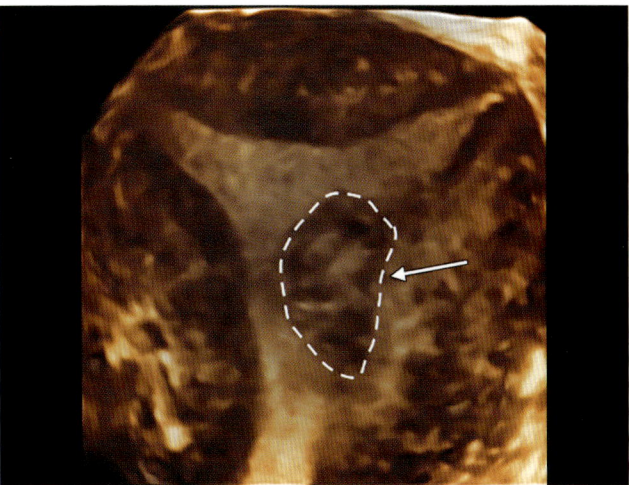

Fig. 18.18: 3D ultrasound rendered image of submucous fibroid as marked by dotted line showing distortion of the endometrial cavity.

location, which is distorting the endometrial cavity, causes stretching of the endometrium and in turn compression of the blood vessels inside also. This hampers the endometrial blood flow required for the development of estrogen receptors and implantation and may cause subfertility. 3D US shows endometrial distortion by the fibroid very clearly **(Fig. 18.18)**. This not only helps in deciding that the fibroid can be a cause of fertility problem or not but also helps to decide the route of surgery. A fibroid, the major part of which is popping in the endometrial cavity, can be removed hysteroscopically and that of which only small part is projecting in the endometrial cavity has to be removed through the external surface of the uterus, either laparoscopically or by laparotomy.

Lasmar's score for submucous fibroids and STEPW classification that evaluates the size, topography, extension, penetration, and lateral wall involvement is being used widely for the same. The scoring system is demonstrated in the pictures below **(Figs. 18.19A and F)**.

Submucous fibroids are a common cause of menstrual abnormalities. 3D saline contrast hysteroscopy provides important information about the size and location of these fibroids. Submucous fibroid protrusion ratio, fibroid diameter, and size of fibroid's intramural component are significantly associated with likelihood of successful hysteroscopic fibroid resection.[6]

Using 2D US and color Doppler, usually fibroids can be differentiated from adenomyomas as the former shows peripheral vascularity, whereas the latter shows translesional vascularity **(Figs. 18.20A and B)**. The edge shadows are seen in fibroids apart from the fan-shaped

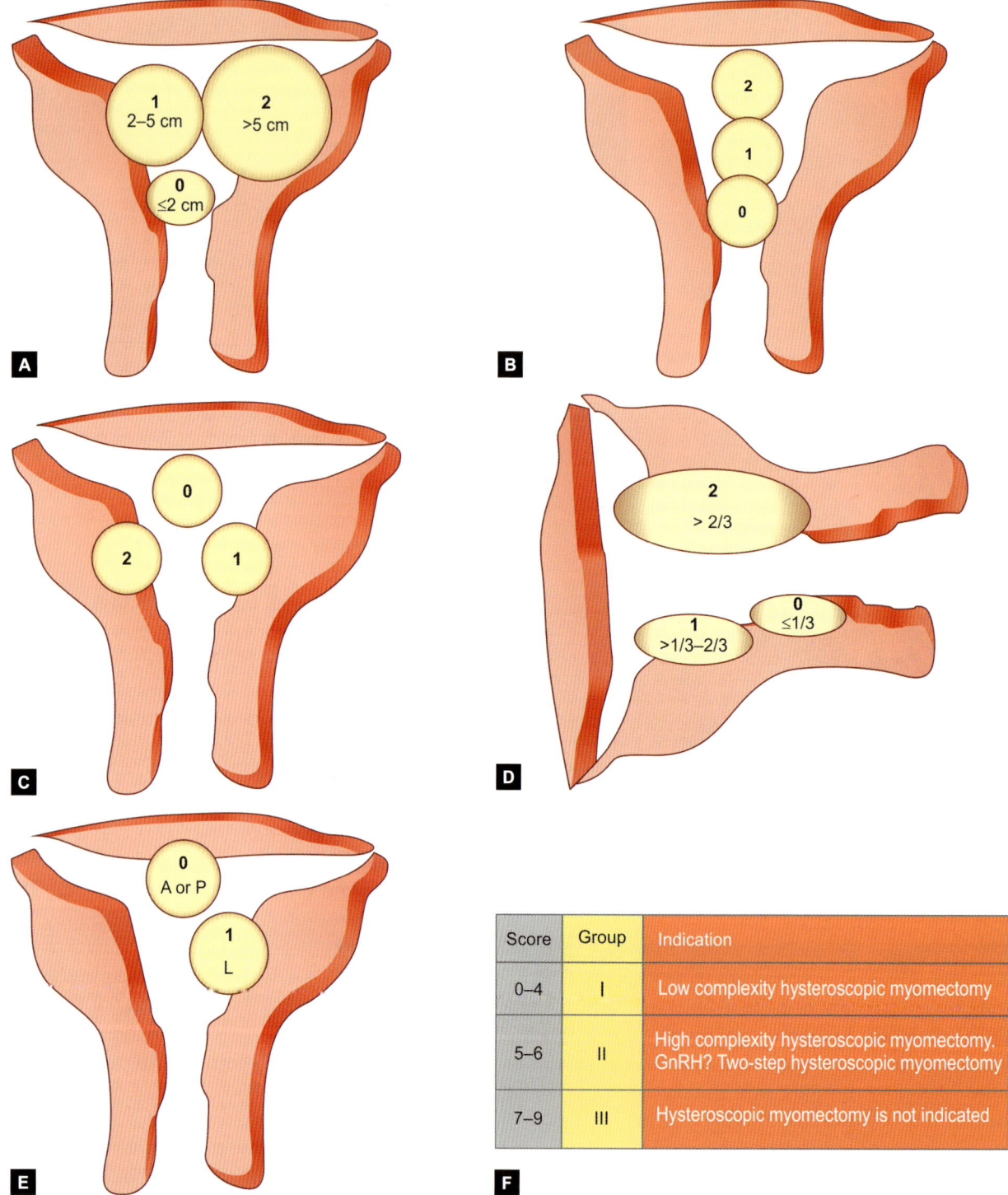

Figs. 18.19A to F: (A to E) STEPW classification features for scoring size, topography, extension, penetration, and lateral wall involvement; (F) Treatment protocol suggestions against a particular score. (STEPW: Size, topography, extension, penetration, wall).

shadows that are not seen in adenomyomas **(Figs. 18.21A and B)**. Differentiation is difficult when adenomyomas are relatively more defined or the fibroids show internal vascularity because of degeneration. 3D power Doppler can be used here to define the vascular arrangement in the lesion. A radial or irregular arrangement is suggestive

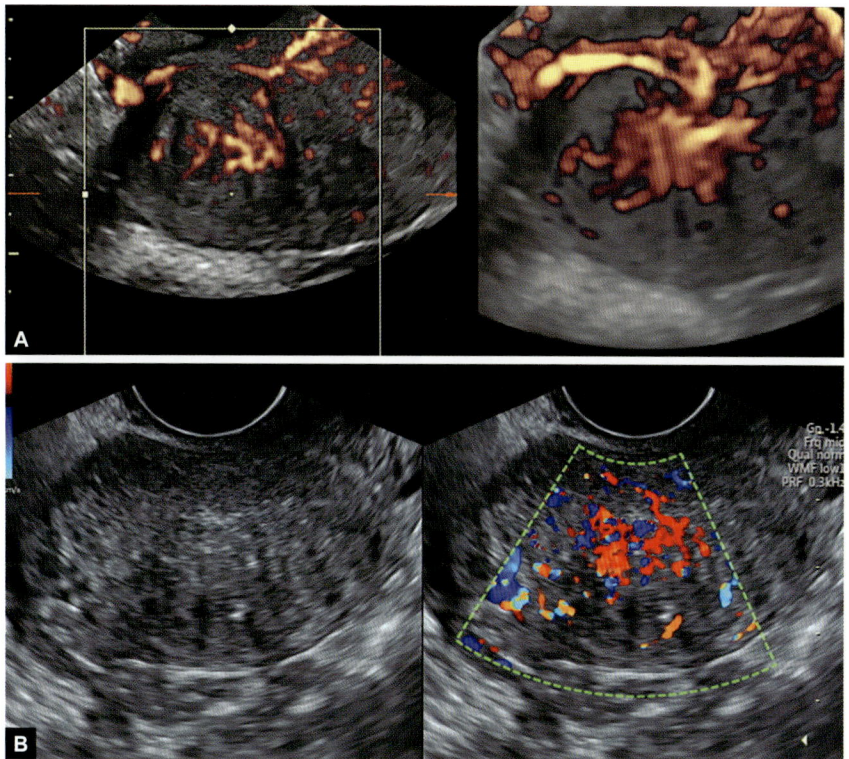

Figs. 18.20A and B: (A) Power Doppler and 3D power Doppler image of a degenerated fibroid showing peripheral and intralesional vascularity; (B) B mode and color Doppler image of adenomyoma showing translesional vascularity.

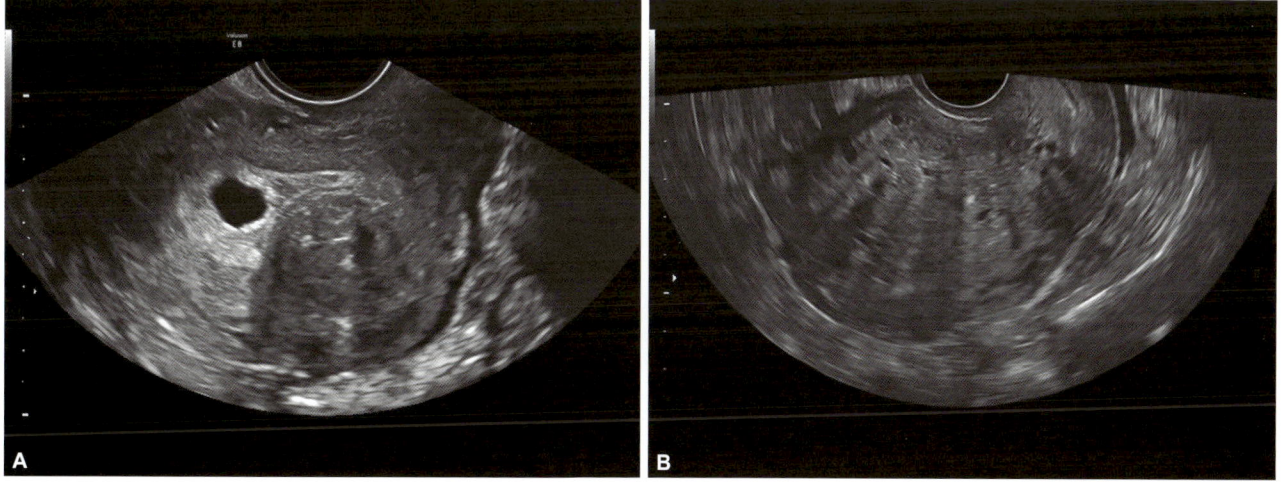

Figs. 18.21A and B: (A) B mode ultrasound image showing fibroid with fan shadows and edge shadows; (B) Adenomyoma showing fan shadows.

of adenomyoma, whereas a circular arrangement is suggestive of a fibroid **(Figs. 18.22A and B)**.

Fibroids may undergo malignant change, when these are named as leiomyosarcoma. The pseudocapsule then shows discontinuity or is completely absent. It becomes difficult to define the extent of the lesion. It may invade the endometrium or may also extend not only up to serosa. 3D is a reliable tool to define the extent of the lesion, breaking of tissue planes and involvement of other structures, using either rendering mode or tomographic US imaging in the scanning plane and in coronal plane **(Fig. 18.23)**. Moreover, extension of the malignant vascular pattern

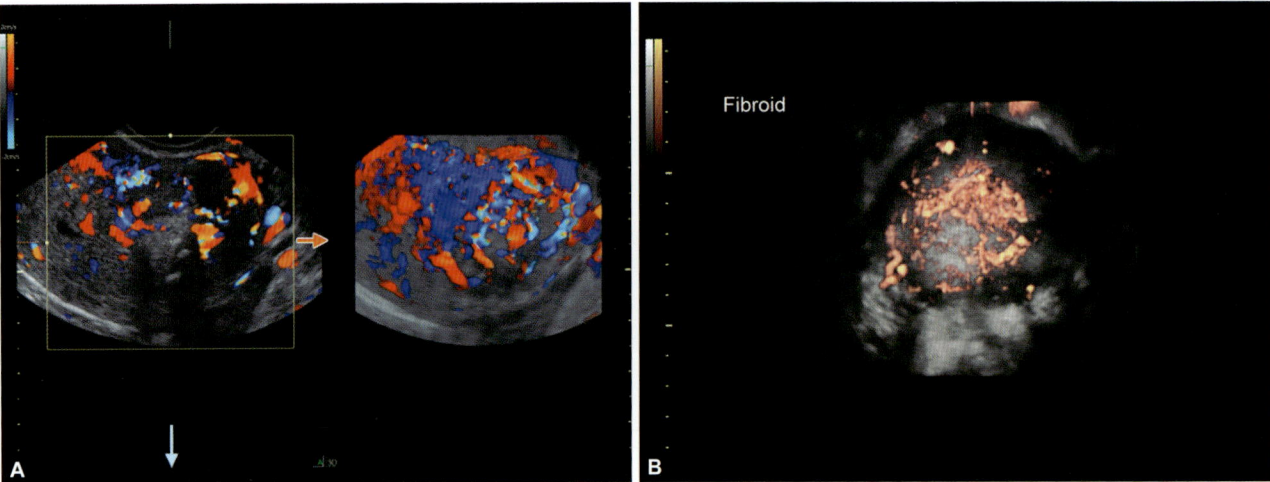

Figs. 18.22A and B: (A) Color Doppler and 3D color Doppler image showing circular arrangement of blood vessels, suggestive of a fibroid; (B) 3D power Doppler glass body angio image of adenomyoma showing irregular arrangement of the vessels.

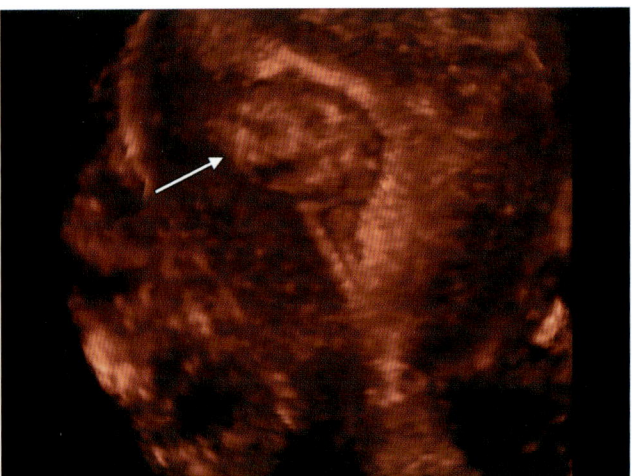

Fig. 18.23: 3D ultrasound rendered image of the uterus showing submucous fibroid with ill-defined lateral margin.

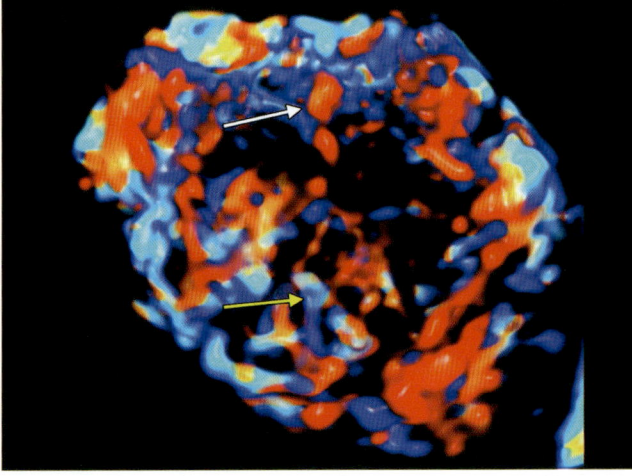

Fig. 18.24: 3D angiography showing vessels with irregular caliber (white arrow), and vascular communications (yellow arrow) suggestive of malignant features of the vascular tree.

in the surrounding tissues may also be a reliable guide for the extension of the tumor.

A malignant lesion has neoangiogenesis, and the vascular pattern is evidently different from the physiological angiogenesis. These are fast developing vessels and therefore do not have muscularis layer in their walls and therefore show a low-resistance flow. These vessels distend/break easily under pressure, thus forming microaneurysms and arteriovenous malformations. To cope up with the fast-growing tumor, it also gives dichotomous branches. This creates a typical malignant chaotic pattern

on 3D-power Doppler which can be a very useful tool to differentiate benign from malignant lesions.

Three-dimensional power Doppler signs of malignancy[7] (**Fig. 18.24**) are as follows:

- Loss of tree-like branching of vessels
- Sacculation of arteries and veins
- Focal narrowing of arteries
- Internal shift of velocities within arterial lumen
- Beach ball finding of abnormally increased and disorganized peripheral flow (combination of above four characteristics). Beach ball appearance with crowded

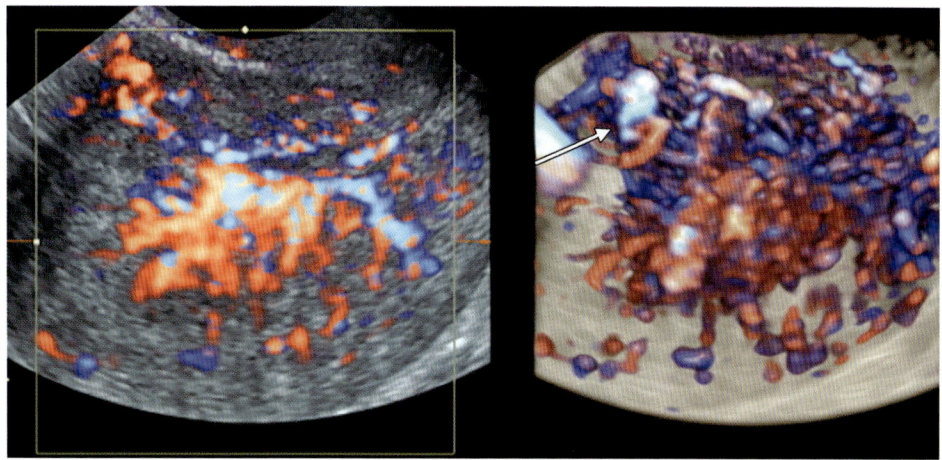

Fig. 18.25: High definition flow and 3D HD flow image of the endometrial carcinoma extending into the anterior myometrium as diagnosed by extension of the malignant vascular pattern into myometrium as marked by arrow.

haphazard interwoven matrix of arteries and veins suggests malignancy.

- Increased flow to the center of solid lesion
- Crowding of vascularity
- Start and stop arteries: Arteries appear to start and stop within a mass in a disjointed fashion, losing the tree-like expected appearance of a benign mass.

Apart from leiomyosarcomas, this vascular pattern may also be useful guide for the diagnosis and extension of endometrial carcinoma also **(Fig. 18.25)**.

ADNEXAL LESIONS

Most adnexal lesions are diagnosed by B mode and Doppler and 3D is not required. Though 3D is used for the demonstration of typical vascular pattern of endometrioma **(Fig. 18.26A)**. Endometriomas are known to have short coursed vessels in the periphery of the lesion. And this vessel tree when seen on 3D US, it typically shows a "bird's nest appearance"[8] **(Fig. 18.26B)**.

This is of course a supportive sign and not a diagnostic sign for endometrioma. Endometriomas on B mode usually show ground glass echogenicity, thick shaggy walls, and hyperechoic flecks in the walls due to hemosiderin or cholesterol deposit[9] **(Fig. 18.27A)**. But endometriomas may appear as lesions with internal echogenicities other than like ground glass. Layering effect is commonly seen in endometriomas **(Fig. 18.27B)**, due to blood in different forms due to new fresh bleeds and degeneration. Acoustic streaming is also often seen in endometriomas due to thick fluid content.[10] Tenderness on probe pressure and

adhesions are considered additional important supportive signs for the diagnosis of endometriomas.

As for the uterine malignancies, 3D power Doppler qualitative analysis of tumor angiogenesis allows accurate detection of earliest appearance of ovarian malignancy— stage IA.

Differentiation between benign and malignant lesions by contrast-induced 3D PD:[11,12]

- Sensitivity—100%
- Specificity—93.9%
- Positive predictive value (PPV)—85.7%
- Negative predictive value (NPV)—100%.

Tubal pathologies also are adnexal lesions. The one that is most commonly found in the infertile population is hydrosalpinx. Hydrosalpinx is distention of the fallopian tube due to inflammatory fluid and secretions as a result of obstruction at the fimbrial end most commonly but sometimes also involving the cornual end. This obstruction is due to adhesions, and the most common causes are infection, endometriosis, and surgery. Hydrosalpinx may present as an extraovarian cystic lesion. It typically changes its shape on rotation of the probe. It appears round in transverse section but sausage or retort shaped in the longitudinal section **(Fig. 18.28)**. It shows thicker walls in acute inflammation **(Fig. 18.29)**, often with ascites. Chronic inflammations show thinner walls, and adhesions may also be seen. At times in chronic inflammation, tubes may appear rigid **(Fig. 18.30)**. When the tube is markedly distended and tortuous, it may appear like multiple cystic areas. It is in these cases that 3D US aids

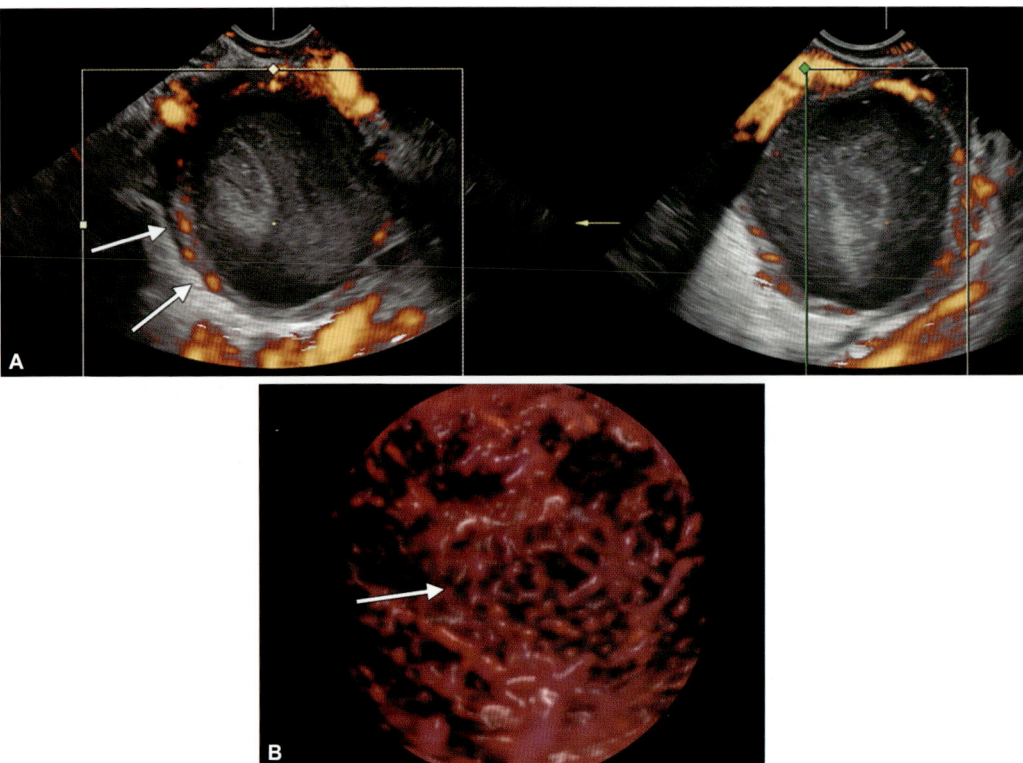

Figs. 18.26A and B: (A) Power Doppler image of endometrioma showing short coursed vessels; (B) 3D power Doppler of the endometrioma showing bird's nest appearance.

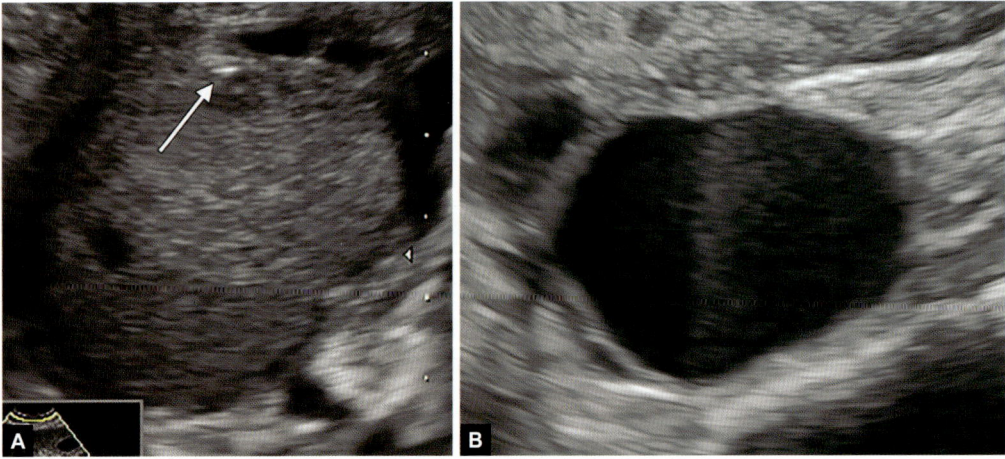

Figs. 18.27A and B: (A) B mode ultrasound image of endometrioma with ground glass echogenicity and hyperechoic fleck (arrow) in the wall; (B) Vertical fluid–fluid level of the endometrioma as seen on B mode image.

to establish the continuity between these cystic areas and confirm the diagnosis of hydrosalpinx. Though coronal plane imaging either on multiplanar view or omni-view **(Fig. 18.31A)** may be of help but in these cases rendering on minimum mode or inversion mode are the best alternatives **(Fig. 18.31B)** to establish the continuity between the cystic lesions and confirm the diagnosis of hydrosalpinx.

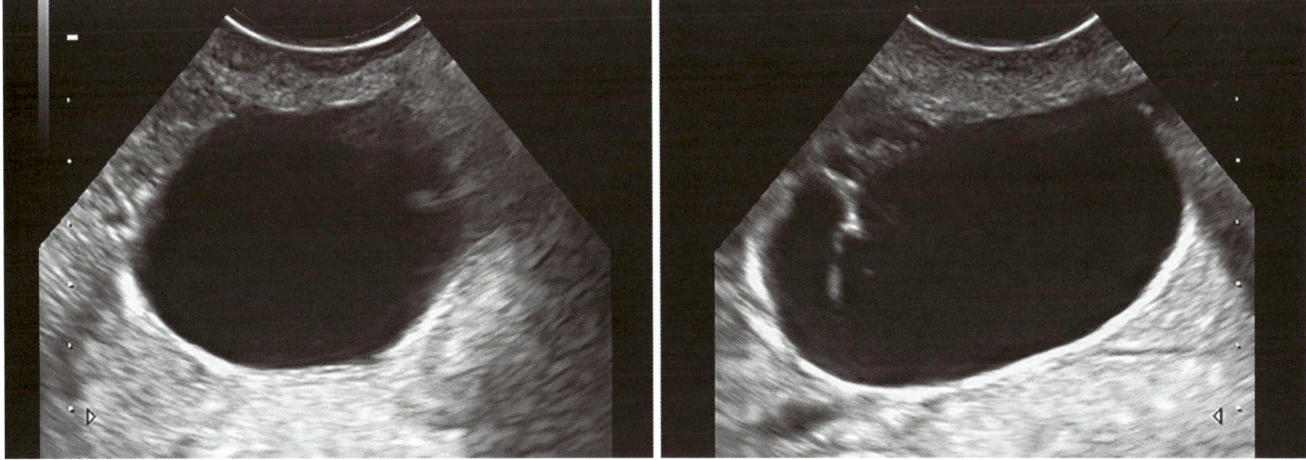

Fig. 18.28: B mode ultrasound image of hydrosalpinx in transverse and longitudinal sections.

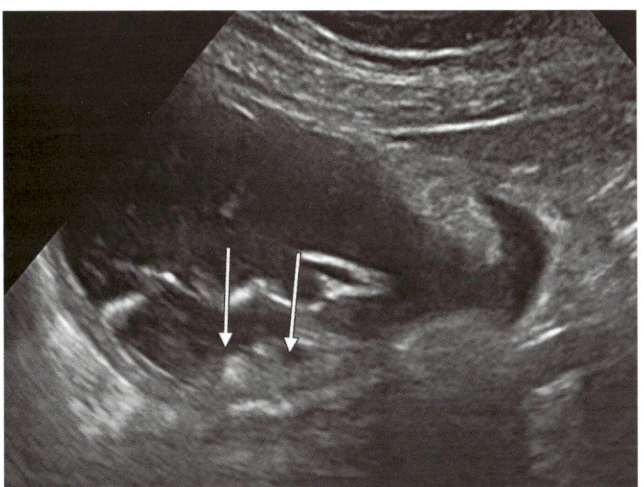

Fig. 18.29: B mode image of acute hydrosalpinx showing thick walls due to acute inflammatory edema.

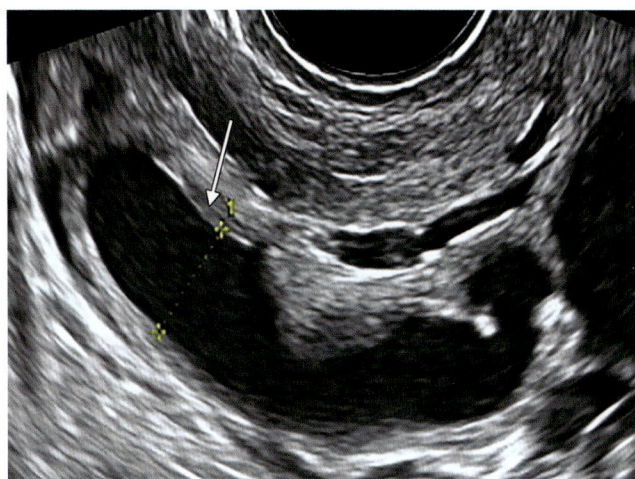

Fig. 18.30: Chronically inflamed tube with hydrosalpinx showing thin walls and only mild dilatation due to rigid walls.

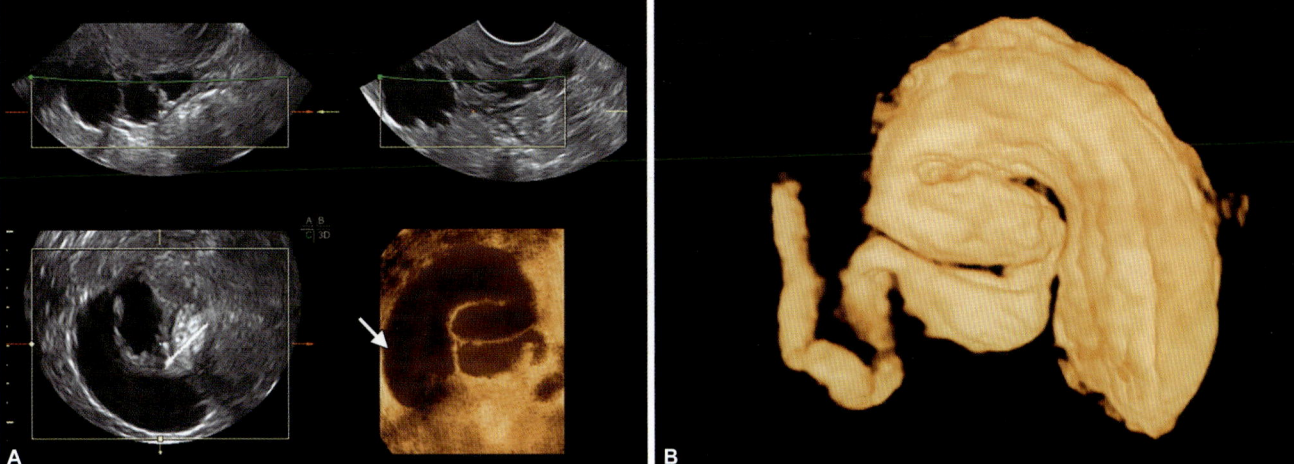

Figs. 18.31A and B: (A) 3D ultrasound acquired multiplanar image of hydrosalpinx seen as multiple cystic lesions on the acquired plane, but on the coronal plane, the continuity of these lesions is seen as marked by white arrow and on minimum mode imaging the entire tube is seen (yellow arrow); (B) The same lesion as mentioned in Figure A is shown in inversion mode.

TUBAL PATENCY ASSESSMENT

Tubal pathology is a cause of subfertility in 25–35% of subfertile couples. Evaluation of fallopian tubes therefore forms an essential part of evaluation of a subfertile female. Various nonsurgical and surgical investigative modalities have been reported to assess fallopian tubes. While nonsurgical techniques, such as hysterosalpingogram (HSG) (Carey, 1914) and US-based techniques, such as saline infusion sonography (Corfman and Taylor, 1966), and hysterocontrast sonosalpingography (HyCoSy) (Deichert, 1993) are less invasive and associated with less serious risks than surgical technique, such as laparoscopy and dye test (chromopertubation). Demonstration of the lumen of tubes requires visualization of movement of fluid using highly echogenic medium.[13]

Hyperechogenic contrast medium enhances echo signals and allows detection of the flow, both by B mode and Doppler US. HyCoSy is a safe outpatient procedure with a relatively low cost, and its accuracy has been assessed in a meta-analysis, which compared the results of HyCoSy and laparoscopy and dye tests in 428 infertile women. Sensitivity was 93.3%, and specificity was 89.7%.[14]

Study by Exacoustos et al. has also shown that HSG and HyCoSy had the same high concordance as laparoscopy, 86.7% and 86.7%, respectively.[15] 3D power Doppler was therefore tried to visualize the whole tube and spill. This technique has shown to be superior to conventional HyCoSy and demonstrated free spill from fallopian tubes in 91% of tubes as compared to only 46%

by conventional HyCoSy, and the contrast agent required was almost half for 3D PD in one of these studies[16] **(Fig. 18.32)**.

There are various advantages with 3D HyCoSy techniques that allow simultaneous visualization of the uterine cavity and whole tube, short procedure time and reduced patient discomfort, requirement of less amount of contrast and storage of the 3D volume, which allows off-line review and reassessment **(Fig. 18.33)**.

Advantages of 3D Hysterocontrast Sonosalpingography

- Uterine cavity and whole tube can be seen together
- Condition of lumen and fimbriae can be studied
- Shortens procedure time and patient discomfort
- Less amount of contrast is required
- Storage of volumes allows reassessment and reviews
- Spill is better appreciated
- More accurate.

Technique of 3D Hysterocontrast Sonosalpingography

SonoVue (Bracco) is used as the contrast agent. Patient preparation, catheter placement, and preparation of contrast media were done according to the method described earlier. Scanning is performed using a 3D US machine (e.g. Voluson E8 Expert BT12; GE Medical Systems). A high-frequency transvaginal volume probe

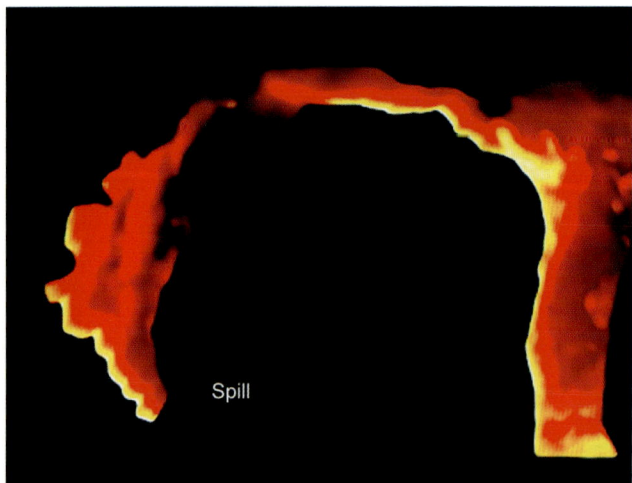

Fig. 18.32: 3D power Doppler hysterocontrast sonosalpingography, showing uterus and right fallopian tube.

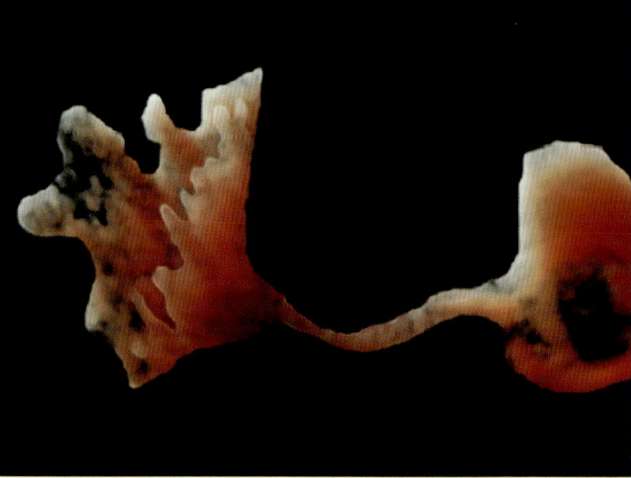

Fig. 18.33: 3D hysterocontrast sonosalpingography rendered in high definition live mode shows the uterus, right fallopian tube with the fimbrial end.

(6–9 MHz) is used for pelvic evaluation. Contrast mode is switched on the machine. As the contrast is slowly injected through the balloon catheter into the uterus, transvaginal probe is so oriented that uterine cornu and ovaries are seen on the same plane. Having defined the contrast filling in the tubes, 3D is switched on, and volumes are acquired for each side independently **(Fig. 18.34)**.

Rendering is done in front back viewing direction. Surface-enhanced mode is used. Threshold is set to make the contrast path more obvious. Magicut (electronic scalpel) is then used to cut all shadows other than the contrast path. Then HDlive rendering mode is switched on, and direction of the light is adjusted to visualize the fimbriae and spill to its best. After the final picture is ready, both the halves are matched and put together to make a complete picture of uterus and both tubes **(Fig. 18.35)**.

Hysterocontrast sonosalpingography with automated 3D-coded contrast imaging technology retains the advantages of conventional 2D HyCoSy while overcoming the disadvantages. 2D HyCoSy is highly observer dependent and is only accurate in the hands of experienced investigators; by obtaining a volume of the uterus and tubes, automated 3D volume acquisition permits visualization of the tubes in the coronal view and of the tubal course in 3D space and should allow less experienced operators to evaluate tubal patency status relatively easily.[17]

Large studies have reported that 3D HyCoSy is highly accurate with 100% sensitivity, 67% specificity, 89% PPV, and 100% NPV for tubal patency and concordance rate with laparoscopy of 91%.[18]

In a study by Kupesic et al., 3D HyCoSy (sensitivity, specificity, PPV, and NPV of 97.9, 100, 97.9, and 100%, respectively) was found to be marginally superior to 2D HyCoSy (sensitivity, specificity, PPV, and NPV of 93.6, 97.3, 98.2, and 97.3%, respectively) for tubal assessment.[19]

Three-dimensional SonoVue-HyCoSy had a sensitivity of 93.5%, specificity of 86.3%, PPV and NPV of 87.8% and 92.6%, respectively, and diagnostic accuracy of 90.0%. The test-positive rates of 3D SonoVue-HyCoSy versus lap and dye were not significantly different (82/150 vs 77/150, $P > 0.05$).[20]

Yet another study by Chan et al. has shown that the sensitivity of 3D-HyCoSy for detecting tubal patency was 100% with a specificity of 67%. The PPV and NPV were 89% and 100%, respectively; the concordance rate was 91%. The mean duration ($\pm$SD) for the 3D-HyCoSy was 13.4 ± 5.5 minutes.[18] Color-coded 3D power Doppler imaging (PDI) with surface rendering allowed visualization of the flow of contrast through the entire tubal length, and free spill of contrast was clearly identified in the majority of cases. The 3D-PDI method appeared to have advantages over the conventional HyCoSy technique, especially in terms of visualization of spill from the distal end of the tube, which was achieved twice as often with the 3D technique. The 3D-PDI technique allowed better storage of the information for reanalysis and archiving than conventional HyCoSy. The mean duration of the imaging procedure was less with 3D-PDI, but the operator time which included

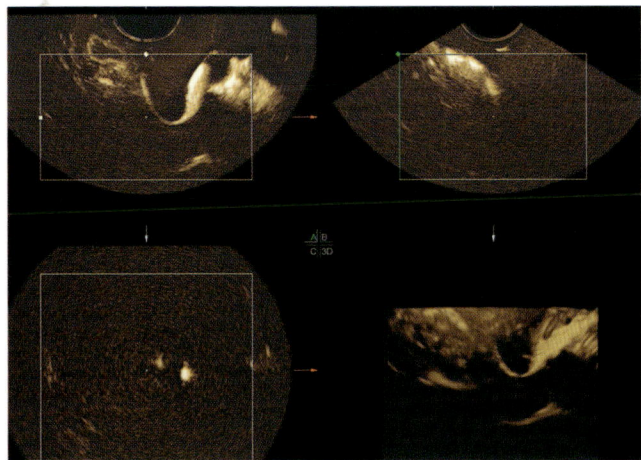

Fig. 18.34: 3D ultrasound acquired image of the uterus and tubes with hysterocontrast sonosalpingography and contrast mode.

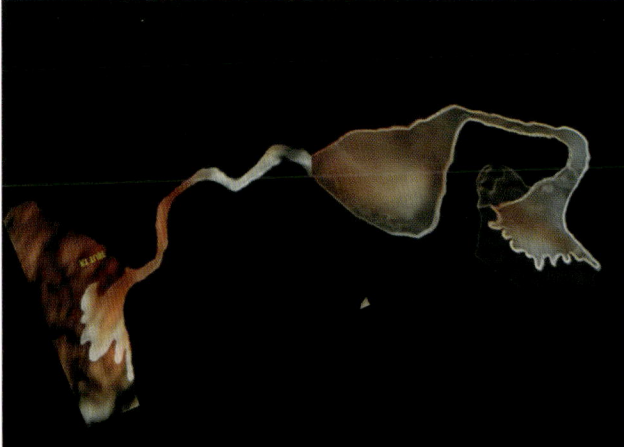

Fig. 18.35: HD live rendered image of the 3D hysterocontrast sonosalpingography, reconstructed for one tube and uterus at a time and pasted together on the computer.

post-procedure analysis of the stored information was similar. A significantly lower volume of contrast medium (5.9 ± 0.6 mL) was used for 3D-PDI in comparison with that (11.2 ± 1.9 mL) used for conventional 2D HyCoSy.[21]

POLYCYSTIC OVARIES

According to the European Society for Human Reproduction/American Society of Reproductive Medicine consensus 2018, the polycystic ovarian disease consists of various different phenotypes and in majority US showing polycystic ovaries was important.

Polycystic ovary on US according to this consensus is an ovary that is 10 cc in volume and/or has more than 20 antral follicles of 2–9 mm in diameter. But this criteria of >10 cc would fail to identify a group of ovulatory, normoandrogenic women still at risk of complications associated with polycystic ovary (PCO) syndrome (PCOS), such as ovarian hyperstimulation syndrome (OHSS), failed implantation, miscarriage, and hyperinsulinemia.[22] Ovarian volume (OV) of *6.6 cc has 91% sensitivity and 91% specificity for PCOS.*[23] Jonard et al. have also suggested that lowering the OV to 7 cc has allowed 67.5% sensitivity and 91.2% specificity for PCOS. And the mean OV in normal ovaries was suggested as 4.5 cc in this study.[24] But it is important to assess the correct OV, and this can be done by 3D US. After the volume of the ovary is acquired by 3D US, VOCAL (virtual organ computer-aided analysis) software is used to calculate the OV. VOCAL calculates volume of any structure by rotating it 180°. A rotating step of 6–30 can be selected. A circumference is drawn around the structure of interest at every step of rotation, and at the end of 180° rotation, total volume is calculated by the scanner computer **(Fig. 18.36)**.

But size is not the only important criteria. Histologically and biochemically polycystic ovaries can be of normal size, and a wide overlap is seen between the size of normal and polycystic ovaries. Polycystic ovarian morphology (PCOM) has been found to be a better discriminator than OV between polycystic ovarian syndrome and control women.[25] Among the morphological features of polycystic ovaries are the follicular number per ovary (FNPO) of more than 12 according to the old consensus and more than 20 per ovary according to new consensus, the follicular arrangement that may be peripheral or generalized and stromal abundance.

The mean FNPO of follicles 2–5 mm in size was significantly higher in polycystic ovaries than in controls,

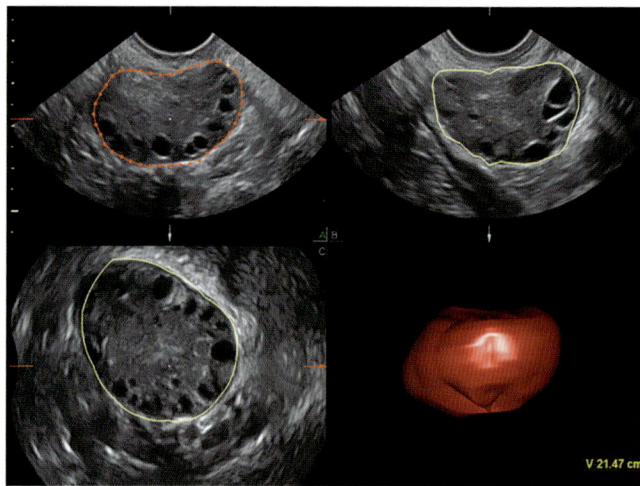

Fig. 18.36: Virtual organ computer-aided analysis calculated volume of the ovary on 3D ultrasound acquired volume of ovary.

while it was similar within 6–9 mm range. Within 2–5 mm range, significant relationship was found between FNPO and androgens but FNPO in the range of 6–9 mm was significantly and negatively related to body mass index and fasting serum insulin level. It is believed that androgen leads to early follicular development but further progression is not normal due to hyperinsulinemia and/or other metabolic influence linked to obesity.[26] Androgen is the cause, and anti-Müllerian hormone is the result of multiple antral follicles. An average value of 26 or more follicles per ovary is a reliable threshold for detecting polycystic ovaries in women with frank manifestation of PCOS. Sensitivity and specificity for the diagnosis of PCOS for FNPO (26) was 85% and 94% and for OV (10 cc) was 81% and 84%.[27]

These antral follicles that are more than 12–20 can be confidently counted only by 3D US and SonoAVC (sonographic automated volume calculation) **(Fig. 18.37A)**. SonoAVC is based on the inversion mode and color codes the follicles this allowing more correct calculation of the number. More exact value of antral follicle count (AFC) was acquired when counted by 3D US. Number of follicles more than 12 mm on the day of oocyte retrieval correlated significantly with AFC counted by 3D US rather than 2D US. Inversion mode is most convenient method for counting antral follicles when they are multiple.[28] SonoAVC measured less number of follicles on AFC, though it took significantly less time to measure the size and record the number of antral follicles (132 ± 56.23 vs. 324.47 ± 162.22 seconds).[29] Postprocessing can be used for the follicles that are missed out on automated counting.

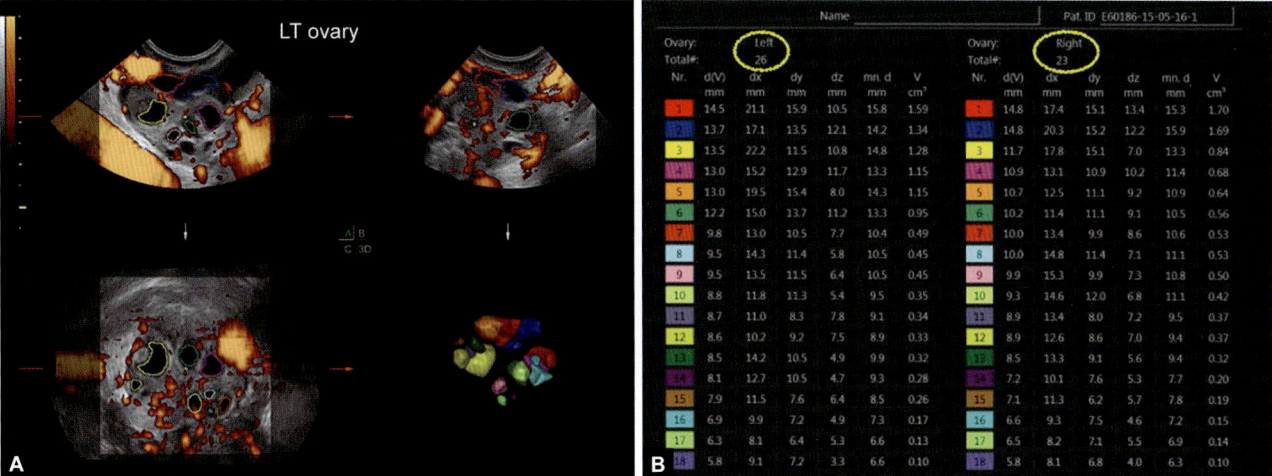

Figs. 18.37A and B: (A) 3D ultrasound acquired volume of the ovary, with SonoAVC showing color-coded follicles; (B) Result sheet of sonoAVC showing total number of follicles in either ovary (circles) and all three diameters, mean diameter and volume of individual follicle marked by the relevant color in the box.

Apart from this, SonoAVC also calculates the size of each follicle and that is important for the understanding of the variable biochemical derangement in various patients with PCOS **(Fig. 18.37B)**.

Stromal abundance is another important feature of polycystic ovaries. Earliest description of polycystic ovaries appears to date from 1845 as "sclerocystic ovaries".[30] To identify women with *milder form of PCOS*, further information, particularly about the ovarian stroma and the degree of vascularization, is required.[21] Patients having long-standing PCOS and long-standing anovulation have more dense stroma, and a cardinal feature has been shown to be the presence of a bright, highly echogenic stroma on transvaginal US.[31] Stromal hypertrophy was recognized as a frequent and specific feature in ovarian androgenic dysfunction.[32] PCOM (stromal echogenicity) in normal women is not a morphological variant of normal ovaries but rather represent a functional entity—a silent form of PCOS.[33] Stromal abundance and echogenicity is one of the major features that discriminate PCO from MCO. This can be assessed by stromal echogenicity, stromal area, and stromal volume. *Polycystic ovaries show a* hyperechoic[34] stroma and by ovarian area: 5.5 cm² (93% sensitivity and 91% specificity)—strict longitudinal ovarian section and by stromal area: 4.6 cm² (91% sensitivity and 86% specificity).[35] But the most accurate assessment of stromal abundance can only be with ovarian and stromal volume by 3D US. 3D US has the potential to address these points and improve the sensitivity and specificity of US in the diagnosis of PCOS.[36]

Both total OV and stromal volume during the early follicular phase are significantly higher in women with PCOS.[36] Stromal volume was positively correlated with serum androstenedione concentrations in patients with polycystic ovarian syndrome.[37] Statistically significant relationship was reported between OV and stroma echogenicity with serum luteinizing hormone and testosterone concentrations.[38] OV can be calculated by VOCAL as mentioned earlier and applying threshold volume to this can calculate the stromal volume. After the volume is calculated by VOCAL when threshold volume is activated, pigment appears on the VOCAL calculated volume. The threshold is so adjusted that the pigmented area fills up all the follicles and only follicles. On the screen, above threshold and below threshold volumes are displayed. Below threshold is the follicular volume, and above threshold is the stromal volume **(Fig. 18.38)**. In PCOS patients, a strong and similar correlation is seen between ovarian and stromal volumes to fasting and postprandial insulin levels.[39]

Three-dimensional US not only permits improved spatial awareness and volumetric and quantitative vascular assessment but also provides a more objective tool to examine stromal echogenicity through the assessment of the mean grayness (MG) of the ovary **(Fig. 18.39)**.[40] Stromal index (stromal echogenicity/total ovarian echogenicity) was significantly higher in PCOS than controls.[31]

Moreover, 3D US has clearly shown higher AFC (median 16.3 vs. 5.5 per ovary), OV (12.56 vs. 5.6 mL), stromal volume (10.79 vs. 4.69 mL), and stromal

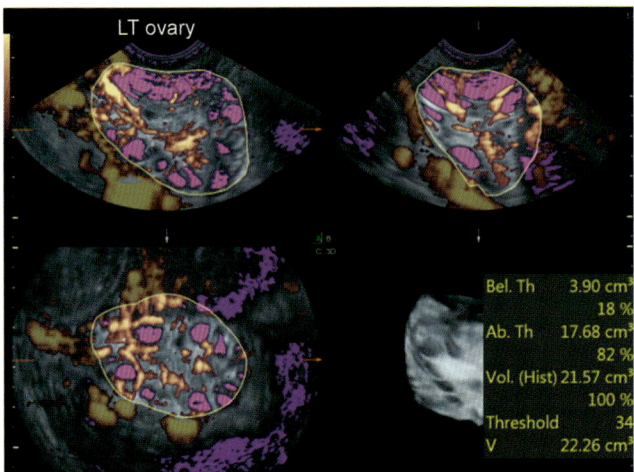

Fig. 18.38: 3D ultrasound acquired, virtual organ computer-aided analysis calculated ovarian volume with threshold volume used to calculate stromal volume of the ovary.

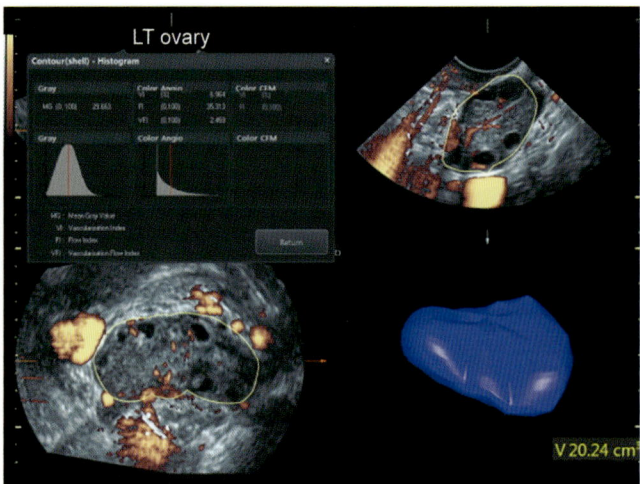

Fig. 18.39: 3D ultrasound acquired, virtual organ computer-aided analysis calculated ovarian volume with volume histogram, showing vascularity index, flow index, and vascular flow index values of the ovary.

vascularization [vascularity index (VI) 3.85 vs. 2.79%, vascular flow index (FI) (VFI) 1.27 vs. 0.85] in PCO patients.[41] Ovarian stromal FI is higher (33.94 vs. 29.30) in hirsuties than in normoandrogenic PCOS women. But in PCOS women with obesity the vascularity was lower than in normal weight women (VI 3.25 vs. 4.51%, VFI 1.22 vs. 1.56).[41] It is this vascularity that is responsible for hyperstimulation in the patients with PCOS.

To summarize the morphological features of PCO that correlate the most with the biochemical derangements of PCOS, OV, stromal volume, and AFC can all be better and more precisely assessed by and correlated with by 3D US.

FOLLICULAR MONITORING

- Assessment of ovarian reserve and response
- Assessment of follicular maturity and endometrial receptivity.

Assessment of Ovarian Reserve and Response

Three-dimensional US is also being used to predict the ovarian response in patients on assisted reproductive techniques.

Predictors of ovarian response are enumerated as follows:[42]

- Number of antral follicles
- Stromal flow: stromal FI
- Total ovarian stromal area
- Total OV

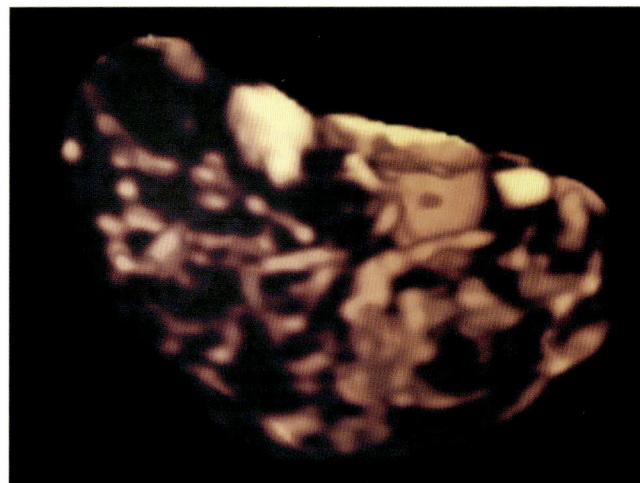

Fig. 18.40: 3D ultrasound acquired, VOCAL calculated ovarian volume rendered in 3D power Doppler angio-mode showing ovarian global vascularity. (3D: three-dimensional; VOCAL: Virtual organ computer-aided analysis)

Antral follicle count can be used reliably for the assessment of ovarian response. More exact value of AFC can be acquired by 3D US. Number of follicles more than 12 mm on the day of oocyte retrieval correlated significantly with AFC counted by 3D US rather than 2D US.[28]

Measurement of ovarian stromal flow in early follicular phase is related to subsequent ovarian response in IVF treatment[43] **(Fig. 18.40)**. 3D power Doppler with histogram can also be used to assess stromal vascularity on baseline scan. Kupesic et al. have shown a correlation between the ovarian stromal FI and number of mature oocytes retrieved in an IVF cycles and pregnancy rates. (Stromal FI <11 low responder, 11–14 good, >15 risk of OHSS).[42] *Another group has demonstrated that VI, FI, and VFI of the ovary were significantly related to ovarian response to stimulation.*[44]

Pretrigger Evaluation of Follicle and Endometrium

Assessment of Follicular Maturity

A follicle that is 16–18 mm in diameter and shows perifollicular vascularity covering three fourths of the circumference of the follicle with RI of less than or equal to 0.48 and PSV of 10 cm/s or more is known to be functionally mature. 3D US and 3D power Doppler have been used for further assessment of these follicles.

On 3D the follicular volume of 3–7.5 cc has been found to be optimum in our study[5] **(Fig. 18.41)**.[45] Follicular volumes of between 3 cc and 7 cc are optimum for oocyte retrieval by VOCAL. The limits of agreement between the volume of the follicular aspirate and 3D volume of the follicle were +0.96 to –0.43 with 3D and +3.47 to –2.42 by 2D volume estimation.[46]

This is because 3D US measurement is not affected by the follicular shape as the changing contours are outlined serially to obtain the specific volume measurement. Though the follicles of <10 mm in diameter cannot be assessed accurately by 3D US because limits of agreement are too wide in this range.

After the volume calculation, the follicle is seen plane by plane in the acquired volume by translation and rotation that is walking through the volume and rotating the volume. Using the surface smooth or light gradient mode for rendering with high threshold can show beautiful cumulus **(Fig. 18.9)**. Feichtinger et al. in their study have shown the presence of cumulus in follicles more than 15 mm by 3D US **(Fig. 18.42)**.[47]

Follicles without visualization of cumulus in all three planes are not likely to contain mature oocytes. Poehl et al. also found a significant correlation between the number of detected cumuli by 3D US and the number of retrieved oocytes (P <0.0001), mature oocytes (P <0.0001), and number of fertilized oocytes (P < 0.0001).[48]

It has also been suggested that the follicles containing oocytes capable to produce a pregnancy have a perifollicular vascular network more uniform and distinctive.[49] Although it is possible to assess the follicular flow as expressed by the peak systolic velocity and perifollicular color map.[42] it is the 3D power Doppler which proves the most precise information about the vascularization and follicular blood flow. 3D power Doppler gives global assessment of the vascularity, or follicular perfusion, both qualitatively and quantitatively.

The pulse repetition frequency settings for 3D power Doppler are fixed at 0.3 always, and a 3D volume with power Doppler is taken. For the assessment of the perifollicular vascularity, the vascularity is assessed in the outside shell with the wall thickness of 2 mm, which has been found to be the most appropriate to include the perifollicular vessels **(Fig. 18.43A)**. Volume histogram of this shell will give VI, FI, and VFI values of the perifollicular vessels **(Fig. 18.43B)**.

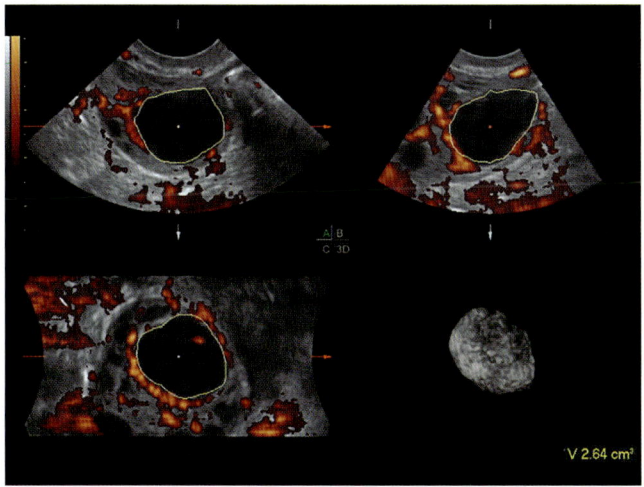

Fig. 18.41: 3D ultrasound acquired, virtual organ computer-aided analysis calculated follicular volume.

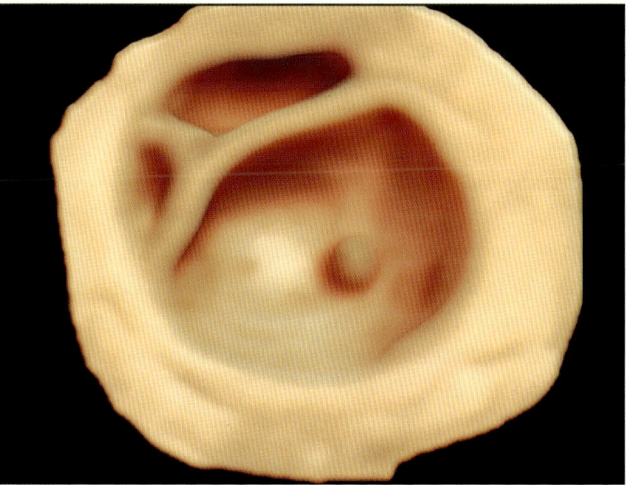

Fig. 18.42: 3D ultrasound acquired follicular volume and rendered on high definition live mode, showing the cumulus.

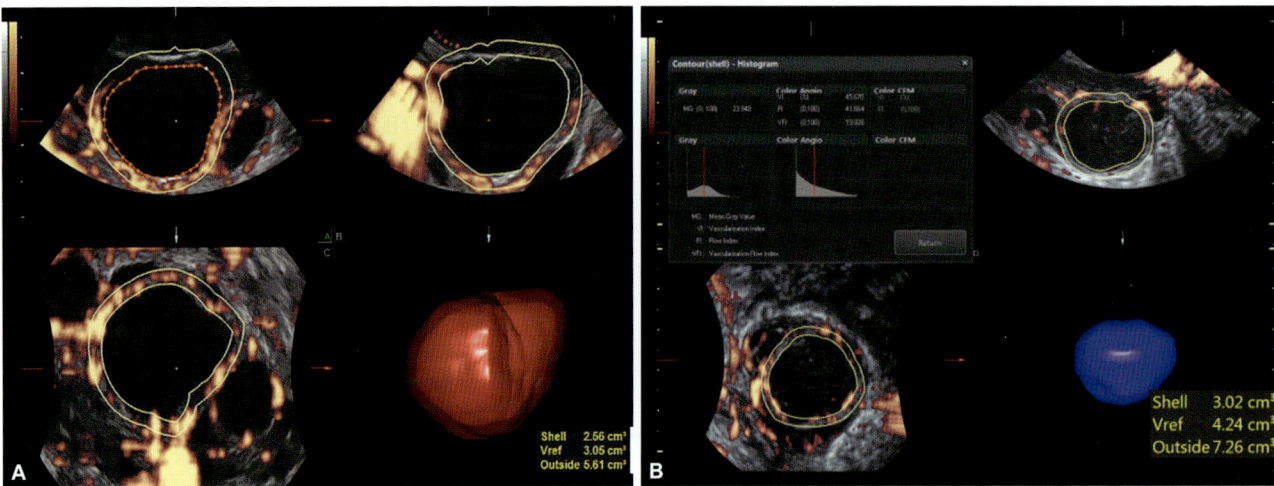

Figs. 18.43A and B: (A) 3D power Doppler ultrasound acquired follicular volume, with VOCAL calculated volume of the follicle with shell of 2 mm; (B) Volume histogram applied on the shell volume of follicle showing vascularity index, flow index, and vascular flow index values of the perifollicular flow.

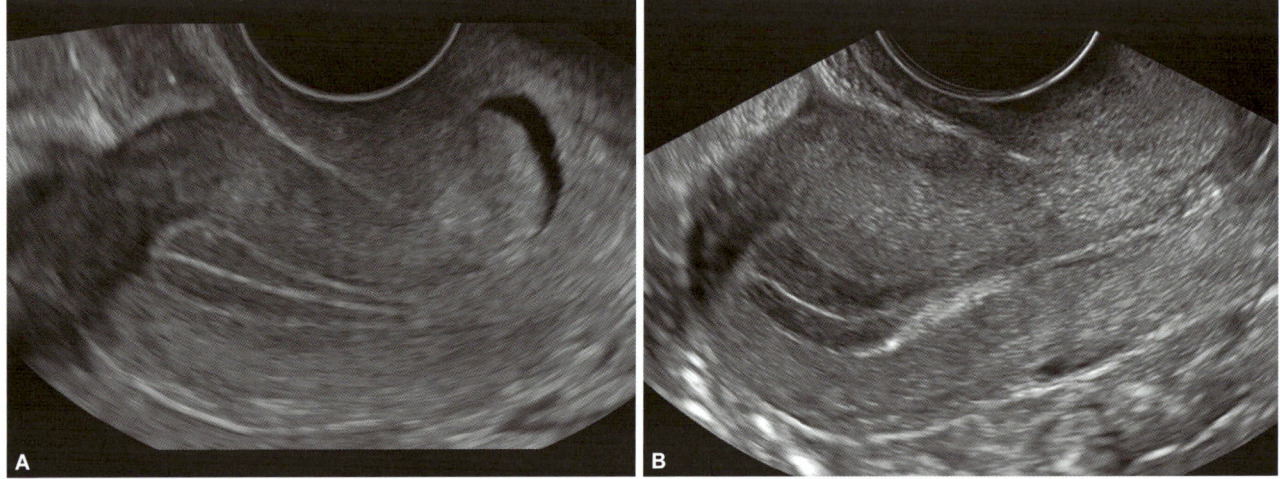

Figs. 18.44A and B: B mode ultrasound image of the uterus showing grade A and grade B endometrium, respectively.

We, in our study, have found perifollicular VI of between 6 and 20 and perifollicular FI more than 35 as most optimum for fertilizable oocyte. 68.4% of patients conceived when VI was between 6% and 18% and 50% when it was between 18 and 20. However, the pregnancy rates were less than 25% when VI was less than 6 and only 7.4% when VI was more than 20.[45]

Meaning that even when the follicle appeared mature according to the 2D US and color and pulse Doppler parameters, the pregnancy rates were significantly better only when the follicular volume was between 3 cc and 7.5 cc, cumulus was present, the perifollicular VI was between 6 and 20, and FI was more than 27.

A study by Kupesic and Kurjak shows that when the ratio of follicular volume to blood FI (FV/FI) is between 0.4 and 0.6, the pregnancy rates are 39%, if more than 0.6, it is 52% and when less than 0.4 is only 21%.[42]

Assessing Endometrial Receptivity

Endometrium, such as follicle, is assessed by transvaginal 2D US and color Doppler. Endometrial thickness of minimum 6 mm is required on the day of human chorionic gonadotropin (hCG), but 8 mm is optimum with a multilayered morphology, preferably grade A or B[50] **(Figs. 18.44A and B)**.

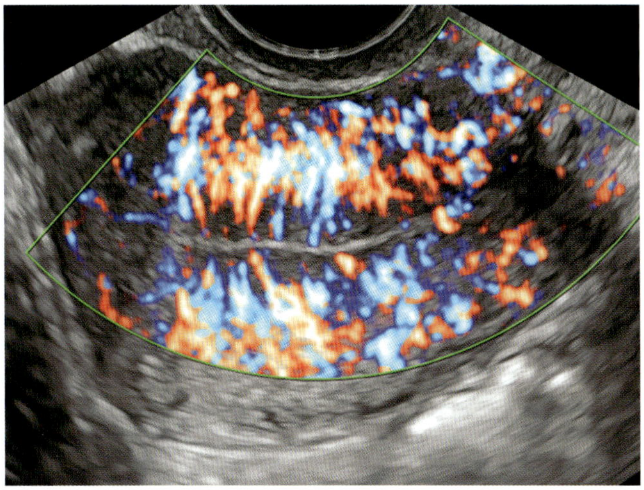

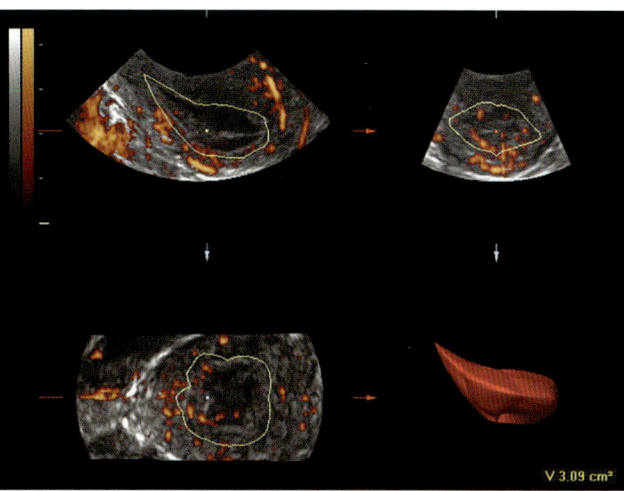

Fig. 18.45: High definition flow image showing zones 3 and 4 vascularity of the endometrium.

Fig. 18.46: 3D power Doppler acquired, virtual organ computer-aided analysis calculated volume of the endometrium.

Segmental uterine artery perfusion demonstrates significant correlation with hormonal and histological markers of uterine receptivity, reaching the highest sensitivity for subendometrial blood flow.[51] On color Doppler the endometrium which is mature shows vascularity in zones 3 and 4 or may be said in subendometrial and endometrial layers[52] **(Fig. 18.45)**. Zaidi et al. found that the absence of flow in the endometrial and subendometrial zones on the day of hCG indicate total failure of implantation. The vessels that reach the endometrium are the spiral arteries.[53]

Our study[37] showed that at endometrial volume of <2 cc, no pregnancies occurred. With endometrial volume of 2–3 cc, only 16.66% of patients conceived, between 3 cc and 5 cc 47%, and when the endometrial volume was between 5 cc and 7 cc, 61.5% patients conceived.[46] Endometrial volume by 3D US volume calculation of the endometrium may help to correlate the cycle outcome with quantitative parameter rather than endometrial thickness[53] **(Fig. 18.46)**. For endometrial volume the inter CC definition of internal os (interobserver variation) was 0.82 and intra CC (intraobserver variation) was 0.90, the chief source of error being definition of endometrial margins.[46]

A study by Raga et al.[54] shows pregnancy and implantation rates were significantly lower when endometrial volume was less than 2 mL, while no pregnancy was achieved when endometrial volume was less than 1 mL. Study by Kupesic et al. also shows no pregnancy when endometrial volume was less than 2 mL, or when

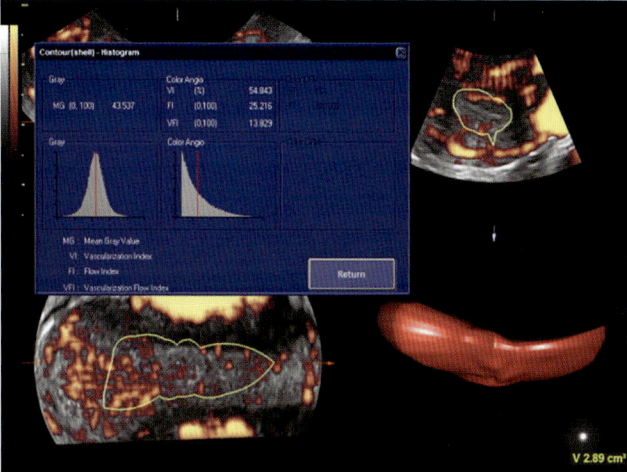

Fig. 18.47: 3D power Doppler acquired, virtual organ computer-aided analysis calculated volume of the endometrium with volume histogram showing global vascularity indices vascularity index, flow index, and vascular flow index values of the endometrium.

exceeded 8 mL.[55] For the same calculated volume, volume histogram is switched on, and it calculates the endometrial VI, FI, and VFI **(Fig. 18.47)**.

A scoring system reported by Kupesic et al., for uterine receptivity, done on the day of embryo transfer, shows that subendometrial FI less than 11 was a cutoff limit (Subendometrial indices are calculated in the same way from the endometrial volume as we calculate the perifollicular indices from the follicular volume, i.e. by shell volume of 2-mm thickness). No pregnancies occurred when it was less than 11, and the conception group showed its values of 13.2 ± 2.2.[55]

Contrary to this, Ng et al. documented a low endometrial VI and VFI in pregnant group on the day of oocyte retrieval and also a nonsignificant trend of higher implantation and pregnancy rates in patients with absent subendometrial and endometrial flow.[56] Though they concluded that number of embryos replaced and the endometrial VFI were the only two predictive factors for pregnancy. Wu et al.[57] reported that endometrial VFI was more reliable than VI and FI, and best prediction rate was achieved by VFI cutoff value of more than 0.24.

Collectively the evidence from various studies suggest that adding 3D and 3D-power Doppler for the assessment of follicular maturity and endometrial receptivity improves the outcome of the fertility treatment by the assessment of global vascularity.

ECTOPIC PREGNANCY

Gestational sac that has implanted at places other from the upper body of the endometrial cavity. It can be in the fallopian tube (95%), abdominal cavity, ovary, broad ligament, uterine cornu, myometrium, cervix, or scar. It is suspected when in a female with a missed period and beta hCG level of more than 1,500 IU/mL on US does not show an intrauterine gestational sac. In the case of an early intrauterine pregnancy, the endometrial lips are asymmetrical **(Fig. 18.48A)**, and in the case of ectopic pregnancy, the lips of endometrium are symmetrical **(Fig. 18.48B)**. This may be easily appreciated also on B mode US. True gestational sac is eccentric in the sac and shows peripheral vascularity. Any adnexal lesion in such a female that is tender on probe pressure or shows peripheral ring of vascularity is an ectopic **(Figs. 18.49A and B)**. Tubal pregnancies can be diagnosed by B mode and color Doppler. 3D ultrasound helps to demonstrate the surrounding anatomy and thus the exact location of the tubal ectopic pregnancy in relation to uterus and ovary **(Fig. 18.49C)**. It is the differentiation between interstitial pregnancy and angular pregnancy, diagnosis of cervical pregnancy and scar pregnancy, for which 3D plays an important role. Interstitial pregnancy on coronal plane of the uterus clearly shows a myometrial gap between the gestational sac and the endometrial cavity, unlike the angular pregnancy in which the endometrium covers one side of the gestational sac but not the other side **(Figs. 18.50A and B)**. Cervical pregnancy typically leads to expansion of the cervix due to progressing pregnancy and leads to hourglass uterus, with gestational sac placed eccentrically in the cervix **(Fig. 18.51)**. Scar pregnancies may be in the sac or over the scar, and the prognosis for both is significantly different. Scar over the pregnancy leads to growth of the pregnancy in the uterus, and the risk is only adherent placenta. But for the pregnancy in the scar, the risk of rupture of the uterus is significantly high and requires immediate intervention **(Figs. 18.52A to D)**.

Apart from this, even when conservative or interventional treatment is planned, with the onset of the medical line of treatment, there is first decrease in the

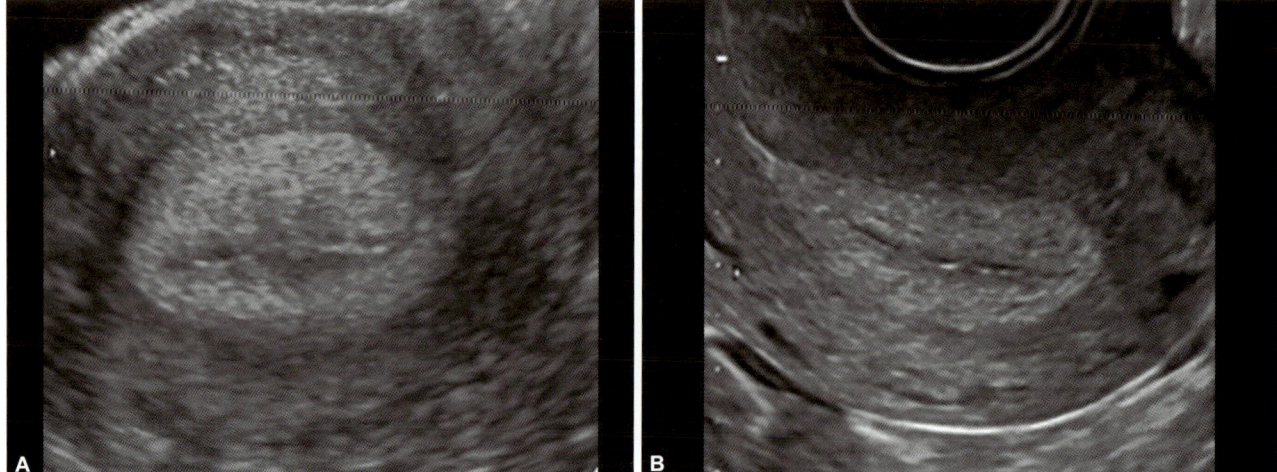

Figs. 18.48A and B: (A) B mode ultrasound image of the endometrium showing asymmetrical thickness of the endometrial lips; (B) B mode ultrasound image of the endometrium showing symmetrical thickness of the endometrial lips.

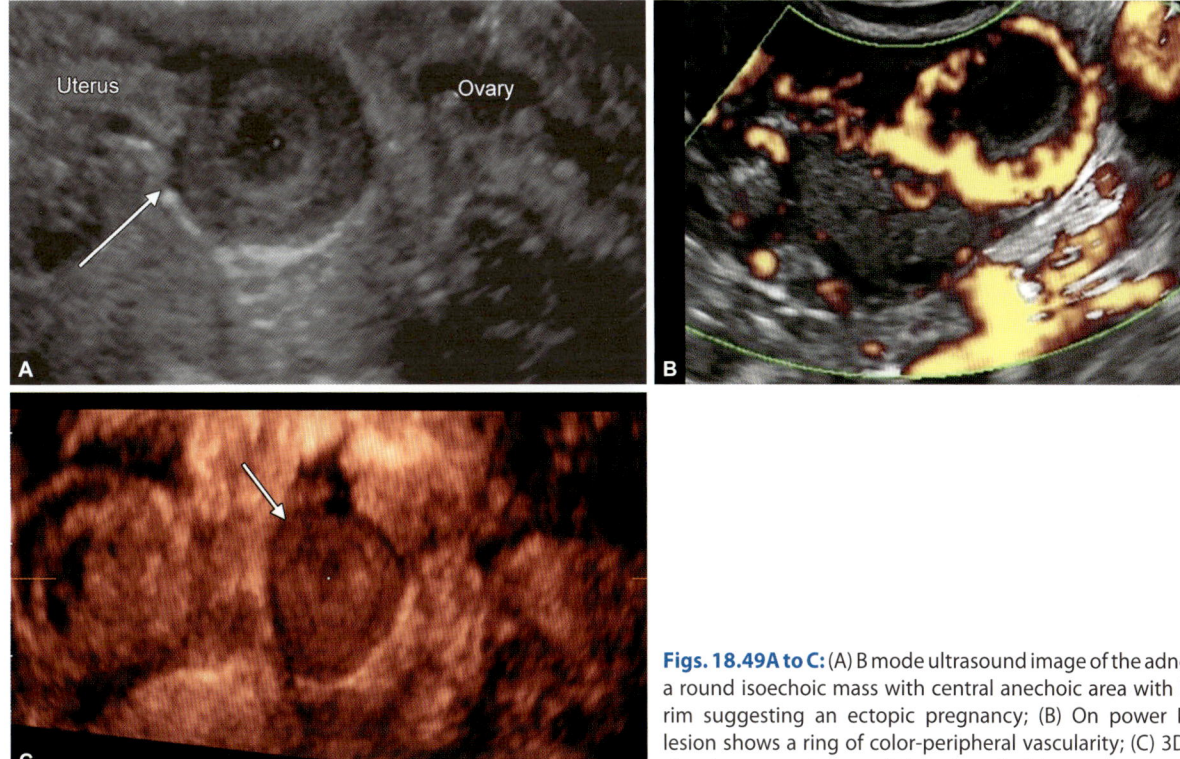

Figs. 18.49A to C: (A) B mode ultrasound image of the adnexa showing a round isoechoic mass with central anechoic area with hyperechoic rim suggesting an ectopic pregnancy; (B) On power Doppler the lesion shows a ring of color-peripheral vascularity; (C) 3D ultrasound showing coronal plane of the adnexal with ectopic pregnancy mass.

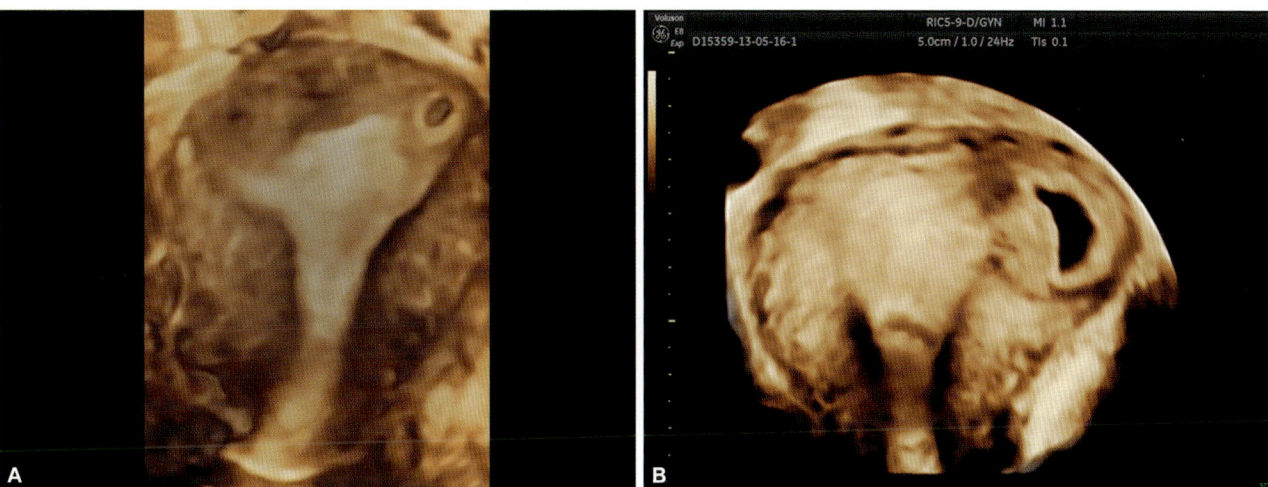

Figs. 18.50A and B: (A) 3D rendered image of the uterus showing left angular pregnancy; (B) 3D rendered image of the uterus showing interstitial pregnancy.

vascularity and that 3D and 3D PD will be a useful tool to diagnose that the regression of the lesion even before the size of the lesion decreases. Reduction in VI, FI, and VFI values is useful to assess the regression of the ectopic pregnancy quantitatively **(Fig. 18.53)**.

CONCLUSION

Three-dimensional US can better demonstrate the uterine lesions, such as polyps, endometrial synechiae, and fibroids. Better delineation of endometrio–myometrial

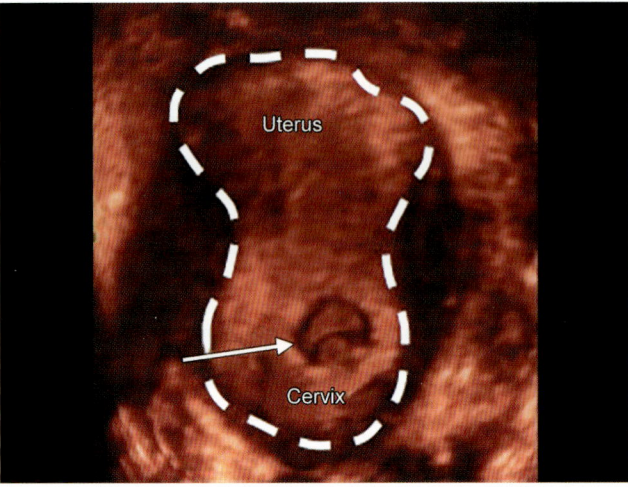

Fig. 18.51: 3D rendered image of the uterus showing cervical pregnancy and hourglass uterus.

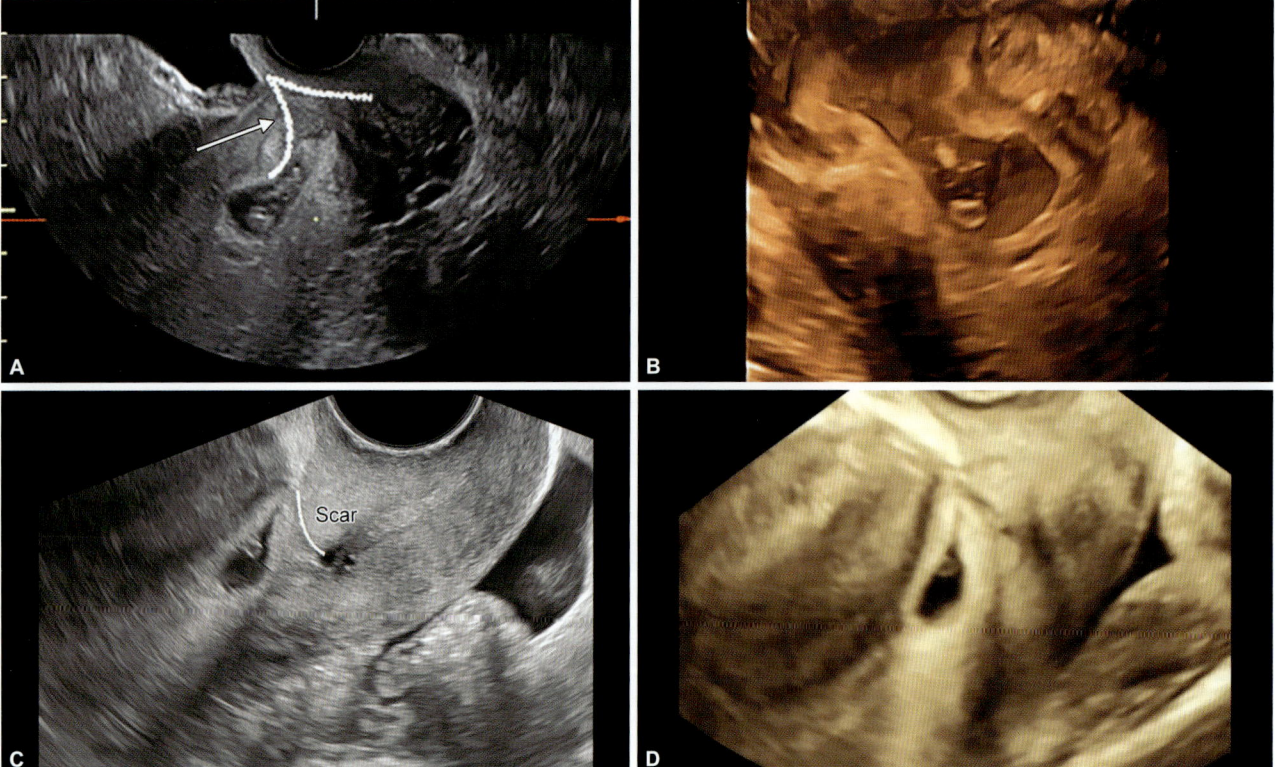

Figs. 18.52A to D: (A) Pregnancy in the scar on B mode; (B) Pregnancy in the scar on 3D ultrasound; (C) B mode ultrasound image showing gestational sac over the scar; (D) 3D ultrasound with volume contrast imaging A confirming the diagnosis of pregnancy in the scar.

junction helps in the diagnosis of adenomyosis, comparable to MRI. Tubal assessment can be made more effective by adding 3D to HyCoSy. 3D US is accurate for volume assessment both for follicle and the endometrium that are much more reliable parameters than follicular diameter or endometrial thickness. The presence of cumulus, the presence of which can be confirmed by 3D US more easily than with B mode and increases the

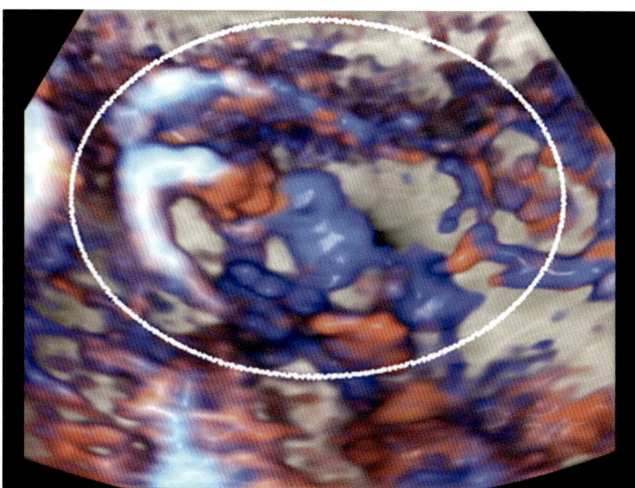

Fig. 18.53: 3D high definition flow volume showing global vascularity of the ectopic pregnancy.

surety of the presence of a mature ovum in the follicle. 3D-power Doppler gives idea about the global vascularity of the follicle and the endometrium. Though still larger studies are needed to establish more precise values for follicular and endometrial VI, FI, and VFI, the results are fairly promising.

REFERENCES

1. Cil AP, Tulunay G, Kose MF, et al. Power Doppler properties of endometrial polyps and submucosal fibroids: preliminary observational study in women with known intracavitary lesions. Ultrasound Obstet Gynecol. 2010;35: 233-7.
2. de Souza NM, Brosens JJ, Schwieso JE, et al. The potential value of magnetic resonance imaging in infertility. Clin Radiol. 1995;50(2):75-9.
3. Exacoustos C, Brienza L, Di Giovanni A, et al. Adenomyosis: three-dimensional sonographic findings of the junctional zone and correlation with histology. Ultrasound Obstet Gynecol. 2011;37:471-9.
4. Van Den Bosch T, Dueholm M, Leone FP, et al. Terms, definitions and measurements to describe sonographic features of myometrium and uterine masses: a consensus opinion from the Morphological Uterus Sonographic Assessment (MUSA) group. Ultrasound Obstet Gynecol. 2015;46(3):284-98.
5. Lasmar RB, Barrozo PRM, Dias R, Oliveira MAP. Submucous fibroids: A new presurgical classification (STEP-w) Minim Invasive Gynecol. 2005;12(4):308-11.
6. Mavrelos D, Naftalin J, Hoo W, et al. Preoperative assessment of submucous fibroids by three-dimentional saline contrast sonohysterography. Ultrasound Obstet Gynecol. 2011;38:350-4.
7. Crade M. Tissue block ultrasound and ovarian cancer—a pictorial presentation of findings. Ultrasound Obstet Gynecol. 2009;3(1):41-7.
8. Raine-Fenning N, Jayaprakasan K, Deb S. Three-dimensional ultrasonographic characteristics of endometriomata. Ultrasound Obstet Gynecol. 2008;31:718-24.
9. Patel MD, Feldstein VA, Chen DC, et al. Endometriomas: diagnostic performance of US. Radiology. 1999;210: 739-45.
10. Van Holsbeke C, Zhang J, Van Belles V, et al. Acoustic streaming cannot discriminate reliably between endometriomas and other types of adnexal lesion: a multicenter study of 633 adnexal masses. Ultrasound Obstet Gynecol. 2010;35:349-53.
11. Kurjak A, Kupesic S, Sparac V, et al. The detection of stage I ovarian cancer by three dimensional sonography and power Doppler. Gynecol Oncol. 2003;90:258-64.
12. Kupesic S, Kurjak A. Contrast enhanced three dimensional power Doppler sonography for the differentiation of adnexal masses. Obstet Gynecol. 2000;96:452-8.
13. Jeanty P, Besnard S, Arnold A, et al. Air-contrast sonohysterography as a first step assessment of tubal patency. J Ultrasound Med. 2000;19(8):519-27.
14. Holz K, Becker R, Schürmann R. Ultrasound in the investigation of tubal patency: a meta-analysis of three comparative studies of Echovist-200 including 1007 women. Zentralbl Gynakol. 1997;119:366-73.
15. Exacoustos C, Zupi E, Carusotti C, et al. Hysterosalpingo-contrast sonography compared with hysterosalpingo-graphy and laparoscopic dye pertubation to evaluate tubal patency. J Am Assoc Gynecol Laparosc. 2003;10(3): 367-72.
16. Balen FG, Allen CM, Gardener JE, et al. 3-dimensional reconstruction of ultrasound images of the uterine cavity. Br J Radiol. 1993;66:588-91.
17. Exacoustos C, Di Giovanni A, Szabolcs B, et al. Automated three-dimensional coded contrast imaging hystero-salpingo-contrast sonography: feasibility in office tubal patency testing. Ultrasound Obstet Gynecol. 2013;41(3): 328-35.
18. Chan CC, Ng EH, Tang OS, et al. Comparison of three-dimensional hysteron-contrast-sonography and diagnostic laparoscopy with chromopertubation in the assessment of tubal patency for the investigation of subfertility. Acta Obstet Gynecol Scand. 2005;84(9):909-13.
19. Kupesic S, Plavsic MB. 2D and 3D hysterosalpingocontrast-sonography in the assessment of uterine cavity and tubal patency. Eur J Obstet Gynecol Reprod Biol. 2007;133(1): 64-9.
20. Zhou L, Zhang X, Chen X, et al. Value of three-dimensional hysterosalpingo-contrast sonography with SonoVue in the assessment of tubal patency. Ultrasound Obstet Gynecol. 2012;40(1):93-8.
21. Sladkevicius P, Ojha K, Campbell S, et al. Three-dimensional power Doppler imaging in the assessment of Fallopian tube patency. Ultrasound Obstet Gynecol. 2000;16(7):644-7.

22. Lam PM, Raine-Fenning N. The role of three-dimensional ultrasonography in polycystic ovary syndrome. Hum Reprod. 2006;21(9):2209-15.

23. Kupesic S. Sonographic imaging in infertility. In: Donald school textbook of transvaginal ultrasound, 1st edition. New Delhi: Jaypee Brothers Medical Publishers (P) Ltd.; 2005. pp. 357-83.

24. Jonard S, Robert Y, Dewailly D. Revisiting the ovarian volume as a diagnostic criterion for polycystic ovaries. Hum Reprod. 2005;20(10):2893-8.

25. Legro RS, Chiu P, Kunselman AR, et al. Polycystic ovaries are common in women with hyperandrogenic chronic anovulation but do not predict metabolic or reproductive phenotype. JCEM. 2005;90(5):2571-9.

26. Jonard S, Robert Y, Cortet-Rudelli C, et al. Ultrasound examination of polycystic ovaries: is it worth counting the follicles?. Hum Reprod. 2003;18(3):598-603.

27. Lujan ME, Jarrett BY, Brooks ED, et al. Updated ultrasound criteria for polycystic ovary syndrome: reliable thresholds for elevated follicle population and ovarian volume. Hum Reprod. 2013;28(5):1361-8.

28. Ng EH, Chan CC, Yeung WS, et al. Effect of age on ovarian stromal flow measured by three-dimensional ultrasound with power Doppler in Chinese women with proven fertility. Hum Reprod. 2004;19:2132-7.

29. Deb S, Campbell BK, Clewes JS, et al. Quantitative analysis of AFC and size: a comparison of 2D & automated three-dimensional ultrasound techniques. Ultrasound Obstet Gynecol. 2010;35:354-60.

30. Thatcher. Defining PCOS—a perspective. The American Infertility Association News Letter, February 2001.

31. Buckett WM, Bouzayeb R, Watkin KL, et al. Ovarian stromal echogenicity in women with normal and polycystic ovaries. Hum Reprod. 1999;14(3):618-21.

32. Falghesu A, Angioni S, Frau E, et al. Ultrasound in polycystic ovary syndrome—the measuring of ovarian stroma and relationship with circulating androgens: results of a multicentric study. Hum Reprod. 2007;22: 2501-8.

33. Franks S, Webber LJ, Goh M, et al. Ovarian Morphology is a marker of heritable biochemical traits in sisters with polycystic ovaries. J Clin Endocrinol Metab. 2008;93: 3396-402.

34. Robert Y, Dubrulle F, Gaillandre L, et al. Ultrasound assessment of ovarian stroma hypertrophy in hyperandro-genism and ovulation disorders: visual analysis versus computerized quantification. Fertil Steril. 1995;64: 307-12.

35. Dewailly D, Robert Y, Helin I, et al. Ovarian stromal hypertrophy in hyperandrogenic women. Clin Endocrinol (Oxf). 1994;41:557-62.

36. Raine-Fenning NJ, Campbell BK, Clewes JS, et al. The reli-ability of virtual organ computer-aided analysis (VOCAL) for the semiquantification of ovarian, endometrial and subendometrial perfusion. Ultrasound Obstet Gynecol. 2003;22:633-9.

37. Kyei-Mensah AA, LinTan S, Zaidi J, et al. Relationship of ovarian stromal volume to serum androgen concentrations in patients with polycystic ovary syndrome. Hum Reprod. 1998;13:1437-41.

38. Pache TD, de Jong FH, Hop WC, et al. Association between ovarian changes assessed by transvaginal sonography and clinical and endocrine signs of the polycystic ovary syndrome. Fertil Steril. 1993;59:544-9.

39. Panchal S, Nagori CB. Assessing correlation between ovarian & stromal volumes and fasting & postprandial insulin levels in PCOS patients. Int J Infertil Fetal Med. 2014;5(1):12-4.

40. Jarvela IY, Mason HD, Sladkevicius P, et al. Characterization of normal and polycystic ovaries using three dimensional power Doppler ultrasonography. J Assist Reprod Genet. 2002;19:582-90.

41. Lam PM, Johnson IR, Rainne-Fenning NJ. Three dimen-sional ultrasound features of the polycystic ovary and the effect of different phenotypic expressions on these parameters. Hum Reprod. 2007;22(12):3116-23.

42. Kupesic S, Kurjak A. Predictors of IVF outcome by three dimensional ultrasound. Hum Reprod. 2002;17(4): 950-5.

43. Zaidi J, Barber J, Kyei-Mensah A, et al. Relationship of ovarian stromal blood flow at baseline ultrasound to subsequent follicular response in an in vitro fertilization program. Obstet Gynecol. 1996;88:779-84.

44. Merce LT, Barco MJ, Bau S, et al. Prediction of ovarian response and IVF/ICSI outcome by three-dimensional ultrasonography and power Doppler angiography. Eur J Obstet Gynecol Reprod Biol. 2007;132(1):93-100.

45. Panchal SY, Nagori CB. Can 3D PD be a better tool for assessing the pre hCG follicle and endometrium? A randomized study of 500 cases. Presented at 16th World Congress on ultrasound in obstetrics and gynecology, 2006, London. Ultrasound Obstet Gynecol. 2006;28(4): 504.

46. Kyei-Mensah A, Zaidi J, Pittrof R, et al. Transvaginal three dimensional ultrasound. accuracy of follicular volume measurements. Fertil Steril. 1996;65:371-6.

47. Feichtinger W. Transvaginal three dimensional imaging for evaluation and treatment of infertility. In: Merz E (Ed). 3D Ultrasound in Obstetrics and Gynecology. Philadelphia, PA: Lippincott Williams and Wilkins; 1998. pp. 37-43.

48. Poehl M, Hohlagschwandtner M, Doerner V, et al. Cumulus assessment by three dimensional ultrasound for in vitro fertilization. Ultrasound Obstet Gynecol. 2000;16: 251-3.

49. Vlaisavljevic V, Reljic M, Gavric Lovrec V, et al. Measurement of perifollicular blood flow of the dominant preovulatory follicle using three-dimensional power Doppler. Ultrasound Obstet Gynecol. 2003;22(5):520-6.

50. Smith B, Porter R, Ahuja K, et al. Ultrasonic assessment of endometrial changes in stimulated cycles in an in vitro fertilization and embryo transfer program. J In Vitro Fertil Embryo Transf. 1984;1:233-38.

51. Merce LT, Barco MJ, Kupesic S, et al. 2D and 3D power Doppler ultrasound from ovulation to implantation. In: Kurjak A, Chervenak F (Eds). Textbook of Perinatal Medicine. London: Parthenon Publishing; 2005.

52. Applebaum M. The 'steel' or 'teflon' endometrium— ultrasound visualization of endometrial vascularity in IVF patients and outcome. Presented at the third World Congress of ultrasound in obstetrics and gyneacolgy. Ultrasound Obstet Gynecol. 1993;3(Suppl 2):10.

53. Zaidi J, Campbell S, Pittrof R, et al. Endometrial thickness, morphology, vascular penetration and velocimetry in predicting implantation in an in vitro fertilization program. Ultrasound Obstet Gynecol. 1995;6:191-8.

54. Raga F, Bonilla-Musoles F, Casan EM, et al. Assessment of endometrial volume by three-dimensional ultrasound prior to embryo transfer: clues to endometrial receptivity. Hum Reprod. 1999;14:2851-4.

55. Kupesic S, Bekavac I, Bjelos D, et al. Assessment of endometrial receptivity by transvaginal color Doppler and three-dimensional power Doppler ultrasonography in patients undergoing in vitro fertilization procedures. J Ultrasound Med. 2001;20:125-34.

56. Ng EH, Chan CC, Tang OS, et al. The role of endometrial and subendometrial blood flows measured by three-dimensional power Doppler ultrasound in prediction of pregnancy during IVF treatment. Hum Reprod. 2006;21(1): 164-70.

57. Wu HM, Chiang CH, Huang HY, et al. Detection of subendometrial vascularization flow index by three-dimensional ultrasound may be useful for predicting pregnancy rate for patients undergoing in vitro fertilization-embryo transfer. Fertil Steril. 2003;79(3):507-11.

Advantage of 3D Ultrasound in Exact Diagnosis of Normal and Abnormal Fetal Corpus Callosum

Sonila Pashaj, Eberhard Merz

INTRODUCTION

Direct visualization of the fetal corpus callosum can be performed with two-dimensional (2D) and three-dimensional (3D) ultrasound.[1-3] However, 2D ultrasound allows visualization of the corpus callosum only in a fetal position in which anterior fontanel or sagittal suture can be used as acoustic windows. 3D ultrasound does not only facilitate the demonstration of the corpus callosum but also enables precise measurements.

The aim of this chapter is to explain the benefits of 3D ultrasound in the demonstration of the normal corpus callosum and its pathology and how 3D ultrasound can be correctly used for corpus callosum demonstration.

WHY IS THE DEMONSTRATION OF THE CORPUS CALLOSUM IMPORTANT?

Corpus callosum is an important landmark in the fetal brain development. It is the largest connective pathway of the human brain that allows controlling movement and feeling in the opposite half of the body, as well as in processing certain types of information such as language or spatial patterns.

In a targeted ultrasound examination, particularly in neurosonography, the demonstration of the corpus callosum plays an important role.

Abnormal corpus callosum may result in somatic complaints, attention problems, aggressive behavior, social problems, and thought problems.[4,5]

The demonstration of the corpus callosum is not part of a routine ultrasound examination, but it is necessary in a targeted ultrasound examination. Early detection of corpus callosum malformations allows better genetic counseling and a better decision making of the parents.

WHAT IS THE NORMAL SONOGRAPHIC APPEARANCE OF THE CORPUS CALLOSUM AND WHEN CAN IT BE DISPLAYED?

The corpus callosum is fully developed when it overlies the quadrigeminal plate of the mesencephalon in the median view of the fetal brain.[6] In 2D ultrasound, the corpus callosum can be demonstrated as early as 18–20 weeks of gestation with its four anatomical parts, but only if the fetus is in an appropriate position. The corpus callosum is displayed as an anechoic band, demarcated superiorly and inferiorly by two echoic lines **(Figs. 19.1A and B)**.

Clear sonographic visualization of the corpus callosum requires scanning planes that are often difficult to obtain in utero with 2D ultrasound, due to an unfavorable position of the fetus. A cephalic presentation enables the use of endovaginal probes to demonstrate the fetal brain, but even with this technique the 2D ultrasound examination can be difficult in case of asynclitism of the fetal head. Furthermore, this approach has a limited range in terms of lateral movement of the intravaginal probe. In the presence of breech presentation, the corpus callosum can be demonstrated only with an abdominal scan.

When color or power Doppler is added, the pericallosal arteries (there are two of them, one on each hemisphere) can be seen superior to the corpus callosum following their upper margin **(Fig. 19.2)**.[2]

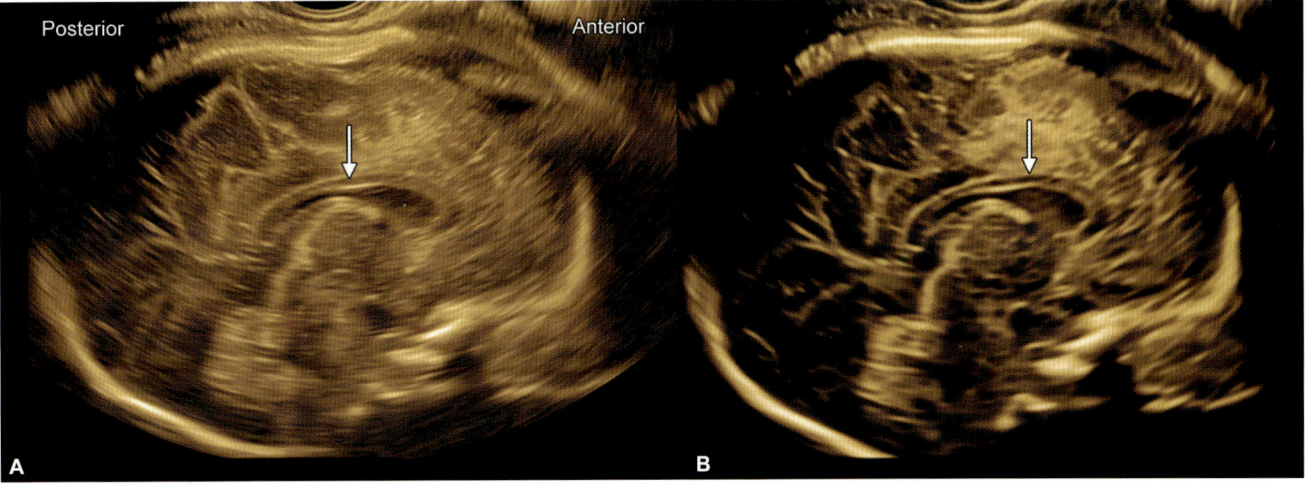

Figs. 19.1A and B: Demonstration of the corpus callosum as a hypoechoic structure in the median plane (→). (A) 2D plane, (B) 3D surface-rendered image.

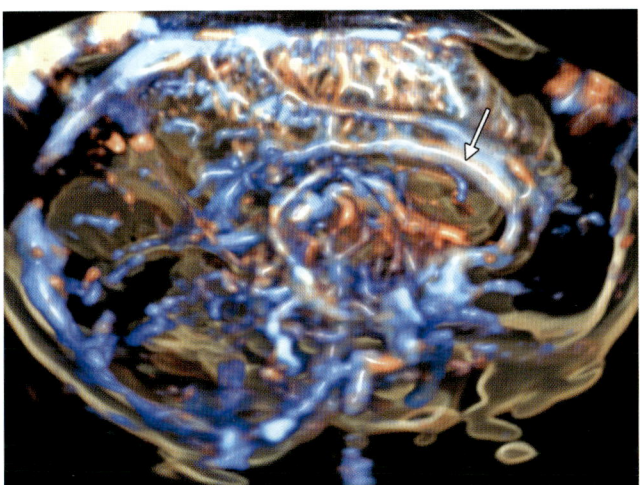

Fig. 19.2: Volume acquisition of the brain with the glass body mode, showing the pericallosal artery in the median plane (→).

ADVANTAGES OF THREE-DIMENSIONAL ULTRASOUND IN THE DEMONSTRATION OF THE CORPUS CALLOSUM

In comparison to 2D ultrasound, 3D ultrasound has several advantages for the visualization of the corpus callosum:

- 3D ultrasonography has the potential to acquire a volume of the fetal head. The acquisition of such a volume can be initiated from the median plane as well as from a tilted parasagittal plane **(Figs. 19.3A and B)**. The simultaneous demonstration of the three orthogonal planes is used to visualize the brain in all three planes, while the user can navigate through the volume in a continuous fashion.[7] By rotating the volume into a standard orientation of the fetal head, it is possible to achieve a symmetric demonstration of the fetal brain in the axial and coronal views. This enables also a precise demonstration of the correct median plane with exact demonstration of the entire corpus callosum structure in all cases.[8,9]

- In case of an unfavorable position of the fetal head, the operator can use the free hand to manipulate the fetal head from outside of the abdomen to achieve the acquisition of the brain volume in a sagittal plane.

- 3D ultrasound reduces the time for obtaining the correct sagittal and coronal planes.

- 3D ultrasound enables even the less experienced sonographer to visualize the corpus callosum in the correct median plane.

- Volume scanning facilitates the consultation with an expert. The sonographic information can be stored as a volume dataset and the volume can be reloaded for offline analysis.

SCANNING TECHNIQUES WITH THREE-DIMENSIONAL ULTRASOUND AND OFFLINE ANALYSIS

Depending on the fetal position, the acquisition of the brain volume can be performed transabdominally or transvaginally. However, not all acoustic windows of the fetal head enable a precise demonstration of the corpus callosum.

If the acquisition plane is acquired from the anterior fontanelle or the sagittal suture, the anterior midline

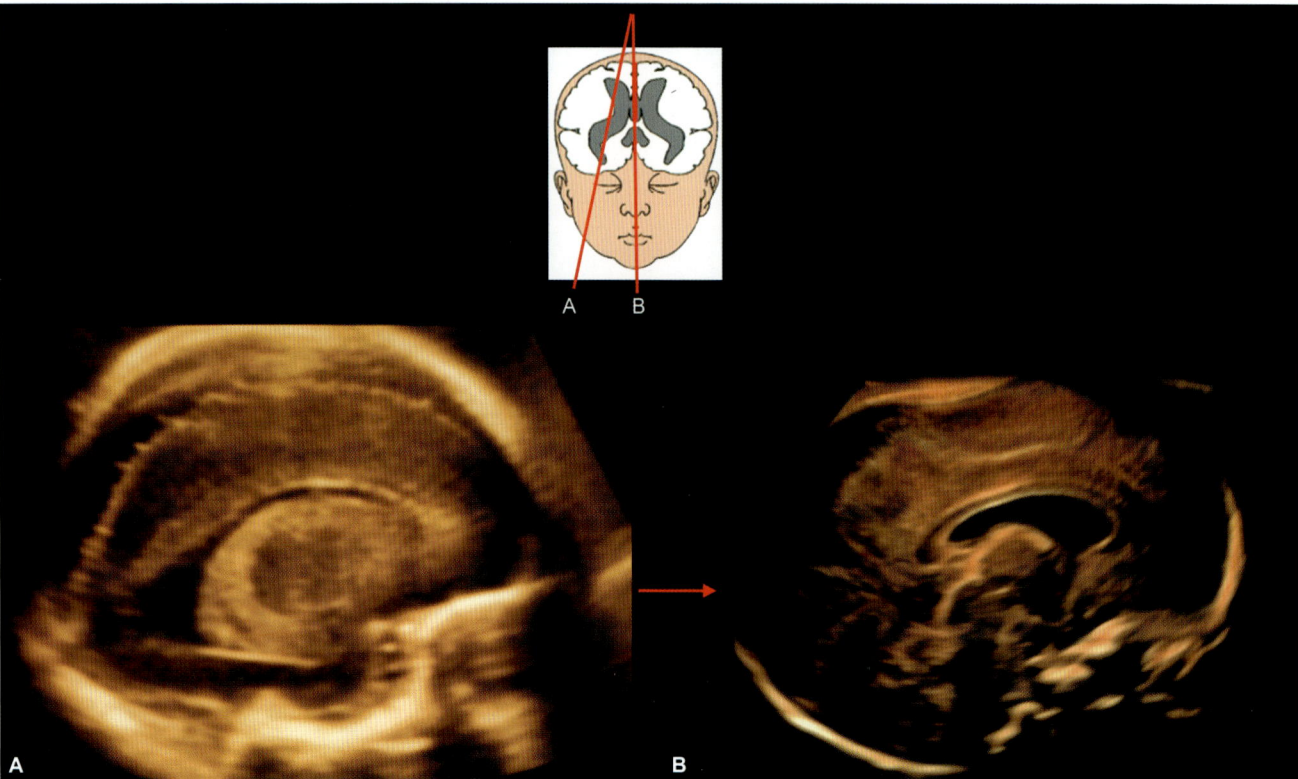

Figs. 19.3A and B: (A) Volume acquisition starting from the three-horn view. (B) After placement of the "reference dot" at the interhemispheric fissure and rotation of plane A to plane B it is possible to demonstrate the corpus callosum in the median plane.

structures, such as the superior subarachnoid cistern, the surface of the brain hemispheres, corpus callosum, and lateral ventricles are demonstrated with a better resolution than the posterior midline structures in the fossa posterior. In contrast, volumes taken from the small posterior fontanelle allow a good demonstration of the posterior fossa, but not of the corpus callosum. This is due to the shadow caused by the ossified parts of the fetal head.

The best initial plane for volume acquisition of the corpus callosum is a sagittal plane. It can be the median plane or an oblique sagittal plane, such as the plane of the three-horn view **(Figs. 19.3A and B)**. Depending on the gestational age, the sweep angle for volume acquisition can be set between 45° and 120°, to include most of the fetal head. In case of fetal movements, this angle should be set as low as possible (20–30°), to get at least the corpus callosum included in the volume.

Offline analysis can be conducted using dedicated 3D/4D software (4D View, General Electric) on a laptop computer. A systematic volume manipulation can be performed in the multiplanar display mode until a standard orientation of the orthogonal planes is achieved.

Placement of the "reference dot" at the interhemispheric fissure and rotation of the axis helps to find the correct axial plane **(Figs. 19.4A to D)**.[3]

When the median plane is displayed in plane A, the coronal plane in plane B and the axial plane in plane C, the entire corpus callosum can be seen in plane A and in the surface rendered image. A morphologic analysis can then be performed with correlation to the coronal and axial planes **(Figs. 19.5A to C)**.

Several display modes may be used to demonstrate the corpus callosum in the stored volumes:

- Tomographic display mode which allows visualization of multiple parallel slices at different distances on the screen, similar to those seen in computed tomography (CT) or magnetic resonance imagining (MRI) **(Fig. 19.6)**.[10]
- Thick slice display enhances the margins of the corpus callosum by selecting a number of successive slices with their sequential information and "collapse" them into a single rendered plane **(Fig. 19.7)**.[9]
- Omniview allows defining of any plane in the volume dataset and simultaneous display of the perpendicular plane **(Figs. 19.8A and B)**.[11]

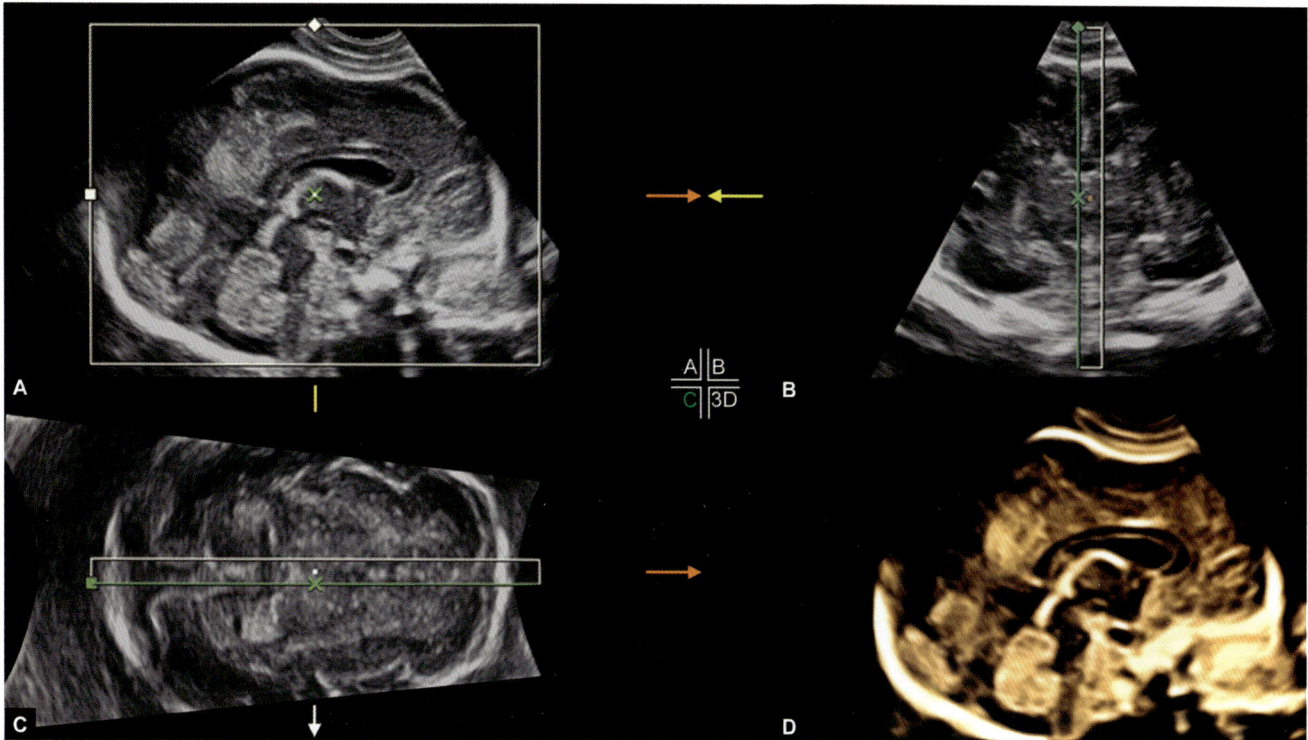

Figs. 19.4A to D: Multiplanar demonstration of corpus callosum. (A) Sagittal plane, (B) coronal plane, and (c) axial plane. The reference dot in plane B and C is exact between the two hemispheres. (D) Surface-rendered image of the median plane.

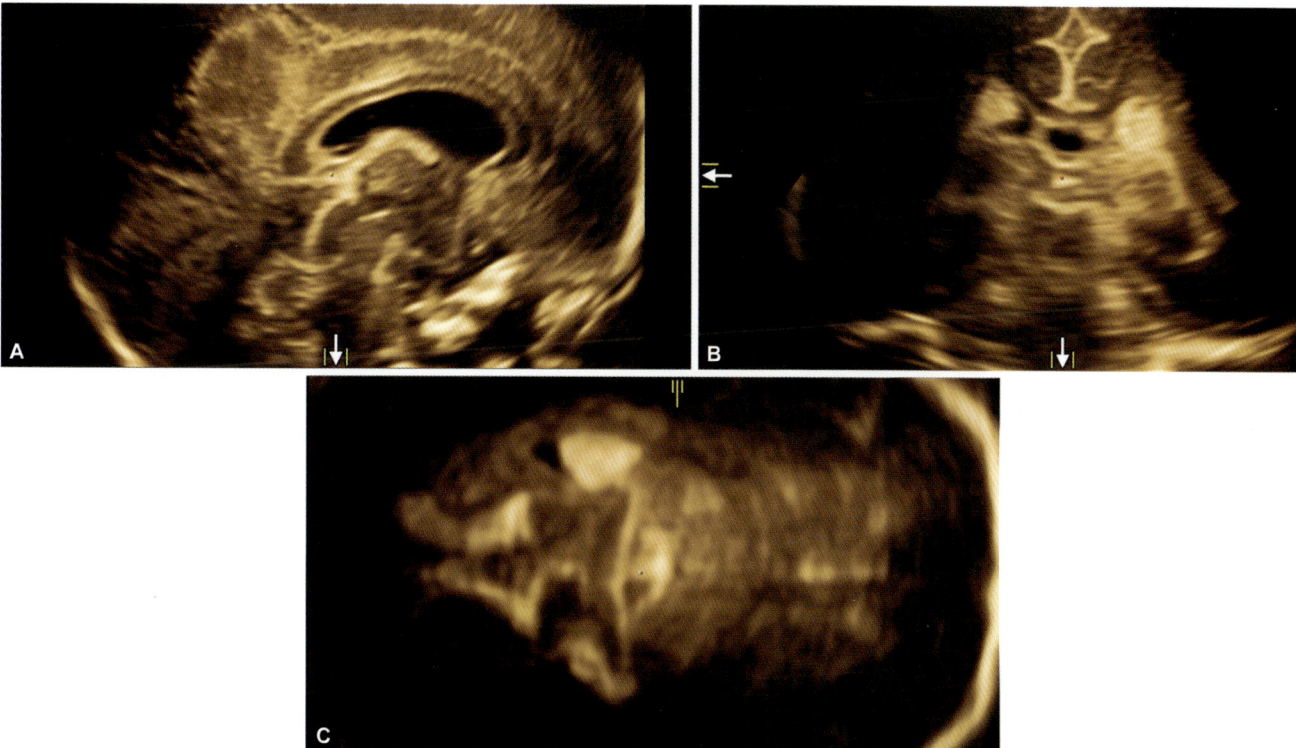

Figs. 19.5A to C: Multiplanar display of the corpus callosum. (A) Median plane, (B) coronal plane, and (C) axial plane of the fetal brain.

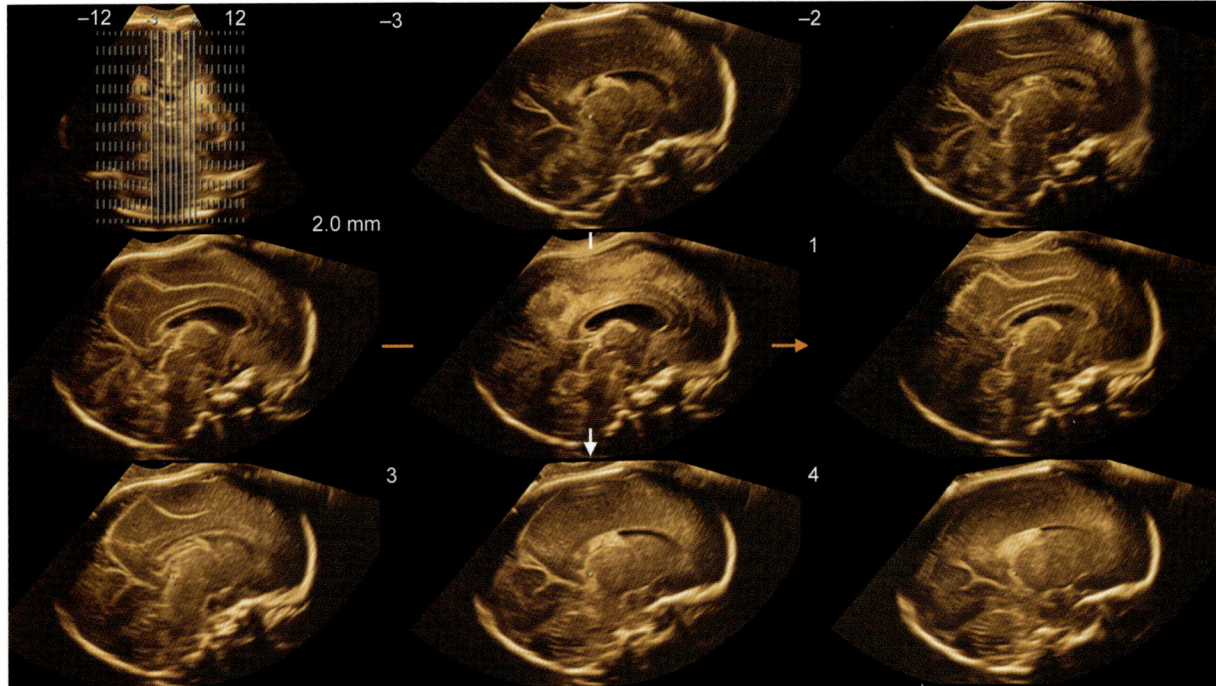

Fig. 19.6: The tomographic display of the fetal brain shows the corpus callosum within several parallel sagittal planes at 2 mm spacing similar to computed tomography (CT) or magnetic resonance imaging (MRI).

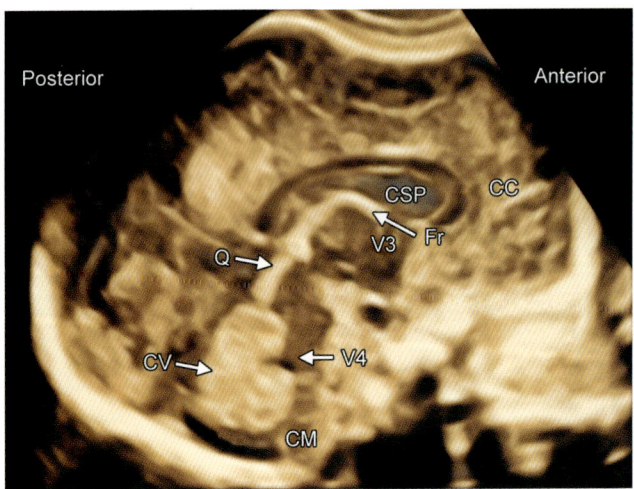

Fig. 19.7: Thick slice view of a volume acquired from a sagittal plane. Structures visualized in this plane are corpus callosum (CC), cavum septi pellucidi (CSP), fornix (Fr), quadrigeminal plate (Q), third (V3) and fourth (V4) ventricle, cerebellar vermis (CV), and cisterna magna (CM).

- The surface mode allows surface demonstration of the median cut plane **(Fig. 19.9A)**. The surface mode HDlive improves 3D images by using adjustable light sources and software that calculates the propagation of the light direction through the surface. Light and shadow enable better understanding of the surface **(Fig. 19.9B)**.[12]

- HDlive silhouette is a new technology that creates a gradient at organ boundaries, fluid-filled cavity and vessel wall, where an abrupt change of the acoustic impedance exists within the tissues.[13] This technique provides vitreous-like clarity demonstration of the different tissues.

HDlive silhouette is the latest modality that can be used in the demonstration of the corpus callosum, but yet there is no additional clinical advantage in comparison with the other modes **(Fig. 19.9C)**.

HOW NOT TO RENDER THE FETAL CORPUS CALLOSUM?

In different publications, it is recommended to reconstruct the corpus callosum from a volume that was acquired from the fronto-occipital plane.[14-18] This always results in a very blurry and hyperechoic demonstration of the corpus callosum, which cannot be assessed precisely. Therefore, 3D reconstruction of sagittal planes from a volume acquired in the fronto-occipital plane or the use of Omniview in the fronto-occipital plane are not recommended **(Figs. 19.10 and 19.11)**.

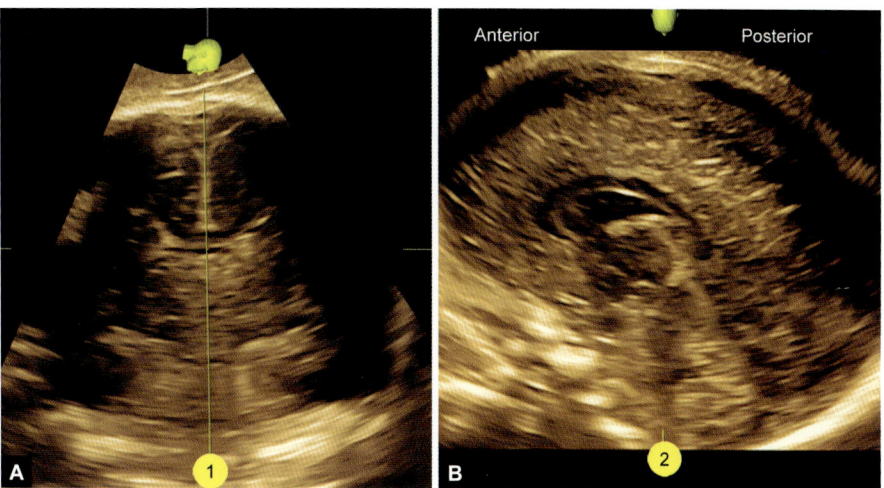

Figs. 19.8A and B: Omniview in a volume acquired from a sagittal plane. (A) Drawing a line between the hemispheres in the coronal plane; (B) demonstrates the corpus callosum as a hypoechoic structure in the perpendicular plane (→).

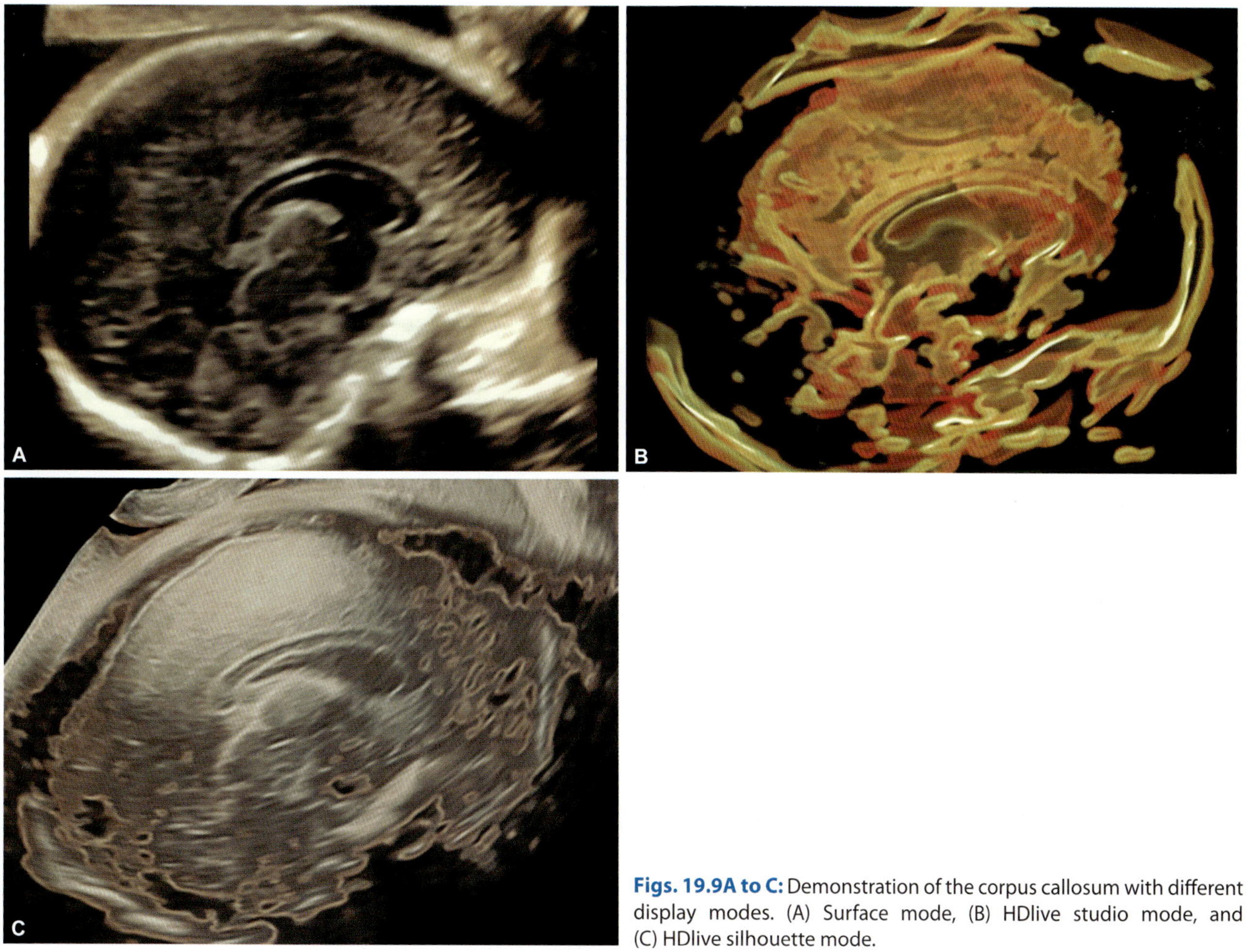

Figs. 19.9A to C: Demonstration of the corpus callosum with different display modes. (A) Surface mode, (B) HDlive studio mode, and (C) HDlive silhouette mode.

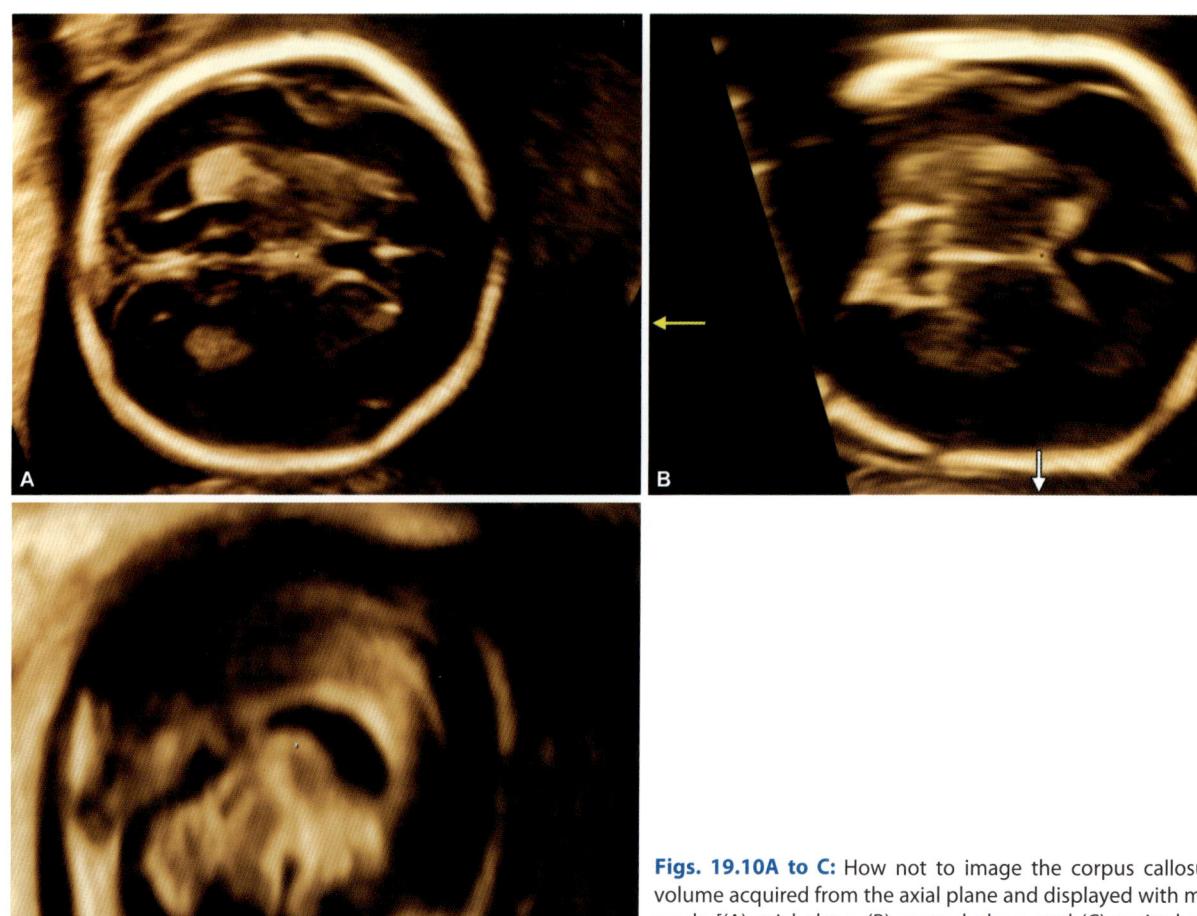

Figs. 19.10A to C: How not to image the corpus callosum? Brain volume acquired from the axial plane and displayed with multiplanar mode [(A) axial plane, (B) coronal plane, and (C) sagittal plane]. The reconstructed sagittal plane (C) reveals the corpus callosum as a hyperechoic instead of hypoechoic structure.

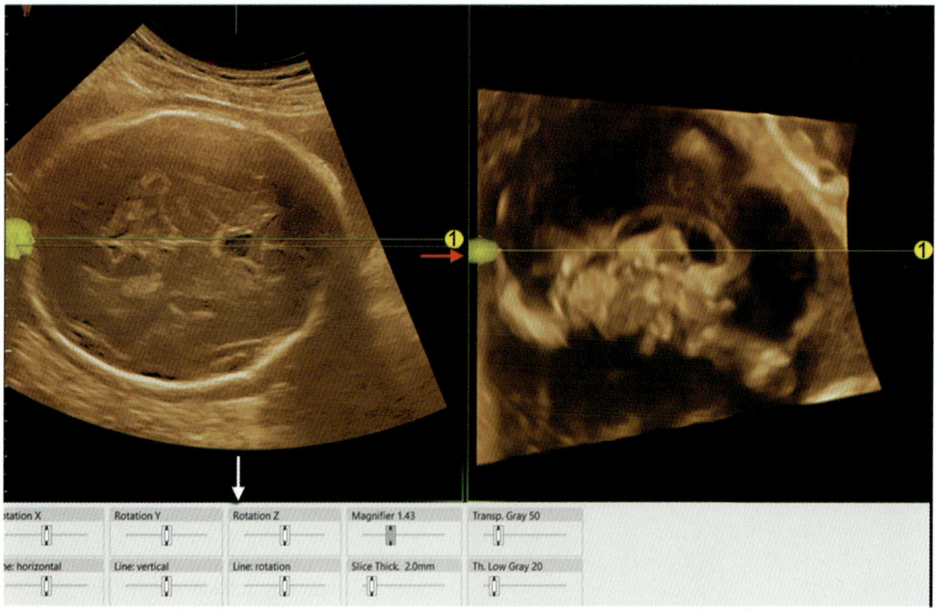

Fig. 19.11: How not to image the corpus callosum? Brain volume acquired from the axial plane. The Omniview + volume contrast imaging (VCI) mode shows the corpus callosum as a hyperechoic instead of hypoechoic structure. 28 weeks gestation.

MEASUREMENTS OF THE CORPUS CALLOSUM

Measurements of the corpus callosum include three different lengths and height (= thickness) of the segments rostrum, genu, body, and splenium.

The rostrum has been defined as a bill-shaped posteriorly or posteroinferiorly oriented segment located at the front part of the corpus callosum. The genu is described as the curved anterior portion of the corpus callosum projecting anteriorly to a line drawn parallel to the posterior part of the fornix and the quadrigeminal plate and starting at the most anterior part of the fornix. The body is defined as a hypoechoic slightly curved horizontal structure, while the splenium is described as the posteriorly oriented portion located at the rear of the corpus callosum.

All measurements of the corpus callosum lengths are performed in the median plane (**Fig. 19.12A**):[3]

- *Curved or traced corpus callosum length (CCL-C)*: Along the length of the corpus callosum by using a trace measurement.
- *Inner–inner corpus callosum length (CCL-II)*: Measurement from the top part of the rostrum to the innermost part of the splenium.
- *Outer–outer corpus callosum length (CCL-OO)*: Measurement from the most anterior part of the genu to the most posterior part of the splenium

Measurements of the height (= thickness) of the different corpus callosum segments can also be performed in the median plane (**Fig. 19.12B**).[3]

A cross-shaped caliper with 0.1 mm resolution is necessary for the described measurements.[3]

PATHOLOGIES OF THE CORPUS CALLOSUM

Disorders of the corpus callosum are among the most complicated neurological birth defects, because many developmental processes are involved until the entire corpus callosum structure is fully formed.[4]

Pathologies of the corpus callosum include complete agenesis of the corpus callosum, partial agenesis of the corpus callosum, hypoplasia, hyperplasia and lipoma of the corpus callosum.[19]

COMPLETE AGENESIS OF CORPUS CALLOSUM

Complete agenesis of corpus callosum (ACC) is the most reported malformation of the corpus callosum in the literature.[20-24] Complete ACC is a nondevelopment of the corpus callosum structure as early as 12 weeks of gestation.[25] Prenatal diagnosis of corpus callosum agenesis includes direct and indirect signs. The indirect signs are the so-called tear drop-shaped ventricles[26] or

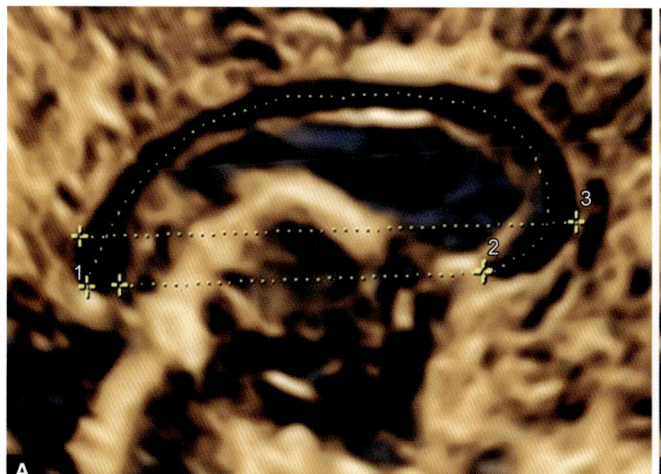 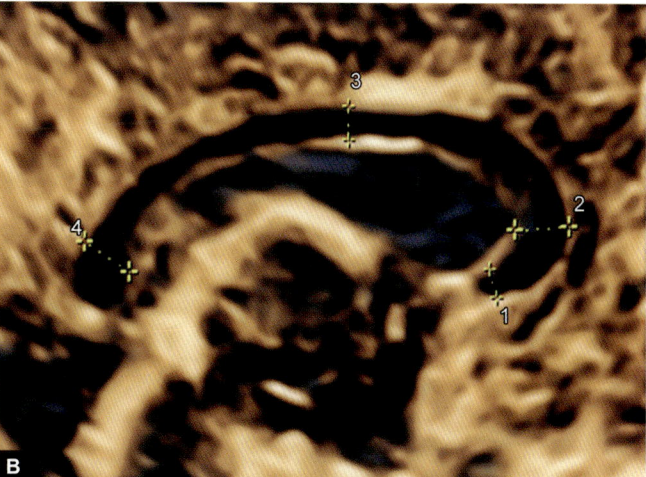

Figs. 19.12A and B: Demonstration of the different corpus callosum measurements in the median plane (27 weeks gestation). (A) Different corpus callosum lengths: (1) Traced (curved) corpus callosum length (CCL-C), (2) inner–inner corpus callosum length (CCL-II), and (3) outer–outer corpus callosum length (CCL-OO). (B) Demonstration of the height (thickness) measurements of the four corpus callosum segments: (1) Rostrum, (2) genu, (3) body, and (4) splenium.

colpocephaly,[27] absent cavum septi pellucidi, viking helmet sign in the coronal plane, high riding third ventricle, and widely separated frontal horns.[28,29] The direct signs include the missing of the corpus callosum in the median plane, as well as in the axial and coronal views **(Fig. 19.13)**.[19]

PARTIAL AGENESIS OF CORPUS CALLOSUM

Partial ACC is diagnosed if at least one of the anatomical segments is missing, while the heights of the present segments are within the normal range and all three

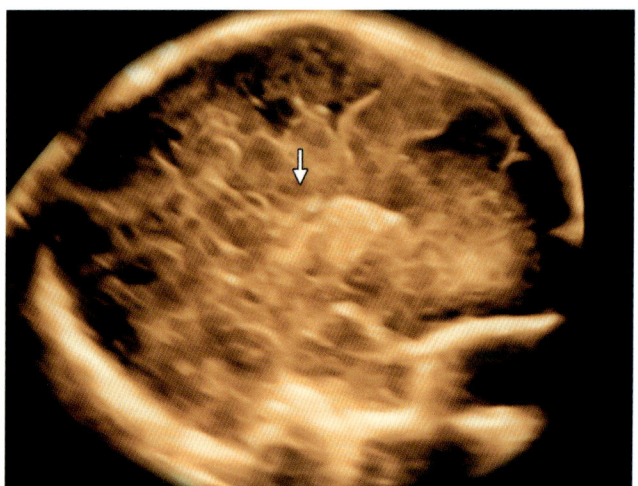

Fig. 19.13: Agenesis of corpus callosum. The surface-rendered image of the median plane shows no corpus callosum (→).

lengths of the corpus callosum are less than the 5th percentile.[3] Partial corpus callosum agenesis can be observed in the anterior part with missing rostrum or genu, in the posterior part with missing body or splenium as well as in middle part with missing body **(Figs. 19.14A to D)**. The indirect signs of the corpus callosum agenesis can be missing. Moreover, a interhemispheric fluid collection, can indicate in some cases the missing posterior part of the corpus callosum. Using 3D ultrasound, this supratentorial fluid collection can be easily differentiated from other midline cystic structures such as cavum veli interpositi or archnoidal cysts.

HYPOPLASIA OF CORPUS CALLOSUM

Hypoplasia is diagnosed when all anatomical segments are present and the height of at least one corpus callosum segment is less than the 5th percentile according to growth charts **(Fig. 19.15)**,[3] while all three lengths are normal or reduced.

HYPERPLASIA OF CORPUS CALLOSUM

Hyperplasia is defined when all anatomical segments are present and the height of at least one corpus callosum segment is found above the 95th percentile according to growth charts,[3] while all three lengths are normal or out of normal range **(Figs. 19.16A to C)**.[19]

Hypoplasia and hyperplasia of the corpus callosum require a precise demonstration of the structure and a proper measurement of the different anatomical parts.

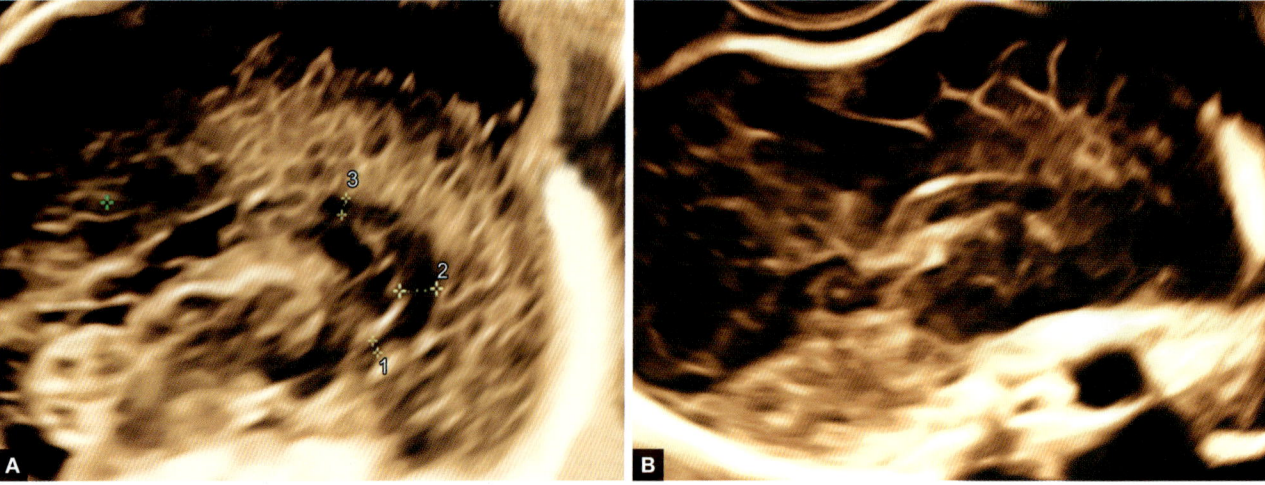

Figs. 19.14A and B

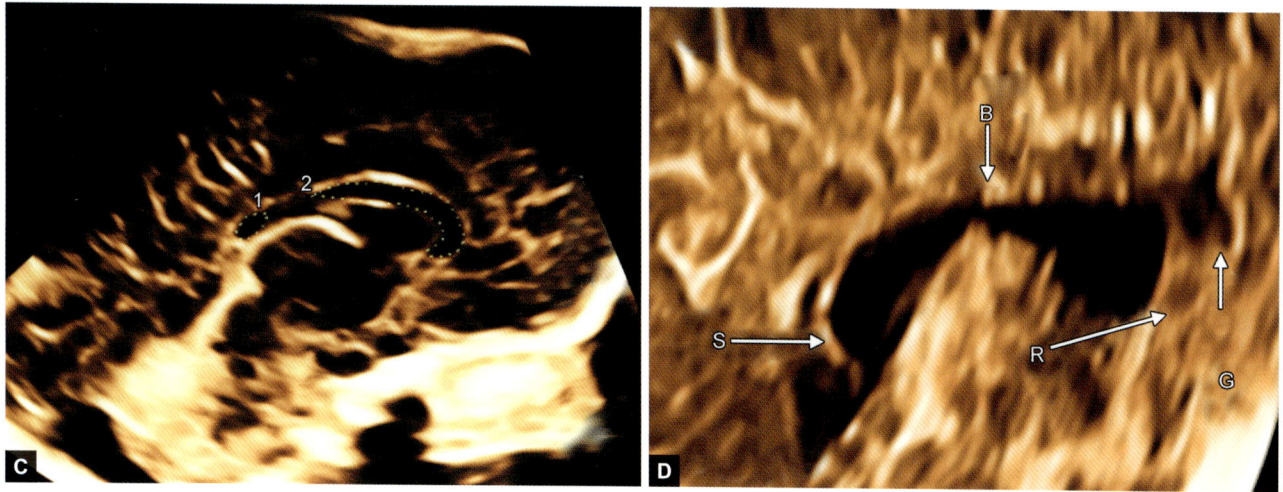

Figs. 19.14C and D

Figs. 19.14A to D: Different types of partial agenesis of corpus callosum. (A) Missing splenium. (B) Missing rostrum and genu. (C) Missing the posterior part of body. (D) Missing the entire body of the corpus callosum (R = rostrum, G = genu, B = missing body, and S = splenium).

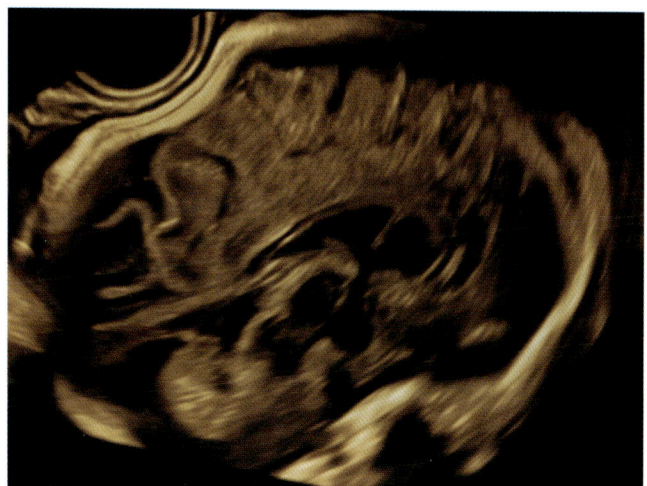

Fig. 19.15: Hypoplasia of the corpus callosum in a case with Apert syndrome. The corpus callosum is too thin.

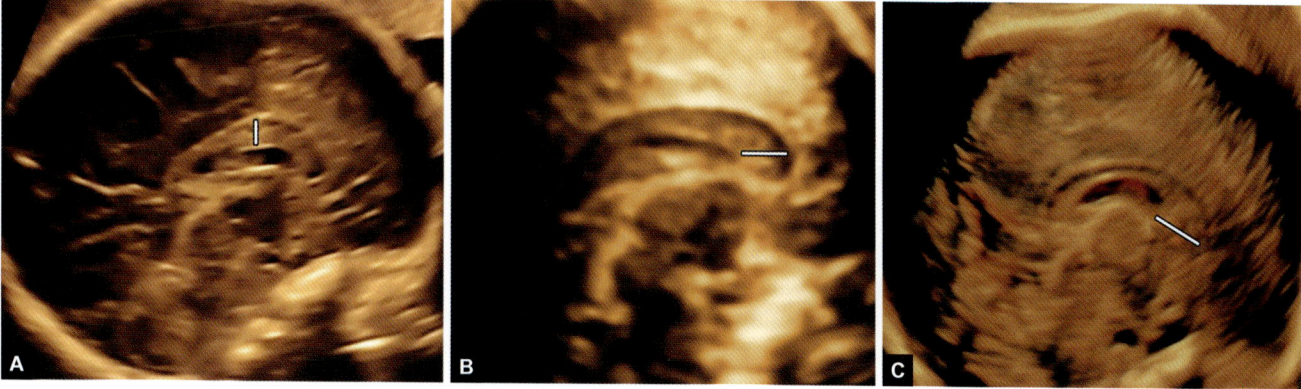

Figs. 19.16A to C: (A) Hyperplasia of the corpus callosum demonstrating thick body, (B) thick genu, and (C) thick genu-rostrum.

CONCLUSION

Corpus callosum is an important landmark of the fetal brain. 3D ultrasound enables an exact demonstration of the normal and abnormal corpus callosum. However, a proper training of examiners, exact use of 3D modalities and a correct image interpretation are needed to avoid diagnostic mistakes in corpus callosum pathologies.

REFERENCES

1. Monteagudo A, Reuss ML, Timor-Tritsch IE. Imaging the fetal brain in the second and third trimester using transvaginal sonography. Obstet Gynecol. 1991;77:27-32.
2. Monteagudo A, Timor-Tritsch IE. Normal sonographic development of the central nervous system from the second trimester onwards using 2D, 3D and transvaginal sonography. Prenat Diag. 2009;29:326-39.
3. Pashaj S, Merz E, Wellek S. Biometric measurements of the fetal corpus callosum by three-dimensional ultrasound. Ultrasound Obstet Gynecol. 2013;42:691-8.
4. Paul LK, Brown WS, Adolphs R, et al. Agenesis of the corpus callosum: genetic, developmental and functional aspects of connectivity. Nat Rev Neurosci. 2007;8:287-99.
5. Paul LK. Developmental malformation of the corpus callosum: a review of typical callosal development and examples of developmental disorders with callosal involvement. J Neurodev Disord. 2011;3:3-37.
6. Ghi T, Carletti E, Cera E, et al. Prenatal diagnosis and outcome of partial agenesis and hypoplasia of the corpus callosum. Ultrasound Obstet Gynecol. 2010;35:35-41.
7. Merz E, Benoit B, Blass GH, et al. Standardization of three-dimensional images in obstetrics and gynecology: consensus statement. Ultrasound Obstet Gynecol. 2007;29:697-703.
8. Monteagudo A, Timor-Tritsch IE, Mayberry P. Three-dimensional transvaginal neurosonography of the fetal brain: "navigating" in the volume scan. Ultrasound Obstet Gynecol. 2000;16:307-13.
9. Timor-Tritsch IE, Monteagudo A, Mayberry P. Three-dimensional ultrasound evaluation of the fetal brain: the three horn view. Ultrasound Obstet Gynecol. 2000;16:302-6.
10. Merz E. Current 3D/4D ultrasound technology in prenatal diagnosis. Eur Clinics Obstet Gynecol. 2005;1:184-93.
11. Rizzo G, Capponi A, Pietrolucci ME, et al. An algorithm based on OmniView technology to reconstruct sagittal and coronal planes of the fetal brain from volume datasets acquired by three-dimensional ultrasound. Ultrasound Obstet Gynecol. 2011;38:158-64.
12. Nebeker J, Nelson R. Imaging of sound speed reflection ultrasound tomography. J Ultrasound Med. 2012;31:1389-404.
13. Pooh R. First trimester scan by 3D, 3D HDlive and HDlive Silhouette/Flow ultrasound imaging. Donald School J Ultras Obstet Gynecol. 2015;9:361-71.
14. Correa FF, Lara C, Bellver J, et al. Examination of the fetal brain by transabdominal three-dimensional ultrasound: potential for routine neurosonographic studies. Ultrasound Obstet Gynecol. 2006;27:503-8.
15. Miguelote FR, Vides B, Santos FR, et al. The role of three-dimensional imaging reconstruction to measure the corpus callosum: comparison with direct mid-sagittal views. Prenat Diagn. 2011;31(9):875-80.
16. Rizzo G, Pietrolucci ME, Capponi A, et al. Assessment of corpus callosum biometric measurement at 18 to 32 weeks' gestation by 3-dimensional sonography. J Ultrasound Med. 2011;30:47-53.
17. Pilu G, Segata M, Ghi T, et al. Diagnosis of midline anomalies of the fetal brain with the three-dimensional median view. Ultrasound Obstet Gynecol. 2006;27:522-9.
18. Youssef A, Ghi T, Pilu G. How to image the fetal corpus callosum. Ultrasound Obstet Gynecol. 2013;42:718-20.
19. Pashaj S, Merz E. Detection of fetal corpus callosum abnormalities by means of 3D Ultrasound. Ultraschall Med. 2016;37:185-94.
20. Comstock CH, Culp D, Gonzalez J, et al. Agenesis of the corpus callosum in the fetus: its evolution and significance. J Ultrasound Med. 1985;4:613-6.
21. Bedeschi MF, Bonaglia MC, Grasso R, et al. Agenesis of the corpus callosum: clinical and genetic study in 63 young patients. Pediatr Neurol. 2006;34:186-93.
22. Fratelli N, Papageorghiou AT, Prefumo F, et al. Outcome of prenatally diagnosed agenesis of the corpus callosum. Prenat Diagn. 2007;27:512-7.
23. Moes P, Schilmoeller K, Schillmoer G. Physical, motor, sensory and developmental features associated with agenesis of the corpus callosum. Child Care Health Dev. 2009;5:656-72.
24. Sotiriadis A, Makrydimas G. Neurodevelopment after prenatal diagnosis of isolated agenesis of the corpus callosum: an integrative review. Am J Obstet Gynecol. 2012;206:337.e1-337.c5.
25. Paupe A, Bidat L, Sonigo P, et al. Prenatal diagnosis of hypoplasia of the corpus callosum in association with non-ketotic hyperglycinemia. Ultrasound Obstet Gynecol. 2002;20:616-9.
26. Oh KY. Absent cavum septi pellucidi. In: Woodward P, Kennedy A, Sohaey R, Byrne J, Oh K, Puchalski M (Eds). Diagnostic Imaging: Obstetrics. Salt Lake City, UT: Amirsys, Inc.; 2006. pp. 54-5.
27. Filly RA, Cardoza JD, Goldstein RB, et al. Detection of fetal central nervous system anomalies: a practical level of effort for a routine sonogram. Radiology. 1989;172:403-8.
28. Barkovich AJ. Congenital malformations of the brain and skull. Pediatric Neuroimaging. 3rd edition. Philadelphia: Lippincott Williams & Wilkins; 2000. pp. 251-381.
29. Pilu G, Sandri F, Perolo A, et al. Sonography of fetal agenesis of the corpus callosum: a survey of 35 cases. Ultrasound Obstet Gynecol. 1993;3:318-29.

Three-dimensional Ultrasound and Maternal Bonding

Leonid M Rovner, Katelyn T Horton, Mishella I Perez, Dolores H Pretorius

INTRODUCTION

Maternal–fetal bonding is a natural phenomenon that develops over the course of the pregnancy and peaks shortly after the child is born.[1] This process is believed to have been accelerated through modern technologies, such as the popular use of ultrasound in obstetrical and perinatal care **(Fig. 20.1)**.[2] This earlier start to the maternal–fetal bonding originates through earlier interaction and visualization of the fetus.[3] This process is increasingly important, as a strong correlation exists between the development of a secure relationship with the parent in the early years of life and better cognitive outcomes, social acuity, and school performance.[4] As a result of this phenomenon, studies into the factors that affect an increase in bonding and effectiveness of

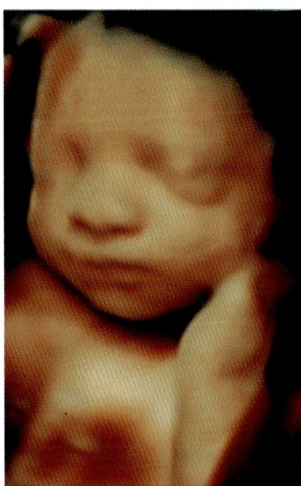

Fig. 20.1: Normal fetal face at 29 weeks of gestational age. 3D US-rendered image of fetal face. A three-dimensional ultrasound fetal face image provides an understandable picture to the parents and allows a mental image to be formed of their child.

increased bonding in altering the mother's behavior for health reasons have become more prevalent.

"Attachment" and "bonding" are terms that are often used interchangeably in both colloquial and scientific and literary settings, especially those concerning ultrasound and fetal psychology. In actuality, "bonding" refers to the parental bond for the child, whereas "attachment" is the child's bond with the parents or primary caregivers, which develops gradually over time.[5] Conversely, "bonding" tends to occur more quickly, specifically within the first few hours or days after birth; today the bonding process begins during pregnancy. To follow this convention, within this paper, "bonding" will refer to the parent's relationship with the fetus.

Three-dimensional ultrasound (3D US) imaging not only impacts parents but also siblings, grandparents, extended family, and friends. Patients, family, and friends often feel like they received a "state-of-the-art" exam when 3D images were performed during diagnostic exams. The purpose of this chapter is to review the effectiveness of 3D/4D US on bonding of parents to their fetuses in comparison to 2D US.

BACKGROUND OF ULTRASOUND TECHNOLOGY

As the central obstetric tool, ultrasound has undergone various improvements that have affected the dynamic of bonding between parent and the child. 2D US is the technique of using single slice images, sometimes in a video clip, to display a single plane of fetal anatomy. The transducer must be moved in various planes and through multiple angles to allow for the viewer to imagine how the fetus appears **(Figs. 20.2A and B)**. This method is the fundamental use of diagnostic imaging, and its

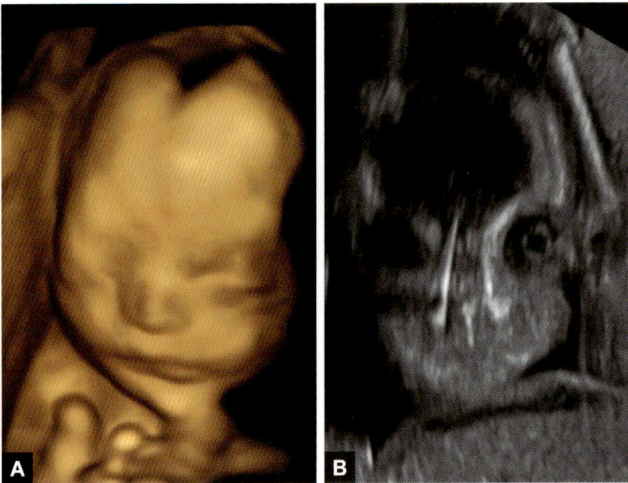

Figs. 20.2A and B: Normal fetal face at 22 weeks of gestational age. (A) 3D ultrasound-rendered image of fetal face provides a more understandable picture to the parents and allows a mental image to be formed of their child more easily in comparison to 2D ultrasound. (B) 2D ultrasound face image of same fetus.

functionality remains such that it will continue to remain in use well into the future. 3D US is the use of a mechanical scanning system to recreate a 3D image **(Fig. 20.1)** by compiling multiple 2D images with a computer in real time. This method has potential to be of additional benefit to 2D US due to easier recognition of physical deformities, easier understanding by laypeople and the possibility of increase in parental bonding **(Figs. 20.2A and B)**. 4D US is functionally very similar to 3D US; it displays a 3D volume that is consistently updated, creating the appearance that the object is moving.[6] This process is similar to a film, thus videos of the fetus can be seen, allowing easier and more accurate documentation of fetal movement.

Various 3D US images of the fetus impact the parents. Although the fetal face **(Figs. 20.3A to G)** is most commonly commented on by parents, other anatomies such as the spine, hands, and feet **(Figs. 20.4A and B)** are also important in the bonding process.

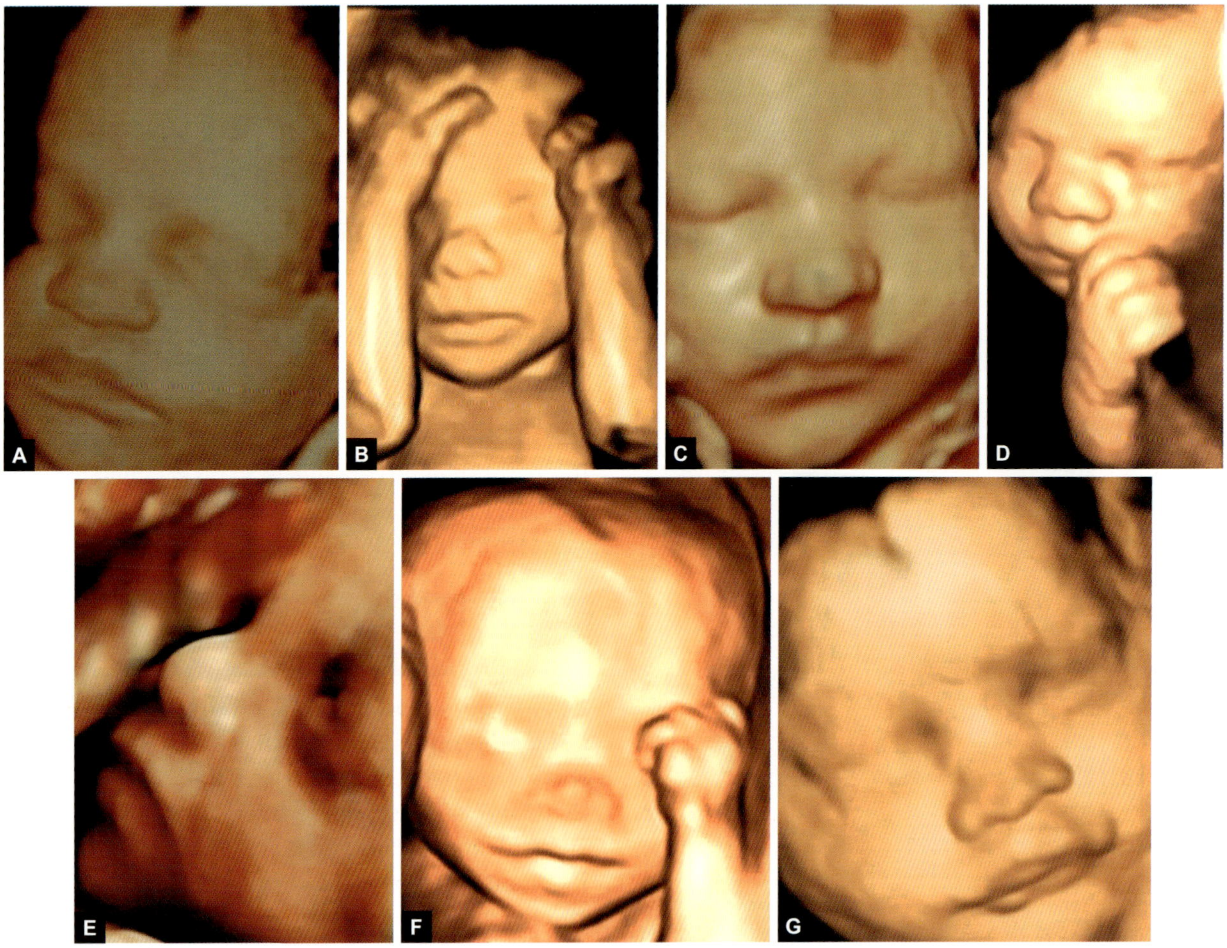

Figs. 20.3A to G: Collage of 3D-rendered images of fetal faces showing clarity of images that allows bonding between parents and fetus.

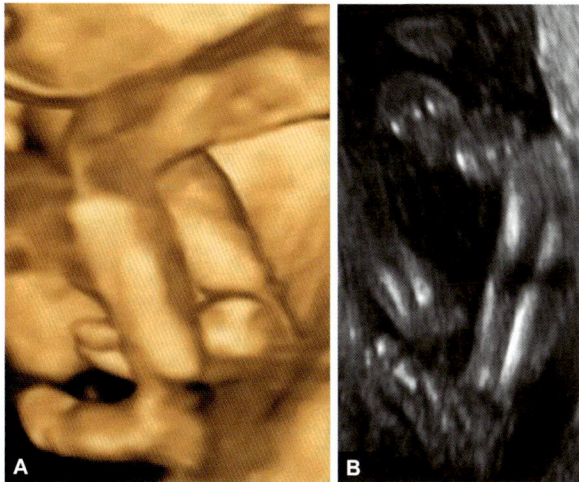

Figs. 20.4A and B: Normal fetal legs at 14 weeks. (A) 3D ultrasound-rendered image of normal fetal ankles. The ankles are understandable to the layperson and may reduce anxiety to ensure that the fetus is healthy. (B) 2D ultrasound image of normal fetal ankle. Such images are standard images obtained to evaluate for fetal anomalies.

TWO-DIMENSIONAL ULTRASOUND

Two-dimensional ultrasound and its effect on bonding has been studied by multiple investigators over the years. In 1980, Kohn et al. showed that out of 100 women who had received 2D US, the majority felt that they were more attached to their fetus, and some also reported that there was a greater degree of vulnerability to the possible outcomes of the pregnancy.[7] Milne and Rich reported that midwives found through small observational studies, an increase in maternal–fetal bonding in mothers after being shown 2D US of the fetus.[8]

In 1986, Hyde (1986) studied the impact of selective ultrasound (patients opted into having an ultrasound study) and routine ultrasound (scans performed as part of routine care) scanning and its effect on maternal expectations and maternal–fetal bonding.[9] The authors compared one hospital (Hospital R) with routine scanning (100 subjects) and another hospital (Hospital S) with selective scanning (315 subjects). In Hospital R with routine scanning, women placed higher expectations for reassurance in the ultrasound scan, seeing it as essential, whereas the women in the selected scanning group at Hospital S were less significantly affected by unimpressive results. The study found that an increased number of ultrasound exams per patient had no statistically significant effect on the maternal–fetal bonding process. In addition, a major source of reassurance for women was

the confirmation of the physical well-being of the child. In regard to reassurance, 87% of the scanned patients from Hospital S had positive responses on attitudes to scanning in comparison to unscanned patients of whom only 45% had reassurance from a manual examination at an office visit; in Hospital R, 85% of the scanned patients had positive responses, whereas 91% had a positive response with only a manual examination.[9]

In 2002, Whynes reported the largest single study cohort of 384 pregnant women (989 ultrasound scans over pregnancy), and 98% of the women having had at least two scans performed, that 94% showed positive responses to 2D US images, 63% of women input the highest satisfaction score, and only 6.4% had any negative feelings about the scans.[10]

Feedback from the sonographer or medical provider performing the scan is important. In a study performed in London of 129 mothers, Reading and Cox found that in low-risk pregnancies "high-feedback" examinations were more effective in reducing anxiety in the mothers and ensuring adherence to the prescribed regimen of medical tests, whereas a low-feedback examination was in danger of providing the opposite effect, i.e. providing a lack of reassurance to the mother.[11] It should be noted, however, that no long-term statistically significant effect was found between the two groups in anxiety after the examinations.[11] Hyde's (1986) study corroborates this effect with finding 72 of 243 women being dissatisfied with their scan, with a noncommunicative operator.[9]

Multiple other variables have been studied in their effect on maternal/fetal bonding. Kemp and Page found in a study of 85 women during their third trimester that attachment (bonding) levels had no significant differences between women in high- and low-risk pregnancies.[12] In addition, no correlation was found between attachment scores and age, race, education level, or whether the fetus was planned. Due to the small sample size and the nature of high-risk pregnancies, the authors mention that the results could have been affected with women being more attached due to being confident in the survival of their fetus, and they may have been in denial about possible concerns. Finally, Kemp and Page suggested that early involvement may hasten the prenatal bonding with the fetus, but ultimately, the effect will not be different in the long term.[12]

Regular screening was shown to result in multiple fetal health benefits due to mothers' reduced participation in activities harmful to the fetus (e.g. smoking, drugs), after seeing the fetus on screen. In a cohort of 2,482 pregnant women with no planned elective ultrasound at 12 gestation weeks, the researchers found that screening reduced the rate of inductions of labor by 2% (3.7% to 1.7%),[13] mean birth weight was higher, and fewer children were born with low birth weights. This change was attributed to women reducing the amount of smoking performed, as they "were strongly affected by watching their fetus on screen."[13]

2D US VERSUS 3D US

Whilst comparing 2D US with 3D US in respect to maternal–fetal bonding, studies have had mixed results. As early as 1998, Nelson and Pretorius remarked on the positive features of 3D US in cardiology, and how it was likely to expand into obstetrics with its ability to view fetal structures, especially the fetal face.[2] 3D US provided a more recognizable image to the layperson and a grander range of identifiable anomalies in the fetus **(Fig. 20.3)**. In addition, occasionally multiplanar imaging allowed anomalies to be seen on 3D US that were not visible on 2D US. They found that 3D US could "demonstrate normal development and reassure parents that all was well."[2]

In a comparison between 2D and 2/3D US of 100 second and third trimester high-risk pregnancies, statistical significances favoring 3D US were found in various categories by Ji et al. **(Fig. 20.2)**.[14] The majority of mothers felt that seeing their child on the scan had "created a closer relationship with their child"; the data also suggested that this feeling was slightly more common in the 3D US group (88%) than the 2D US group (83%). Both groups had an overall positive ultrasound experience with both 2D US (68%) and 3D US (84%). No significant difference was found between these two groups, but women from the 3D US were more exclamatory with their remarks, and these women were more likely to share these images. The frequency of photograph sharing (3D US—median 27 people vs. 2D US—median 11 people) and verbalized similarities between mother and fetus by those who saw the images showed a significant difference favoring 3D US. Furthermore, 82% of 3D US-scanned mothers formed a mental image of their baby, compared with 39% of 2D US subjects. Moreover, 70% of mothers felt that they "knew their baby" after the scan, compared with 56% of mothers after a 2D US scan. The researchers found that gestational age had no impact on maternal bonding. However, some mothers experienced dissatisfaction with the images, in which 8% of the 3D US and 5% of the 2D US groups expressed negative comments with the chief complaint of the images being suboptimal.[14]

De Jong-Pleijj et al. (2012) also found benefits of 3D US in comparison with 2D US. In the third trimester, 160 Caucasian women were evaluated before and after seeing a fetal face with either 2D or 3D/4D US using the maternal antenatal attachment score (MAAS). The groups were separated into MAAS1 (before US) and MAAS2 (after US). Within both groups, MAAS2 scores rose, with a statistically significant increase in visibility and recognition after 3D US, in comparison with 2D US. In addition, the MAAS2 scores were conflicting for 3D US, and no statistically significant effect was observed between 2D US and 3D US in the reduction of anxiety.[15]

In 2006, Pretorius et al. studied the effect of 3D/4D US on 65 fathers and 124 mothers and found a statistically significant increase in bonding after the ultrasound.[16] This effect was discovered using Cranley's MFA questionnaire before and after the appointment (with blinding of the initial score), the Likert scale to test for positive feelings, and a line test denoting excitement before and after the 3D/4D US appointment. Both mothers and fathers indicated a statistically significant increase in bonding after the examination; however, fathers showed a significant difference for only two questions, while mothers had five such questions. While this suggests that mothers and fathers bond with the fetus differently, all five of the questions were Type 1, which the study denoted as questions relating to the parent's imagination, curiosity, and wonder toward the fetus. Men experienced a statistically significant increase in excitement with the line test, whilst women did not, but this was due to the median response of women already being at the maximum reading preexamination.[16]

In 2005, Rustico et al. reported similar findings in a study of 100 women of a mean of 21 gestational weeks comparing 2D US and 2D/4D results using MAAS scores.[17] There was no statistically significant difference between the overall satisfaction of the scan, or a positive change in the perception of the fetus between the two groups, even though over 90% of patients were satisfied with the scan in both groups. Group 2 (2D/4D US) had larger scores in the categories of positive perception change, quality, intensity, and global attachment scores, with the last three almost doubling in comparison to the solely 2D US group, but no statistically significant relationship was present between the two groups in these scores. In addition, while 4D US had clear visual impact, the images obtained could be inferior to maternal expectations which would result in disappointment or additional anxiety.[17]

A 2007 study of 60 second and third trimester mothers found that 87.5% of mothers preferred 3D US over 2D US, even though 2D US had slightly better quality of images performed. In addition, mothers had difficulty in visualizing the fetus in 2D US compared to 3D US which was statistically significant. However, no significant impact in maternal–fetal bonding after 3D US was detected, despite mothers preferring 3D US. This effect may be due to a high preexisting level of attachment to the fetus, which would lessen the effect.[18]

In addition, Hull et al. found no significant difference in increases of maternal–fetal bonding between 3D US and 2D US in a sample cohort of 36 patients, despite the fact that both 2D US and 3D US increased bonding postexamination.[19] In fact, bonding steadily increased throughout pregnancy in all patients.

As well as gaining an increased acuity for how the fetus appears, parents showed a statistically significant difference in drawings of their fetuses before and after 3D/4D US.[20] Out of 100 parents (32 males, 68 females) who drew their fetuses before and after the 3D US examination, 23–56% were identified as statistically significant by reviewers, 41–64% showed a slight difference, and 2–22% showed no significant difference. Differences were related to "extremity positioning, personalized uterine environment, and artistic nature." Reviewers familiar with ultrasonography could predict which drawing was drawn first in 78%, and reviewers unfamiliar with ultrasonography correctly predicted which drawing was drawn first in 35% to 51%. No statistically significant difference was identified between mothers and fathers in their drawings.[20]

PATERNAL BONDING

Current studies into paternal bonding with their children are few in number, with the majority of research focusing on the expectant mothers. Out of 28 studies reviewed, 11% studied paternal bonding.[21] This disproportionality may be, in part, due to the more difficult nature of recording paternal bonding and that different criteria may be needed. The extent of the development of the relationship

of the father with the fetus is unclear during pregnancy; and thus, it is unclear how much of it can be changed. However, the lack of social support and harmful behaviors to the fetus exerted by the mother (e.g. smoking) have shown to negatively affect the formation of such a bond, whereas emotional maturity and a marital satisfaction both increased the level of bonding for both parents.[21]

Various qualitative studies have suggested that ultrasound scans may have an equally large effect in paternal bonding as maternal bonding with the fetus.[22] Draper suggests that ultrasound may be an effective platform to increase paternal bonding as it eliminates the abstract nature of the fetus.[23] Thus, the ultrasound can be the father's first "real" interaction with the fetus, and it may be the most memorable event of the pregnancy. Draper concludes that this ubiquitous feeling exhibited by men is due to a lack of interaction with the fetus through touch, instead substituting it through vision. Therefore ultrasound could act as both a medical and a social event by allowing further parental participation. Walsh et al. (2014) concludes that ultrasound can be used as a major event to enhance paternal feelings toward the fetus.[22]

However, Righetti et al. found in a study of 44 couples that maternal–fetal bonding increased after 2D and 4D US, similar to many other studies.[24] However, the fathers actually had a decrease in bonding after the 2D US scan and experienced a significant increase in bonding only after the 4D US scan.

Certain groups appear to receive extremely beneficial levels of reassurance after a 3D US scan, in our experience at University of California San Diego (UCSD). These cases are seen in hospice patients, surrogate patients, and their intended parents, patients with infertility or mothers whose children have had prior or current anomalies and have a family history of anomalies or even experienced a previous fetal death.

CONFOUNDING FACTORS

Johnston and Vögele note that the ceiling effect can obscure differences between groups in terms of pain and levels of satisfaction that differences between groups become indifferentiable.[25] Johnston and Vögele found that psychological methods, such as measuring patient's assessments on helpfulness, communication, nursing care, and nursing, provided with a clear effort to repeat the pattern of care. All of these methods showed an increase in satisfaction and could be used to confirm and reproduce the studies performed, and account for differences in patient care for reproducibility.[25]

In Kowalcek et al.'s study, 140 pregnant women, and in 108 cases, their partners were surveyed for stress ratings before and after screening procedures, both invasive (amniocentesis) and noninvasive (ultrasound).[26] It was found that on average, men had statistically significant smaller levels of stress in comparison with the mothers, and after the operations, both men and women in both groups had significant decreases in stress.[26] Glover and Capron (2017) have shown that maternal stress increases the likelihood of altered neurodevelopmental outcomes, with mothers of stress levels in the top 15th percentile doubling the risk for negative consequences.[27] This further shifts the necessity of fully understanding 3D US impact on maternal–fetal bonding, since any psychological impact could turn into medical realities, and preventing those would be extremely beneficial.

In addition, these studies could also be affected by the parents' upbringings and current mental state. Lindgren studied a cohort of 252 adult pregnant women and found that those with higher education and in relationships had higher levels of maternal–fetal bonding, but those with high levels of depression developed the inverse, with lower levels of prenatal bonding.[28] A Swedish study of 100 pregnant women found that women with positive emotions expressed from their mothers during their childhood had a positive association in developing the same bond with their children.[29]

Scharf et al. found that out of 433 ultrasounds on fetuses, 3D US was able to provide a distinguishable image to identify gender in 7.9% of cases, compared to 2D US 95%, and in only one case did 3D US provide a superior image to that of 2D US in identifying a malformation.[30] However, in a cohort of 3,472 fetuses where 2D US and 3D US were used in adjunct to identify fetal anomalies, of which 1,012 were found; Merz et al. found that 3D US was advantageous in 60.8% of cases, compared with 42 out of 1,012 found solely via 3D US.[31] Thus, it was concluded that 3D US should best be used in conjunction with 2D US, instead of a replacement. We suspect that the maximal effect on bonding of 3D US would be to use in conjunction with 2D US, instead of as a replacement.

PUBLIC OPINION ABOUT 3D US

Overall, there are many supporting points for using 3D US medically and to help facilitate maternal, and paternal bonding prenatally. The reassurance that couples gain from looking at realistic images of their growing fetuses has been shown to decrease stress in the parent and increase bonding to the infant and has positive psychological effects that are virtually unmatched during a time where so little of the growth and health can otherwise be visually observed. The current research briefly assesses the perceived psychological effect of 3D US on nonpregnant college students and a convention of doctors and sonographers.

In a study conducted at UCSD, 137 nonpregnant college students viewed a video tape of both 3D US and 2D US on a 30-week-old fetus.[32] The rationale for this substudy was to gain a better understanding of the impact of 3D US versus 2D US from an objective perspective. Of these 137 participants, 72% reported that they felt 3D US would have a positive effect on parental fetal bonding, while 18% said that 3D US would have either no effect or a negative effect, and 9% were uncertain as to whether 3D US would affect parental bonding. No significant difference in responses between men and women within this sample was found. Importantly, 83% of this sample reported that they would personally request a 3D US in their future pregnancy due to reasons that include having the unique ability to visualize a detailed image of their fetus, increasing their chances for more accurate anomaly detection, gaining reassurance during pregnancy, and filling the curiosity of what is going on within their own or their partners' bodies. Finally, 97% reported that they believed 3D US was an important diagnostic tool. These reports of unbiased and uninvolved adults help show that 3D US fetal scans would likely have a positive effect on parental bonding, participants prefer themselves to have a 3D (vs. 2D) scan during pregnancy, and that 3D US is an important diagnostic tool.[32]

To further investigate the need for 3D US, 520 sonographers and sonologists were surveyed after a 45-minute lecture on 3D US in obstetrics using slides and multimedia videos given at several national meetings.[32] Of these 520, 314 were medical doctors, 184 were sonographers, and 22 were classified as something other than a doctor or sonographer. When asked whether they thought that 3D US would contribute to providing reassurance to pregnant women, 74% felt that it would. When asked about a future pregnancy, 57% reported a desire to have a 3D US themselves (or on their partner), and 32% of the sample did not respond. Rationale for the desire to have the scan included both medical reasons and reassurance.

Gender, age, or career did not have a significant effect on the perception of 3D US.[32]

One of the most remarkable and touching outcomes of 3D US, however, has been observed in parents who have a fetus with an anomaly. 3D US has allowed families at UCSD who have affected fetuses to gain a more comprehensive understanding of the anomaly itself, from a cleft lip and palate to clubfeet. Through this scan, the family can visually observe the other normal aspects of the fetus which can help reduce stress and heighten bonding. Some mothers find comfort in connecting with the baby during pregnancy through these special images when they otherwise could not have seen the fetal face and may have otherwise felt negatively toward the fetus. Some mothers noted that the anomaly sounded much worse than it actually appeared via 3D US. This aspect of 3D US alone has alleviated much worry and pain in families who can only think of the abnormality in their child without having the opportunity to understand how otherwise healthy and beautiful their infant will be.

While it can be difficult to truly assess parental bonding to their fetuses, the current research proposes many valuable reasons to consider including 3D US as a routine diagnostic tool, as well as providing psychological relief and reassurance. While there are some points supporting 2D over 3D scans, the overwhelmingly positive responses to 3D US from many investigators speaks to the impact that 3D US could have if adopted and used as an adjunct to 2D US. Therefore, as the public becomes further aware of this technology, and with growing trends of "scanning for entertainment,"[33] the utilization of 3D US and its effects should be better understood diagnostically and psychologically.

NEGATIVE ASPECTS OF 3D US

Despite the influential applications of 3D US in familial reassurance and stimulating parental bonding, it is important to acknowledge the negative reactions toward both 3D US and 2D US to adequately consider potential pitfalls. Importantly, negative factors related to each technique are discussed below.

First, 3D US has been growing in commercial popularity which facilitates a seemingly nonmedical environment, but which also lacks highly trained sonographers, and brings to light many safety and productivity issues. As previously mentioned, there are many problems with this as it is not advised to have an ultrasound conducted by uncertified medical providers. Potential negative effects of the sonographic equipment must also be considered. In order to obtain the 3D US images, energy is released from the ultrasound machine as heat,[34] and because it has potential to cause rare birth effects, extending the duration of the scan in order to obtain clearer and better images for the parents or family could increase risk to the fetus.[35] Of note, 3D US has similar power levels as 2D US. It is important to remember that pulsed and color Doppler have higher power levels than grayscale imaging; this can be important if sonographers spend too much time scanning the fetal heart with color Doppler when they cannot see other structures (e.g. face) due to poor image quality.

Second, 3D US can be difficult to reach image perfection, or even satisfaction resulting from fetal ultrasound. According to Campbell, problems in visualization result during early gestational age, when adjacent structures cast shadows on other parts of the fetal body, and when there is inadequate amniotic fluid adjacent to the fetus.[33] Potential problems with these factors could include misdiagnoses, misidentifications, and falsely negative interpretations of the fetus by the mother or family based solely on appearance. It would be important to notify the family of these potential drawbacks prior to conducting a 3D US scan to help reduce stress. According to Ciatti, in today's day and age, images seen on a television screen are perceived as absolute truth and all other parts of the fetus that cannot be seen on the screen are doubted or perceived as missing.[36] Interestingly, this demonstrates the gravity of showing a very real 3D image to a mother or family because everything seen will be acknowledged as true and everything missing will be doubted. This is unfortunate for the cases where there are other biological interferences that affect the way the image output appears and can bring stress or fear to a mother. Campbell remedies this issue by supporting 4D US as opposed to 3D US and claims that it is more successful in obtaining adequate photos,[33] which would result in less psychological distress due to faulty images. When transducer pressure on the maternal abdomen is excessive, which is often necessary to make sure that the sonographer obtains a "perfect" image of the fetus, considerations for maternal and fetal health may lose priority.

Third, some investigators claim that 3D US did not offer any additional psychological benefits not offered by 2D US.[37] This finding reflects controversy from various

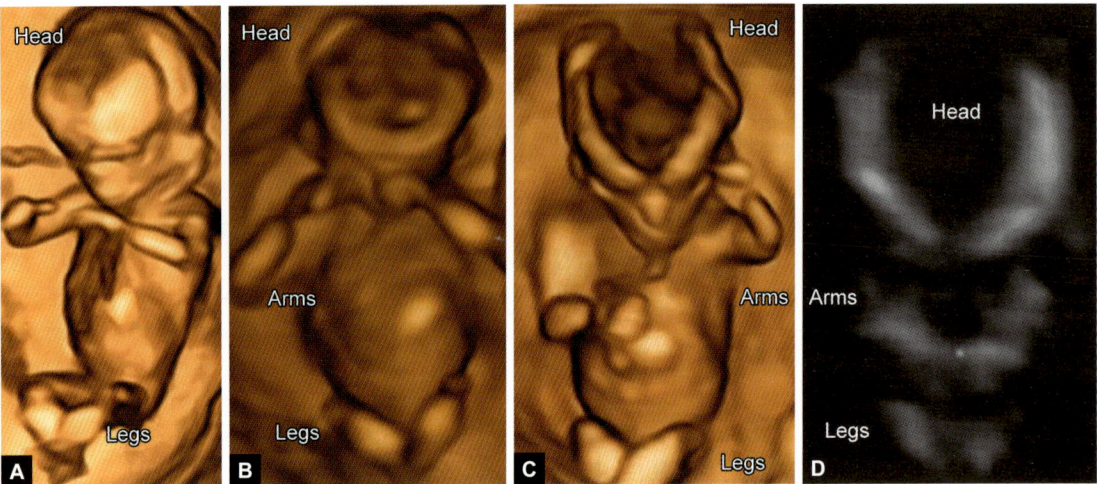

Figs. 20.5A to D: Devil-like images of normal fetuses at 12–13 weeks of gestational age. (A) 3D ultrasound of fetus at 12 weeks 3 days. (B) 3D ultrasound of fetus at 12 weeks 2 days. (C) 3D ultrasound of fetus at 12 weeks 3 days. (D) 2D ultrasound of fetus at 13 weeks 2 days. Many patients declare that their fetus may resemble a devil due to the cranium producing a horned or V-shaped structure. This may induce additional anxiety and fear in the mother if not prefaced or explained by the medical practitioner as images appear on the screen.

authors who have found 3D US to offer benefits in parental bonding (see above).

Fourth, some 3D US images can be interpreted by parents as scary or worrisome. For example, in the first trimester, the fetal cranium has a "V-shaped" appearance, and many parents comment that it appears like the devil (**Figs. 20.5A to D**); this can be prevented by the sonographer performing the study commenting on the beautiful appearance of the fetus and noting how the cranial bones are normally formed.

Fifth, when 3D US is conducted in a medical setting, professionals are asked to conduct extended and extensive viewing sessions of the fetus, and this cuts time that they could be serving other patients in need.[38]

Sixth, 3D US and fertility spotlights the polarizing argument for or against women's reproductive freedom.[39] 3D US brings the fetus out of the dark and into an image; in doing this, the perception of the fetus changes to a patient itself because of the ability to visualize it.[40] Uniquely, 3D US generates a more anatomically realistic image of the growing fetus,[41] which creates visual rhetoric for the pro-life opinion that abortion is murder and makes it difficult for pregnant mothers to overcome threats and additional stress-inducing barriers.[40] This aspect of 3D US could cause emotional and familial distress for a mother who may want to abort but feels pressure against it. Further, this could lead to more births of unwanted infants with severe cultural, social, and medical implications.

NEGATIVE ASPECTS OF 2D US

Two-dimensional ultrasound, while widely used and accepted, has still received some negative backlash. These arguments range from the technological aspects of the scan to the need for standardization.

First, based on the nature of the 2D scan, some added degree of difficulty is required in obtaining a 2D image of a 3D object because a challenge arises in attempting to imagine the flat computerized image inside of a human body.[42] Any form of dimension transformation from the real world to a flat image can pose problems in diagnosis, treatment, and spatial understanding.

Second, a lack of standardization in scanning techniques across the United States implies that different sonographers potentially produce very different images; this, in turn, could make for extreme difficulty in obtaining adequate diagnoses and understanding.[43] With the first medical use of an ultrasound machine dating back to 1942, the continued lack of standardization forms an argument against 2D US and supporting a newer technique.[44]

Third, discrepancies between measurements acquired by 3D US and 2D US have been reported.[45] Some 3D US volumetric measurements of the fetal lung may be less accurate than routine 2D US measurements.[45] These are important factors in understanding other considerations that could promote or deter medical professionals from prioritizing bonding.

These contrasting viewpoints show that there may not be a clear-cut, unanimous preference for 3D over 2D US. There may be situations where each method is favored as the primary diagnostic technique depending on the health of the fetus and mother, as well as on the need for parental bonding.

CONTROVERSY OF DOING 3D FOR ENTERTAINMENT VERSUS REASSURANCE

As 3D US has become increasingly common in medical diagnosis, controversies about the extent of its proper usage in other realms emerged. These contentions range across various fields from marketing and safety[3] to culture and politics.[46] The American Institute of Ultrasound in Medicine (AIUM) and Food and Drug Administration (FDA) take especially standout stances against using ultrasound for entertainment. The AIUM "strongly discourages the nonmedical use of ultrasound for psychosocial or entertainment purposes" in a press release in April 2004.[47] The two main risks that the AIUM addresses are predominantly related to (1) possible negative bioeffects related to ultrasound power levels on both grayscale and color Doppler imaging, and prolonged scanning by insufficiently trained technicians (e.g. technicians that perform entertainment ultrasound often have 2 weeks of training, whereas diagnostic sonographers have at least 1 year of training and certification from the American Registry for Diagnostic Medical Sonography) and (2) potential for a false sense of security since patients often think of these "entertainment" exams as diagnostic.[47] Similarly, the FDA suggests limiting 3D US solely to serve medical needs, recognizing its contribution to bonding.[48]

Both organizations concretely oppose fetal keepsake videos lacking medical necessity due to undefined scan length and risk of operational misuse when outside of a strictly clinical setting. While commercial and lengthy scans have received strong opposition from these organizations, 3D US images used to alleviate patient anxiety could provide a sense of reassurance. Outward expression of support and calming from the medical examiner to the patient can have very positive effects on reducing anxiety. Mattson et al. found that patient reassurance was actually a more influential benefit than physical improvement from medications found in a cardiac study.[49] Specifically, in regard to pregnancy, prenatal anxiety can have negative biomedical and developmental implications.[50] Similarly,

3D US has been shown to decrease prenatal anxiety through reassurance which could have positive effects that can reduce other biomedical problems. This psychological and biomedical convergence may increase the need to address the advantages and disadvantages of 3D US display to the patient and immediate family.

In summary, images are provided to patients as part of most 2D US diagnostic examinations today. These images are "reassuring" to patients. It is not surprising that 3D US images are also reassuring. The research performed to date is conflicting although favoring 3D US; for those who do prenatal diagnostic ultrasound on a routine basis, it is obvious that there is some positive impact of 3D US fetal images on most of our patients.

REFERENCES

1. Leckman JF, Feldman R, Swain JE, et al. Primary parental preoccupation: circuits, genes, and the crucial role of the environment. J Neural Transm. 2004;111(7): 753-71.
2. Nelson TR, Pretorius DH. Three-dimensional ultrasound imaging. Ultrasound Med Biol. 1998;24(9):1243-70.
3. Grzesiak M, Nowakowska D, Wilczyński, J. 3D and 4D ultrasonography—review of doubts and controversies. Arch Perinat Med. 2009;15(1):12-6.
4. Thompson RA. Relationships, regulation, and early development. In: Handbook of child psychology and developmental science. US: John Wiley & Sons; 2015. pp. 1-46.
5. Carlson EA, Sampson MC, Sroufe LA. Implications of attachment theory and research for developmental-behavioral pediatrics. J Dev Behav Pediatr. 2003;24(5): 364-79.
6. Timor-Tritsch IE, Platt LD. Three-dimensional ultrasound experience in obstetrics. Curr Opin Obstet Gynecol. 2002;14(6):569-75.
7. Kohn CL, Nelson A, Weiner S. Gravidas' responses to realtime ultrasound fetal image. J Obstet Gynecol Neonatal Nurs. 1980;9(2):77-80.
8. Milne LS, Rich OJ. Cognitive and affective aspects of the responses of pregnant women to sonography. Matern Child Nurs J. 1981;10(1):15-39.
9. Hyde B. An interview study of pregnant women's attitudes to ultrasound scanning. Soc Sci Med. 1986;22(5):587-92.
10. Whynes DK. Receipt of information and women's attitudes towards ultrasound scanning during pregnancy. Ultrasound Obstet Gynecol. 2002;19(1):7-12.
11. Reading AE, Cox DN. The effects of ultrasound examination on maternal anxiety levels. J Behav Med. 1982;5(2): 237-47.
12. Kemp VH, Page CK. Maternal prenatal attachment in normal and high-risk pregnancies. J Obstet Gynecol Neonatal Nurs. 1987;16(3):179-84.

13. Waldenström U, Nilsson S, Fall O, et al. Effects of routine one-stage ultrasound screening in pregnancy: a randomized controlled trial. Lancet. 1988;332(8611):585-8.

14. Ji EK, Pretorius DH, Newton R, et al. Effects of ultrasound on maternal–fetal bonding: a comparison of two- and three-dimensional imaging. Ultrasound Obstet Gynecol. 2005;25(5):473-7.

15. De Jong-Pleij EAP, Ribbert LSM, Pistorius LR, et al. Three-dimensional ultrasound and maternal bonding—a third trimester study and a review. Prenat Diagn. 2013;33(1):81-8.

16. Pretorius DH, Gattu S, Ji EK, et al. Pre-examination and post-examination assessment of parental-fetal bonding in patients undergoing 3-/4-dimensional obstetric ultrasonography. J Ultrasound Med. 2006;25(11);1411-21.

17. Rustico MA, Mastromatteo C, Grigio M, et al. Two-dimensional vs. two-plus four-dimensional ultrasound in pregnancy and the effect on maternal emotional status: a randomized study. Ultrasound Obstet Gynecol. 2005;25(5):468-72.

18. Lapaire O, Alder J, Peukert R, et al. Two-versus three-dimensional ultrasound in the second and third trimester of pregnancy: impact on recognition and maternal–fetal bonding. A Prospective Pilot Study. Arch Gynecol Obstet. 2007;276(5):475-9.

19. Hull AD, Pretorius DH, James G, et al. Three-dimensional ultrasound (3DUS) does not enhance maternal bonding during pregnancy. Ultrasound Obstet Gynecol. 2001;18:CEO-05.

20. Pretorius DH, Hearon HA, Hollenbach KA, et al. Parental artistic drawings of the fetus before and after 3-/4-dimensional ultrasonography. J Ultrasound Med. 2007;26(3):301-8.

21. Cataudella S, Lampis J, Busonera A, et al. From parental-fetal attachment to a parent-infant relationship: a systematic review about prenatal protective and risk factors. Life Span Disabil. 2016;19(2):185-219.

22. Walsh TB, Tolman RM, Davis RN, et al. Moving up the "magic moment": fathers' experience of prenatal ultrasound. Fathering. 2014;12(1):18-37.

23. Draper J. 'It was a real good show': the ultrasound scan, fathers and the power of visual knowledge. Soc Health Illn. 2002;24(6):771-95.

24. Righetti PL, Dell'Avanzo M, Grigio M, et al. Maternal/paternal antenatal attachment and fourth-dimensional ultrasound technique: a preliminary report. Br J Psychol. 2005;96(1):129-37.

25. Johnston M, Vögele C. Benefits of psychological preparation for surgery: a meta-analysis. Ann Behav Med. 1993;15(4):245-56.

26. Kowalcek I, Mühlhoff A, Bachmann S, et al. Depressive reactions and stress related to prenatal medicine procedures. Ultrasound Obstet Gynecol. 2001;19(1):18-23.

27. Glover V, Capron L. Prenatal parenting. Curr Opin Psychol. 2017;15:66-70.

28. Lindgren K. Relationships among maternal-fetal attachment, prenatal depression, and health practices in pregnancy. Res Nurs Health. 2001;24(3):203-17.

29. Siddiqui A, Hägglöf B. Does maternal prenatal attachment predict postnatal mother–infant interaction? Early Hum Dev. 2001;59(1):13-25.

30. Scharf A, Ghazwiny MF, Steinborn A, et al. Evaluation of two-dimensional versus three-dimensional ultrasound in obstetric diagnostics: a prospective study. Fetal Diagn Ther. 2001;16(6):333-41.

31. Merz E, Abramovicz J, Baba K, et al. 3D imaging of the fetal face–recommendations from the International 3D Focus Group. Ultraschall Med. 2001;33(02):175-82.

32. Lee S, Pretorius DH, Asfoor S, et al. Prenatal three-dimensional ultrasound: perception of sonographers, sonologists and undergraduate students. Ultrasound Obstet Gynecol. 2007;30(1):77-80.

33. Campbell S. 4D or not 4D: that is the question. Ultrasound Obstet Gynecol. 2002;19(1):1-4.

34. U.S. Food and Drug Administration. (2014). Consumer updates—avoid fetal "Keepsake" images, heartbeat monitors. [online] Available from https://www.fda.gov/ForConsumers/ConsumerUpdates/ucm095508.htm [Retrieved July, 2018].

35. Horsager-Boehrer R. (2016). Why to avoid 'keepsake' 3-D and 4-D ultrasounds. In: Your pregnancy matters. UT Southwestern Medical Center. [online] Available from https://utswmed.org/medblog/3d-4d-ultrasound/ [Retrieved August, 2018].

36. Ciatti S. (2003). Part 1: The psychological impact of 3-D ultrasound on pregnant women. [online] Available from: www.auntminnie.com/index.aspx?sec=ser& sub=def&pag=dis&ItemID=60472 [Accessed August, 2018].

37. Sedgmen B, McMahon C, Cairns D, et al. The impact of two-dimensional versus three-dimensional ultrasound exposure on maternal–fetal attachment and maternal health behavior in pregnancy. Ultrasound Obstet Gynecol. 2006;27(3):245-51.

38. Chudleigh T. Scanning for pleasure. Ultrasound Obstet Gynecol. 1999;14(6):369-71.

39. Moen E. Women's rights and reproductive freedom. Hum Rights Q. 1981;3(2):53-60.

40. Zechmeister I. Foetal images: the power of visual technology in antenatal care and the implications for women's reproductive freedom. Health Care Anal. 2001;9(4):387-400.

41. Hata T, Hanaoka U, Tenkumo C, et al. Three-and four-dimensional HD live rendering images of normal and abnormal fetuses: pictorial essay. Arch Gynecol Obstet. 2012;286(6):1431-5.

42. Bajura M, Fuchs H, Ohbuchi R. Merging virtual objects with the real world: seeing ultrasound imagery within the patient. ACM SIGGRAPH Comput Graph. 1992;26(2):203-10.

43. Benacerraf BR, Minton KK, Benson CB, et al. Proceedings: beyond ultrasound first forum on improving the quality of ultrasound imaging in obstetrics and gynecology. J Ultrasound Med. 2018;37(1):7-18.

44. Fanello W (Ed). History of ultrasound. Ultrasound Schools Info. [online]. Available from https://www.ultrasound-schoolsinfo.com/history/ [Retrieved August, 2018].

45. Moeglin D, Talmant C, Duyme M, et al. Fetal lung volumetry using two- and three-dimensional ultrasound. Ultrasound Obstet Gynecol. 2005;25(2):119-27.

46. Roberts J. The visualised foetus: a cultural and political analysis of ultrasound imagery. Routledge; 2016.

47. AIUM Opinion. (2004). The AIUM reaffirms its opposition to entertainment ultrasound. [online] Available from https://www.aium.org/press/viewRelease.aspx?id=66; Using ultrasound for entertainment purposes. [online]. Available from https://www.aium.org/patients/entertainment.aspx [Retrieved August, 2018].

48. FDA Opinion. (2014). Avoid fetal "keepsake" images, heartbeat monitors. [online] Available from https://www.fda.gov/ForConsumers/ConsumerUpdates/ucm095508.htm [Retrieved August, 2018].

49. Mattson ME, Curb JD, McArdle R. Participation in a clinical trial: the patients' point of view. Control Clin Trials. 1985;6(2):156-67.

50. Mulder EJ, De Medina PR, Huizink AC, et al. Prenatal maternal stress: effects on pregnancy and the (unborn) child. Early Hum Dev. 2002;70(1-2):3-14.

First-trimester Placenta Volume and Three-dimensional Vascularization

Giuseppe Rizzo, Victoria Bitsadze, Alessandro Quarto, Alexander Makatsarya

INTRODUCTION

The placenta plays a central role in the pathogenesis of most adverse pregnancy outcomes, such as fetal growth restriction (FGR), gestational hypertension, and pre-eclampsia (PE).[1,2] Quantitative assessment of placental vascularization may be therefore useful for predicting or early diagnosing such complications.

The advent of three-dimensional (3D) ultrasound has allowed to evaluate placental volume as well as its vascularization status using power Doppler (PD) sonography.[3-5] There are evidences that 3D placental vascular indices are already altered at 11 – 0 to 13 + 6 weeks of gestation in pregnancies that will later develop adverse pregnancy outcome.[6,7]

In this chapter, we will review the technique of obtaining placental volume, the methodology of analysis of acquired volume and the potential clinical applications.

TECHNIQUE OF ACQUISITION

The entire view of the placenta needs to be identified transabdominally using a volumetric probe by two-dimensional ultrasound as shown the volume box was adjusted to include the entire placenta. The angle of volume acquisition varied from 45° to 90° according to placental size **(Fig. 21.1)**.[8] The volume acquisition should be obtained in "maximum" quality and setting the duration between 10 seconds and 15 seconds. For posteriorly and laterally located placentas, a slight lateral inclination of the transducer is performed to acquire the entire placenta. The same preestablished instrument settings should be used in all the acquisition as reported in **Table 21.1**.

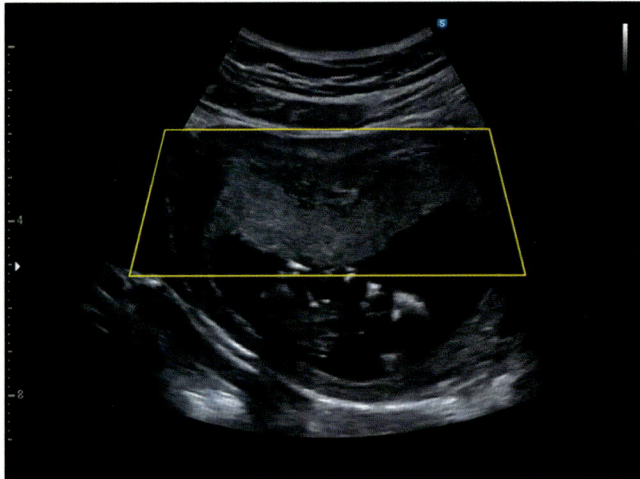

Fig. 21.1: Example of the first-trimester placental visualization. The region of interest (ROI) is superimposed to cover the whole placenta (yellow box).

Table 21.1: Standard setting of ultrasound equipment to record placental volume.

Power	96%
Frequency	Low
Quality	Normal
Density	6
Ensemble	16
Balance	150
Filter	2
Smooth	3/5
Pulse repetition frequency	0.9 kHz
Gain	−0.2

After the acquisition from the real-time images, PD is superimposed **(Fig. 21.2)** and a second volume is acquired.[9] In order to obtain reproducible results, the gain is set in all the cases respectively at –0.2 for PD and –0.8 if high-definition flow is used.

Volume Analysis

After acquisition, the placental volumes were stored for later analysis. The software virtual organ computer-aided analysis is used to evaluate placental volume by obtaining a sequence of 12 sections of the placenta, separated by successive rotations of 15°. In each plane, the contour was traced manually and the organ was then reconstructed automatically by the software **(Figs. 21.3 and 21.4)**.

After estimation of the placental volume, the 3D PD histogram was used to determine the following vascular indices from computer algorithms:[4] (1) vascularization index which refers to the color voxel/total voxel ratio, i.e. the color percentage within the volume of interest (placenta), and provides an indication of how many vessels can be detected within the placenta (vascularity); (2) flow index (FI), which refers to the weighted color voxel (on a scale of 0–100)/total color voxel ratio and provides an amplitude value for the color signal, thus giving infor-

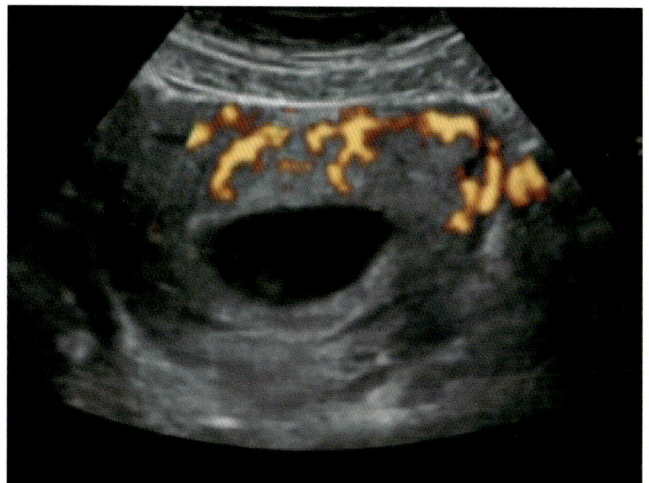

Fig. 21.2: Same example as in Figure 21.1 with power Doppler activated.

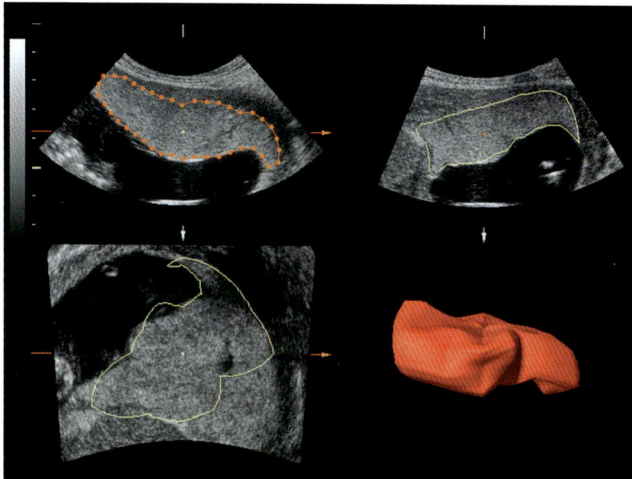

Fig. 21.3: Example of placental manual tracing and subsequent reconstructed volume.

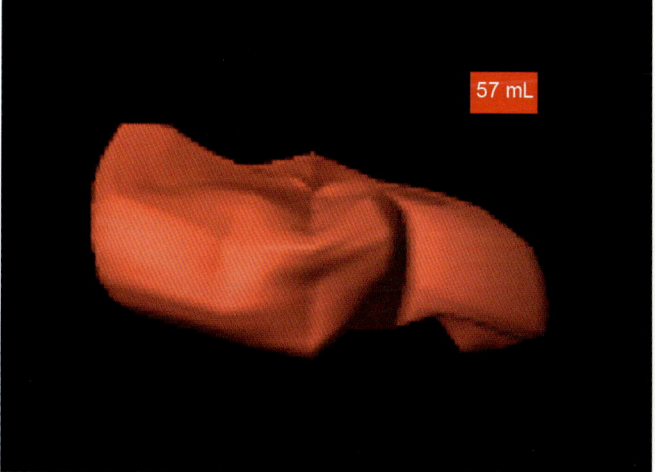
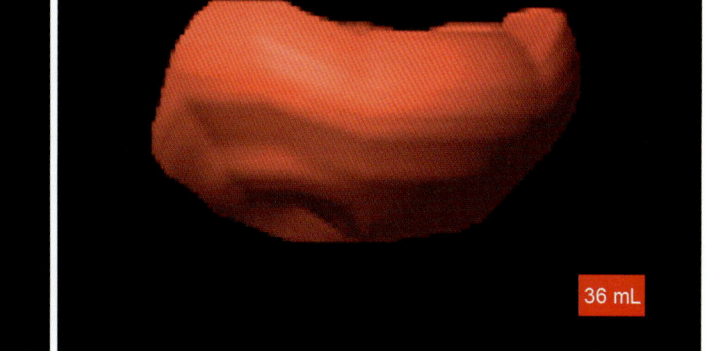

Fig. 21.4: Placentas of different sizes at 12 weeks.

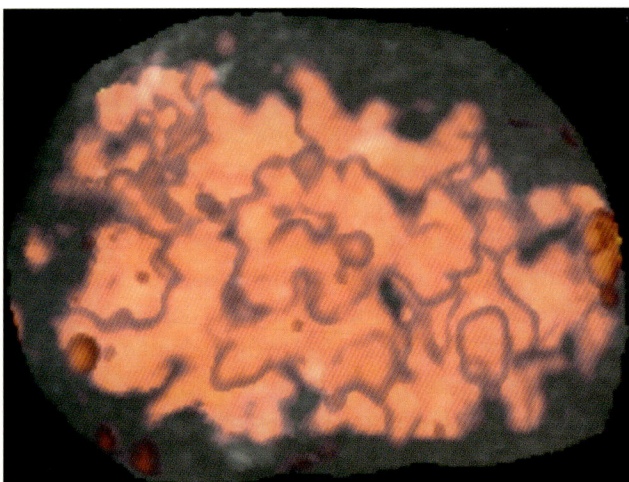

Fig. 21.5: Example of placental volume with 3D flow vascularization.

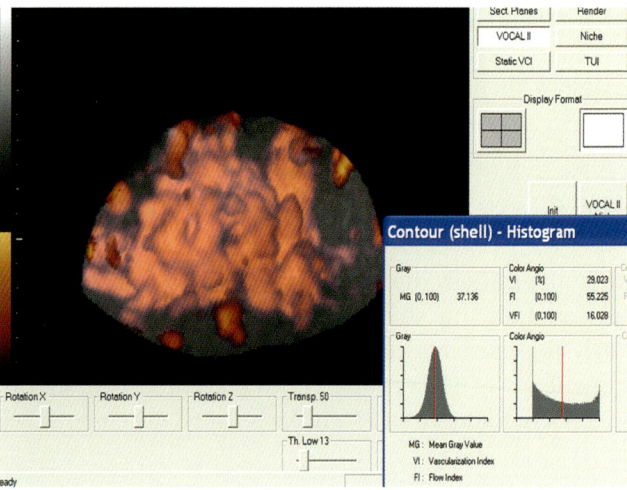

Fig. 21.6: Example of quantification of vascular indices.

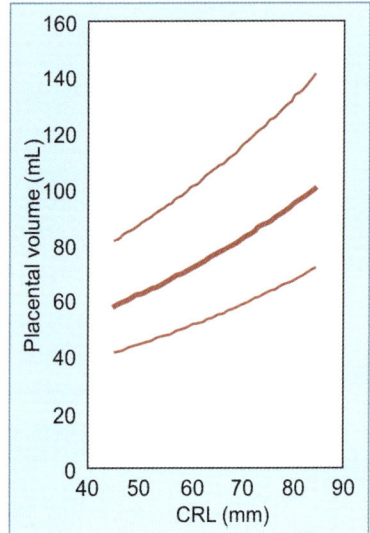

Fig. 21.7: Reference limits for crown–rump length of placental volume.[8]

mation on how many blood cells are being transported at the time of the 3D sweep (placental blood flow); and (3) vascularization FI, which refers to the weighted color voxel/total voxel ratio, combining the information of vessel presence (vascularity) and amount of transported blood cells (blood flow) **(Figs. 21.5 and 21.6)**.

Reference Limits for Gestation

Since placental volume increases with gestational age, we constructed reference limits for crown–rump length (CRL) in order to allow proper comparison **(Fig. 21.7)**.[8] Similarly indices of vascularization change with advancing

gestation and reference limits for CRL were constructed[9] **(Fig. 21.8)**.

Significance of Placental Vascular Indices

Although caution is necessary in relation to 3D Doppler measurements to anatomical placental characteristics, we related histomorphological analysis of chorionic villi to ultrasonographic evaluation of 3D placental volume and vascularization in pregnancies undergoing chorionic villus sampling (CVS).[10] A direct relationship was evidenced between the number of capillaries and the 3D Doppler placental vascularization demonstrating of a direct relationship between histological results and 3D ultrasound evaluation of placental vascularization.

CHANGES OF PLACENTAL VOLUME AND VASCULARIZATION IN ABNORMAL PREGNANCIES

Aneuploid Fetuses

In pregnancies affected by trisomies 13 and 18, the placental volume does not differ from that of euploid fetuses but the vascular indices were significantly lower than the norm.[9] This confirms histological findings in ongoing pregnancies affected by trisomies 13 and 18 that show decreased vascularization and trophoblastic hypoplasia in placental samples obtained by CVS.[9] In spite of a tendency toward lower vascularization indices in the placentae of trisomy 21 fetuses, there were no statistical differences compared with normal fetuses. One possible

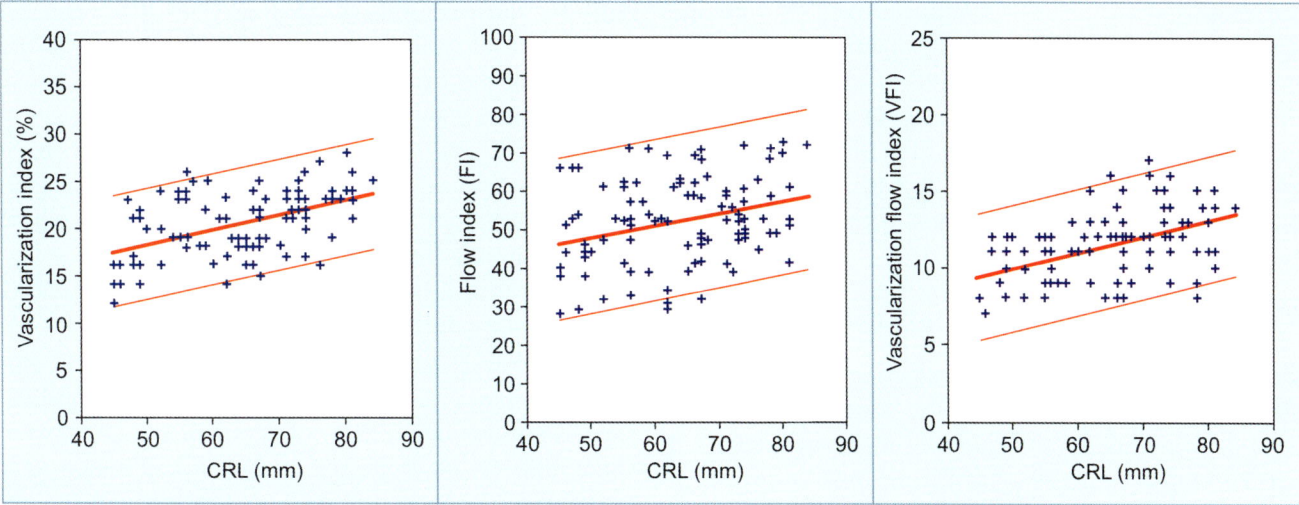

Fig. 21.8: Reference limits for crown–rump length of vascular indices.[9]

explanation for the low vascular indices values found in such fetuses is delayed development of placental vascularization. Indeed, histomorphological studies on CVS material from ongoing trisomy 21 pregnancies have shown delayed development of the structure of the chorionic villi.[9] Since placental vascular indices increase with advancing gestation, the lower values found in the trisomy 21 cases may simply reflect a temporal delay in changes in the villi. Irrespective of the underlying mechanisms, there appears to be less difference (from normal) in placental vascularization in the cases of trisomy 21 compared with the cases of trisomies 13 and 18. As a consequence, it seems unlikely that the study of placental vascularization as assessed by 3D Doppler ultrasound might be incorporated into the first-trimester screening of trisomy 21. Similarly, it is difficult to suggest that these vascular indices may further increase the high detection rate for trisomies 13 and 18, already achieved by using a combination of nuchal translucency.

Maternal Smoking

We have investigated the effects of smoking on placental volume and its Doppler measured vascularization.[11] Smoking less than 10 cigarettes/day did not induce any evident changes in the 3D Doppler placental vascular indices considered, while in mothers who smoked heavily, there was a significant reduction of all these indices suggesting a reduced placental vascularization already present at 11 + 0 to 13 + 6 weeks of gestation. We did not evidence any dose-dependent effect of maternal smoking

more than 10 cigarettes/day on placental vascularization. Possible explanations are the absence of a dose-dependent effect of smoking on placental angiogenesis as suggested by in vitro studies. Of interest is that placental vascular indices are significantly related to birth weight, and this relationship resulted stronger when the analysis was restricted to heavy smokers.

Prediction of Preeclampsia

We tested the role of uterine artery Doppler, placental volume assessed by 3D ultrasound, and their combined use in the first trimester for the prediction of PE in an unselected population of nulliparous pregnancies.[8] We demonstrated how both abnormal uterine artery and reduced placental volume resulted in independent risk factors to develop PE. Of interest is the lack or relationship found in our study between uterine Doppler and placental volume suggesting their independent role as risk factors. The lack of relationship may reflect two different pathophysiological mechanisms involved in the genesis of PE. Pregnancies with abnormal Doppler uterine waveforms may reflect an inadequate tropho-blastic invasion of the maternal spiral arteries that may occur in the presence of a normal size placenta. On the other hand, despite the presence of a normal trophoblastic invasion as indicated by normal uterine Doppler indices, a small placenta, for example by producing a smaller amount of vasoactive substances or antioxidative agents, may act as distinct genesis of PE. Irrespective of the underlying mechanisms, our data suggest that combining the first-trimester uterine Doppler screening with the assessment of placental volume by 3D ultrasound may improve the detection rate of PE to values similar to those found for the late second trimester. These data encourage further research on uterine Doppler combined with placental volume as well as with other potential biochemical markers in the attempt to detect pregnancies at risk of PE in the first trimester.

Prediction of Fetal Growth Retardation

We tested the efficiency of the assessment of placental volume and its vascularization in pregnancies characterized by low maternal serum of pregnancy-associated plasma protein A (PAPP-A) at 11 – 0 to 13 + 6 weeks of gestation,[12] a condition associated with a higher incidence of low birth weight.[13] An interesting aspect of this study was the evidence that among pregnancies with low serum PAPP-A levels, only those resulting in the birth of FGR neonates showed a significant decrease of the 3D PD indices of placental vascularization at 11 + 0 to 13 + 6 weeks of gestation. On the other hand, pregnancies with low PAPP-A concentrations delivering newborns of appropriate weight or healthy low birth-weight neonates did not show differences in placental vascularization during the first trimester. A second finding of this study is the significant association between the degree of reduction in 3D placental Doppler indices and the severity of the growth defect at birth. Although caution is necessary in the interpretation of these Doppler indices as the experimental design of this study does not allow to investigate direct links between vascular indices and histomorphometric parameters, the relationships found between the changes in placental vascular indices and birth weight support the hypothesis that the Doppler parameters measured reflect a reduced placental vascularization already present in the first trimester.

Maternal Type I Diabetes Mellitus

We investigated placental volume and vascularization assessed by 3D ultrasound in a population of type I diabetes mellitus (DM).[14] We demonstrated that while diabetic condition does not affect placental volume, its vascularity is significantly increased. An interesting result of this study is the evidence that among pregnancies with diabetes, those with a poorer glycemic control, as expressed by hemoglobin A1c concentrations more than or equal to 7%, exhibited significantly higher values of placental vascular indices. This suggests that placental vascular development in women with diabetes can be affected by the first-trimester maternal hyperglycemia. Although associations between the first-trimester glycemic control and placental angiogenesis have been already recognized by stereological studies on human placentas at term showing an increased capillary volume in DM with poor metabolic control, our data are the first to provide an in vivo evidence of an increased vascularity already present during the first trimester.

The clinical significance of the modification of placental vascular indices in DM remains to be established. However, there are some evidences that the phenotypic changes in the placental microvascular bed may extend to umbilical vascular cells and even to fetal vasculature and heart, which might produce an overt pathological response in the offspring later life if challenged with additional cardiovascular stresses. The presence of abnormalities in fetal cardiac function occurring already in early gestation in fetuses of type I DM supports this hypothesis.

In conclusion, placentas of diabetic mothers exhibited evidence of the first-trimester increased vascular indices, and these changes become more evident with worsening glycemic control. The ability to document placental vascular changes so early in pregnancy potentially opens new avenues to understand the range of fetal developmental consequences of maternal glycemic status.

Pregnancies from in Vitro Fertilization[15,16]

Pregnancies achieved with in vitro fertilization (IVF) are at increased risk of obstetrical complications, such as PE. Further, the incidence of this disease is significantly higher in pregnancies obtained with donor oocytes than in pregnancies achieved with autologous IVF. We analyzed three groups of pregnancies (naturally conceived, autologous IVF, and heterologous IVF); when the two IVF groups are considered, the incidence of PE was three-fold higher in donor oocytes recipient pregnancies thus suggesting the coexistence of other causative factors. No relationships were found between placental volume and maternal age, and multivariate logistic regression evidenced an independent role of placental volume. Of interest is the significant contribution in the prediction of PE given from donor IVF in association with maternal age and placental volume.

An impaired trophoblastic invasion is considered to be the major etiological factor in the development of PE, particularly when at early onset. Indeed there are several evidences showing that an abnormal impedance to flow in the uteroplacental circulation, manifested by an increased uterine artery pulsatility index (PI), already present at 11 weeks of gestation in pregnancies, will develop PE. Despite the high prevalence of PE in IVF pregnancies found in this study, we did not evidence any differences in mean uterine PI values. This is in agreement with other reports and suggests that the mechanism causing the increased incidence of PE in IVF pregnancies is unlikely to be related to impaired uteroplacental perfusion.

The presence, in IVF pregnancies, of reduced placental volume, particularly marked in donor oocytes recipients and its association with the development of PE despite the presence of normal uterine artery PI values found in this study must be pointed out. One different hypotheses that has been suggested to explain the increased incidence of PE in IVF pregnancies is a different immune response of the mother to trophoblastic antigens. This abnormal immune response may be either secondary to the different maternal endocrine characteristics of women undergoing IVF or to the presence of foreign antigens as it is the case with donor oocytes (since placental development is influenced by maternal immune response); this hypothesis may well explain the reduced volume hereby found in IVF pregnancies.

The importance of the first-trimester identification of IVF pregnancies at higher risk to develop PE should be underlined since this condition is associated with an increased risk of perinatal mortality and morbidity and both short- and long-term maternal complications that deserve targeted antenatal care and surveillance. However, the degree of overlap in placental volume, multiples of median values evidenced in this study between pregnancies who did or did not develop PE suggest a limited role in its isolated use as a screening tool. In naturally conceived pregnancies, effective screening for PE was achieved only with the combined use of maternal variables, uterine artery Doppler, and biochemical markers. A similar approach should also be applied to IVF pregnancies adding placental volume data. The results obtained in the multiple logistic models constructed support this hypothesis by showing a potential combined role of placental volume with maternal characteristics, such as age or type of conception.

We also analyzed placental volume in IVF pregnancies divided according to the use of fresh or frozen–thawed embryos. We found a reduced placental volume, particularly evident when fresh embryos are used, and it was associated with a higher incidence in the development of PE.

The lower placental volume found in IVF with fresh embryos is probably secondary to the inferior endometrial receptivity occurring in these pregnancies rather in naturally conceived and cryopreservation groups. Indeed the use of ovarian stimulation in the former group is associated with an altered endometrial development that may impair its receptivity and therefore the subsequent placental development. Although the role of endometrial receptivity seems to play a pivotal role, it is not possible to exclude others factors that may explain our findings. A possibility is that the freeze–thawed procedure may filter out flawed embryos thus selecting a higher percentage of more viable blastocysts to be transferred. A second possibility is that freezing and thawing the embryos may improve their biological ability in reaching a normal implantation. Irrespective of the underlying cause, which is out of the objectives of this work, we demonstrated that placental volume is reduced in IVF pregnancies achieved with fresh embryos and these pregnancies are at higher risk of PE.

In conclusion, during the first-trimester placental volume in IVF pregnancies is lower than in naturally conceived pregnancies, and it is particularly reduced in donor oocytes recipients and fresh embryos. Placental volume assessment at 11 + 0 – 13 + 6 weeks may be therefore useful to identify among IVF pregnancies those destined to develop PE.

CONCLUSION

In this chapter, we tried to improve our knowledge regarding early placentation and subsequent placental function in normal early pregnancy and in complicated pregnancies using 3D ultrasound datasets. We developed methods to measure the success of early placentation and subsequent placental function and their association with fetal growth and abnormal pregnancy outcome. This may be a first step toward implementation of a technique in clinical practice for identifying women at risk for the development of placenta-related pregnancy complications in the future. Fully automating the segmentation process would potentially allow a wider use of placental volume to screen for pregnancies at increased risk of complications.[17]

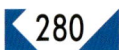

REFERENCES

1. Salafia CM, Charles AK, Maas EM. Placenta and fetal growth restriction. Clin Obstet Gynecol. 2006;49:236-56.
2. Meekins JW, Pijnenborg R, Hanssens M, et al. A study of placental bed spiral arteries and trophoblast invasion in normal and severe pre-eclamptic pregnancies. Br J Obstet Gynaecol. 1994;101:669-74.
3. Pretorius DH, Nelson TR, Baergen RN, et al. Imaging of placental vasculature using three-dimensional ultrasound and color power Doppler: a preliminary study. Ultrasound Obstet Gynecol. 1998;12:45-9.
4. Pairleitner H, Steiner H, Hasenoehrl G, et al. Three-dimensional power Doppler sonography: imaging and quantifying blood flow and vascularization. Ultrasound Obstet Gynecol. 1999;14:139-43.
5. Mercé LT, Barco MJ, Bau S. Reproducibility of the study of placental vascularization by three-dimensional power Doppler. J Perinat Med. 2004;32:228-33.
6. Guiot C, Gaglioti P, Oberto M, et al. Is three-dimensional power Doppler ultrasound useful in the assessment of placental perfusion in normal and growth-restricted pregnancies? Ultrasound Obstet Gynecol. 2008;31:171-6.
7. Odibo AO, Goetzinger KR, Huster KM, et al. Placental volume and vascular flow assessed by 3D power Doppler and adverse pregnancy outcomes. Placenta. 2011;32:230-4.
8. Rizzo G, Capponi A, Cavicchioni O, et al. First-trimester uterine Doppler and three-dimensional ultrasound placental volume calculation in predicting pre-eclampsia. Eur J Obstet Gynecol Reprod Biol. 2008;138:147-51.
9. Rizzo G, Capponi A, Cavicchioni O, et al. Placental vascularization measured by three-dimensional power Doppler ultrasonography at 11 to 13 + 6 weeks in normal and aneuploid fetuses. Ultrasound Obstet Gynecol. 2007;30:259-62.
10. Rizzo G, Silvestri E, Capponi A, et al. Histomorphometric characteristics of first trimester chorionic villi in pregnancies with low serum pregnancy-associated plasma protein-A levels: relationship with placental three-dimensional power Doppler ultrasonographic vascularization. J Matern Fetal Neonatal Med. 2011;24(2):253-7.
11. Rizzo G, Capponi A, Pietrolucci ME, et al. Effects of maternal cigarette smoking on placental volume and vascularization measured by 3-dimensional power Doppler ultrasonography at 11+0 to 13+6 weeks of gestation. Am J Obstet Gynecol. 2009;200(415):e1-5.
12. Rizzo G, Capponi A, Pietrolucci ME, et al. First-trimester placental volume and vascularization measured by 3-dimensional power Doppler sonography in pregnancies with low serum pregnancy-associated plasma protein A levels. J Ultrasound Med. 2009;28:1615-22.
13. Spencer K, Cowans NJ, Avgidou K, et al. First-trimester biochemical markers of aneuploidy and the prediction of small-for-gestational age fetuses. Ultrasound Obstet Gynecol. 2008;31:15-9.
14. Rizzo G, Capponi A, Pietrolucci ME, et al. First trimester placental volume and three-dimensional power Doppler ultrasonography in type I diabetic pregnancies. Prenat Diagn. 2012;32:480-4.
15. Rizzo G, Aiello E, Pietrolucci ME, et al. Placental volume and uterine artery Doppler evaluation at 11+0 to 13+6 weeks of gestation in pregnancies conceived with in vitro fertilization: comparison between autologous and donor oocyte recipients. Ultrasound Obstet Gynecol. 2016;47(6):726-31.
16. Rizzo G, Aiello E, Pietrolucci ME, et al. Are there differences in placental volume and uterine artery Doppler in pregnancies resulting from the transfer of fresh versus frozen-thawed embryos through in vitro fertilization? Reprod Sci. 2016;23:1381-6.
17. Looney P, Stevenson GN, Nicolaides KH, et al. Fully automated, real-time 3D ultrasound segmentation to estimate first trimester placental volume using deep learning. JCI Insight. 2018;3(11).

Fetal Cognitive Functions and Three-dimensional/ Four-dimensional Ultrasound

Aida Salihagić Kadić, Anja Šurina, Oliver Vasilj, Sanja Tomasović, Asim Kurjak

INTRODUCTION

In the past decades, advances in modern imaging methods, especially three-dimensional/four-dimensional ultrasound (3D/4D US), functional magnetic resonance imaging (MRI) (fMRI) and fetal magnetoencephalography (fMEG), enabled the studies of the important neurodevelopmental events and opened the field of the investigation of fetal cognitive functions. Prenatal structural, functional, and behavioral development, including the development of the central nervous system (CNS), and cognitive functional development are nowadays accessible to a better assessment due to the implementation of these methods.[1,2] 3D/4D US imaging provides many important information about the fetus. It can detect various malformations and clarify suspicious findings, improve diagnostic accuracy, display fascinating fetal activity, and also it supports the advancements in fetal neurobehavioral and cognitive science.[3] Apart from the US, fMRI and fMEG are also methods worth mentioning, as they offer an assessment of fetal brain function, notably the fetal response to the auditory and visual stimuli by fMRI, and the direct measurement of fetal neuronal activity by fMEG.[4]

Data on cognitive functions of the fetus could be important in clinical practice for the management of fetal pain, treatment of preterm infants, and improvement of the neurological outcome of the fetuses from high-risk pregnancies. Furthermore, some of the cognitive deficits and impairments in childhood and adult age, such as impaired learning and memory, deficits in attention, delayed language development, and intellectual disability may originate in the prenatal period.[1]

This chapter will serve as a brief review of 3D/4D US-assessed insights in the field of fetal neurodevelopment, particularly the development of fetal cognitive functions: sensory perception, motor action, emotions, learning and memory, as well as the role of the fetal stress in cognitive development.

STRUCTURAL AND FUNCTIONAL BRAIN DEVELOPMENT AND COGNITIVE FUNCTIONS

Prenatal and postnatal sensory and motor experience shapes and changes the structure and function of the cerebral cortex. Functional brain development begins in utero, and more than 99% of the human neocortex is already formed prenatally, resulting in amazing diversity of fetal abilities.[5] The maturation of the cerebral cortex is a very complex and dynamic process influenced by intrinsic and extrinsic factors, stimuli, and the environment.[6] Contemporary models of brain development portray a dynamically developing system which relies on genetic, systemic, and experiential factors that interact in complex ways. An understanding of how brain systems emerge through the interaction of all of these factors is important to unlock the mystery of neurocognitive development.[7] In this section, neurodevelopmental processes and the emergence of cognitive functions will be described.

The CNS begins its development in an early embryonic period from the ectodermal germinative layer, and its differentiation and maturation continue postnatally. The neural plate, thickened ectodermal layer, is formed at the beginning of the third week as a precursor of the future brain and the spinal cord. Process of neural tube formation is called primary neurulation. The forebrain (prosencephalon), midbrain (mesencephalon), and hindbrain (rhombencephalon) are three dilations which are distinguished in the rostral part of the neural tube around the 22nd day of the embryonic life as three primary brain vesicles. After the neural tube closes completely, cephalic flexure appears in the midbrain region and cervical flexure at the junction of the hindbrain and the spinal cord. Later on, the forebrain region divides into two parts: (1) the diencephalon, characterized by outgrowing of the optic vesicles, and (2) the telencephalon, basis for the future cerebral hemispheres. In the fetal period the hemispheres continue to grow and develop into lobes, gyruses, and sulci. The rhombencephalon is the fundament of the pons, cerebellum, and myelencephalon.[8] Caudal part of the neural tube, future spinal cord, develops in the process called secondary neurulation.[9]

Histogenetic processes lead to the growth of the neural tube and changes in its wall's shape and structure. Those are very complex overlapping processes divided into neurogenesis, migration, and cytodifferentiation. Production of neurons starts at week 3 of gestation with 125,000 and increases at 7 weeks at a pace of 250,000 per minute.[10] It is important to note that by 20 weeks, the cortex has acquired its full complement of neurons. Between the 24th gestational week and 34th gestational week (GW), cortical area differentiation begins and continues until the end of gestation.[11]

Histologically, there are three zones of the neural tube: ventricular, intermediary, and marginal zone. Along with these three zones, the telencephalon also has the subventricular and subplate zone. In the ventricular and subventricular zone of the telencephalon, all of the future neurons and glial cells are generated, i.e. the neurogenesis is taking place in there. Final targets of the neurons and the glia cells, the cortical plate, brainstem, diencephalon, and basal ganglia nuclei, are genetically predisposed. During their migration, transitional zones are being created, representing temporary forms of the cerebral cortex organization. Hence, during the embryonic and fetal period, the brain is formed not only of adult structures but also of transitional structures which are not found in the adult human brain.[12]

The subplate zone is a key zone for the development of the cerebral cortex because it is a place where early synaptogenesis, a creation of temporary synapses of afferent axons and neurons, is carried out. It is formed between the 15th week and 17th week of gestation when a number of cortical synapses grow. A six-layered lamination of cerebral cortex appears after the 32nd GW, proceeding the process of neuronal differentiation and laminar allocation of the thalamocortical axons. However, this does not represent the end of the cerebral cortex development. It continues intensively after the birth, especially in the association regions of the cortex.[11,13] In other words, even though the neurons and the pathways are present already at the neonates, their quantitative and qualitative features and their connections still need fine tuning so the development continues during the postnatal life in the permanent interaction with the environment. Postnatal synapse generation is the most intensive between 8 months and 2 years of life, and it antecedes the development of more advanced cognitive functions, such as speech.[14]

Cognitive functions are mediated by specialized areas of neocortex. Large areas of association cortex, which develop gradually during the fetal life, are contained within each of the four lobes and contribute to the cognition.[15] Building up synapses in these regions enlarge its activity recorded by fMRI. This imaging technique, which enables investigation of fetal brain function, has shown low activity in the association regions of the neonate's brain in comparison with the adult brain. The highest activity was detected in the somatosensory, auditory, and visual cortex of the newborn's brain.[16] Recent study has indicated that deficits in the complex interneural connections can presage cognitive impairments.[17] fMRI also enables examining functional connectivity development of the human fetus. It provides information about the spatial distribution and interaction of neural processing networks. By applying resting-state fMRI to the fetal brain, it is possible to noninvasively examine fetal functional brain circuits.[18] Resting-state studies in full-term[19] and preterm infants[20] have suggested the existence of a "proto," or partial, default mode network (DMN) in the early newborn. The DMN is an organized, baseline default mode of brain activation that is observed in adults and children.[21] Fetal resting-state fMRI examination offers the first opportunity to confirm the prenatal origins of this network and to evaluate processes by which it becomes organized prior to birth. Recent studies have shown that primitive forms of functional networks, including a primitive form of the DMN, appear to be present by midgestation.[18,22] In utero MRI has significantly increased our knowledge of early fetal brain development and has the potential of generating biomarkers for developmental prognosis in the future.[4]

White matter myelination is a complex and long-lasting process. The development of the myelin sheath provides synchronized communication across the neural systems responsible for higher order cognitive functioning.[17] One of the substantial parts of cerebral white matter, the corpus callosum, is fashioned around the 20th GW. The corpus callosum integrates sensory, motor, cognitive, and emotional functions from both cerebral hemispheres. It represents the major interhemispheric commissure. Abnormalities of the corpus callosum include agenesis, partial agenesis, and thickness variations: hypoplasia and hyperplasia. These malformations are diagnosed in a large number of conditions that interfere with early cerebral development. An abnormal volume of the corpus callosum has been associated with different learning and behavioral difficulties, speech and language delays, cognitive and motor impairments, including cerebral palsy.[17,23] Moreover, there is a correlation of splenial structure of corpus callosum with language skills. Over- or underdevelopment of the splenium results in the impairment of visuospatial skills, attention, and motor coordination. Further, reduced posterior callosal connections have been associated with impaired social skills, diminished processing speed during complex tasks and impairments in the excitatory interhemispheric transfer.[24] 3D US enables a precise visualization of the normal **(Fig. 22.1)** and abnormal corpus callosum. By correlating the prenatal corpus callosum abnormalities with the known functions of its structures, we are stepping

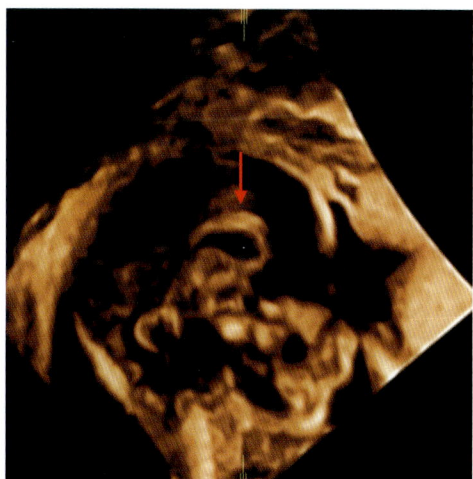

Fig. 22.1: Three-dimensional ultrasound image of the corpus callosum (displayed by an arrow, 19 + 6 weeks of gestation).

forward into a more meaningful understanding of the prenatal neurological development of the white matter and postnatal neurological outcomes.[23]

PRENATAL NEUROMOTOR DEVELOPMENT AND FETAL INTENTIONAL MOVEMENTS

The repertoire of fetal activities and functions during pregnancy increases as the CNS develops. Understanding of fetal neuromotor development enables assessment of the fetal neural system integrity. Fetal behavior, a product of the functioning CNS, represents all the activities of the fetus which can be observed or recorded by US or other imaging techniques. Fetal behavioral patterns and its variations during the gestational period correspond to the development and maturity of the fetal CNS. Aberrations from the normal fetal behavior in certain gestational period can refer to the presence of neurological disorders as well as other organ system abnormalities.[2,14]

The synapses, interneuronal connections, and innervated muscle fibers are prerequisites for fetal mobility which is important for development of the fetus. The earliest synapses in the spinal cord are detected between the 6th week and 7th week of gestation.[25] The first movements that can be seen, vermicular movements at 7–7.5 weeks, are a result of the neural activity of spinal motoneurons.[26] Simultaneously with the onset of spontaneous movements, the earliest motor reflex activity appears, indicating the existence of the first afferent–efferent circuits in the spinal cord.[27] General movements (GMs), seen from the 8th to 9th weeks of gestation onward, are the earliest complex and well-organized movement pattern. Those movements express a supraspinal control on motor activity and include the head, trunk, and limbs.[28,29]

It has been well known that neural cells begin to generate and propagate action potentials as soon as they interconnect. This intrinsic property of neurons explains recognizable temporal sequences of embryonic and fetal movements. What is more, studies have shown that neurons are able to communicate through the non-synaptic mechanism even before the onset of synaptogenesis.[14] The medulla oblongata, pons, and midbrain (the brainstem) develop around the 7th GW, while the diencephalon and main parts of the cerebral hemispheres are formed by the end of the 8th GW.[30,31] The medulla matures earlier than other brainstem structures, so activities under its control, breathing-like movements, heart rate alternations, and reflexive movements of the head, trunk, and limbs appear prior to other functions. Facial movements, also controlled by cranial nerves V and VII, emerge around the 10th week and 11th week.[30] After the 10th GW, number, frequency, and diversity of fetal movements increase. GMs, which used to be slow and of limited amplitude, become more pronounced.[32] The earliest signs of right- or left- "handedness" are present from the 10th GW when the fetus starts demonstrating signs of lateralized behavior. Stimulation of the brain is known to influence the brain organization, and it is considered that fetal motor activity may eventually stimulate the brain to develop lateralization of function.[14] From GW 13 onward, a "goal-orientation" of hand movements appears, and a target point can be recognized for each hand movement.[33] Finally, at 13–14 weeks, isolated finger movements can be observed.[34]

General movements were found to be the most frequent movement pattern in the first trimester of normal pregnancies.[35] These movements are big and slow, lasting from a few seconds to 1 minute. Intensity, force, and velocity of these movements vary, and sequence of the head, neck, trunk, and extremities movements is undefined. Those characteristics are analyzed after the US recording when their qualitative aspect: complexity, variations, and fluency are being described.[14] Gestalt perception, an overall assessment of GMs, is also a part of their analysis.[29,36] Predictive value of GMs appears to be important for detection of neurodevelopmental disorders, cerebral palsy, for example.[37]

In the second trimester, fetal motor activity and fetal behavior are very diverse as a consequence of the development of neural connections, axons, synaptogenesis, and dendrite proliferation. Structures of the brainstem continue to mature, causing an increase in the complexity of fetal behavioral patterns and activities. Moreover, the second half of the pregnancy is characterized by a gradual organization of fetal movement patterns. The periods of fetal quiescence increase, and the rest-activity cycles become recognizable.[2,14] However, cerebral pathways are still not mature enough, and the cerebral cortex cannot be considered responsible for motor activity and behavioral patterns.[11] The brainstem, on the other side, gradually matures and begins to take over control of fetal movements and behavioral patterns.[30] Wide repertoire of fetal activity has been observed during the second trimester, including GMs, isolated movements of the extremities, retroflexion, anteflexion, rotation of the

head and facial movements, such as yawning, hiccupping, thumb sucking, swallowing, and mouthing.[28] Between the 16th week and 18th week, sporadic eye movements appear as a result of the midbrain maturation. In the midbrain, structures important for eye movement control: cranial nerves III, IV, and, V and medial longitudinal fasciculus are situated.[30] Further, 4D US imaging in the second and third trimester of pregnancy shows that fetuses change facial expressions, such as smiling, grimacing, and crying.[38] Recent data have indicated that fetal movements serve not only to express different orientations but also emotional states and manifestations of intentions.[39] The spatial and temporal characteristics of fetal movements are not uncoordinated or unpatterned. Furthermore, a kinematic study has shown a presence of a recognizable form of intentional fetal hand movements **(Fig. 22.2)**, which can be detected by the 22 GW, with kinematic patterns that depend on the goal of the action. This suggests that there is a surprisingly advanced level of fetal motor planning.[40] It is important to stress that fetal motor behavior reflects the development of diverse cognitive, sensory, and motor systems. Recent study has shown that primary sensorimotor and affective integration errors and poorly regulated motor intentions might underline autistic spectrum disorders.[41]

The subplate zone, as already mentioned, is formed in the second trimester, and after this process the first cortical electrical activity can be registered as a result of an increase in a number of cortical synapses.[12] Intensive synaptogenesis and establishment of the spinothalamic

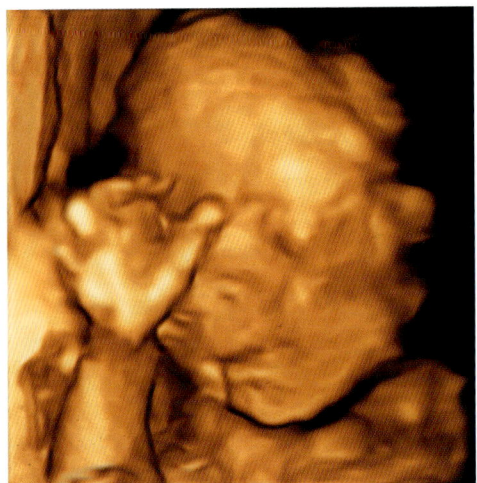

Fig. 22.2: Fetal hand-to-face movement, recorded by three-dimensional/four-dimensional ultrasound (23 + 4 weeks of gestation).

tract occur between the 15th GW and 20th GW, but the myelinization of the spinothalamic tract continues until the 29th GW.[42] Studies conducted on monkey's and human's brain have shown that the thalamocortical connections develop between the 24th GW and 26th GW.[43,44] The cerebellum start to mature at the 24th GW, and the brainstem and cerebellum become accessible to clinical assessment around the 28th GW.[45]

In the third trimester of pregnancy the CNS continues its development. Regarding the motor development, there is a decrease in the number of the GMs, and the head and the arm movements. On the other hand, these movements are becoming more and more complex. It was thought that the reason for this decrease in fetal movement number is a smaller volume of amniotic fluid, thus less space for the bigger fetus to move. Now we know that this is a consequence of the maturation of the medulla oblongata and more stable intrinsic activity of the brainstem, which includes control of the spontaneous fetal movements. During the third trimester, the frequency of facial movement patterns shows a decreasing or stagnant developmental trend, and the complexity of the fetal facial movements increases.[2,14] There is a possibility that these are consequences of the establishment of control of more cranial brain structures, not only of a maturation of the brainstem.[5,14] The fetal face reflects the brain development very well and that is the important reason for its investigation during the gestation. Ultrasonographic examination of the fetal face can also provide information that may lead to the diagnosis of anomalies in other organs or systems. Many genetic disorders affecting the CNS are characterized by dysmorphology and dysfunction of facial structures. Therefore, the fetal face represents a "diagnostic window" for fetal diseases and syndromes.[38]

From the beginning of the third trimester, evoked potentials can be registered from the cerebral cortex, indicating that the functional connection between the periphery and cortex operates from that time onward.[46] At the 30th GW, by means of electroencephalography, fetal sleep/awake patterns may be recorded, also as a result of the brainstem maturation.[47]

It is unclear whether infants might have a "memory" for the movements they produced in utero. However, it has been found that fetal experiences, e.g. exposure to sounds and language,[48-50] are remembered postnatally, so it might be possible that the infant also remembers prenatal movement patterns.[51] By all means, fetal

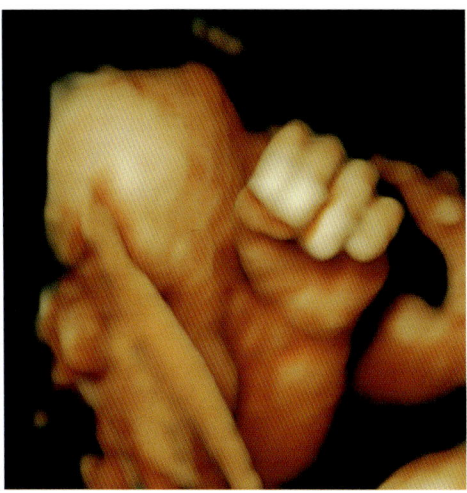

Fig. 22.3: High definition three-dimensional ultrasound image of fetal neurological thumb in a clenched fist (29 + 3 weeks of gestation).

movements provide the brain with sensory input that spurs its development.[1]

Fetal spontaneous movements, assessed by 4D US, are important part of the Kurjak Antenatal Neurodevelopmental Test (KANET)[52] which has proved its usefulness in prenatal assessment of the neurological outcome. This test has been used to asses almost 2,000 fetuses, and the results have indicated that KANET has the ability to recognize normal, borderline, and abnormal behavior in fetuses from normal and pathological pregnancies.[53] Some of the studies that implemented this prenatal neurological scoring test have shown that fetuses with abnormal KANET demonstrate a deficiency in the repertoire of the movements, abnormal GMs, a fetal face, such as a mask or a neurological thumb **(Fig. 22.3)**,[54,55] a sign of upper control motor system damage (the cerebral hemispheres and basal ganglia), which can indicate that the fetus suffered from severe hypoxia.[45] Comprehension of normal patterns of prenatal behavior is important as it is the foundation for differentiation of pathological aberrations, which may be indicators of prenatal neurological impairment.[56]

PRENATAL NEUROSENSORY DEVELOPMENT AND FETAL PERCEPTION OF STIMULI

Information enters the neural system by means of sensory receptors which register sensory stimuli: sound, light, touch, pain, cold, and heat. Sensory information from the somatic body segments enters into the spinal cord through the dorsal roots of spinal nerves. Then they travel up to the CNS through the dorsal column of the medial lemniscus and anterolateral tract, the thalamus to the somatosensory part of the cerebral cortex. Vision, hearing, and chemical senses are special sensory systems.[57] The fetus is able to process tactile, vestibular, taste, olfactory, auditory, and visual sensations. When the thalamocortical connections are generated, tactile sensations can be processed at the cortical level. A minimum level of consciousness, by some studies, emerges after the 25th GW.[58] This section will provide a review of insights of fetal sensory perception with an emphasis on somatosensory, visual, and auditory systems, and the role of different sensory stimuli in the development of fetal cognitive functions.

Touch and pain are the first senses that develop in utero. Nociceptors are pain receptors, free nerve endings, present since the seventh GW. That is the time after which the fetus gives the earliest response to pain, a motor reflex, which can be induced in various ways. This motor reflex emerges in the middle of the seventh GW, and it is controlled by the spinal cord. It resembles a withdrawal reflex, but it is still very nonspecific. In this early phase of development, there is no perception or processing of the pain in the higher parts of the brain.[59] Further, from the middle of the seventh GW, perioral region is touch sensitive. The fetus reflexively moves his head in the opposite direction if this region is touched. Reflexive movements of the extremities in response to touch arise later. Upper extremities move if stimulated in the middle of the 10th GW, while lower extremities produce this response at the 14th GW.[14] Studies on twin pregnancies were useful in research of the touch and pain. It was detected that monochorionic twins react by moving when stimulated by touch after the 10th GW. Bichorionic twins, on the other side, react to touch after the 12th GW.[60,61] At the 14th GW, all parts of the fetal body, with exception of the back and scalp, are sensitive to touch.[62]

Fetal pain is a neural process and a sense. Taking into account its direct and permanent consequences, fetal pain has to be evaluated and explained in detail, considering different fetal answers to painful stimuli. Pain has an important effect on the CNS development, and it can leave long-term cognitive, emotional, and behavioral consequences.[63] Fetal reaction to painful stimulus includes the neuroendocrine answer, activation of the hypothalamus–hypophysis axis, and autonomic nervous system. However, it needs to be emphasized

that these responses do not reach the cerebral cortex. The ability to sense pain requires developed neural pain system, from nociceptors to sensory areas in the cerebral cortex. Perception of sensory impulses is possible after they reach the somatosensory cortex around the 25th GW when the thalamocortical pathways and the cerebral cortex are connected.[12] Moreover, somatosensory-evoked potentials can be registered from the cortex at the 29th week of gestation. That is the evidence of pain processing in the somatosensory cortex.[46] The way how the fetus reacts to pain was observed during invasive intrauterine procedures. During these procedures, in the second trimester, between the 16th GW and 18th GW, cerebral blood flow increases.[64,65] Intrauterine transfusion through the innervated hepatic vein leads to an increase in plasma cortisol, noradrenaline, and beta-endorphin levels in the fetus at the 23rd GW. On the other hand, there is no increase in levels of these hormones if the needle is inserted in the noninnervated umbilical cord.[66,67] Fetal pain is a very important issue, especially considering the advances in intrauterine procedures and fetal surgery. It is necessary to take into account the knowledge about fetal pain and the effects of fetal stress response to prevent pain during invasive intrauterine procedures.[42] We are still uncertain if the fetus is fully aware of the pain and if there is any memory of fetal pain.[68] The cerebral cortex is necessary for pain perception, meaning the fetus cannot experience pain prior to reaching of connections from the periphery to the cortex. According to recent findings, the cortical pain response has been recorded by near-infrared spectroscopy from about 25 weeks of gestation. Preterm infants after 25 weeks of gestation are thus probably conscious of pain. On the other hand, there is an opinion that the fetus may not be conscious of pain even after the 25th GW due to high endogenous sedative and analgesic substances.[16] Nowadays, it is considered that fetal adaptation to stress and stress hormone secretion, which can enormously change developmental processes and leave lifelong consequences, are probably more dangerous and serious problem of the fetus than potential bad memories.[5,69]

Oftentimes, intrauterine life is described as living in darkness and silence, but the intrauterine environment is not fully deprived of the light and sound. Moreover, auditory and light stimulations are necessary for the development of fetal visual and auditory system.[70] Postnatal stimulation is also very important as the development of the visual system lasts until the 8th month after delivery.[71] Studies have revealed the developmental processes of the eye and their timeline. Visual connections between the retina, lateral geniculate nucleus and visual cortex begin their development in the mid-gestation. The thalamic projections reach the visual cortex between the 23rd GW and 27th GW. Maturation of the visual cortex can be registered by surface evoked potentials after the 36th GW.[14] It has been shown that the amplitude of visually evoked potentials can be used in the assessment of fetal habituation to light stimuli.[72] Moreover, from the 28th GW onward, a flash stimulus over the maternal abdomen can cause the visually evoked brain activity in the human fetus, recorded by megnetoencephalography.[73] Fetal eye motility is very important in retinal (neuronal) cell differentiation and in the eye functional maturation.[74,75] Eye movements **(Fig. 22.4)** are, in addition to facial movements and expressions, an important indicator of healthy development because they can predict postnatal eye function.[75] Stimulative intrauterine environment, as well as postnatal environmental enrichments, fosters the development of the visual system on the molecular, physiological, and behavioral level.[76-78]

Along with the visual, tactile, and motor stimuli, sound and vibration also affect neurodevelopment, in particular, the auditory system development. Studies have shown that the fetus reacts to exogenous acoustic stimulation and as the pregnancy progresses, fetal response to these stimuli changes.[79] These findings have opened many questions about fetal auditory system development. What is the connection between structural and functional development and what is the role of acoustic stimuli? The answer to these questions needs to be elaborated in studies of transmission of sound to the fetus, factors which influence fetal sound perception and fetal answer to acoustic stimuli.[80] The cochlear function develops between the 22nd GW and 25th GW, and its maturation continues in the first 6 months postnatally. Neural structures important for auditory system development are cochlear nuclei in the medulla oblongata and pons, auditory collicles in mesencephalon and primary auditory cortex. The pons and mesencephalon are later to mature in comparison with the structures of the medulla oblongata. For this reason the selective answer to sound and vibration arises later. The fetus reacts to strong sound stimuli delivered to the maternal abdomen by reflexive rotation of the trunk, head, and with lateral eye movements. This response of the fetus to sound appears later in the gestation. Fetal reactions to very loud sounds have been detected at 26 weeks, and progressive development of hearing has been observed in the third trimester.[30] At around 33 weeks of gestation, there is a change in the processing of complex sounds, such as music. In the younger fetuses the response is limited to the acoustic properties of music. In older fetuses, on the other hand, it seems that attention plays a role.[81] Due to tonotopic organization of cochlear nuclei and maturation of the brainstem, the fetus is capable of distinguishing different sounds by the end of gestation. Moreover, the existence of preference to mother's voice and other familiar voices has been proved. Repeated sound stimulus, or lack of it, forms neural networks and tracts in the medulla oblongata. After that, these structures selectively react to the same stimulus that formed them. This indicates that the brainstem already at that time possesses the activity connected with learning, and the brainstem nuclei and auditory pathways show synaptic plasticity and sensitivity to exogenous stimuli.[30] There are some factors that are known to affect the development of the auditory system and those are smoking,[82] intrauterine growth restriction (IUGR),[83] and hypertension in pregnancy.[84] Marshall et al.[85] noted that neonates of mothers who suffer from speech and hearing impairments, interestingly may have delayed development of the auditory system.

FETAL LEARNING AND MEMORY

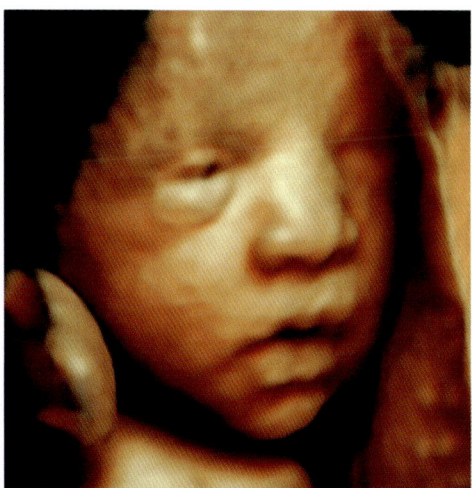

Fig. 22.4: High definition three-dimensional ultrasound image of fetal face with opened eyelid (30 + 2 weeks of gestation).

Studies of fetal cognitive functions are just at the beginning, but it is already found that the possibilities of fetal learning are astonishing. Furthermore, it has been shown that prenatally acquired memory lasts longer than it was initially considered.[86] Fetal learning and memory have been investigated by employing habituation methods, classical conditioning, and exposure learning.[1]

Habituation is a decrement in response following repetition of the same stimulus from the 22nd GW onward.[87] This phenomenon is one of the most well-documented and fundamental forms of nervous system plasticity. A major role of habituation is to limit the utilization of attentional resources for stimuli that are no longer salient.[88] Habituation can be distinguished from receptor adaptation as it requires an immediate recovery of the response on presentation of a different stimulus as well as faster response decrement upon representation of the original stimulus.[89,90] The first study of fetal habituation was reported in 1925. Subsequent studies showed that repeated stimulation of fetuses with the same stimulus resulted in a decrement of their response,[91,92] which was assessed by fetal heart rate alternations[93] or fetal movements. It has been noticed that younger fetuses require more exposure to the stimulus than older ones to register developmental trends. It should be mentioned that fetal habituation can be affected in a negative way by the presence of maternal stress and depression. This can result in developmental delays linked to the impaired function of the cerebral cortex.[94]

Classical conditioning involves the pairing of two stimuli: a conditioned and an unconditioned stimulus. Conditioned stimulus does not elicit response when presented alone, while unconditioned stimulus elicits one. After repeated paired exposure to these two stimuli the conditioned stimulus also elicits a response termed "conditioned response." This method of fetal learning has been demonstrated in 32–39-week-old fetuses.[95] However, it could also be demonstrated on anencephalic fetuses. Studies conducted on chimpanzees have shown that fetuses can learn and retain obtained information for at least 2 months after birth.[96]

Exposure learning is the third method used in the investigation of fetal memory and learning. It is used in such way where the fetus is reexposed to a stimulus after a number of exposures, and then this response is compared to the "unfamiliar" stimulus or to the response of an unexposed fetus to the same stimulus. Exposure learning confirmed that fetuses are able to hear and learn mother's voice before birth, and this gave insight to the fetal

preference of the mother's voice over an unacquainted one as well as mother's voice in utero over her voice after delivery.[97] At 34 weeks of gestation, selective fetal cortical processing for the voice of the mother over an unfamiliar voice has been reported.[98] The fetus is able to learn and remember familiar auditory stimuli and retain this information over the birth period.[99] Rudimentary capacity for retention of information may be expressed very early, at 30 weeks of gestation while prenatally acquired auditory memory can last even 6 weeks. The long-term auditory memory might have a role in the developmental psychobiology of attention and perception as well as early speech perception.[86]

The fetus is able to distinguish pleasant from an unpleasant taste of amniotic fluid, and it seems that sweet taste is the favorite taste even in utero.[5] The fetus can also learn different tastes and acquire taste preference as well as learn through smell.[16] Behavioral responses to pleasant and unpleasant smells can be recorded in preterm infants from about the 29th week. Furthermore, it has been shown that the preference for a certain food may be acquired during fetal life.[100]

Moreover, the process of prenatal language acquiring may be possible when the fetus starts discriminating different speeches in utero.[97,101] Presumably, fetal memory begins to develop prenatally. It probably functions in some rudimentary form and gradually develops as the fetus and child mature. Prenatal learning and memory may have a role in the development of maternal recognition, attachment, establishment of breastfeeding, language acquisition, and social recognition.[95] A study conducted on 93 pregnant women to assess fetal learning and memory, based on habituation to repeated vibroacoustic stimulation of fetuses of 30–38 weeks of gestational age, has shown that fetal learning and short-term (10 minutes) memory is present at 30th GW. Moreover, there is evidence that at the 34th GW, fetuses are able to store information and retrieve it 4 weeks later.[102] The fetus can detect, respond, and remember for a relatively long time the stimuli experienced during the prenatal period. It is important to point out that recent investigation has shown experience-dependent plasticity in the primary auditory cortex before the brain has reached full-term maturation. Extremely premature infants exposed to maternal sounds had significantly larger auditory cortex compared with control infants receiving standard care.[103]

EMOTIONAL DEVELOPMENT OF THE FETUS

Emotions are being born in fetal life. Recent data reported on ability of fetal movements to express different emotional states of the fetus.[39] Facial expressions represent one of the external signs of emotion. It is possible that facial movements demonstrate endogenously generated physiologic reflex patterns.[104] In fact, smiling as well as crying can be induced by the brainstem stimulation even with complete forebrain transection or destruction.[30] Using 4D US during the second and the third trimester of pregnancy has revealed a full range of different fetal facial expressions **(Figs. 22.5 and 22.6)**, similar to an adult's facial expressions.[38] As the pregnancy progresses, fetal facial expressions become more complex and some of them, such as facial expressions of pain or distress, are considered to be an adaptive process useful postnatally.[51] High-resolution 4D scans allow us to study fetal facial features in detail, their development over the gestation[38,105,106] and coordination of movements to form recognizable facial gestalts. "Cry-face gestalt" or "laughter-face gestalt" appear in the third trimester. This might be beneficial for fetal and maternal communication and postnatal bonding.[107] In addition, it is assumed that the facial expressions and emotion-like behaviors represent some kind of fetal emotion and awareness.[108]

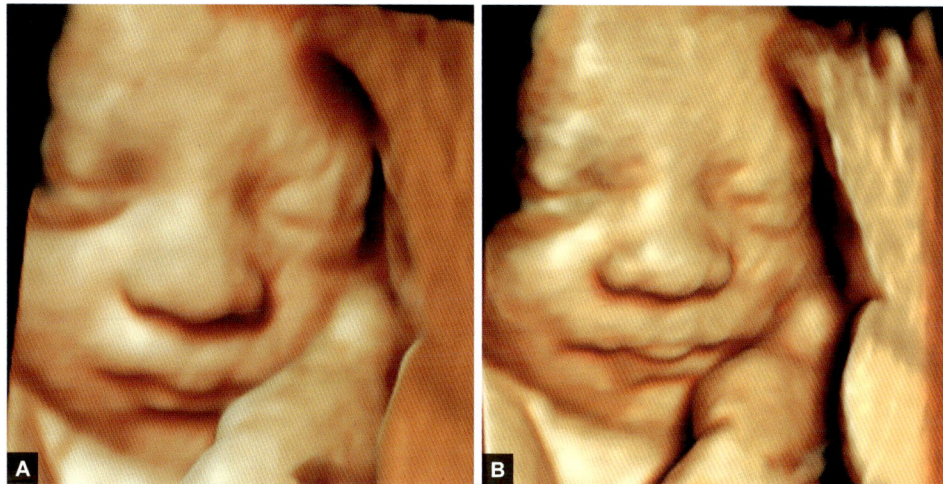

Figs. 22.5A and B: Sequence of four-dimensional high definition live mode ultrasound images of fetal calm and satisfied face (31 + 2 weeks of gestation).

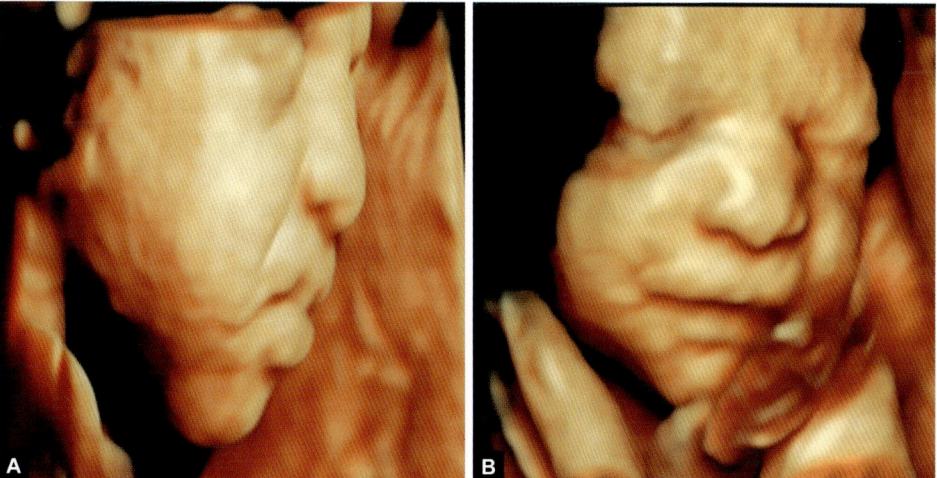

Figs. 22.6A and B: Sequence of four-dimensional high definition live mode ultrasound images of fetal face with dissatisfied and gloomy facial expression (30 + 22 weeks of gestation).

The limbic system, particularly the amygdala, is responsible for the experience and the expression of emotions.[109] The amygdala begins its development in early embryonic life[110] and has a great role in the mediation of emotional memory, attention, arousal, and the experience of different emotions: love, fear, pleasure, and joy. It contains facial recognition neurons which discern the emotional significance of different facial expressions. The evaluation of faces in social processing is an area of cognition specific to the amygdala.[109] The amygdala is essential for evaluating the biological relevance of sensory information and initiating behavioral responses based on the initial assessment of the presented stimulus. Facial expressions represent biologically important visual stimuli, and the amygdala neurons are very responsive to them.[88] An interesting finding is that affective problems in girls, exposed to high levels of maternal cortisol in early pregnancy, are linked with larger amygdala volume measured by MRI.[111]

ROLE OF FETAL STRESS IN COGNITIVE DEVELOPMENT

Physiological conditions in the intrauterine environment have an extremely important role in fetal growth and development. The emphasis is on balance, which enables the fetus to develop in its full potential. The fetus has to be protected in an environment where there are no harmful stimuli and where optimal conditions for growth and development are conserved. Though the role of stress is primarily protective, because it induces different adaptations of the organism and allows survival, fetal stress can leave negative consequences on the structure and function of the organism, especially the nervous system. The most important stressful factors are mother's malnutrition, IUGR, painful stimuli, and severe emotional stress of the mother as well as stressful life events.[69]

Stressful response stimulates fetal neuroendocrine axis which is active since the mid-gestation. This includes the production and secretion of the corticotropin-releasing hormone (CRH), adrenocorticotropic hormone (ACTH), and cortisol. Fetal hypothalamic–pituitary–adrenal response to stress is independent of mother's.[112] In addition, it has been determined that the fetus secretes noradrenaline, cortisol, and beta-endorphin between the 18th GW and 23rd GW in response to painful stimuli. Adaptation of the fetus to stress includes accelerated maturation, notably the maturation of the lungs and brain.

Unfortunately, even though this is a protective adaptation, interfering with the normal development of the CNS and other organ systems, it can leave long-term adverse sequels.[14,69] Cortisol, on one hand, initiates accelerated maturation of the brain and lungs, but also it has negative effects on growth of the fetal organism in a whole, as well as on the brain development. The hippocampus and parahippocampal region, the brain structures that contribute greatly to learning and memory, contain a large concentration of cortisol and CRH receptors. Consequently, these regions are susceptible to accelerated brain maturation, which can cause different structural changes in the developing brain. Apart from structural changes, behavioral changes were also noticed. Stress-induced changes in the hippocampus include decreased number of neurons and corticosteroid receptors, decreased a level of serotonin, and decreased synaptic density on distinct hippocampal regions. These changes are associated with memory impairment and learning disabilities later in life. Behavioral changes associated with accelerated brain development include hyperalertness and impaired fetal responsiveness to novel stimuli. Fetal ACTH may also be a cause of irritability and diminished attention. In addition, ACTH affects movement coordination and muscle tonus, which can be disturbed due to great exposure to this hormone. Fetal CRH influences the timing of the birth, which means that the fetus has an active role in the initiation of the delivery. A high serum level of cortisol and CRH is correlated to pregnancies complicated with IUGR, preeclampsia, infectious diseases, diabetes, and twin pregnancies. Many neuropsychiatric disorders [attention-deficit/hyperactivity disorder (ADHD), sleep disturbances, unsociable and inconsiderate behavior, schizophrenia, depressive and neurotic symptoms, drug abuse, and anxiety] are marked as potential neurodevelopmental consequences of prenatal stress exposure.[69] Increased maternal stress during pregnancy can influence an infant's temperament and cognitive functions,[113-115] and it may leave adverse effects on the child's learning and memory at age of 6.[116] However, it should be emphasized that infant cognitive development can be moderated enormously by increased mother's care and developed emotional mother–infant attachment.[115]

Etiology of many chronic diseases, diabetes, hypertension, and coronary disease[117] as well as psychiatric diseases, ADHD, cognitive impairments in children and later in adult life, can be found in the prenatal period.[118]

These conditions and diseases may be the consequences of the fetal adaptations, which happen due to suboptimal intrauterine conditions and change homeostatic regulation mechanisms, metabolism, or organ structure and function. This is called early life programming or developmental programming.[117,119]

High maternal cortisol in pregnancy is associated with programmed outcomes even in childhood, such as hypertension, behavioral disorders, and altered brain structure.[118] Programming and fetal stress might have different effects on female and male fetuses.[120,121] Prenatal exposure to stress can create a greater risk of depressive symptoms, schizophrenia, and ADHD in boys than in girls.[118] On the other side, high levels of maternal cortisol in early pregnancy are associated with more affective problems in girls. This was linked with the larger right amygdala volume measured by MRI, as mentioned in the previous section.[111]

CONCLUSION

Prenatal period is annotated with an opportunity for prosperous development of the fetus (including fetal cognitive development) but also it is a fragile period of great vulnerability to environmental effects. The fetus is exposed to numerous stimuli (e.g. tactile, chemical, auditory, etc.) which differently shape the brain structure and guide the brain's functional development. Prenatal 3D/4D US imaging has improved prenatal assessment of fetal structural, functional, behavioral development and assists in puzzle solving of fetal cognitive development.[122] In addition to US technology, recent advancements in fMRI and fMEG have made it possible to examine functional neurodevelopment as well. All of these tools should be used in the best possible way to learn more about the fetal neurodevelopmental events and provide the most stimulative environment for the cognitive development of the fetus.

Primary cortical areas and subcortical formations are fully developed and high active in a newborn, thus cognitive functions at the end of the gestation rely on them. At term, there is also low activity in the association cortical areas.

Early action planning development and fetal motor learning are recognized in the second trimester. Progression in fetal activity and behavior complexity reflexes the maturational processes in the brainstem and later on, in the forebrain structures (the diencephalon and cerebrum). It starts with the emerging of the spontaneous movements and culminates with the presumed preference for the sound of the mother's voice.

Functional thalamocortical and corticocortical connections are required for the linkage between the periphery and the cerebral cortex. That is needed for the establishment of the fetal awareness of noxious as well as other sensory stimuli and higher order sensory perception begins in fetal life.

Fetal learning and fetal memory possibilities are impressive. Even though considered rudimentary, fetal memory is lasting longer than it was previously thought. A remarkable property of synaptic plasticity is shown in the primary auditory cortex even before the brain has reached full-term maturation.

Studies conducted by 4D US indicate that emotion-like behaviors and roots of emotions appear during fetal life. It has been suggested that facial expressions and emotion-like behaviors may represent some kind of fetal emotion and awareness.

Roots of many disorders and chronic diseases of adult age have been linked to adverse events and effects on the fetus. Cognitive impairments and deficits in childhood and adulthood (impaired learning and memory, intellectual disabilities, attention deficits, etc.) may also originate in the prenatal life.

Investigation of fetal cognitive functions is still in its beginning, but it is certain that future advances in the application of new imaging methods, such as different 3D/4D US modes and fMRI, will enable a better understanding of the cognitive abilities and functions of the fetus. These techniques can help in early detection of abnormal brain development, i.e. to allow early diagnosis and prevention of the brain dysfunctions and damage and to assure in due time intervention and habilitation of affected children. Finally, it is of great importance to emphasize again that infant cognitive development can be moderated enormously by increased mother's care and developed emotional mother–infant attachment.

REFERENCES

1. Kadic AS, Kurjak A. Cognitive functions of the fetus. Ultraschall Med. 2018;39(2):181-9.
2. Salihagić-Kadić A, Glavac F, Vasilj O. Advances in understanding of neurophysiological function of the fetus. Donald Sch J Ultrasound Obstet Gynecol. 2018;2(1):23-31.
3. Merz E. 25 years of 3D ultrasound in prenatal diagnosis. Ultraschall Med. 2015;36:3-8.

4. Schopf V, Langs G, Jakab A. Functional imaging of prenatal brain. In: Reissland N, Kisilevsky B (Eds). Fetal Development: Research on Brain and Behavior, Environmental Influences, and Emerging Technologies. New York, NY: Springer International Publishing; 2016. pp. 429-39.

5. Salihagić Kadić A, Predojević M. Fetal neurophysiology according to gestational age. Semin Fetal Neonatal Med. 2012;17(5):256-60.

6. Huttenlocher P. Synaptogenesis in human cerebral cortex. In: Dawson G, Fisher K (Eds). Human Behavior and the Developing Brain. New York, NY: Guilford; 1994. pp. 137-52.

7. Stiles J, Brown T, Haist F, et al. Brain and cognitive development. In: Lerner M (Ed). Handbook of Child Psychology and Developmental Science, 7th edition. New York, NY: John Wiley & Sons, Inc.; 2015. pp. 1-54.

8. Sadler T. Central nervous system. In: Sadler T (Ed). Langman's Medical Embryology, 9th edition. Philadelphia, PA: Lippincott and Wilkins; 2004. pp. 433-80.

9. Saitsu H, Yamada S, Uwabe C, et al. Development of the posterior neural tube in human embryos. Anat Embryol (Berl). 2004;209(2):107-17.

10. Nelson CA. Neural development and lifelong plasticity. In: Keating P. (Ed). Nature and Nurture in Early Child Development. Cambridge: Cambridge University Press; 2011. pp. 45-69.

11. Kostović I, Judaš M, Petanjek Z, et al. Ontogenesis of goal-directed behavior: anatomo-functional considerations. Int J Psychophysiol. 1995;19(2):85-102.

12. Kostovic I, Judas M. The development of the subplate and thalamocortical connections in the human foetal brain. Acta Paediatr. 2010;99(8):1119-27.

13. Kostovic I. Laminar organization of the human fetal cerebrum revealed by histochemical markers and magnetic resonance imaging. Cereb Cortex. 2002;12(5):536-44.

14. Salihagić-Kadić A, Predojević M, Kurjak A. Advances in fetal neurophysiology. In: Pooh RK, Kurjak A (Eds). Fetal Neurology. New Delhi: Jaypee Brothers; 2009. pp. 160-204.

15. Olson CR, Colby CL. Organization of cognition. In: Kandel ER, Schwartz JH, Jessell TM, Siegelbaum SA, Hudspeth AJ (Eds). Principles of Neural Science. New York, NY: McGraw-Hill; 2013. pp. 392-411.

16. Lagercrantz H. The emergence of consciousness: science and ethics. Semin Fetal Neonatal Med. 2014;19(5): 300-5.

17. Qiu A, Mori S, Miller MI. Diffusion tensor imaging for understanding brain development in early life. Annu Rev Psychol. 2015;66:853-76.

18. Anderson A, Thomason ME. Functional plasticity before the cradle: a review of neural imaging in the human fetus. Neurosci Biobehav Rev. 2013;37:2220-32.

19. Fransson P, Skiöld B, Horsch S, et al. Resting-state networks in the infant brain. Proc Natl Acad Sci U S A. 2007;104:15531-6.

20. Doria V, Beckman CF, Arichi T, et al. Emergence of resting state networks in the preterm human brain. Proc Natl Acad Sci U S A. 2010;107:20015-20.

21. Thomason M, Chang CE, Glover GH, et al. Default-mode function and task-induced deactivation have overlapping brain substrates in children. NeuroImage. 2008;41: 1493-503.

22. Jakab A, Schwartz E, Kasprian G, et al. Fetal functional imaging portrays heterogeneous development of emerging human brain networks. Front Hum Neurosci. 2014;8:852.

23. Pashaj S, Merz E. Detection of fetal corpus callosum abnormalities by means of 3D ultrasound. Ultraschall Med. 2016;37(2):185-94.

24. Paul L. Developmental malformation of the corpus callosum: a review of typical callosal development and examples of developmental disorders with callosal involvement. J Neurodev Disord. 2011;3:3-27.

25. Okado N, Kakimi S, Kojima T. Synaptogenesis in the cervical cord of the human embryo: sequence of synapse formation in a spinal reflex pathway. J Comp Neurol. 1979;184(3):491-517.

26. Okado N, Kojima T. Ontogeny of the central nervous system: neurogenesis, fibre connection, synaptogenesis and myelination in the spinal cord. In: Prechtl H (Ed). Continuity of Neural Function from Prenatal to Postnatal Life. Oxford: Blackwell Science; 1984. pp. 31-5.

27. Okado N. Onset of synapse formation in the human spinal cord. J Comp Neurol. 1981;201(2):211-9.

28. de Vries JIP, Visser GHA, Prechtl HFR. The emergence of fetal behaviour. I. Qualitative aspects. Early Hum Dev. 1982;7(4):301-22.

29. Einspieler C, Prechtl HF. Prechtl's assessment of general movements: a diagnostic tool for the functional assessment of the young nervous system. Ment Retard Dev Disabil Res Rev. 2005;11(1):61-7.

30. Joseph R. Fetal brain behavior and cognitive development. Dev Rev. 2000;20(1):81-98.

31. Pomeroy S, Volpe J. Development of the nervous system. In: Polin R, Fox W (Eds). Fetal and Neonatal Physiology. Philadelphia–London–Toronto–Montreal–Sydney–Tokyo: WB Saunders Company; 1992. pp. 1491-509.

32. Lüchinger AB, Hadders-Algra M, Van Kan CM, De Vries JIP. Fetal onset of general movements. Pediatr Res. 2008;63(2):191-5.

33. Kurjak A, Azumendi G, Veček N, et al. Fetal hand movements and facial expression in normal pregnancy studied by four-dimensional sonography. J Perinat Med. 2003;31(6):496-508.

34. Pooh RK, Ogura T. Normal and abnormal fetal hand positioning and movement in early pregnancy detected by three- and four-dimensional sonography. J Perinat Med. 2003;31:496-508.

35. Andonotopo W, Medić M, Salihagić-Kadić A, et al. The assessment of fetal behaviour in early pregnancy: comparison between 2D and 4D sonographic scanning. J Perinat Med. 2005;33(5):406-14.

36. Prechtl HFR. Qualitative changes of spontaneous movements in fetus and preterm infant are a marker of neurological dysfunction. Early Hum Dev. 1990;23(3):151-8.

37. Einspieler C, Prechtl HFR, Ferrari F, et al. The qualitative assessment of general movements in preterm, term and young infants—review of the methodology. Early Hum Dev. 1997;50(1):47-60.

38. Kurjak A, Azumendi G, Andonotopo W, et al. Three- and four-dimensional ultrasonography for the structural and functional evaluation of the fetal face. Am J Obstet Gynecol. 2007;196(1):16-28.

39. Delafield-butt J, Trevarthen C. Theories of the development of human communication. Theories and models of communication. In: Cobley P, Schutz PJ (Eds). Handbook of Communication Science. Berlin: De Gruyter Mouton; 2013. pp. 199-221.

40. Zoia S, Blason L, D'Ottavio G, et al. Evidence of early development of action planning in the human foetus: a kinematic study. Exp Brain Res. 2007;176(2):217-26.

41. Trevarthen C, Delafield-butt J. Autism as a developmental disorder in intentional movement and affective engagement. Front Integr Neurosci. 2013;7:49-73.

42. Anand KJS, Carr DB. The neuroanatomy, neurophysiology, and neurochemistry of pain, stress, and analgesia in newborns and children. Pediatr Clin North Am. 1989;36(4): 795-822.

43. Kostovic I, Rakic P. Development of prestriate visual projections in the monkey and human fetal cerebrum revealed by transient cholinesterase staining. J Neurosci. 1984;4(1):25-42.

44. Kostovic I, Goldman-Rakic P. Transient cholinesterase staining in the mediodorsal nucleus of the thalamus and its connections in the developing human and monkey brain. J Comp Neurol. 1983;219:431-47.

45. Amiel-Tison C, Gosselin J. From neonatal to fetal neurology: some clues for interpreting fetal findings. In: Pooh R, Kurjak A. (Eds). Fetal neurology. New Delhi: Jaypee Brothers Medical Publishers (P) Ltd; 2009. pp. 373-99.

46. Klimach VJ, Cooke RWI. Maturation of the neonatal somatosensory evoked response in preterm infants. Dev Med Child Neurol. 1988;30(2):208-14.

47. Groome LJ, Swiber MJ, Atterbury JL, et al. Similarities and differences in behavioral state organization during sleep periods in the perinatal infant before and after birth. Child Dev. 1997;68(1):1-11.

48. Kawai N. Towards a new study on associative learning in human fetuses: fetal associative learning in primates. Infant Child Dev. 2010;19:55-9.

49. Kisilevsky B, Hains S, Lee K, et al. Effects of experience on fetal voice recognition. Psych Sci. 2003;14:220-4.

50. Kisilevsky B, Hains S. Exploring the relationship between fetal heart rate and cognition. Infant Child Dev. 2010;19: 60-75.

51. Reissland N, Francis B, Mason J. Can healthy fetuses show facial expressions of "pain" or "distress"? PLoS One. 2013;8(6):e65530.

52. Kurjak A, Miskovic B, Stanojevic M, et al. New scoring system for fetal neurobehavior assessed by three- and four-dimensional sonography. J Perinat Med. 2008;36(1):73-81.

53. Salihagić-Kadić A, Stanojević M, Predojević M. Assessment of the fetal neuromotor development with the New KANET Test. In: Reissland N, Ksilevsky B (Eds). Fetal Development: Research on Brain and Behavior, Environmental Influences, and Emerging Technologies. Heidelberg, New York, Dordrecht, London: Springer International Publishing Switzerland; 2016. pp. 177-89.

54. Kurjak A, Abo-Yaqoub S, Stanojevic M, et al. The potential of 4D sonography in the assessment of fetal neurobehavior—multicentric study in high-risk pregnancies. J Perinat Med. 2010;38(1):77-82.

55. Predojević M, Talić A, Stanojević M, et al. Assessment of motoric and hemodynamic parameters in growth restricted fetuses—case study. J Matern Neonatal Med. 2014;27(3):247-51.

56. Tomasovic S, Predojevic M. Neurodevelopment disorders and possibility of their prenatal detection. Acta Med Croat. 2015;69(5):415-20.

57. Hall J, Guyton A. Textbook of Medical Physiology, 13th edition. Philadelphia, PA: Elsevier; 2016. pp. 577-688.

58. Lagercrantz H. The emergence of the mind: a borderline of human viability? Acta Paediatr. 2007;96:327-8.

59. Vanhatalo S, Van Nieuwenhuizen O. Fetal pain? Brain Dev. 2000;22(3):145-50.

60. Arabin B, Bos R, Rijlaarsdam R, et al. The onset of inter-human contacts: longitudinal ultrasound observations in early twin pregnancies. Ultrasound Obstet Gynecol. 1996;8(3):166-73.

61. Piontelli A, Bocconi L, Kustermann A, et al. Patterns of evoked behaviour in twin pregnancies during the first 22 weeks of gestation. Early Hum Dev. 1997;50(1): 39-45.

62. Hepper P. Prenatal development. In: Slater A, Lewis M (Eds). Introduction to Infant Development. New York, NY: Oxford University Press; 2007. pp. 39-101.

63. Gupta A, Giordano J. On the nature, assessment, and treatment of fetal pain: neurobiological bases, pragmatic issues, and ethical concerns. Pain Physician. 2007;10(4): 525-32.

64. Teixeira JMA, Glover V, Fisk NM. Acute cerebral redistribution in response to invasive procedures in the human fetus. Am J Obstet Gynecol. 1999;181(4): 1018-25.

65. Smith RP, Gitau R, Glover V, et al. Pain and stress in the human fetus. Eur J Obstet Gynecol Reprod Biol. 2000;92(1):161-5.

66. Giannakoulopoulos X, Glover V, Sepulveda W, et al. Fetal plasma cortisol and β-endorphin response to intrauterine needling. Lancet. 1994;344(8915):77-81.

67. Giannakoulopoulos X, Teixeira J, Fisk N, et al. Human fetal and maternal noradrenaline responses to invasive procedures. Pediatr Res. 1999;45(4 Pt 1):494-9.

68. White MC, Wolf AR. Pain and stress in the human fetus. Best Pr Res Clin Anaesthesiol. 2004;18(2):205-20.

69. Kadić AS. Fetal neurology: the role of fetal stress. Donald Sch J Ultrasound Obstet Gynecol. 2015;9:30-9.

70. Magoon EH, Robb RM. Development of myelin in human optic nerve and tract. A light and electron microscopic study. Arch Ophtalmol. 1981;99:655-9.

71. Huttenlocher P, de Courten C. The development of synapses in striate cortex of man. Hum Neurobiol. 1987;6(1):1-9.

72. Sheridan CJ, Preissl H, Siegel ER, et al. Neonatal and fetal response decrement of evoked responses: a MEG study. Clin Neurophysiol. 2008;119(4):796-804.

73. Eswaran H, Wilson J, Preissl H, et al. Magnetoencephalographic recordings of visual evoked brain activity in the human fetus. Lancet. 2002;360(9335):779-80.

74. Kablar B. Determination of retinal cell fates is affected in the absence of extraocular striated muscles. Dev Dyn. 2003;226(3):478-90.

75. Baguma-Nibasheka M, Reddy T, Abbas-Butt A, et al. Fetal ocular movements and retinal cell differentiation: analysis employing DNA microarrays. Histol Histopathol. 2006;21:1331-7.

76. Sale A, Cenni MC, Clussi F, et al. Maternal enrichment during pregnancy accelerates retinal development of the fetus. PLoS One. 2007;2(11):e1160.

77. Sale A, Putignano E, Cancedda L, et al. Enriched environment and acceleration of visual system development. Neuropharmacology. 2004;47(5):649-60.

78. Landi S, Sale A, Berardi N, et al. Retinal functional development is sensitive to environmental enrichment: a role for BDNF. FASEB J. 2006;21(1):130-9.

79. Hepper PG, Shahidullah B. The development of fetal hearing. Fetal Matern Med Rev. 1994;6(3):167-79.

80. Lecanuet JP, Schaal B. Fetal sensory competencies. Eur J Obstet Gynecol Reprod Biol. 1996;68(1-2):1-23.

81. Kisilevsky BS, Hains SMJ, Jacquet AY, et al. Maturation of fetal responses to music. Dev Sci. 2004;7(5):550-9.

82. Cowperthwaite B, Hains SMJ, Kisilevsky BS. Fetal behavior in smoking compared to non-smoking pregnant women. Infant Behav Dev. 2007;30(3):422-30.

83. Kisilevsky BS, Davies GAL. Auditory processing deficits in growth restricted fetuses affect later language development. Med Hypotheses. 2007;68(3):620-8.

84. Lee CT, Brown CA, Hains SMJ, et al. Fetal development: voice processing in normotensive and hypertensive pregnancies. Biol Res Nurs. 2007;8(4):272-82.

85. Marshall J. Infant neurosensory development: considerations for infant child care. Early Child Educ J. 2011;39(3):175-81.

86. Granier-Deferre C, Bassereau S, Ribeiro A, et al. A melodic contour repeatedly experienced by human near-term fetuses elicits a profound cardiac reaction one month after birth. PLoS One. 2011;6(2):e17304.

87. Yamaguchi S. Rapid prefrontal–hippocampal habituation to novel events. J Neurosci. 2004;24(23):5356-63.

88. Wright CI, Fischer H, Whalen PJ, et al. Differential prefrontal cortex and amygdala habituation to repeatedly presented emotional stimuli. Neuroreport. 2001;12(2):379-83.

89. Jeffrey WE, Cohen LB. Habituation in the human infant. Adv Child Dev Behav. 1971;6:63-97.

90. Thompson RF, Spencer WA. Habituation: a model phenomenon for the study of neuronal substrates of behavior. Psychol Rev. 1966;73(1):16-43.

91. Van Heteren CF, Boekkooi PF, Jongsma HW, et al. Fetal learning and memory. Lancet. 2000;356(9236):1169-70.

92. Shalev E, Weiner E, Serr DM. Fetal habituation to sound stimulus in various behavioral states. Gynecol Obstet Invest. 1990;29(2):115-7.

93. Gagnon R, Hunse C, Carmichael L, et al. Human fetal responses to vibrator acoustic stimulation from twenty-six weeks to term. Am J Obstet Gynecol. 1987;157(6):1375-81.

94. Morokuma S, Fukushima K, Kawai N, et al. Fetal habituation correlates with functional brain development. Behav Brain Res. 2004;153(2):459-63.

95. Hepper P. Fetal memory: does it exist? What does it do? Acta Paediatr. 1996;416:16-20.

96. Kawai N, Morokuma S, Tomonaga M, et al. Associative learning and memory in a chimpanzee fetus: learning and long-lasting memory before birth. Dev Psychobiol. 2004;44(2):116-22.

97. Hepper PG, Scott D, Shahidullah S. Newborn and fetal response to maternal voice. J Reprod Infant Psychol. 1993;11(3):147-53.

98. Jardri R, Houfflin-Debarge V, Delion P, et al. Assessing fetal response to maternal speech using a noninvasive functional brain imaging technique. Int J Dev Neurosci. 2012;30(2):159-61.

99. Hepper P. Fetal "soap" addiction. Lancet. 1988;331(8598):1347-8.

100. Mennella JA, Jagnow CP, Beauchamp GK. Prenatal and postnatal flavor learning by human infants. Pediatrics. 2001;107(6):e88.

101. DeCasper AJ, Spence MJ. Prenatal maternal speech influences newborns' perception of speech sounds. Infant Behav Dev. 1986;9(2):133-50.

102. Dirix CEH, Nijhuis JG, Jongsma HW, et al. Aspects of fetal learning and memory. Child Dev. 2009;80(4):1251-8.

103. Webb A, Heller H, Benon C. Mother's voice and heartbeat sounds elicit auditory plasticity in the human brain before full gestation. Proc Natl Acad Sci U S A. 2015;112(10):3152-7.

104. Merz E. Fetal facial expressions: demonstrations of the smiling, the sad and the scowling fetus with 4D-ultrasound. Ultraschall Med. 2015;36(1):1-2.

105. Kurjak A, Andonotopo W, Hafner T, et al. Normal standards for fetal neurobehavioral developments—longitudinal quantification by four-dimensional sonography. J Perinat Med. 2006;34(1):56-65.

106. Hata T, Dai SY, Marumo MG. Ultrasound for evaluation of fetal neurobehavioural development: from 2-D to 4-D ultrasound. Infant Child Dev. 2010;19:99-118.

107. Reissland N, Francis B, Mason J, et al. Do facial expressions develop before birth? PLoS One. 2011;6(8):e24081.

108. Hata T, Kanenishi K, AboEllail MAM. Fetal consciousness: four-dimensional ultrasound study. Donald Sch J Ultrasound Obstet Gynecol. 2015;9(4):471-4.

109. Joseph R. Environmental influences on neural plasticity, the limbic system, emotional development and attachment: a review. Child Psychiatry Hum Dev. 1999;29(3): 189-208.

110. Humphrey T. The development of the human amygdala during early embryonic life. J Comp Neurol. 1968;132(1): 135-65.

111. Buss C, Davis EP, Shahbaba B, et al. Maternal cortisol over the course of pregnancy and subsequent child amygdala and hippocampus volumes and affective problems. Proc Natl Acad Sci U S A. 2012;109(20):E1312-9.

112. Gitau R, Fisk NM, Teixeira JMA, et al. Fetal hypothalamic–pituitary–adrenal stress responses to invasive procedures are independent of maternal responses. J Clin Endocrinol Metab. 2001;86(1):104-9.

113. Buitelaar JK, Huizink AC, Mulder EJ, et al. Prenatal stress and cognitive development and temperament in infants. Neurobiol Aging. 2003;24:S53-60.

114. Davis EP, Glynn LM, Schetter CD, et al. Prenatal exposure to maternal depression and cortisol influences infant temperament. J Am Acad Child Adolesc Psychiatry. 2007;46(6):737-46.

115. Bergman K, Sarkar P, Glover V, et al. Maternal prenatal cortisol and infant cognitive development: moderation by infant–mother attachment. Biol Psychiatry. 2010;67(11): 1026-32.

116. Gutteling BM, de Weerth C, Zandbelt N, et al. Does maternal prenatal stress adversely affect the child's learning and memory at age six? J Abnorm Child Psychol. 2006;34:789-98.

117. Barker DJ. Fetal origins of coronary heart disease. BMJ. 1995;311(6998):171-4.

118. Reynolds RM. Glucocorticoid excess and the developmental origins of disease: two decades of testing the hypothesis—2012 Curt Richter Award Winner. Psychoneuroendocrinology. 2013;38(1):1-11.

119. Cottrell EC, Seckl JR. Prenatal stress, glucocorticoids and the programming of the adult disease. Front Behav Neurosci. 2009;3(19):1-9.

120. Cottrell EC, Seckl JR, Holmes MC, et al. Foetal and placental 11beta-HSD2: a hub for developmental programming. Acta Physiol. 2014;210(2):288-95.

121. Aiken CE, Ozanne SE. Sex differences in developmental programming models. Reproduction. 2013;145(1):R1-13.

122. Kurjak A, Barisic LS, Stanojevic M, et al. Are we ready to investigate cognitive function of fetal brain? The role of advanced four-dimensional sonography. Donald Sch J Ultrasound Obstet Gynecol. 2016;10(2):116-24.

Three-dimensional Ultrasonographic Evaluation of the Fetal Posterior Fossa

Sertaç Esin, Ebru Tarım, Cihat Şen

INTRODUCTION

Posterior fossa malformations are among the most common brain anomalies. Despite the rapid progress in fetal imaging, the prenatal diagnosis of posterior fossa anomalies remains difficult due to both false-positive and false-negative diagnoses.[1-3] Fetal posterior fossa abnormalities may be broadly divided into hindbrain malformations, including diseases with cerebellar or vermian agenesis, aplasia or hypoplasia, and cystic posterior fossa anomalies; and cranial vault malformations or Chiari malformations.

Evaluation of the fetal posterior fossa is an essential part of routine fetal ultrasonography. Thanks to advances in neuroimaging, the frequency of the evaluation of the posterior fossa has increased significantly over the past 20 years. However, fetal posterior fossa contains complex anatomic structures and therefore conventional two-dimensional (2D) ultrasonography may sometimes have limited value in detecting anomalies, especially in the second trimester of gestation. And when an abnormality is found by standard 2D ultrasonography, there are a number of pathologies, ranging from normal variants to severe anomalies that may look identical or similar. Nevertheless, categorization of posterior fossa anomalies is still controversial, and there is no uniform approach.[4-6] Differential diagnosis of these pathologies may require additional sonographic planes, such as sagittal and coronal planes, and acquiring those may be rather difficult in certain cases. Advanced neuroimaging techniques, such as fetal magnetic resonance imaging (MRI) and three-dimensional (3D) or four-dimensional (4D) ultrasonography, allow detailed evaluation of the complex anatomic structures within the posterior fossa and

improve diagnostic accuracy and diagnostic confidence having a positive clinical impact in a high proportion of cases.[7] Brainstem, cerebellum, fourth ventricle (4V), and cisterna magna are better assessed with these techniques. Having said that, fetal MRI is available only in specialized centers and may not be accepted by the family due to the complexity of the procedure. Another novel option is 3D or 4D evaluation of the fetal brain. Ultrasonographic machines with 3D or 4D capabilities are readily available in most of the perinatology or obstetrics and gynecology centers, and families are more familiar and feel safe with those machines though fetal MRI is superior to ultrasonography in cases with oligohidramnios, maternal obesity, and fetal skull ossification.

By transabdominal ultrasonography, fetal brain anatomy may be visualized fairly in axial sections. However, fetal cranial bone ossification, thick maternal abdominal wall, and anterior placenta may render transabdominal ultrasonography difficult and ineffective. This obstacle may be overcome by high-resolution transvaginal ultrasonography, and high-quality images may be obtained from acoustic window through anterior fontanelle and sagittal sutures. Although it is critically valuable in case of the vertex presentation, acquiring essential sections may be difficult, especially for those who are not acquainted with transvaginal fetal neurosonography. Multidimensional mode in fetal neurosonography by 3D transvaginal probes has several advantages over standard 2D transvaginal probes. Unlimited offline analysis by using three orthogonal planes of the fetal brain, tomographic ultrasound imaging and volume contrast imaging (VCI) may be obtained by a single 3D-acquired data. These neuroimaging modes allow obtaining more precise information on fetal posterior fossa, and the results are comparable to

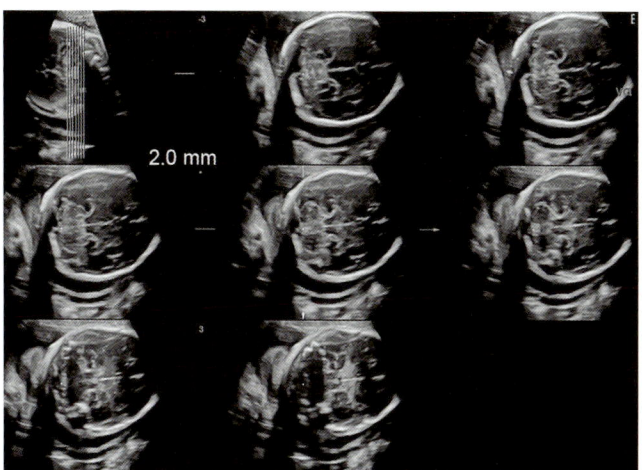

Fig. 23.1: A 3D volume dataset of axial acquisitions of fetal posterior fossa displayed in tomographic mode.

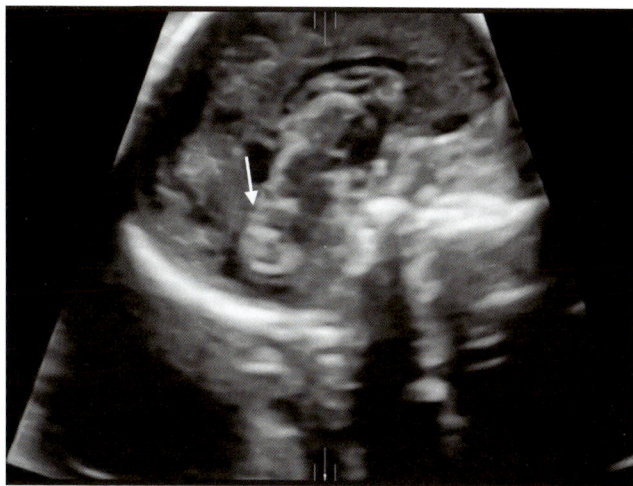

Fig. 23.2: Vermis (arrow) and posterior fossa can be reconstructed after a 3D volume acquisition. In this reconstruction the corpus callosum can also be seen in this midline section.

those obtained with fetal MRI. Paladini et al. showed that the overall accuracy rates of expert neurosonography and fetal MRI were similar (91.3% vs 94.4%), respectively, and fetal MRI was more useful after 24 weeks of gestation.[8]

Cerebellar anatomy is generally assessed in the axial view. This includes the demonstration of the normal shape of both hemispheres with the vermis in between. Inferior part of the vermis should also be visualized and separates the 4V from the cistern (**Fig. 23.1**). Similarly, to the corpus callosum, the cerebellar vermis can also be provided by sagittal 3D acquisitions through the anterior fontanelle, transabdominally when the fetus is in the breech presentation (**Figs. 23.2 and 23.3**).

While examining the axial planes, the demonstration of midsagittal view of vermis with neighboring structures can be so important to diagnose anomalies. In this view the size, shape, and the position of the vermis can be objectively assessed (**Figs. 23.2 to 23.5**).

In this chapter, we would like to summarize the main fetal posterior fossa abnormalities and emphasize the importance and significance of 3D ultrasonography in differential diagnosis of those abnormalities.

Vermian–cerebellar hypoplasia: Vermian–cerebellar hypoplasia refers to varying degrees of incomplete development of the vermis and cerebellum.[9] Ultrasonographic features of vermian–cerebellar hypoplasia include varying degrees of vermian and cerebellar hypoplasia.[9] Vermian hypoplasia may occur without the presence of a fluid collection, further complicating identification of

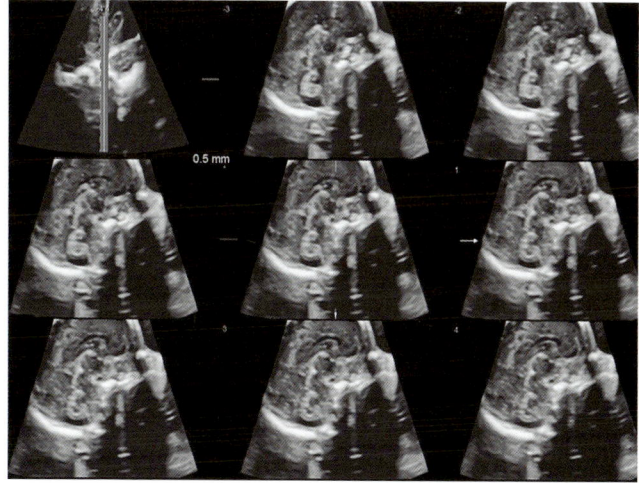

Fig. 23.3: Sagittal and parasagittal sectional planes after a transabdominal 3D acquisition through the fontanelle with a rendering in tomographic mode. The focus is on the midline structures, which are well recognized as the corpus callosum and vermis.

this abnormality.[10] Paladini et al. showed that using 3D ultrasound significant hypoplasia of the cerebellar vermis may be demonstrated, and there is a good correlation between MRI and 3D ultrasound-derived morphometric measurements of the vermis[11] which makes 3D ultrasound an appealing choice.

Dandy–Walker malformation (DWM): DWM is a cerebellar abnormality characterized by the dysgenesis of cerebellar vermis and cystic dilatation of the 4V. The best diagnostic clue for DWM is a large fetal posterior

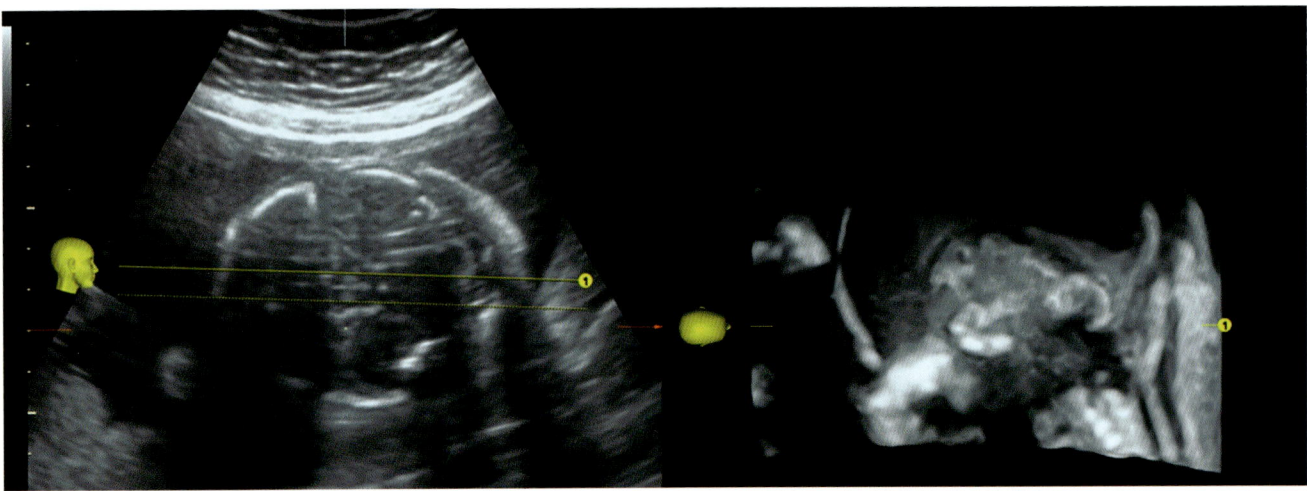

Fig. 23.4: Omniview with volume contrast imaging for the demonstration of vermis and brainstem.

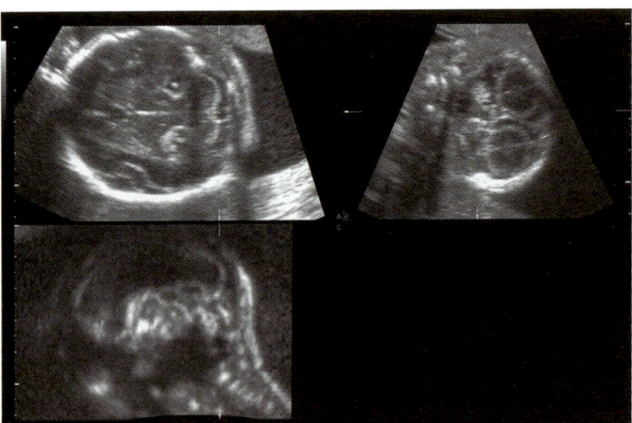

Fig. 23.5: Posterior fossa with multiplanar imaging.

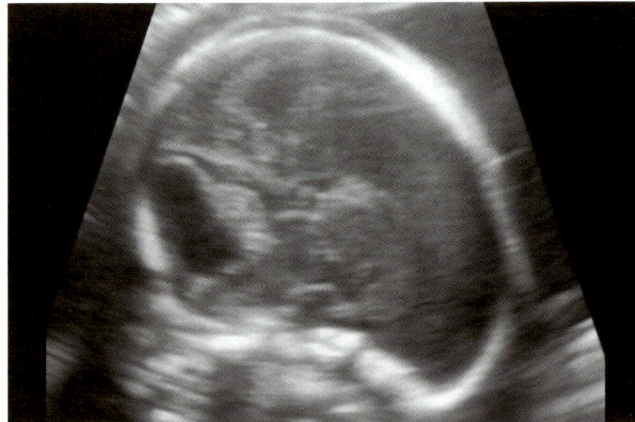

Fig. 23.6: Detailed sonographic demonstration of Dandy–Walker malformation with volume contrast imaging mode.

fossa with big cerebrospinal fluid cyst, and the 4V appears contiguous with the posterior fossa cyst. The tentorium and torcular herophili are elevated. Hydrocephaly, aqueductal stenosis, dysgenesis of the corpus callosum, brainstem dysplasias, migration anomalies, schizencephaly, lipomas, cephaloceles, and lumbosacral meningocele may be associated with DWM. Differential diagnosis of DWM may be difficult and contains Blake's pouch cyst (BPC) and vermian agenesis/hypoplasia. Diagnosis of DWM by using only axial transabdominal ultrasonography may result in erroneous diagnosis.[12] For a proper diagnosis, assessment of the vermis and torcular herophili is essential by a median view.[5,6,13] 3D ultrasonography may be invaluable for those cases due to the ability to control the planes using the orthogonal planes as reference.[14,15] Furthermore, VCI may assist visualization of subtle anatomical details[14,15] **(Fig. 23.6)**.

Blake's pouch cyst: Blake's pouch is a finger-like outpouch of the 4V and is an embryological remnant. Enlargement of this remnant may lead to a slight superior displacement of the vermis and is called BPC. As this gives an impression of 4V contiguous with the posterior fossa cyst, it is an important entity in the differential diagnosis of DWM. In BPC, the cerebellar vermis, cisterna magna, and torcular herophili are in normal position. Assessment of these characteristic features is possible with 3D ultrasonography. Paladini et al. found that the upper wall of the cyst may be visible in 11/19 of the cases.[16]

Megacisterna magna: Megacisterna magna is characterized by abnormal widening of the cisterna magna with a normal-appearing cerebellar vermis and hemispheres. It is usually an isolated finding and in the absence of associated anomalies, the prognosis of megacisterna magna is good.[17] Nevertheless, it is an important entity because it should be differentiated from DWM, BPC, and vermian agenesis/hypoplasia. The key plane is the sagittal one and by 3D ultrasonography, essential median and paramedian planes may be obtained easily.

Spinal dysraphism and Chiari II malformation: Spinal dysraphism refers to a vertebral open defect in which the spinal contents protrude through the bony content. In Chiari II malformation, open spinal dysraphism results in herniation of the cerebellar vermis and brainstem through the foramen magnum.[18] The diagnosis of Chiari II malformations may be achieved by scanning the spine in three planes (axial, sagittal, and coronal) by 2D ultrasound. However, due to maternal body properties and fetal position, not all planes may be accessible in all cases. Using 3D ultrasonography, the spine may be displayed along three orthogonal scanning planes; and therefore, 3D ultrasonography presents obvious advantages.

As a conclusion, different fetal posterior fossa abnormalities may have similar appearances and differential diagnosis is crucial as they have distinct prognosis. 3D ultrasonography is an invaluable instrument for differential diagnosis of these entities. Transabdominal or transvaginal 3D ultrasonography allows detailed evaluation of the complex anatomic structures within the posterior fossa and improves diagnostic accuracy and diagnostic confidence having a positive clinical impact in a high proportion of cases.

REFERENCES

1. Limperopoulos C, Robertson RL, Estroff JA, et al. Diagnosis of inferior vermian hypoplasia by fetal magnetic resonance imaging: potential pitfalls and neurodevelopmental outcome. Am J Obstet Gynecol. 2006;194(4):1070-6.
2. Siebert JR. A pathological approach to anomalies of the posterior fossa. Birth Defects Res A Clin Mol Teratol. 2006;76(9):674-84.
3. Laing FC, Frates MC, Brown DL, et al. Sonography of the fetal posterior fossa: false appearance of megacisterna magna and Dandy–Walker variant. Radiology. 1994;192(1):247-51.
4. Limperopoulos C, Robertson RL, Khwaja OS, et al. How accurately does current fetal imaging identify posterior fossa anomalies? AJR Am J Roentgenol. 2008;190(6):1637-43.
5. Adamsbaum C, Moutard ML, André C, et al. MRI of the fetal posterior fossa. Pediatr Radiol. 2005;35(2):124-40.
6. Barkovich AJ, Millen KJ, Dobyns WB. A developmental and genetic classification for midbrain-hindbrain malformations. Brain. 2009;132(12):3199-230.
7. Griffiths PD, Brackley K, Bradburn M, et al. Anatomical subgroup analysis of the MERIDIAN cohort: posterior fossa abnormalities. Ultrasound Obstet Gynecol. 2017;50(6):745-52.
8. Paladini D, Quarantelli M, Sglavo G, et al. Accuracy of neurosonography and MRI in clinical management of fetuses referred with central nervous system abnormalities. Ultrasound Obstet Gynecol. 2014;44(2):188-96.
9. Kollias SS, Ball WS, Prenger EC. Cystic malformations of the posterior fossa: differential diagnosis clarified through embryologic analysis. Radiographics. 1993;13(6):1211-31.
10. Malinger G, Lev D, Lerman-Sagie T. The fetal cerebellum. Pitfalls in diagnosis and management. Prenat Diagn. 2009;29(4):372-80.
11. Paladini D, Volpe P. Posterior fossa and vermian morphometry in the characterization of fetal cerebellar abnormalities: a prospective three-dimensional ultrasound study. Ultrasound Obstet Gynecol. 2006;27(5):482-9.
12. Carroll SG, Porter H, Abdel-Fattah S, et al. Correlation of prenatal ultrasound diagnosis and pathologic findings in fetal brain abnormalities. Ultrasound Obstet Gynecol. 2000;16(2):149-53.
13. Guibaud L, des Portes V. Plea for an anatomical approach to abnormalities of the posterior fossa in prenatal diagnosis. Ultrasound Obstet Gynecol. 2006;27(5):477-81.
14. Pilu G, Segata M, Ghi T, et al. Diagnosis of midline anomalies of the fetal brain with the three-dimensional median view. Ultrasound Obstet Gynecol. 2006;27(5):522-9.
15. Pilu G, Ghi T, Carletti A, et al. Three-dimensional ultrasound examination of the fetal central nervous system. Ultrasound Obstet Gynecol. 2007;30(2):233-45.
16. Paladini D, Quarantelli M, Pastore G, et al. Abnormal or delayed development of the posterior membranous area of the brain: anatomy, ultrasound diagnosis, natural history and outcome of Blake's pouch cyst in the fetus. Ultrasound Obstet Gynecol. 2012;39(3):279-87.
17. Bolduc ME, Limperopoulos C. Neurodevelopmental outcomes in children with cerebellar malformations: a systematic review. Dev Med Child Neurol. 2009;51(4):256-67.
18. McLone DG, Dias MS. The Chiari II malformation: cause and impact. Childs Nerv Syst. 2003;19(7-8):540-50.

Three-dimensional Sonography in Fetal Syndromes

Lara Spalldi Barišić, Asim Kurjak, Ritsuko Kimata Pooh

INTRODUCTION

Three-dimensional (3D) ultrasound (3D US) has become a very powerful and progressively popular US technique in the last three decades (1989–2019).[1] Today, it is used in regular prenatal assessment in everyday clinical practice as additional method to two-dimensional US (2D US).

Over time, 3D US equipment and technology dramatically enhanced the quality of images, shortened the time of acquisition, and at the same time, improved our ability to assess and visualize the normal and to detect abnormal development of an embryo and fetus in utero.[1-12] Acquired volumes can be stored, reloaded, and reevaluated at any time. Different imaging modalities can be applied for more detailed survey. Particular region of interest, such as small defects, can be displayed in the ideal plane that sometimes cannot be achieved by conventional 2D US technique.[3,4,9,10] This increases the accuracy of the detection and diagnosis of various malformations and *fetal syndromes.*[2]

Diagnosing fetal syndromes is a major challenge both in the prenatal and postnatal period.[2] The syndrome is like a big puzzle whose parts need to be carefully assembled to get a whole picture.[2] Good multidisciplinary approach, proper communication, and collaboration with parents and all physicians involved are required in the diagnostic process. All available resources and tools are needed to increase diagnostic precision in the prenatal diagnosis of fetal syndromes.[4]

The introduction of highly specialized software systems for 3D/(four-dimensional) 4D US enable detailed assessment of the fetal anatomy and the evaluation of the dynamics of structural and functional development of the fetus in real time.[2,4] Owing to this, clinical practice has also gained new functional tests, such as the Kurjak's antenatal neurodevelopmental test (KANET), named in the honor of its author, used for the evaluation of fetal brain function.[2-4,13-20] Prenatal detection and diagnosis of fetal anomalies and syndromes is shifted from the second to the first trimester of pregnancy[2,4,10-12] partly due to technological advances and benefits of imaging quality with 3D/4D US technology, as reported by many authors.

DEFINING A SYNDROME AND WHEN TO SUSPECT A SYNDROME?

Common terminology used to describe fetal syndromes can sometimes be confusing. A wide variety of terms and synonyms are used. Sometimes, there is a lack of good definitions of how many major and minor criteria should be present to diagnose each syndrome. The difference in prenatal detection rates for each region or country can be partly explained by differences in screening policies and follow-up practices, as well as the possible variations in practitioners' skills and available equipment.[4]

Detecting one anomaly should always raise doubts about the presence of other anomalies and should therefore serve as a trigger that will encourage to investigate further and raise awareness of the possible existence of syndromes.[2,4-9]

Other triggers can be positive personal or family history of syndrome, or a child born with a syndrome, consanguinity, exposure to teratogens (drugs, radiation), and other harmful agents [e.g. infections; toxoplasmosis, other agents, rubella, cytomegalovirus (CMV), and herpes simplex; Zika]. Genetic syndromes in children are most commonly diagnosed on the basis of craniofacial dysmorphic features.[5,8,23,24]

Clinical dysmorphology is a branch of clinical genetics devoted to the study of abnormal human development, with emphasis on syndromes that reflect as changes in morphology of the body.[21-24] There are several pathophysiological mechanisms of poor fetal development (fetal maldevelopment), and these include malformation, deformation, disruption, or dysplasia.

Malformations: Due to abnormal embryonic development, commonly defined as single, localized poor formation of tissue, which has genetic etiology. This anomaly then raises a number of other defects (e.g. anencephaly). The recurrence risk for malformations generally ranges from 1% to 5%.[7]

Deformations: Anomalies that are result of extrinsic mechanical forces on otherwise normal tissue and structures (e.g. malposition of the limbs due to prolonged oligohydramnios).

Disruption: Results from an extrinsic insult that destroys normal tissue, altering the formation of affected structure (e.g. amniotic band syndrome).

Dysplasia: When the primary defect is the absence of normal organization of cells into tissue, we speak of dysplasia (e.g. achondroplasia).

Any of the mechanisms of fetal maldevelopment can result in altered morphology of fetal organs and systems, which can result in the formation of a fetal syndrome if many organs are involved. The term "*syndrome*" originates from ancient Greek meaning "running together,"[25] representing a specific pattern of associated signs, symptoms, dysmorphic features, and/or behaviors occurring together in the same person.[2,6,26]

We are currently aware of thousands of syndromes and their variants,[4-8] and this number is rising every day. It is particularly important to learn how to identify and find the right diagnosis in severe cases. In fact, it is estimated for the human genome to have about 80,000 genes, we should probably discover so many rare syndromes. Over 300 syndromes are associated with some type of facial anomaly.[2,4,8,9] The incidence of fetal syndrome varies.[8] It is estimated that the real occurrence of most syndromes is likely to be much greater, but due to natural selection, there is no further development.

Terminology used to describe fetal syndrome can sometimes be very confusing. Namely, different terms and their synonyms are used at the same time. In some cases, it is not well defined how important the main criteria would be, and how many of the subordinate criteria should appear for setting up a particular diagnosis. It is important to point out the difference and to distinguish between the terms: syndrome, sequences, and associations.

Syndrome: The occurrence of anomalies, multiple malformations and/or sequences, together in a recognizable sample. They are mainly the result of one, usually genetic abnormality, and have the same etiology; as for example in trisomy 21 (Down syndrome).

Sequence: The sequence occurs when one developmental disadvantage results in a cascade of secondary deficiencies that cause tertiary and so on, such as *Pierre Robin sequence (PRS)*: primary defect is mandibular hypoplasia, retrognathia that causes glossoptosis, secondary defect, which further disturbs normal, physiological closure of the soft palate and causes a tertiary defect: the palatoschisis of soft palate (retrognathia → glossoptosis → palatoschisis). In 25% of cases, the fetus will have Stickler syndrome (SS).[27] The sequence may be an isolated finding, associated with some other defect or a part of a syndrome.

Association: Connecting random combinations of inherited anomalies that may be the result of numerous pathogenic genetic factors (unlike syndrome). Example: VATER/VACTREL association (acronym for) (anomalies of the vertebrae—V; anal atresia—A; cardiac defects—C; tracheo-esophageal fistula—TE, kidney anomalies—R, anomalies of the limbs—L). This association is typically defined by the presence of at least three of the abovementioned congenital anomalies.[5-8]

Some fetal syndromes can be detected prenatally, while others cannot; some are expressed prenatally, while others are not.[4] In many cases, definitive diagnosis can be made postnatally, many years later.[2] It is estimated that about 1 out of 10 people, or a total of 30 million, live with rare diseases in the United States. Globally, it is about 350 million people who have one of over 7,000 known rare diseases. As already mentioned, the way to diagnosing these children is pretty long and painstaking. It takes about 7 years from symptom to diagnosis, and in that period, the children see at least seven doctors.[24,28,29] All this has a negative impact on the child and his family, representing emotional and financial burden on everyone, and negatively influencing and affecting the quality of life and prognosis of the child. The list of possible differential diagnoses (DDs) of fetal syndromes is extensive.

At present, there are several types of *online databases* that can help in detecting and identifying certain patterns of anomaly in syndromes, sequences, or associations. The most commonly used medical databases are Online Mendelian Inheritance in Man, POSSUMweb (Pictures Of Standard Syndromes and Undiagnosed Malformations) database, London Dysmorphology Database as part of a larger database: London Medical Database (LMD). Some of the larger databases combined their data to enrich them, allowing users a faster and more accurate search. As part of the new Facial Dysmorphology Novel Analysis (FDNA) database, LMD database access is integrated in combination with a brand new technology called Face2Gene.[24,28,29] Namely, with the help of the Face2Gene database, genetic search facilitates detection of dysmorphic facial features and recognizes human malformations from face photos to present a list of the most commonly used syndromes.[29] Patient symptoms, features, and genomic data are analyzed in the network of thousands of genetic experts around the world, providing scientific insights to improve and accelerate diagnosis and therapy. Notwithstanding, all of these network databases are based mainly on the data, symptoms, and features found in newborns and children and are not directly relevant to the recognition of syndromes in the prenatal period. *Phenotip online database*[30] is a database for specialists dealing with prenatal detection of syndromes using ultrasonic technology so that all prenatal sonographic markers and features are involved in data analysis. Data is easily accessed, ultrasonic markers and symptoms are combined, anomaly list that may still appear within the diagnosis is obtained, and some features that are identified in the parents can even be included.[30]

CLINICAL APPLICATION OF THREE-DIMENSIONAL ULTRASOUND IN THE PRENATAL DETECTION OF FETAL SYNDROMES

The systematic approach (according to guidelines) to fetal assessment by 2D US is still a gold standard and should always be followed to avoid mistakes. When evaluating structures, such as the face or brain, the advanced 3D/4D US modalities give a whole range of additional information that cannot be obtained by 2D technique.[3,31]

Systematic review of 525 articles on 3D/4D US by Gonçalves et al.[32] found that 3D US provides additional diagnostic information for diagnosing facial anomalies,

particularly facial clefts, neural tube defects, and skeletal malformation. Merz and Welter[33] examined a large group of 3,472 fetuses with 2D and 3D US intended to detect fetal anomalies. The total number of detected defects was 1,012. Comparing the 2D and 3D techniques, 3D US showed superiority with 60.8% of detected anomalies, which concerned more favorable visualization of target areas in different views (e.g. multiplanar, surface view).[33,34]

Only in recent years, high-frequency probes and high-resolution displays called High-definition live (HD live) technology have revolutionized the quality of sonographic imaging. 3D HD live mode of display uses the advantages of "shadowing effects" to enhance the visualization of the desired details in the image.[34] Unlike the conventional 3D surface display that uses a fixed virtual light source and reflects light from the surface of the skin, HDlive modality calculates the spread of light through the skin and tissue.[10,12,20,31,34] Shadows are created where the light was moved through the dense tissue. The virtual light source can be easily changed and directed from any angle and manipulated in this way to improve segmentation of the tissue structure, define precise contours, and highlight important clinical details.[10,34] This is suitable for observing the surfaces, especially in the face area.[35-39] Any suspicious surface or malformation can be shown and investigated much better than conventional 2D US.

Changing the virtual light angle, it can be perfectly adjusted to highlight something and thus gain a depth perception in the visualization of an area of interest that may be anomalous. Transparent (translucent) effect is obtained if the light source is located behind the object.[34,38] Improved smoothing performance is obtained by applying volume speckle reduction imaging on high-quality multiplanar 3D/4D images using volume (voxel) compared to traditional single-slice imaging (pixels).

The 3D HDlive mode can be used successfully throughout the entire pregnancy.[31] In the first trimester, normal and abnormal development of embryos and fetuses can be monitored and evaluated to the finest details. Only few years ago, new applications in 3D US called HDlive Silhouette (Flow) and HDlive Flow Silhouette were launched. HDlive Silhouette revealed the clinical significance of simultaneous imaging of internal morphology through the outer surface in a transparent manner **(Figs. 24.1 and 24.2)**.

This helps in determining the exact localization and volume of internal structures that may be hyperechoic as bone, or hypoechoic structures **(Figs. 24.2A to D)** such as cysts.[38,39] HDlive flow technology adds more spatial resolution to conventional angiogram. Combining both techniques at the same time (HDlive Silhouette and Flow) can display the exact location of the vascular structure within the body and organs and accurately determine the direction of the vascular flow (3D HDlive bidirectional power Doppler) **(Fig. 24.1C)**. These two new applications allow visualization of blood circulation within the fetus, the various parts of the fetal brain and lung flow.[38,39] Using different color shades of the skin by the HDlive application brought a great news as it gives the impression of a living fetus with even more realistic and impressive imaging illustrations.[31,38-40] Many of the abovementioned innovations in 3D/4D US applications are particularly useful in prenatal detection and visualization of fetal anomalies and discrete details.[41-44]

Together with these sonographic diagnostic tools, we should also mention something new that will greatly assist in accelerating postnatal recognition of rare syndromes. The fascinating combination of science, research, and new technologies is jointly implemented in a new research program titled "Give Face Syndrome." FDNA is a new technology that facilitates the detection of dysmorphic features and recognizable patterns of human malformations in newborns, children, and adults, to provide comprehensive and updated neurogenetic references available to everyone online.[28,29,44]

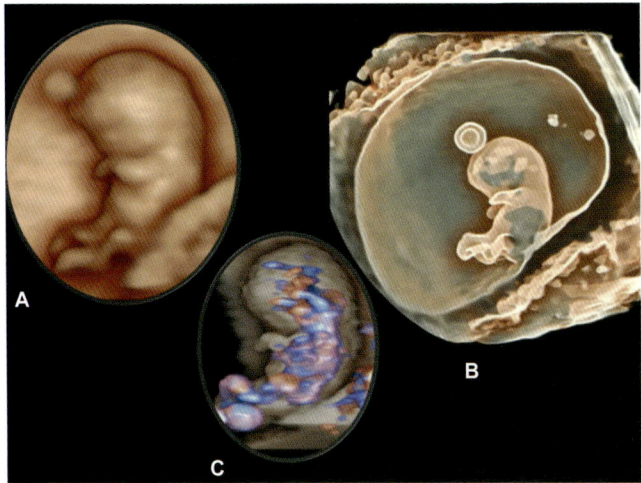

Figs. 24.1A to C: (A and B) 3D HDlive Silhouette fetal presentation at 9 + 3 gestational weeks. With the different intensity of Silhouette mode, we get more or less transparent picture in "see-through fashion." (A) The surface details. (B) See differences in the details of the previous picture (B), see the details of the internal organs filled with fluid, such as a ventricular system in the brain, an egg yolk. (C) 3D HDlive Silhouette and Flow showing the same fetus as above. Facing the details of early fetal circulation in the brain, heart, and umbilical cord.[15] (3D: three-dimensional; HD: high definition)

SYNDROMES FEATURING PRIMARILY CRANIOFACIAL ANOMALIES

In this section, we will describe various syndromes featuring primarily craniofacial anomalies and their associated defects that can be detected by standard 2D US techniques and demonstrate how the recognition is enhanced by advanced 3D/4D techniques in order to increase the accuracy of prenatal diagnosis.

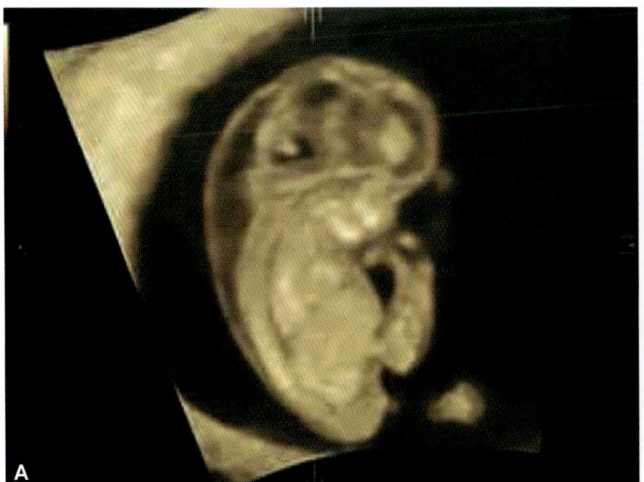
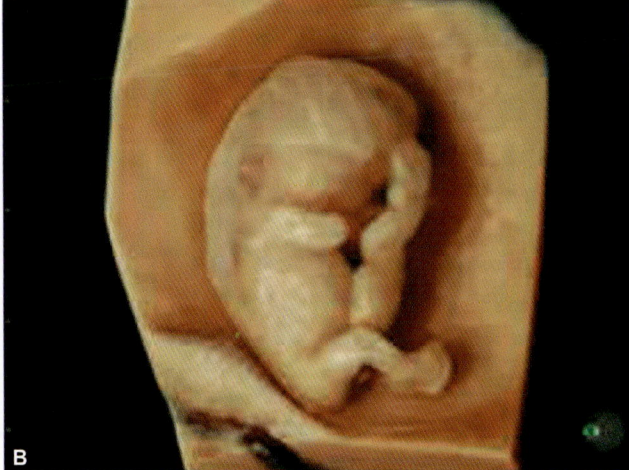

Figs. 24.2A and B

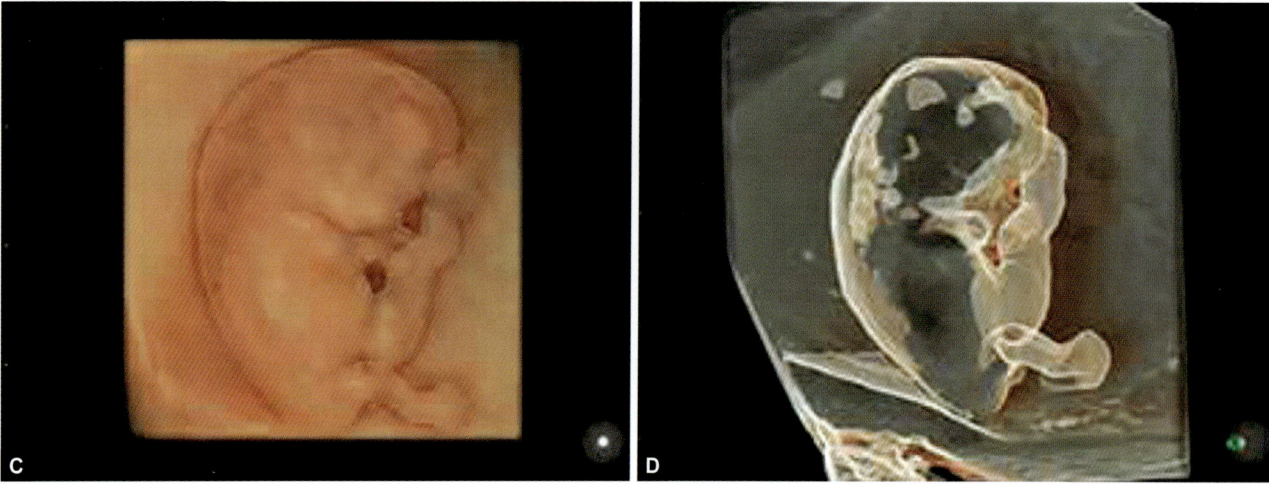

Figs. 24.2C and D

Figs. 24.2A to D: The same fetus at 9 weeks of gestation. Note the difference in imaging details. (A) VCI mode, sagittal image of the fetus with cystic hygroma colli. (B to D) 3D HDlive Silhouette images with the increasing silhouette mode from (B) to (D). Ending up with the transparent view. *Notice:* The increased accumulation of the fluid in the neck area and the cystic structures within: Cystic hygroma colli.[15] (3D: three-dimensional; HD: high-definition; NT: nuchal translucency)

As mentioned earlier, we know more than 300 syndromes associated with some type of facial anomaly, most commonly, with cleft lips (CLs) and/or palate, micrognathia and hypoplasia of the maxilla and the face [Goldenhar syndrome (GS), Treacher–Collins syndrome (TCS), PRSs as part of syndrome, Apert syndrome (AS), and van der Woude (VdW) syndrome].[2,4,8,9] These syndromes can be divided by various features, such as orofacial cleft, craniosynostosis, pharyngeal arch abnormalities, and simply facial dysmorphia. From embryologic point of view, the face is made up of five facial prominences that surround the future mouth and all meet in one point called the philtrum, a small recess above the upper lip.[5,6,45,46]

HOW TO DISTINGUISH WHAT IS NORMAL AND WHAT IS NOT?

Although we all have the same basic features, we also have our own recognizable features. There is evidence that the human brain (fusiform gyrus) has a specialized mental module devoted to processing facial recognition features. Researchers in various parts of the world work on understanding how fusiform gyrus mechanisms follow information: how we recognize faces and interpret their various facial expressions. Fetuses with dysmorphic characteristics are diagnosed, as noted earlier, according to the criteria to be met, which are also used in postnatal assessment. These include head shape and closure of the

skull bones, facial asymmetry, hyper/hypotelorism of the eyes, inclined eyes [mongoloid, antimongoloid position **(Figs. 24.3A to C)**], low-set or abnormal ears, micro or retrograde jaw confirmed by measuring jaw index,[47] CLs and/or palate.[5] In the process of face evaluation, we must also consider ethnic variations and normal differences. For example, epicanthal fold may be normal for Asian and non-Asiatic people but can be considered a dysmorphic feature of syndromes, such as Down, Turner, Noonan, Williams, and Fetal Alcohol syndrome, etc. Different nose forms and shapes is another example (Mediterranean, African, Asian, Latin, and Caucasian) **(Table 24.1)**.

The paramedian CL, cleft palate (CP), or combination of the two —CL and palate (CLP) are one of the most common fetal facial anomalies and one of the most common anomalies of the fetus at all.

This can be an isolated finding **(Fig. 24.4)** in less than 50% of the cases or in combination with associated anomalies as part of diverse syndromes. If this is an isolated finding, it can be elegantly repaired and reconstructed with a professional cranio-maxillo-facial surgeon engagement.

It can be distinguished: A bilateral complete lip and palate cleft that can easily be identified even in the first trimester **(Figs. 24.5 and 24.6)**, and on the other hand, a unilateral complete cleft of the lips and palate, or an incomplete cleft of the lip that has only subtle indications and can easily be overlooked **(Figs. 24.7A to D)**.

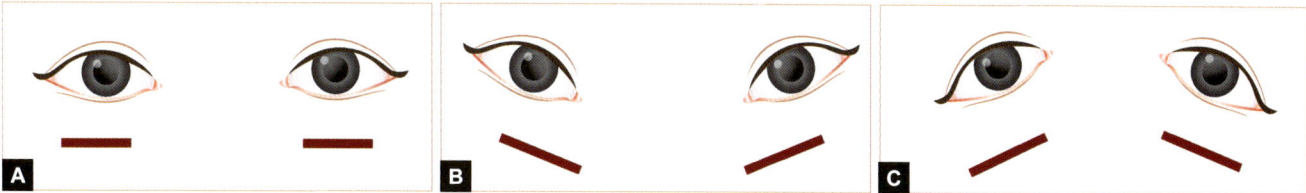

Figs. 24.3A to C: (A) Normal position of the eyes, (B) Mongoloid inclination of the eyes (e.g. trisomy 21), (C) antimongoloid inclination of the eyes (e.g. Treacher Collins syndrome).

Table 24.1: Possibilities of sonographic assessment of fetal face by 3D US in the first trimester of pregnancy.[48]

Anatomy (3 orthogonal planes)	Section	Profile
3D surface rendering	Sagittal view	Forehead, nose, lips, chin
3D transparent rendering	Parasagittal view	Nasal bone yes/no Image angle 45°
3D maximum mode imaging	Coronal view	Forehead, orbits, both nasal bones, maxilla, and mandible
	Transverse view	Forehead, orbits, both nasal bones, maxilla, and mandible
Biometry	Sagittal view	FMF angle (>85°)
Stored images		• Face profile with the nasal bone • FMF, if needed

(FMF: frontomaxillary facial)

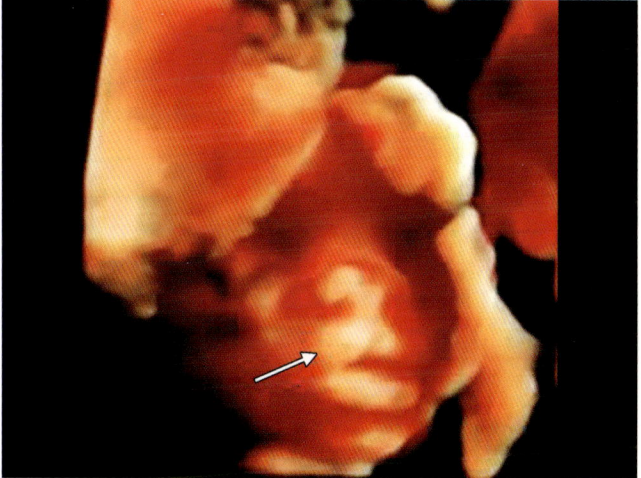

Fig. 24.4: 3D HDlive surface rendering, US imaging of the fetus at 14 weeks of gestation. *Notice:* Subtile, small paramedian cleft lip only.[15] (3D: three-dimensional; HD: high definition; US: ultrasound)

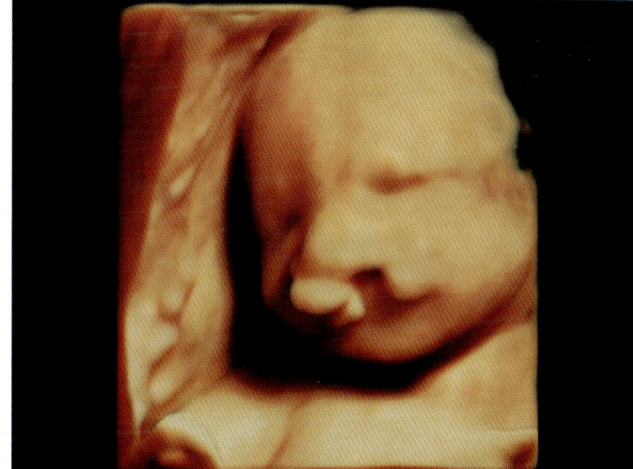

Fig. 24.5: 3D HDlive surface rendering of the fetal face at 23 + 3 weeks of gestation. *Notice:* Bilateral CLP. Because of the protrusion of inner maxillary segment under the nose, anomaly is easily detected.[15] (3D: three-dimensional; CLP: cleft lip and palate; HD: high definition)

The median facial clefts are the most severe anomalies, regularly part of some serious and complex sequences or syndromes, such as holoprosencephaly, *Patau (trisomy 13)* **(Figs. 24.8 to 24.10)**, *Edwards syndrome (trisomy 18), and Aicardi syndrome.*[49] Trisomy 13 is the most common chromosomal abnormality associated with alobar holoprosencephaly (fetal face: cyclopia, cebocephaly, flat nose, facial hypoplasia, and lip clefts) **(Figs. 24.8 to 24.10)**. Nevertheless, it is to be remembered that 75% of fetuses with holoprosencephaly have a normal karyotype **(Figs. 24.6 and 24.11)**! Unfortunately, most of the fetuses with CL, CP, or CLP have a high incidence of chromosomal abnormalities and other related syndromic anomalies.[50]

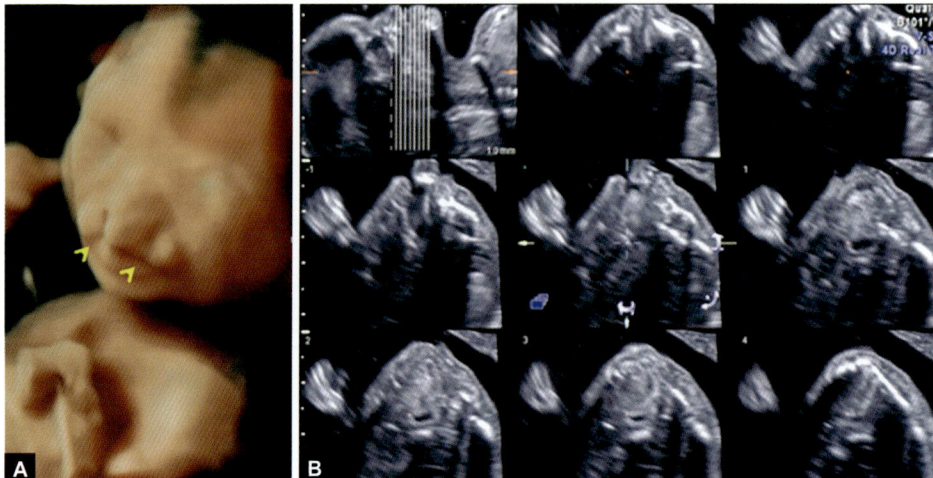

Figs. 24.6A and B: (A) 3D HDlive surface imaging: *bilateral CLP*; fetus with multiple anomalies but normal karyotype! (B) TUI display—*notice:* the extent of the cleft![15] (3D: three-dimensional; CLP: cleft lip and palate; HD: high definition; TUI: tomographic ultrasound imaging technique)

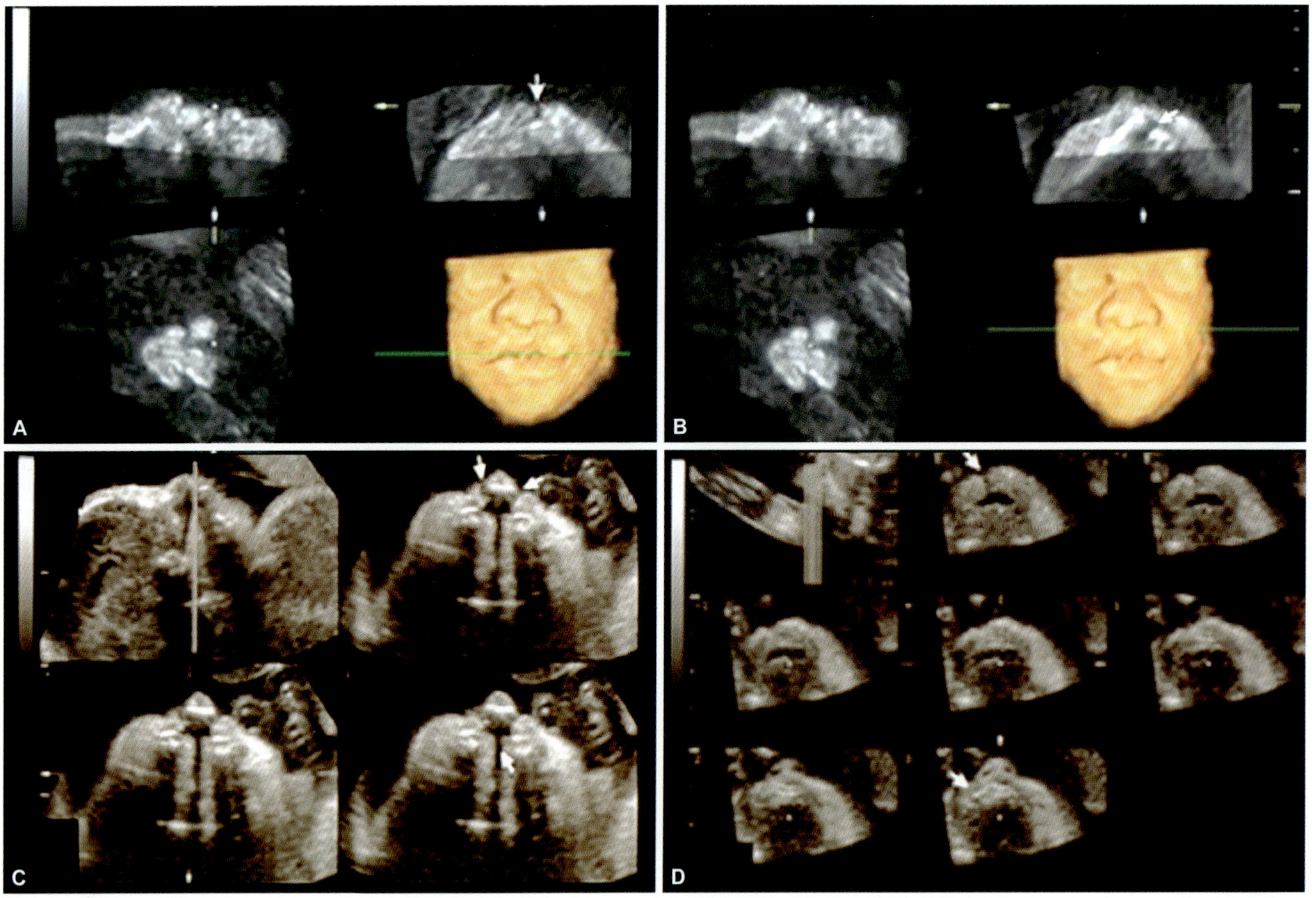

Figs. 24.7A to D: (A) 3D multiplanar imaging, small, only subtile paramedian cleft lip seen on this image but (B) movement of the green dot across the mandible, small alveolar defect becomes evident. (C) Bilateral CLP detected by *TUI*. (D) Isolated cleft lip isolated—integrity of the fetal palate can be obtained by TUI imaging method. (3D: three-dimensional; CLP: cleft lip and palate; TUI: tomographic ultrasound imaging technique).

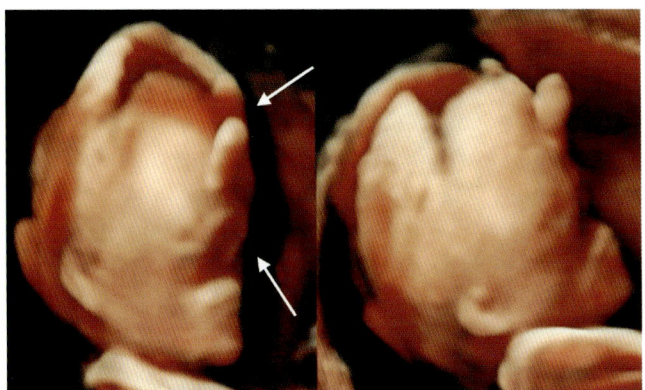

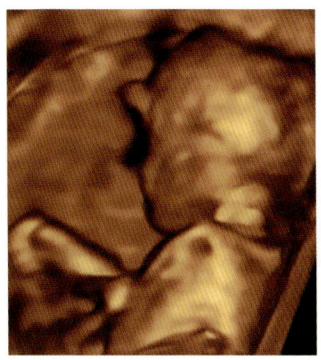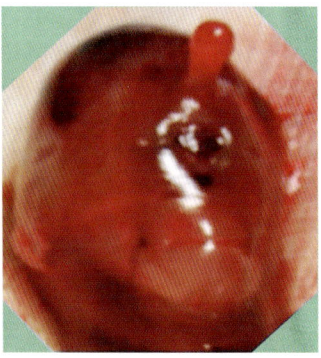

Fig. 24.8: 3D HDlive surface rendering, the same fetus from the front and profile. *Notice:* Abnormal shape of the head, wide open sutures of the skull, anomalies of the midline of the fetal face: cyclopia (lower arrow), proboscis (upper arrow), and holoprosencephaly and low-set ears are seen. All features of trisomy 13—Patau syndrome.[15] (3D: three-dimensional; HD: high definition)

Fig. 24.9: Image on the left: 3D surface-rendering profile. *Notice:* Proboscis! Image on the right: the same fetus after miscarriage. *Notice:* Similarities with the prenatal imaging (proboscis, cyclopia).

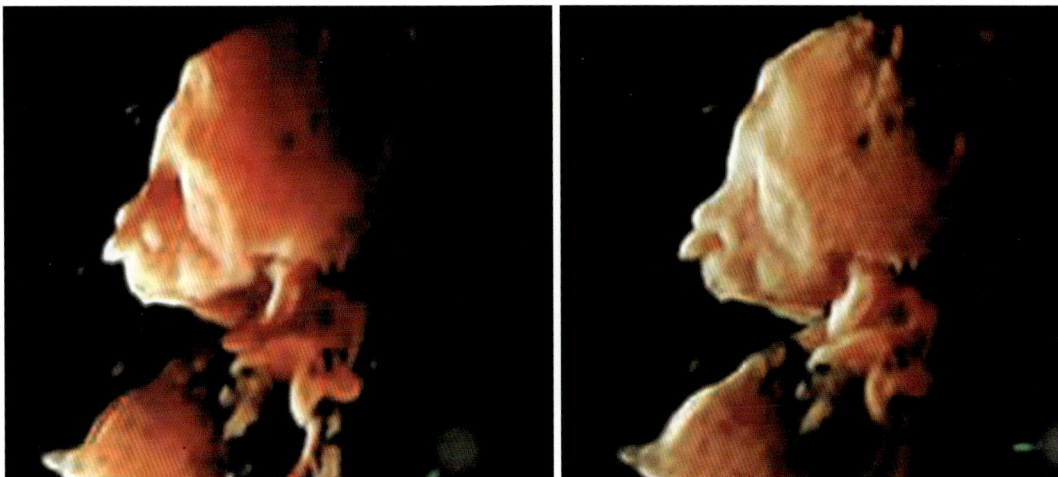

Fig. 24.10: 3D HDlive surface-rendering. *Notice:* CLP and hypoplysia of the mandible. Case of trisomy 13 (Patau syndrome at 21 gestational weeks). (3D: three-dimensional; CLP: cleft lip and palate; HD: high definition)

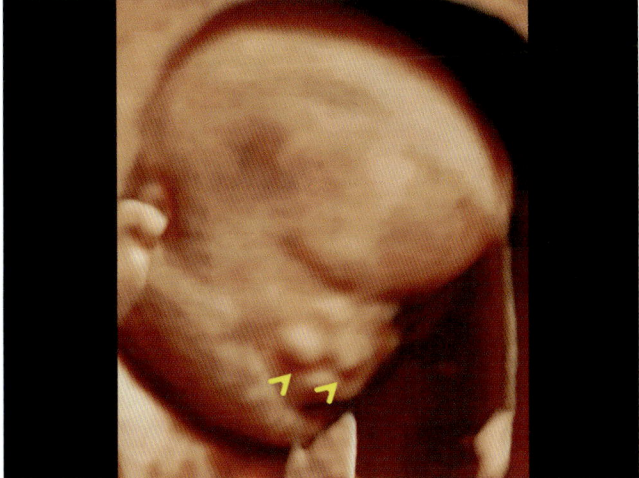

Fig. 24.11: 3D HDlive surface rendering of the fetus at 13 weeks of gestation. *Notice:* Abnormal shape of the head, holoprosencephaly, bilateral CLP, microphthalmia, low-set ears. But normal karyotype! (3D: three-dimensional; CLP: cleft lip and palate; HD: high definition)

Van der Woude syndrome carriers have up to 50% of the cases of facial clefting. VdW syndrome is autosomal dominant mode of inheritance which accounts for about 2% of all cases with CL and CP.[31] A partial one-sided small defect CL can easily be overlooked by the usual 2D US **(Fig. 24.4)**.[31]

Three-dimensional multiplanar display and HDlive surface view is a better method for detecting all forms of clefts and facial malformation. Bilateral CL may sometimes be missed because it does not change the face symmetry. The two-sided complete CL and CP, on the other hand, will most likely be detected due to the protrusion of the inner maxillary segment below the nose **(Figs. 24.5 and 24.6)**, which is an obvious and unusual mass when looking at the face profile.[5] When checking for

cleft of the lip, 3D HDlive techniques are very useful. For detection of cleft palate, the use of tomographic ultrasonic imaging **(Figs. 24.6 and 24.7)** allows better determination of the extent of the cleft in relation to other structures.[31]

Mandibular anomalies (agnathia, micrognathia, and retrognathia) **(Figs. 24.12 to 24.15)** have been described in more than 100 different syndromes.[50] It appears to be very common as isolated anomaly, but also commonly as part of heterogeneous syndromes. By 2D US, abnormal profile **(Figs. 24.10 and 24.12)** is first to be detected. Abnormal fetal profile is noted! With the application of different 3D US modalities, it is possible to investigate in detail and to get a complete impression on the fetal appearance and possible existence of other orofacial anomalies.

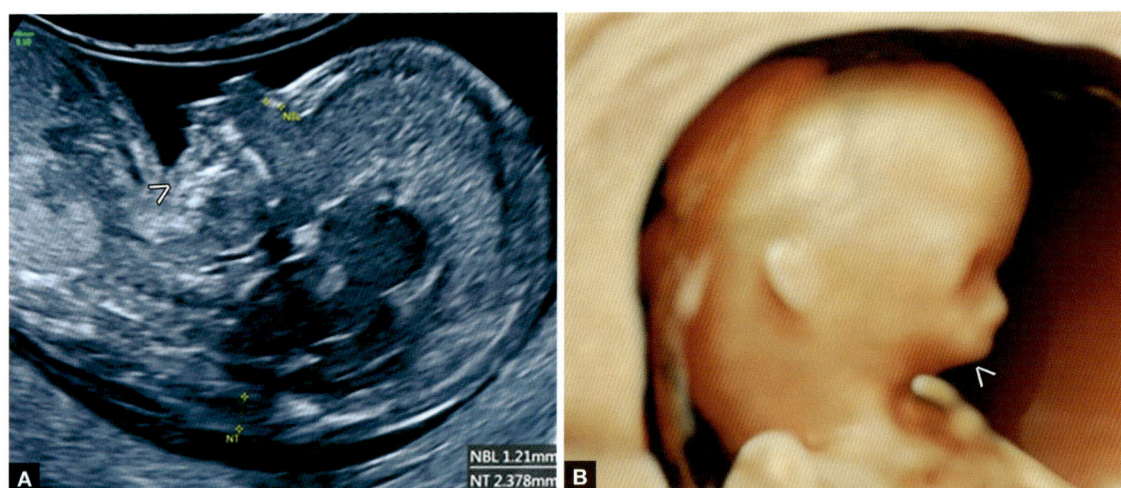

Figs. 24.12A and B: (A) 2D midsagittal view of the fetus, *notice:* abnormal fetal profile and shape of the head, increased NT and prominent micrognathia (arrow). (B) The same fetus as in the left image, 3D HDlive surface rendering modality. Notice all mentioned above and detail of the low-set ears.[15] (2D. two dimensional; 3D; three dimensional; HD: high definition; NT: nuchal translucency)

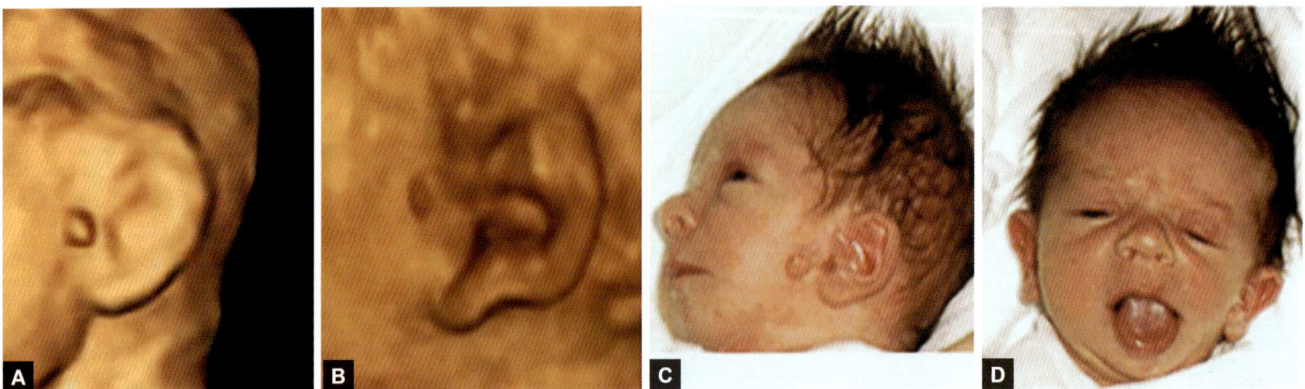

Figs. 24.13A to D: (A and B) *Prenatal:* (A) 3D surface rendering. *Notice:* Preauricular tag. (C and D) *Postnatal:* postnatal images of the baby with Goldenhar syndrome. *Notice:* Hemifacial hypoplasia and microophtalmia.[4]

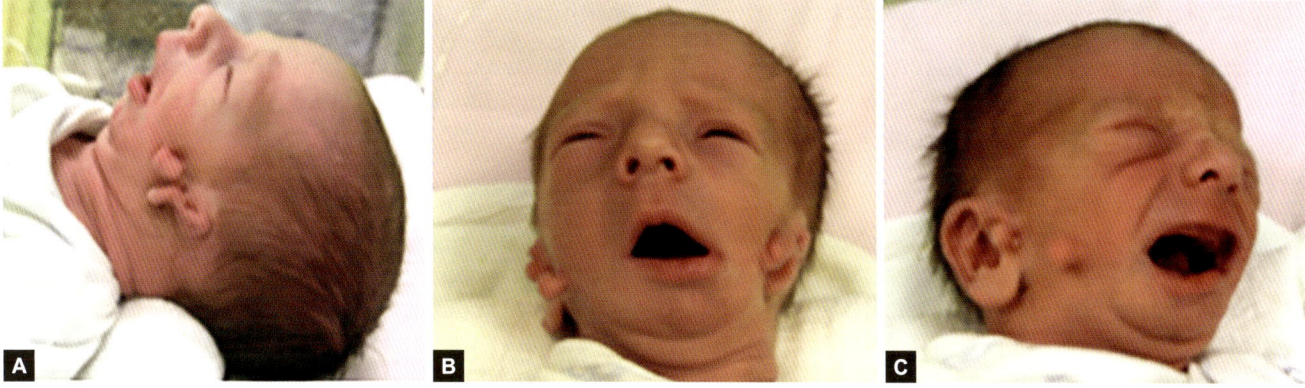

Figs. 24.14A to C: Postnatal images of the baby with Goldenhar syndrome. *Notice:* Hemifacial hypoplasia with microphthalmia, periauricular tags and sinuses, external ear deformity hemihypoplasia of the mandible.[4]

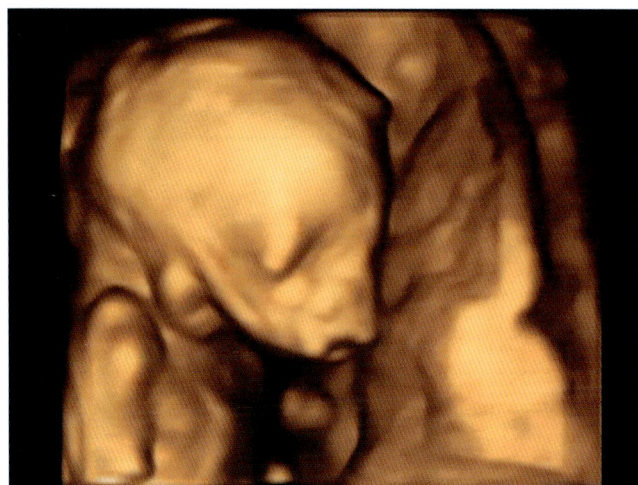

Fig. 24.15: 3D surface rendering of the fetus with. Treacher Collins syndrome. *Notice:* Typical facial dysmorphism: bilateral symmetric otomandibular dysplasia with the hyperplasia of the soft tissue of the face, low-set ears.[4]

Pierre Robin Sequence

It is characterized by a triad of orofacial anomalies consisting of retrognathia, glossoptosis, and median cleft of the soft palate. Mandibular hypoplasia **(Fig. 24.12)** is a primary deficiency that occurs early in pregnancy between the 7th week and 11th week of pregnancy. The tongue maintains high in the oral cavity, which subsequently prevents the normal tongue placement and prevents the soft palate from fusing.[31,51] Prenatal diagnosis of micrognathia in PRS can be set very early in the first trimester of pregnancy, by using 3D US and its applications.[52,53] Micrognathia can be quantified by "jaw index" = the ratio of the anteroposterior mandible and biparietal diameter.

If the ratio is less than 0.23, a micrognathia diagnosis[47] can be set.

More than 40 PRS syndromes have been described, most common of which are *SS and 22q11.2 deletion syndrome (DiGeorge Syndrome).*[54-59]

Pooh and Kurjak published the sequence of images of mandibular hypoplasia and slow development of jaw in the case of PRS during pregnancy.[31] Serial 3D imaging can be used to clearly document the mandibular growth over a few weeks.[31] Accelerated compensatory growth of the lower jaw is expected during the first year of life, and adjustment of the child's profile can be expected from the third to the sixth year of life.[43,60-63]

Isolated PRS (without any other associated malformation) occurs in about 50% of cases; however, in the second half of the cases PRS is part of the syndrome. The clinical manifestations of syndrome depend on the persistence and severity of related anomalies.[5] The nature of these anomalies is diverse, most commonly anomaly of the first pharyngeal arch, various chromosomal disorders (*DiGeorge syndrome*), *collagenopathy* or syndromes associated with the use of toxic substances in pregnancy, such as alcohol [*fetal alcohol syndrome* (*FAS*)], etc. In the study of 115 cases of PRS patients, as expected, 54% had an isolated finding (5%), facial and hemifacial microsomy (3%), other defined (3.5%) and undefined.[58] Other syndromes: *Stickler (18%), Velocardiofacial syndrome (7%), and TCS (9%).*[58]

Facial dysmorphism usually derives from a mixture of migration disorders and poor formation of facial mesenchyme (especially when it is associated with disorders of the first and the second pharyngeal arch).[61,64]

Goldenhar Syndrome

Synonyms are hemifacial microsomy or oculo–auriculo–vertebral syndrome. This is a combination of migration disorder and inadequate formation of facial mesenchyme (disorders of the first and second throat arch).[61,64] GS is characterized by a wide range of main and associated features that can differ in the severity from one to the other case (*see* **Table 24.2**).

The classic feature of GS is asymmetric (mostly unilateral) facial hypoplasia (**Figs. 24.13 and 24.14**). Fetuses with GS have major anomalies such as unilateral mandibular hypoplasia involving the temporomandibular joint, multiple preauricular skin tags (**Figs. 24.13 and 24.14**) around ear, ear hypoplasia/aplasia and/or eye malformations (anophthalmia and microphthalmia), and vertebral anomalies. Typically, these malformations are one sided (70–85%) and give an asymmetric facial appearance. There have been various theories about the emergence of this syndrome. Some authors assumed that the problem could be a one-way blood flow disorder (ischemia) to the first and second pharyngeal arch that could occur during the time period between the 4th and 8th week of pregnancy.[65] Wang et al.[66] analyzed data from a large register of congenital anomalies in Spain and established the association between diabetic mothers and the increased risk of their children born with GS syndrome. It is assumed that poorly controlled mother's diabetes interfere with the migration of cells into the cephalic portion of the neural ridge causing this syndrome.[66]

Table 24.2: Features of Goldenhar syndrome that can be detected by 3D sonographic assessment.

Goldenhar syndrome (GS)	
Asymmetric (unilateral) hypoplasia of the face	70–85%
Mandibular hypoplasia—PRS	
"Skin tags" around the ear	
Hypoplasia of the ear	
Malformation/microphthalmia of the eye Unilateral cleft lip/palate	
Anomaly of vertebrae (hemivertebrae) CHD CNS anomalies—corpus callosum lipoma Malformations of gastrointestinal system	

(CHD: congenital heart defect; CNS: central nervous system; PRS: Pierre Robin sequence)

Prenatal Diagnosis

The first sonographic indicator to detect this syndrome may be the discovery of facial asymmetry due to hemifacial microsomy or a small detail, such as a very typical periauricular skin pendant (tag) (**Figs. 24.13 and 24.14**). This is most commonly diagnosed in the second and third trimesters of pregnancy (**Table 24.3**). With 3D surface rendering, more details can be visualized: unilateral craniofacial anomaly (cerebral hemisphere hypoplasia), eye (micro/anophthalmia), low-set ears with various malformations, face anomalies (soft tissue asymmetry), kidney anomalies (hydronephrosis), etc. Using 3D HDlive imaging technology, even small facial details or other parts of the body can be visualized in a very detailed way,

Table 24.3: Possibilities of sonographic assessment of fetal face by 3D US in the second and third trimester of pregnancy.[48]

Anatomy (3 orthogonal planes)	Section	Visualization
3D surface rendering	Sagittal view	• Forehead, nose, lips, chin • Nasal bone yes/no
3D transparent rendering 3D maximum mode	Coronal view	• Forehead with metopic suture • Orbits with lenses (symmetry) • Lips/palate (3D surface-rendered image) • Transparent (maximum intensity) image
	Transverse view	• Orbits with the lenses • Palate (transparent) • Maxilla • Mandible
Biometry	Sagittal view	• Nasal bone • FMF angle • IFA
	Coronal view	• *Orbital diameter:* – Inner orbital distance – Outer orbital distance
	Transverse view	• Orbital diameter • Inner orbital distance • Outer orbital distance • Maxilla width • Mandible width or jaw index
Stored images		Profile with nasal bone coronal or transverse view with orbits—coronal view

(FmF: frontomaxillary facial; IFA: inferior facial angle)

which can be of great help in counseling the parents. Due to overlapping features, differential diagnosis should be: TCS, Hallermann-Streiff syndrome, Delleman's syndrome, Nager's syndrome, and Townes-Brocks syndrome.

Genetic counseling: GS occurs rarely and sporadically, but for the first-degree relatives, the possibility of repetition (relative risk) is estimated at 2%. Due to the complexity of the clinical picture, multidisciplinary approach to problem is important.[2,4] The combination of micrognathia along with low-set ears is a common occurrence in many syndromes.

Treacher Collins Syndrome (TCS)

The discovery of bilateral symmetrical facial hypoplasia, periauricular tags in combination with micrognathia, may be part of TCS or some other syndrome, such as Nager or Miller syndrome.

Treacher Collins syndrome is the disorder of the first and second pharyngeal arch. This is a congenital disturbance of craniofacial development induced by mutations in the long arm of chromosome 5 (5q32) of *TCOF1* gene.[67] It is depicted by bilateral symmetric otomandibular dysplasia **(Fig. 24.15)**. Furthermore, there is downward slanting of a palpebral fissure, lower eyelid coloboma, lack of medial eyelashes, middle and outer ear malformations, and conductive hearing loss. The frequency of TCS is estimated at 1:50,000 live births per year. The genetic trait is autosomal dominant in 40% of cases with variations of expression. The remaining 60% are the result of new mutations. Cranioskeletal hypoplasia

develops due to insufficient number of neurons as a result of the death of the neuroepithelial progenitor cells.[68] The onset of defects occurs very early between the 4th and 8th week of embryonic development.

Prenatal Diagnosis

Prenatal US TCS is diagnosed mainly in the second trimester of pregnancy,[68-70] but with sophisticated 3D applications and HDlive technology, Pooh reported detection in the first trimester of the pregnancy.[31] With the combination of existing anomalies, the established suspicion of this syndrome is very important to informing geneticists who can order the gene sequencing added to the usual amniocentesis panel to confirm a diagnosis that would otherwise be missed.[70]

Apert Syndrome

Apert syndrome shows autosomal dominant mode of inheritance. There is a congenital mutation in the *FGFR2* gene, chromosome 10q26.13.[67] This syndrome is also associated with the advanced age of the fathers. The syndrome has several characteristic features that can be recognized during a routine US examination. Triad of signs to remember would be strawberry-shaped head, flat face, and "mitten-like" hands (like baby gloves) **(Fig. 24.16)**.[31]

Apert syndrome is characterized by:
- Craniosynostosis is a skull disorder caused by the early fusion of one or more skull bones (early fusion of the sutures). Otherwise, more than 180 different

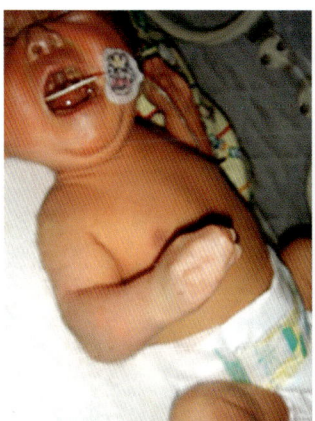 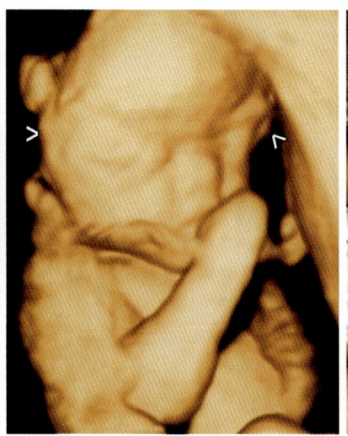 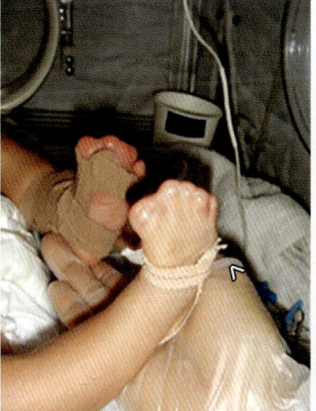 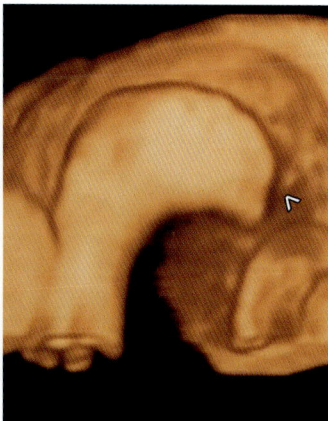

Fig. 24.16: Combination of prenatal and postnatal images of the same baby with the Apert syndrome. Prenatal images with 3D surface mode imaging. *Notice:* The similarities of the images: prenatal and postnatal facial dysmorphism, abnormal shape of the skull, frontal bossing hypertelorism, and "mitten-like hands/feet."[4,31]

syndromes are known, which include craniosynostosis in the diagnosis. Changing shape of the cranial vault varies, depending on the fused sutures, so that the compensating growth occurs in dimensions that are not limited by the fusion. AS occurs in 4.5% of the cases of craniosynostosis **(Fig. 24.16)**.

- In the case of AS, premature fusion of bicoronal suture (metopic suture) occurs and consequently brachycephalic- and acrocephalic-shaped head forms appear. In other words, an abnormal flat-head skull, frontal bossing, midface hypoplasia (flat face), ocular hypertelorism, and swelling of the eyelids (puffy eyes) can be detected **(Fig. 24.16)**.

- *Sonographic assessment:* Combination of conventional 2D US techniques with 3D maximum mode (for bony structure), 3D surface rendering and 3D HDlive surface mode can be used.

- Mild ventriculomegaly can be detected represented by 3D inversion mode or, if available, with the latest HDlive Silhouette display.

- Agenesis of corpus callosum can best be detected by 3D surface imaging in the central (midsagittal) plane with the additional visualization of the 3D sono-angiogram (3D HDlive bidirectional power Doppler) showing the anomaly: the absence of pericallosal artery.

- Very specific for fetuses with AS is a defect at the extremities called "mitten-like hands/feet": syndactyly of the second, third, and fourth finger (soft and bone tissue) in combination with a broad thumb that has the appearance of a child's gloves **(Fig. 24.16)**.

Pooh et al.[43] published prenatally detected case of a fetus with AS by using 3D US diagnostics. Correlation was performed between images taken prenatally by 3D ultrasound and compared by postnatal appearance **(Fig. 24.16)**.[31,53] 3D US images could be used when communicating with the parents for better understanding of the extent of abnormalities of the face, skull, and extremities. DD should include other syndrome with craniosynostosis such as Carpenter, Crouzon, Pfeiffer, and Saethre-Chotzen syndrome.[5] The important difference is that there is no syndactyly for the fingers and toes.[5]

Genetic counseling: AS has autosomal dominant inheritance, but in most cases, it is the case of mosaicism. When the mutation is "de novo," the risk of repetition is unlikely, but if one of the parents is the gene carrier, the recurrence risk is 50%![71]

In order to confirm the diagnosis prenatally, it is necessary to talk to the parents and to offer invasive prenatal testing. Children with AS will need multiple surgical procedures to improve their quality of life. A multidisciplinary approach is required.[2,4]

Some of the Sonographic Signs and their Association with Syndromes

The frontal bossing **(Figs. 24.15 to 24.17)** may be a typical finding in AS **(Figs. 24.15 and 24.16)** with achondroplasia

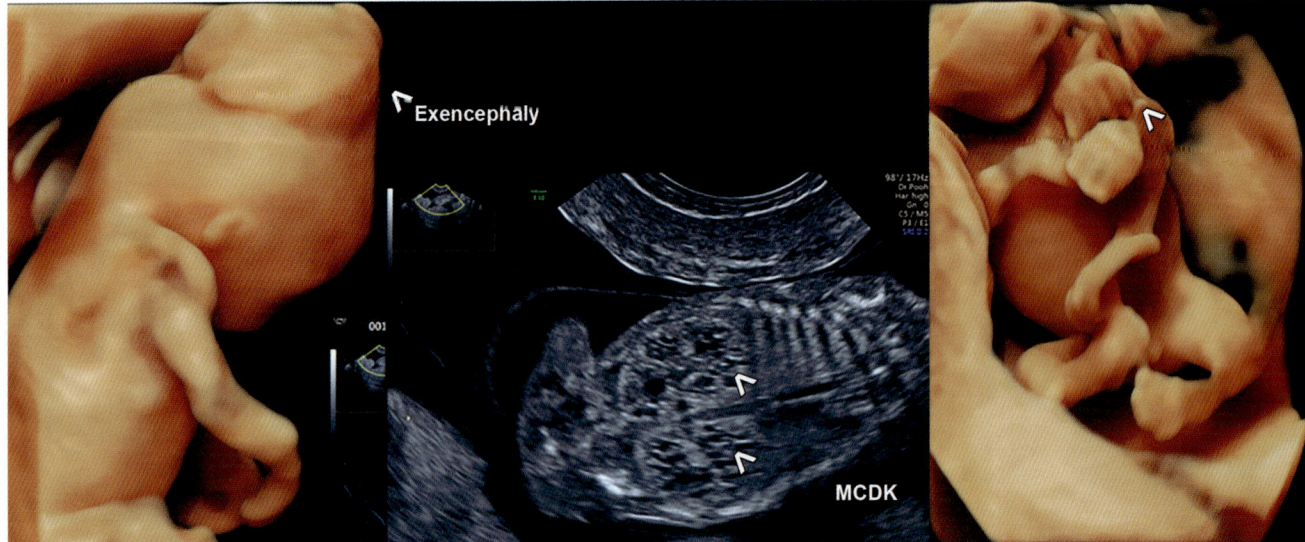

Fig. 24.17: Typical triad of findings: encephalocele (80%), renal cystic dysplasia—bilateral MCDK (95%): polydactyly (75%): Lethal syndrome: Meckel-Gruber syndrome![31] (MCDK: multicystic dysplastic kidney)

(autosomal dominant disease with rhizomelic shortening of extremities) **(Figs. 24.18A to C)**, in Russell–Silver syndrome (poor growth, asymmetric intrauterine growth restriction of the skeleton with normal head size).

Asymmetry of the fetal skull, except for a variety of craniosynostosis which may or may not be associated with syndromes, can also be found in a fetus with amniotic band syndrome (ABS).

Amniotic band syndrome: Because of the rupture of the amnion, which occurs very early in the first trimester of pregnancy, the amniotic band causes a great variety and severity of destructive fetal malformations depending on the fetal parts that come into contact and become trapped in it. When they affect the skull, it is possible to detect asymmetric anencephaly, encephalocele, facial clefts, and micrognathia. Other abnormalities that were also found were limb flaw, constriction rings, and limb amputations.

Other abnormalities of the skull detected by US are microcephaly and macrocephaly.

Microcephaly denotes a group of disorders characterized by a small head and is usually associated with abnormal neurological findings and mental disorders.[5] Microcephaly usually also means microcephaly because the size of the head usually determines the size of the brain. Fetuses with prenatal susceptibility to microcephaly have a head circumference of more than 3 standard deviations below the average for gestational age.[67] The diversity of associated anomalies found by US depends largely on the etiologic factors that cause microcephaly. Precise etiology in most cases of microcephaly is still

unknown. However, this is related to numerous chromosomal abnormalities syndromes, such as Cornelia de Lange, DiGeorge, Wolf–Hirschhorn, CRI du Chat, trisomy 13 and 9, FAS, and exposure to some toxic substances (drugs, clomiphene, methotrexate, and phenylalanine), mothers malnutrition, exposure (of pregnant woman) to certain infections during pregnancy, such as rubella, toxoplasmosis, varices, and CMVs. There are reports of new causes, such as exposure (during pregnancy) to Zika virus and unwanted pregnancy outcomes, such as microcephaly, other brain, and eye anomalies and increase in the loss of pregnancy.[72]

Zika congenital syndrome is generally characterized by *cerebral atrophy* which may interfere with formation and with the neuronal migration during early cerebral embryogenesis.[73] Other features of this syndrome are expressed microcephaly, lissencephaly, microphthalmia, contractures, and arthrogryposis.[67,72,73] Viruses, such as CMV or Zika, have been shown to attack brain cells, particularly neural progenitors, infecting and destroying the primary stem cells (radial glial cell) of the brain, and therefore missing new neuronal "daughters." The severity of depends largely on the time of infection during pregnancy.[51-53,74] Microcephaly is mainly a result of a small cerebral cortex. In addition, the infection can cause scars and calcifications in the brain tissue which can be depicted by US. Infection should be confirmed by a polymerase transcription reaction (real-time reverse transcription polymerase chain reaction).[74] Recent research from the endemic region of Brazil has shown

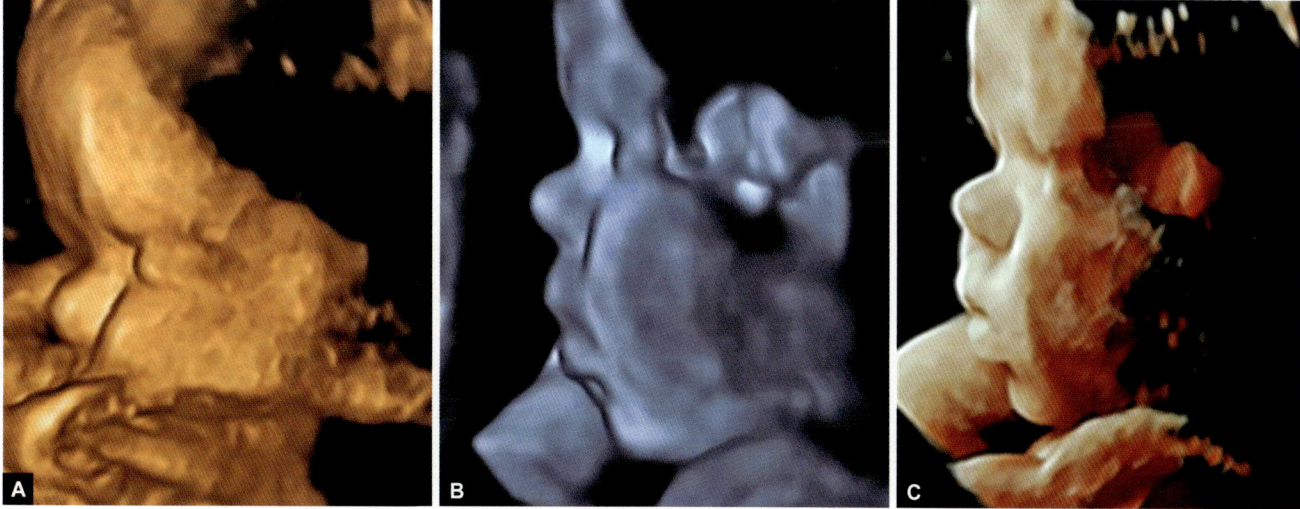

Figs. 24.18A to C: Fetal face profile. 3D ultrasound, surface rendering. Achondroplasia was suspected. *Notice:* Different methods of surface rendering. Frontal bossing and depressed nasal bridge.

that although some babies are born with normal size of head, postnatal development of microcephaly may occur, as well as significant neurological disorders leading to arthrogryposis, conditions leading to deformity of joints and disabilities.[73]

Abnormalities, such as *periventricular and intraparenchymal calcification*, ventricular hypertrophy, secondary cerebral atrophy, cerebellar hypoplasia, and cortical abnormalities, are seen and detected much earlier than the microcephaly itself.[74]

When needed, in addition to the standard US examination by 2D US, 3D/4D US may be used to enhance the accuracy. *Fetal neurosonography* with 3D-advanced US techniques should be included in prenatal assessment if abnormalities are suspected. Different displays of 4D US can be used to evaluate the fetal dynamics and functionality of some organs and different organ systems.[80-83]

Kurjak antenatal neurodevelopmental test can be used to evaluate fetal brain function between 28 gestational weeks and 38 gestational weeks.[15,17,75-78] KANET **(Fig. 24.19)** can be very useful tool, easily performed and used to detect the fetuses at risk for neurological impairment. If score of the test is borderline or abnormal, this test should be repeated at intervals of every 2 weeks until delivery. Prenatal results can be compared with the neonatal ones. Fetuses that are found to be at risk should be followed up during at least first 2–3 years of life, as suggested by pediatricians, to be able to exclude the neurological damage to same extent and cerebral palsy (CP). Clinical usefulness of the KANET test was suggested

by many authors over the past decade, and the exact data of the meta-analysis are underway, nevertheless, preliminary reports are promising.

During the routine US examination**,** *abnormalities of fetal kidneys and bladder* can be detected **(Figs. 24.17 and 24.20)** and *abnormalities of the anterior abdominal wall* in the form of omphalocele **(Figs. 24.21A to H)**. You can see a wide range of structural and functional abnormalities.

Dysplastic kidneys with multiple cysts (multicystic dysplastic kidney—MCDK) **(Figs. 24.17 and 24.20)** that vary in size can be found as an anomaly in some very

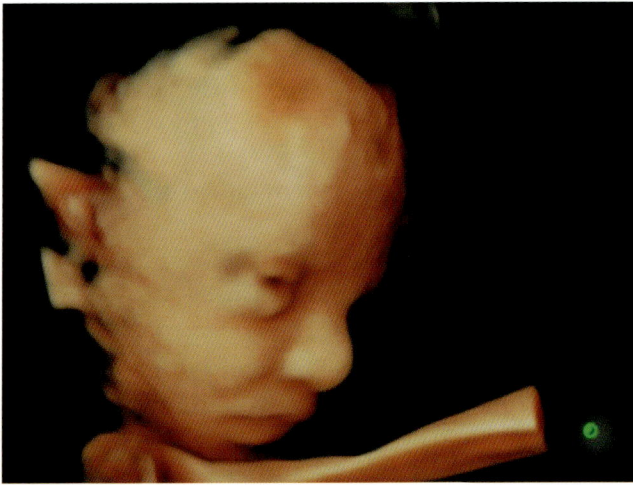

Fig. 24.19: 3D/4D HDlive fetal assessment by KANET: *Notice:* Open eyes of the fetus at 28 gestational weeks.[4] (3D: three-dimensional; 4D: four-dimensional; HD: high definition; KANET: Kurjak's antenatal neurodevelopmental test)

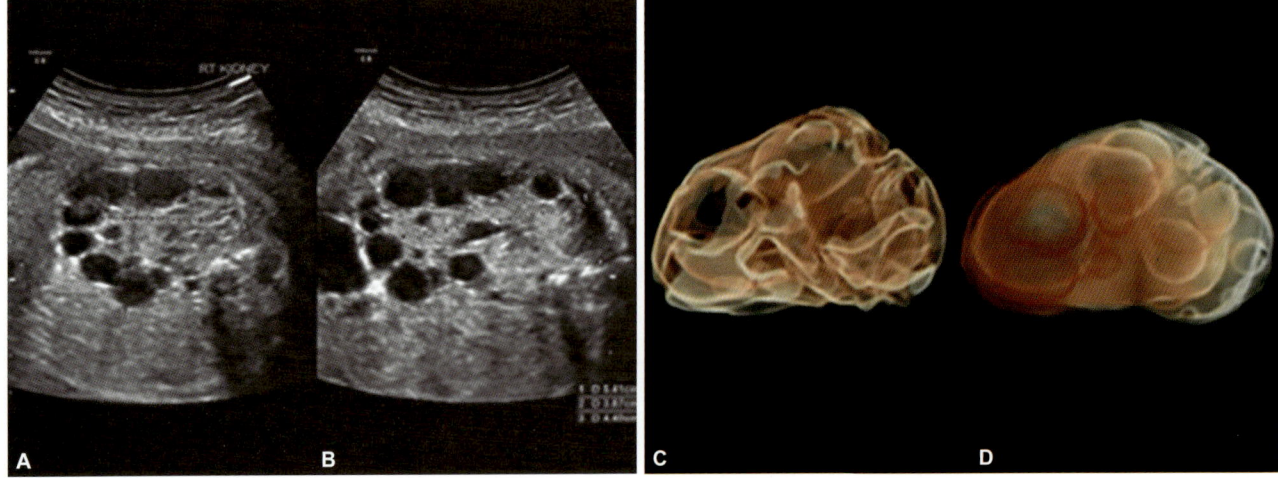

Figs. 24.20A to D: (A and B) MCDK in a fetus of 26 gestational weeks. (C and D) 3D HDlive Silhouette imaging: extraction of the volume of the MCDK kidney.[4,31] (3D: three-dimensional; HD: high definition; MCDK: multicystic dysplastic kidneys)

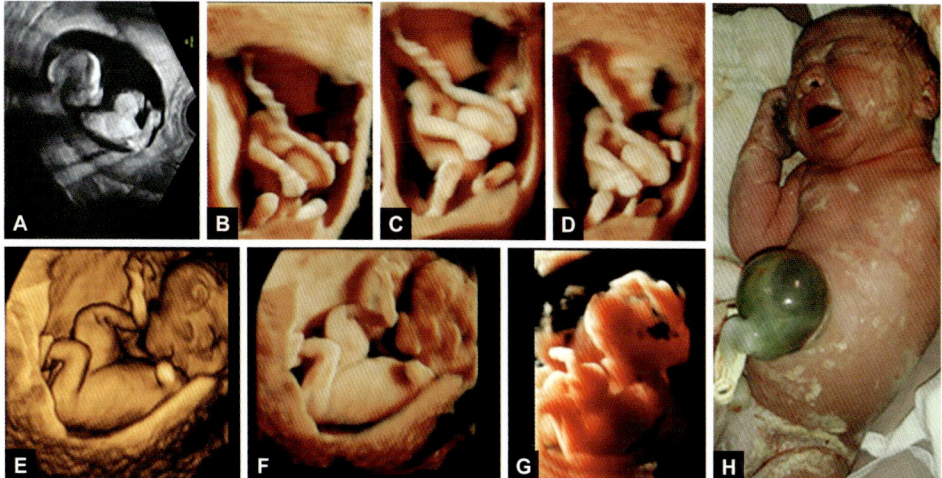

Figs. 24.21A to H: Sequence of images with (A) 2D US: Fetus with the omphalocele in the second trimester, (B to H) 3D HDlive modality in the assessment of the fetus. *Notice:* The difference in image illumination and angle of imaging. *Notice:* The similarities of imaging with post-partum image.[4] (3D: three-dimensional; HD: high definition; 2D US: two-dimensional ultrasound)

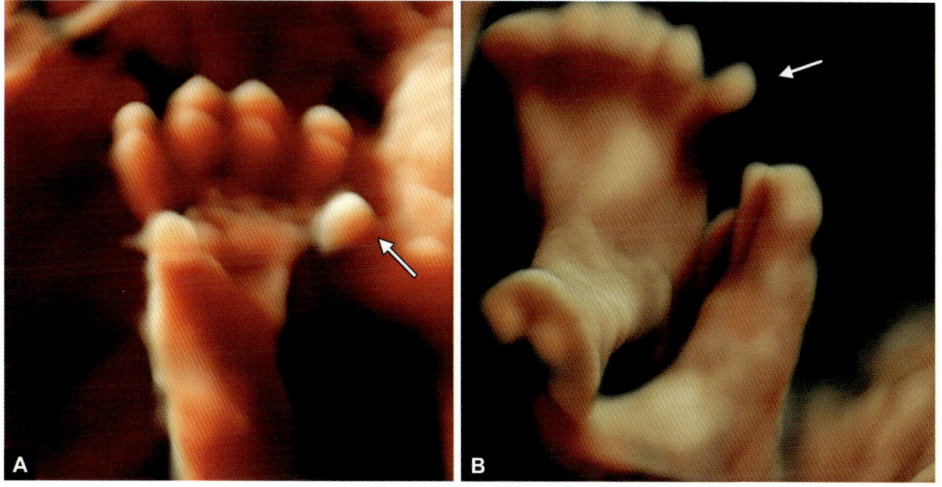

Figs. 24.22A and B: 3D HDlive surface rendering of the fetal hand (A) and the feet (B). *Notice:* The polydactyl in both cases! Fetus with Meckel-Gruber syndrome. (3D: three-dimensional; HD: high definition)

severe syndromes. As MCDK is dysfunctional, if found bilaterally, it indicates a lethal outcome and is often associated with *Meckel–Gruber's syndrome* **(Figs. 24.17 and 24.20)** with autosomal recessive inheritance.[79] Specifically, a triad of anomalies is found: occipital encephalocele, *MCDK* **(Fig. 24.17)**, and polydactyly **(Figs. 24.22A and B)**. A newborn dies in the first few days of life due to lung hypoplasia and kidney failure. Detection of occipital encephalocele in the first trimester is easier because of a better examination and normal amount of amniotic fluid. Later in pregnancy, there is a progressive oligohydramnios which can be the cause that encephalocele is missed. Special attention should be paid to the evaluation of both fetal kidneys because the normal US finding of a kidney excludes lethal Meckel–Gruber syndrome **(Figs. 24.17 and 24.20)**.

CONCLUSION

The 3D US technique with different visualization and manipulation capabilities of stored volume provides a unique opportunity for a detailed view of normal and abnormal fetal development. If facial anomaly is suspected, 3D imaging technique will help in the detailed evaluation. Gained images will give more clues to answer the question about severity and extent of targeted anomalies. This could be particularly handy tool when communicating with the neonatologist, pediatrician, plastic and reconstructive head and neck surgeon and especially when consulting with the parents of the child. However, as in any imaging technique (US, MSCT, and MRI), you need to know the dome and limitations of

3D/4D rendering and to be aware of possible artifacts and traps.

From the first trimester to the next, as soon as it becomes possible to detect congenital anomaly by prenatal US, the question arises—What can and should be done? Many ethical dilemmas present at the time.[2,4] Contemporary medicine faces some major problems when it has the ability to prolong life of severely ill baby with potentially lethal congenital syndromes.

Taking specific ultrasonic diagnostics into account, the idea is to find the balance between the advantages and limitations of sonographic assessment. At the same time, it should be possible to optimize recommendations with the expectations of parents of potentially seriously ill baby. Given the complexity of prenatal diagnosis of syndrome, everything involved in the process is also complex. This includes conformation of prenatal diagnosis postnatally and determination of the short- and long-term prognosis if possible to assist parents who are facing a baby with syndrome.[2,4] It is essential to point out the necessity of complex, lifelong, and costly multidisciplinary care for severely ill baby **(Figs. 24.23 to 24.25)**.

All the aforementioned 3D/4D US techniques promise to improve the accuracy of clinicians in detection of fetal abnormalities and detecting fetal syndromes as early as possible. There are many advantages in prenatal detection of fetal syndromes already described, but there is also a great room for improvement. Since new 3D/4D US technology becomes more available in everyday clinical practice, the clinician should remain well

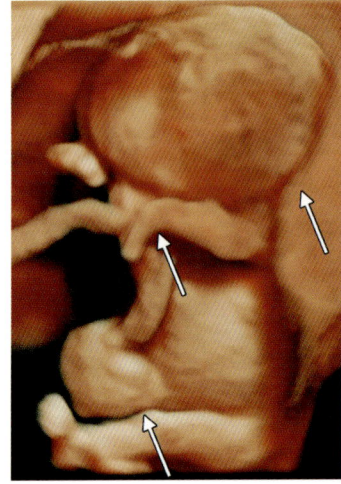

Fig. 24.23: 3D HDlive surface image of the fetus with trisomy 18. *Notice:* The triad of the anomalies: omphalocele, wrist contracture and hygroma colli (arrows).[2,31] (3D: three-dimensional; HD: high definition)

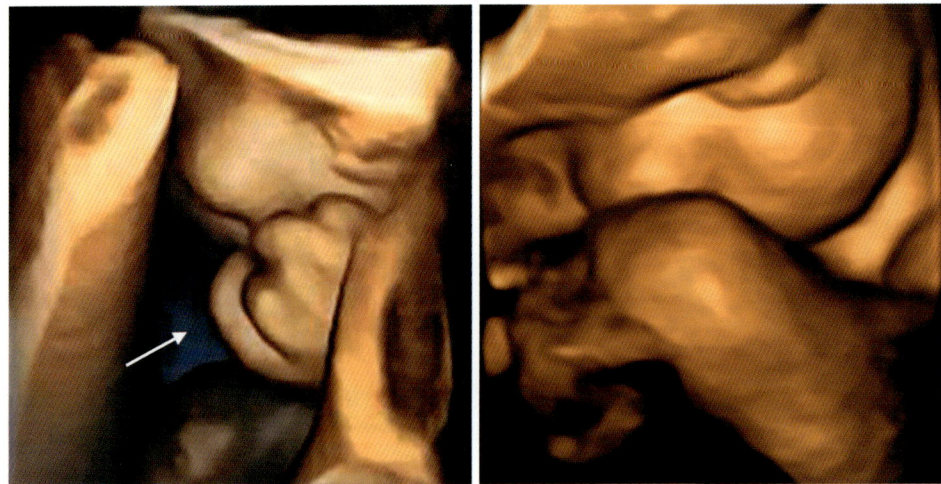

Fig. 24.24: 3D surface rendering; trisomy 18 (Edwards syndrome) in two cases. *Notice:* The clenched hand (arrow) and overlapping fingers in both.

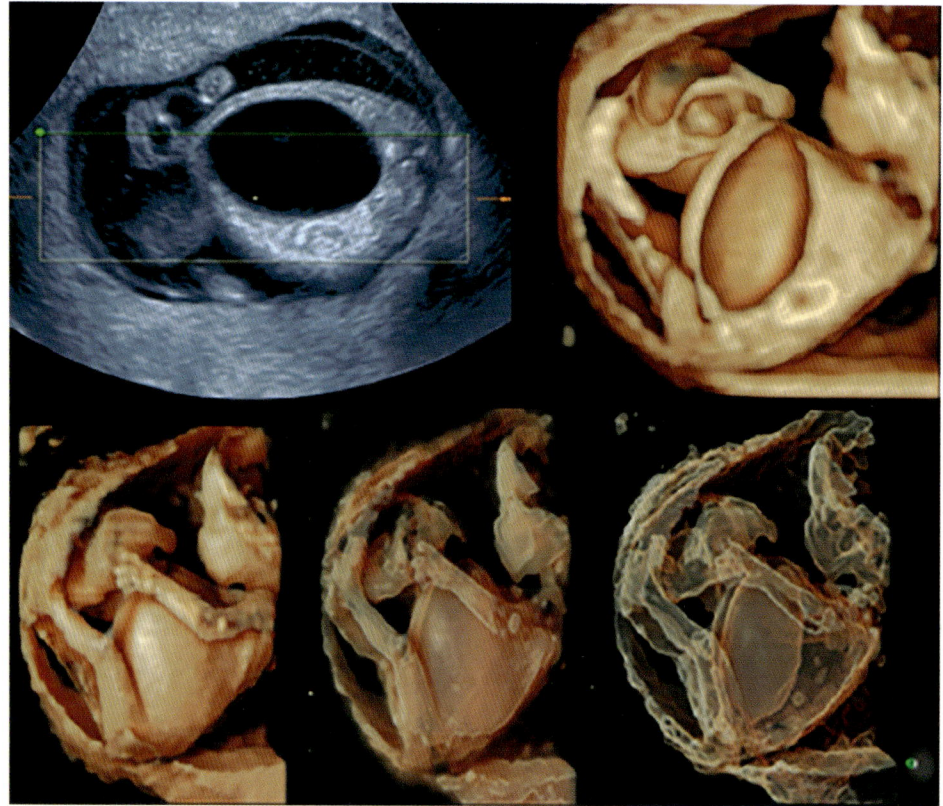

Fig. 24.25: Sequence of images. From 2D to 3D surface and Silhouette display with increasing Silhouette intensity. *Notice:* Megacystic bladder in the fetus with prune belly syndrome.[2,31] (2D: two-dimensional; 3D: three-dimensional)

informed, well trained, and monitor new diagnostic capabilities. Continuous education is necessary. In this way, the number of fetal abnormalities and syndromes detected prenatally will probably be better over time.[4] Auxiliary tools such as network databases (online databases) that integrate all the necessary information should be included and used for better diagnostic precision.[2,4]

REFERENCES

1. Merz E. 25 Years of 3D ultrasound in prenatal diagnosis (1989-2014). Ultraschall Med. 2015;36(1):3-8.
2. Spalldi Barišić L, Kurjak A, Pooh RK, et al. Antenatal detection of fetal syndromes by ultrasound: from a single piece to a complete puzzle. Donald Sch J Ultrasound Obstet Gynecol. 2016;10(1):63-77.
3. Merz E, Abramowicz JS. 3D/4D ultrasound in prenatal diagnosis: is it time for routine use? Clin Obstet Gynecol. 2012;55:336-51.
4. Spalldi Barišić L, Stanojević M, Kurjak A, et al. Diagnosis of fetal syndromes by three- and four-dimensional ultrasound: is there any improvement? J Perinat Med. 2017;45(6):651-65.
5. Benacerraf BR. Ultrasound of fetal syndromes, 2nd edition. Churchill Livingstone; 2008. Chapter 1, Differential Diagnoses; Chapter 2, Syndromes.
6. Lanna M, Rustico MA, Pintucci A, et al. Three-dimensional ultrasound and genetic syndromes. Donald Sch J Ultrasound Obstet Gynecol. 2007;1(3):54-9.
7. Jones, KL. Chapter 1, Introduction including dysmorphology approach and classification. Smith's recognizable patterns of human malformation, 5th edition. Philadelphia, PA: Elsevier Saunders; 1997.
8. Jones, KL. Smith's recognizable patterns of human malformations, 6th edition. Philadelphia, PA: Elsevier Saunders; 2006.
9. Pashaj S, Merz E. Three-dimensional ultrasound for detection of fetal syndromes. In: Kurjak A, Chervenak FA (Eds). Donald School Textbook of Ultrasound in Obstetrics & Gynecology, 4th edition. 2018. pp. 800-16. DOI: 10.5005/jp/books/13058_49
10. Pooh RK, Kurjak A. Novel application of three-dimensional HDlive imaging in prenatal diagnosis from the first trimester. J Perinat Med. 2015;43:147-58.
11. Pooh, RK. Neuroanatomy visualisation by 2D and 3D. In: Pooh RK, Kurjak A (Eds). Fetal neurology. New Delhi: Jaypee Brothers Medical Publisers (P) Ltd; 2009. pp. 15-38.

12. Pooh RK, Kurjak A. 3D/4D sonography moved prenatal diagnosis of fetal anomalies from the second to the first trimester of pregnancy. J Matern Fetal Neonatal Med. 2012;25(5):433-55.

13. Kurjak A, Miskovic B, Stanojevic M, et al. New scoring system for fetal neurobehavior assessed by three- and four-dimensional sonography. J Perinat Med. 2008;36:73-81.

14. Kurjak A, Abo-Yaqoub S, Stanojevic M, et al. The potential of 4D sonography in the assessment of fetal neurobehavior-multicentric study in high-risk pregnancies. J Perinat Med. 2010;38:77-82.

15. Stanojevic M, Talic A, Miskovic B, et al. An attempt to standardize Kurjak's antenatal neurodevelopmental test: Osaka Consensus Statement. Donald Sch J Ultrasound Obstet Gynecol. 2011;5:317-29.

16. Stanojevic M, Antsaklis P, Salihadic-Kadic A, et al. Is Kurjak antenatal neurodevelopmental test ready for routine clinical application? Bucharest consensus statement. Donald Sch J Ultrasound Obstet Gynecol. 2015;9(3):260-5.

17. Kurjak A, Antsaklis P, Stanojević M, et al. Multicentric studies of the fetal neurobehavior by KANET test. J Perinat Med. 2017;45(6):717-27.

18. Kurjak A, Spalldi Barišić L, Stanojević M, et al. Are we ready to investigate cognitive function of fetal brain? The role of advanced four-dimensional sonography. Donald Sch J Ultrasound Obstet Gynecol. 2016;10(2):116-24.

19. Salihagić Kadić A, Kurjak A. Cognitive functions of the fetus. Ultraschall Med. 39(2):181-9.

20. Pooh RK. A new field of 'fetal sono-ophthalmology' by 3D HDlive silhouette and flow. Donald Sch J Ultrasound Obstet Gynecol. 2015;9(3):221-2.

21. Kurjak A, Pooh RK, Merce LT, et al. Structural and functional early human development assessed by three-dimensional and four-dimensional sonography. Fertil Steril. 2005;84:1285-99.

22. Hata T, Mashima M, Ito M, et al. Three-dimensional HDlive rendering images of the fetal heart. Ultrasound Med Biol. 2013;39:1513-7.

23. Hanaoka U, Tanaka H, Koyano K, et al. HDlive imaging of the face of fetuses with autosomal trisomies. J Med Ultrason. 2014;41:339-42.

24. Basel-Vanagaite L, Wolf L, Orin M, et al. Recognition of the Cornelia de Lange syndrome phenotype with facial dysmorphology novel analysis. Clin Genet. 2016;89:557-63.

25. Dorland's illustrated medical dictionary. Elsevier. [online] Available from www.dorlands.com/wsearch.jsp.

26. Lyons KJ, Crandall MJ, del Campo M. Smith's recognizable patterns of human malformation, 7th ed. Philadelphia, PA: Elsevier Saunders; 2013.

27. Shprintzen RJ, Siegl-Sadewitz VL, Amato J, et al. Anomalies associated with cleft lip, cleft palate or both. Am J Med Genet. 1985;29:585-95.

28. Gripp K. Face2Gene RESEARCH for deep phenotyping of novel syndromes. ACMG; 2018. [online] Available from http//www.fdna.com/blog/acmgtalk_gripp.

29. FDNA. Face2Gene. [online] Available from http//www.face2gene.com.

30. Phenotip online database. [online] Available from http://www.phenotip.com.

31. Pooh RK, Kurjak A. Images with the permission of the publisher. Donald school atlas of advanced ultrasound in obstetrics and gynaecology, 1st edition. New Delhi: Jaypee Brothers Medical Publishers (P) Ltd; 2015.

32. Gonçalves LF, Lee W, Espinoza J, et al. Three- and 4-dimensional ultrasound in obstetric practice: does it help? J Ultrasound Med. 2005;24(12):1599-624.

33. Merz E, Welter C. Two-dimensional and three-dimensional ultrasound in the evaluation of normal and abnormal fetal anatomy in the second and third trimesters in a level III center. Ultraschall Med. 2005;26(1):9-16.

34. Benoit B, Levaillant JM. Voluson GE. Healthcare technology. [online] Available from www.volusonclub.net [accessed December 10, 2016].

35. Kagan KO, Pintoffl K, Hoopmann M. First-trimester ultrasound images using HDlive. Ultrasound Obstet Gynecol. 2011;38:607.

36. Hata T. HDlive rendering image at 6 weeks of gestation. J Med Ultrason. 2013;40:495-6.

37. Hata T, Mashima M, Ito M, et al. Three-dimensional HDlive rendering.

38. Pooh RK. Novel application of HDlive silhouette and HDlive flow: clinical significance of the 'see-through fashion' in prenatal diagnosis. Donald Sch J Ultrasound Obstet Gynecol. 2016;10(1):90-8.

39. Pooh RK. Clinical significance of 3D HDlive silhouette/flow in neurosonoembryology and fetal neurosonography. Ultrasound Obstet Gynecol. 2016;48(Suppl 1):51-166.

40. Tonni G, Castigliego AP, Grisolia G, et al. Three-dimensional ultrasonography by means of HDlive rendering in the first trimester of pregnancy: a pictorial review. J Turk Ger Gynecol Assoc. 2016;17(2):110-9.

41. Hata T, Kanenishi K, Akiyama M, et al. Real-time 3-D sonographic observation of fetal facial expression. J Obstet Gynaecol Res. 2005;31:337-40.

42. Kurjak A, Azumendi G, Andonotopo W, et al. Three- and four-dimensional ultrasonography for the structural and functional evaluation of the fetal face. Am J Obstet Gynecol. 2007;196:16-28.

43. Pooh RK, Kurjak A. Three-dimensional ultrasound in detection of fetal anomalies. Donald Sch J Ultrasound Obstet Gynecol. 2016;10(3):376-90.

44. The third cycle of the Give A Face To A Syndrome research program. Research proposals issued at the American College of Medical Genetics and Genomics (ACMG) annual meeting; 2016. [online] Available from http://www.FDNA.com.

45. Sperber GH. Cranifacial embryology, 4th edition. London: Wright; 1989.

46. Johnston MC. Embryology of the fetal head and neck. In: JG. McCarthy (Ed). Plastic surgery, vol. 4. Philadelphia, PA: WB Saunders Co; 1990. pp. 2451-95.

47. Paladini D, Morra T, Teodoro A, et al. Objective diagnosis of micrognathia in the fetus: the Jaw index. Obstet Gynecol. 1999;93(3):382-6.

48. Merz E, Abramovicz J, Baba K, et al. 3D imaging of the fetal face—recommendations from the International 3D Focus Group. Ultraschall Med. 2012;33:175-82.

49. Maarse W, Berge SJ, Pistorius L, et al. Diagnostic accuracy of transabdominal ultrasound in detecting prenatal cleft lip and palate: a systematic review. Ultrasound Obstet Gynecol. 2010;35(4):495-502.

50. Evans KN, Sie KC, Hopper RA, et al. Robin sequence: from diagnosis to development of an effective management plan. Pediatrics. 2011;127(5):936-48.

51. Nowakowski, TJ, Pollen AA, Di Lullo E, et al. Expression analysis highlights AXL as a candidate Zika virus entry receptor in neural stem cells. Cell Stem Cell. 2016;18(5): 591-6.

52. Li, C, Xu D, Ye Q, et al. Zika virus disrupts neural progenitor development and leads to microcephaly in mice. Cell Stem Cell. 2016;19(1):120-6.

53. Society for Maternal-Fetal Medicine (SMFM) Publications Committee. Ultrasound screening for fetal microcephaly following Zika virus exposure. Am J Obstet Gynecol. 2016; 214(6):B2-4. SMFM Statement.

54. Abo-Yaqoub S, Kurjak A, Mohammed AB, et al. The role of 4-D ultrasonography in prenatal assessment of fetal neurobehaviour and prediction of neurological outcome. J Matern Fetal Neonatal Med. 2012;25: 231-6.

55. Talic A, Kurjak A, Ahmed B, et al. The potential of 4D sonography in the assessment of fetal behavior in high-risk pregnancies. J Matern Fetal Neonatal Med. 2011;24: 948-54.

56. Miskovic B, Vasilj O, Stanojevic M, et al. The comparison of fetal behavior in high-risk and normal pregnancies assessed by four-dimensional ultrasound. J Matern Fetal Neonatal Med. 2010;23:1461-7.

57. Andonotopo W, Kurjak A. The assessment of fetal behavior of growth-restricted fetuses by 4D sonography. J Perinat Med. 2006;34:471-8.

58. Talic A, Kurjak A, Stanojevic M, et al. The assessment of fetal brain function in fetuses with ventrikulomegaly: the role of the KANET test. J Matern Fetal Neonatal Med. 2012;25:1267-72.

59. Morokuma S, Fukushima K, Yumoto Y, et al. Simplified ultrasound screening for fetal brain function based on behavioral pattern. Early Hum Dev. 2007;83:177-81.

60. Teoh M, Meagher S. First-trimester diagnosis of micrognathia as a presentation of Pierre Robin syndrome. Ultrasound Obstet Gynecol. 2003;21(6):616-8.

61. Johnson JM, Moonis G, Green GE, et al. Syndromes of the first and second branchial arches, part 2: Syndromes. Am J Neuroradiol. 2011;32:(2):230-7.

62. Breugem CC, Courtemanche DJ. Robin sequence: clearing nosologic confusion. Cleft Palate Craniofac J. 2010;47(2): 197-200.

63. Evans AK, Rahbar R, Rogers GF, et al. Robin sequence: a retrospective review of 115 patients. Int J Pediatr Otorhinolaryngol. 2006;70(6):973-80.

64. Godbout A, Leclerc JE, Arteau-Gauthier I, et al. Isolated versus Pierre Robin sequence cleft palates: are they different? Cleft Palate Craniofac J. 2014;51(4):406-11.

65. Martinelli P, Maurotti GM, Agangi A, et al. Prenatal diagnosis of hemifacial microsomia and ipsilateral cerebellar hypoplasia in a fetus with oculoauriculovertebral spectrum. Ultrasound Obstet Gynecol. 2004;24:199-201.

66. Wang R, Martinez-Frias ML, Graham JM Jr. Infants of diabetic mothers are at increased risk for the oculo-auriculo-vertebral sequence: a case-based and case-control approach. J Pediatr. 2002;141(5):611-7.

67. Chervenak FA, Rosenberg J, Brightman RC, et al. A prospective study of accuracy of ultrasound in predicting fetal microcephaly. Obstet Gynecol. 1987;69(6):908-1043.

68. Paul A Trainor PA, Dixon J, et al. Treacher Collins syndrome: etiology, pathogenesis and prevention. Eur J Hum Genet. 2009;17:275-83.

69. Tsai MY, Lan KC, Ou CY, et al. Assessment of the facial features and chin development of fetuses with use of serial three-dimensional sonography and the mandibular size monogram in a Chinese population. Am J Obstet Gynecol. 2004;190(2):541-6.

70. Jones NC, Lynn ML, Gaudenz K, et al. Prevention of the neurocristopathy Treacher–Collins syndrome through inhibition of p53 function. Nat Med. 2008;14(2):125-33.

71. Toriello HV, Meck JM. Statement on guidance for genetic counseling in advanced paternal age. Genet Med. 2008; 10(6):457-60.

72. De Araújo TV, Rodrigues LC, de Alencar Ximenes RA, et al. Association between Zika virus infection and micro-cephaly in Brazil, January to May, 2016: preliminary report of a case-control study. Lancet Infect Dis. 2016;(16)12: 1356-63.

73. van der Linden V, Pessoa A, Dobyns W, et al. Description of 13 infants born during October 2015–January 2016 with congenital Zika virus infection without microcephaly at birth, Brazil. MMWR Morb Mortal Wkly Rep. 2016; 65(47);1343-8.

74. Melo AS, Aguiar RS, Amorim MM, et al. Congenital Zika virus infection: beyond neonatal microcephaly. JAMA Neurol. 2016;73(12):1407-16.

75. Kurjak A, Miskovic B, Stanojevic M, et al. New scoring system for fetal neurobehavior assessed by three- and four-dimensional sonography. J Perinat Med. 2008;36(1):73-81.

76. Kurjak A, Abo-Yaqoub S, Stanojevic M, et al. The potential of 4D sonography in the assessment of fetal neurobehavior—multicentric study in high-risk pregnancies. J Perinat Med. 2010;38(1):77-82.

77. Stanojevic M, Antsaklis P, Kadic AS, et al. Is Kurjak antenatal neurodevelopmental test ready for routine clinical application? Bucharest consensus statement. Donald Sch J Ultrasound Obstet Gynecol. 2015;9(3): 260-5.

78. Kurjak A, Barisic LS, Stanojevic M, et al. Are we ready to investigate cognitive function of fetal brain? The role of advanced four-dimensional sonography. Donald Sch J Ultrasound Obstet Gynecol. 2016;10(2):116-24.

79. Barišić I, Odak LJ, Loane M, et al. Prevalence, prenatal diagnosis and clinical features of oculo-auriculo-vertebral spectrum: a registry-based study in Europe. Eur J Hum Genet. 2014;22:1026-33.

80. Kurjak A, Carrera JM, Stanojevic M, et al. The role of 4D sonography in the neurological assessment of early human development. Ultrasound Rev Obstet Gynecol. 2004;4: 148-59.

81. Salihagic-Kadic A, Kurjak A, Medić M, et al. New data about embryonic and fetal neurodevelopment and behavior obtained by 3D and 4D sonography. J Perinat Med. 2005;33:478-90.

82. Andonotopo W, Kurjak A, Kosuta MI. Behavior of an anencephalic fetus studied by 4D sonography. J Matern Fetal Neonatal Med. 2005;17:165-8.

83. Bonilla-Musoles F, Raga F, Castillo JC, et al. High-definition real-time ultrasound (HDlive) of embryonic and fetal malformations before week 16. Donald Sch J Ultrasound Obstet Gynecol. 2013;7:1-8.

Three- and Four-dimensional Ultrasound in Fetal Echocardiography: A New Look at the Fetal Heart

Simcha Yagel, Sarah M Cohen, Israel Shapiro, Baruch Messing, Dan V Valsky

BACKGROUND

Three- and four-dimensional (3D/4D) applications in fetal ultrasound (US) scanning have made impressive strides in the past three decades, with particularly dramatic improvement in fetal echocardiography. Recent technological developments in motion-gated scanning allow almost real-time 3D/4D cardiac examination. It appears that 3D/4D US applications will make a significant contribution to our understanding of the developing fetal heart in both normal and anomalous cases, to interdisciplinary management team consultation, to parental counseling, and to professional training. 3D/4D echocardiography may facilitate screening methods and with its offline networking capabilities may improve healthcare delivery systems by extending the benefits of prenatal cardiac screening to poorly served areas. The introduction of "virtual planes" to fetal cardiac scanning has helped sonographers obtain views of the fetal heart not generally accessible with a standard two-dimensional (2D) approach. There is no doubt that 3D/4D gives us another look at the fetal heart.

Three- and four-dimensional cardiac scanning has been extensively applied in clinical practice and investigated as to whether it improves the accuracy of fetal echocardiography. In this chapter, we summarize the 3D/4D acquisition and postprocessing modalities in 3D/4D fetal echocardiography, demonstrating their use through normal and anomalous case examples.

THREE- AND FOUR-DIMENSIONAL TECHNIQUES AND THEIR APPLICATION TO FETAL CARDIAC SCANNING

Acquisition Modalities

Spatiotemporal Image Correlation

Spatiotemporal image correlation (STIC) acquisition is an indirect motion-gated offline scanning mode.[1-5] Briefly, automated volume acquisition is made possible by the array in the transducer performing a slow single sweep, recording a single 3D dataset consisting of many 2D frames, one behind the other. The volume of interest (VOI) is acquired over a period of 7.5 to about 30 seconds at a sweep angle of approximately 20°–40° (depending on the size of the fetus) and frame rate of about 150 frames per second. A 10-second, 25° acquisition would contain 1,500 B-mode images.[3] When using the newer electronic 4D eSTIC acquisitions, the acquisition principle is split into subvolumes, and frame rates are in the range of 800 frames per second.

Following acquisition, mathematical algorithms are applied to the volume data to detect systolic peaks that are used to calculate the fetal heart rate. The B-mode images are arranged in order according to their spatial and temporal domain, correlated to the internal trigger, the systolic peaks that define the heart cycle[3] **(Figs. 25.1A to D)**. The result is a reconstructed complete heart cycle that displays in an endless loop. This cine-like file of a beating fetal heart can be manipulated to display any acquired scanning plane at any stage in the cardiac cycle **(Figs. 25.2A and B)**. This reconstruction takes place directly following the scan in a matter of seconds, allowing the STIC acquisition to be reviewed with the patient still present and repeated, if necessary, and saved to the scanning machine, personal computer, or network.

Spatiotemporal image correlation acquisition can be combined with other applications by selecting the appropriate setting before acquisition (B-flow, color and power Doppler, tissue Doppler, high-definition flow Doppler) or with postprocessing visualization modalities [3D volume rendering, virtual organ computer-aided analysis (VOCAL), inversion mode (IM), tomographic ultrasound imaging (TUI)].

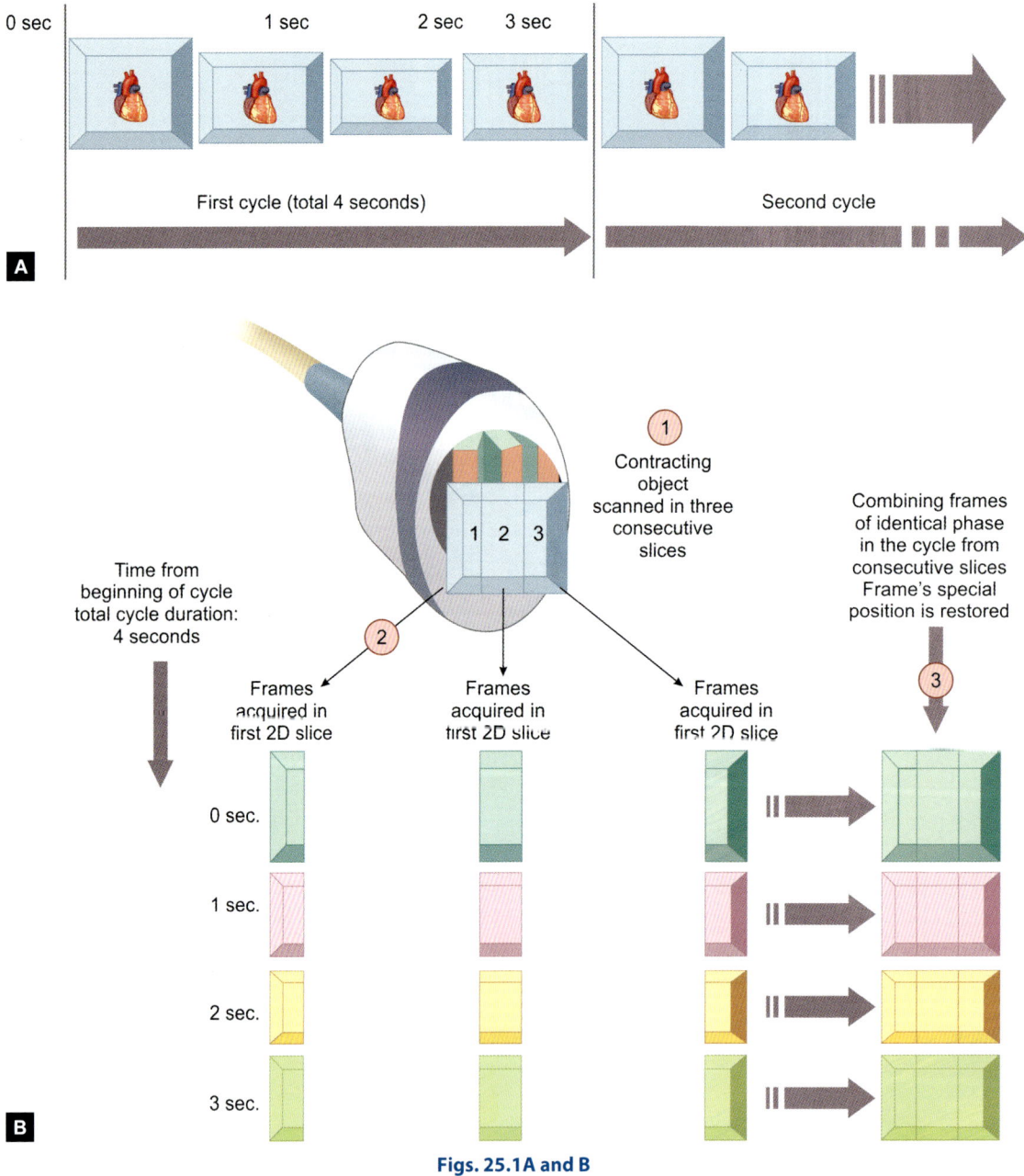

Figs. 25.1A and B

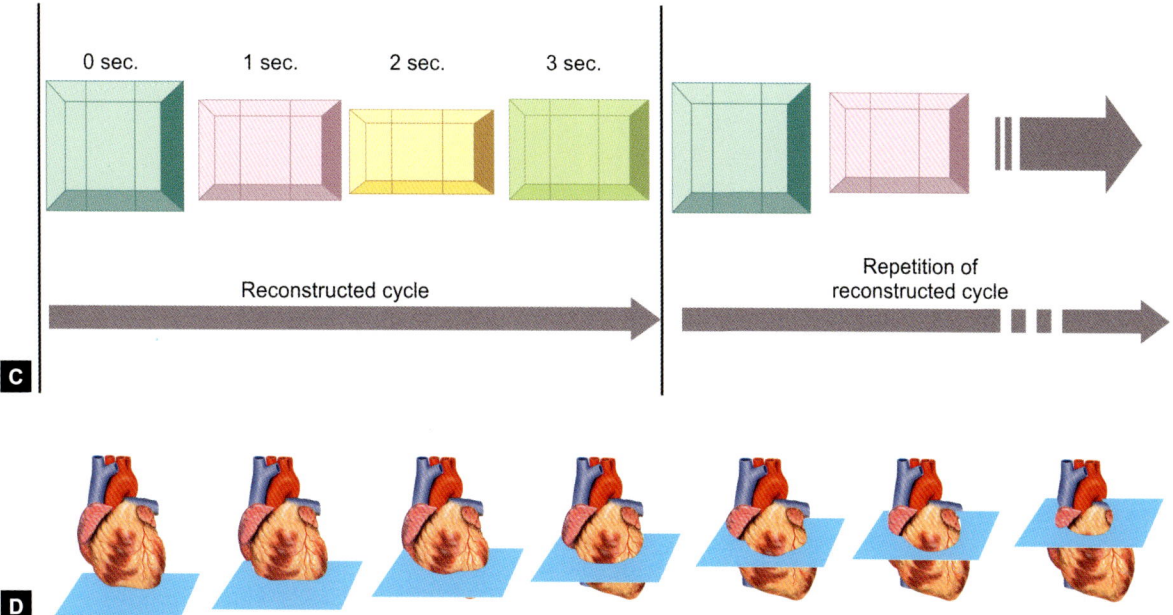

Figs. 25.1C and D

Figs. 25.1A to D: Demonstration of STIC technology. Cycle duration, number of slices, and number of frames per slice were chosen to simplify illustration. The scale applicable to fetal cardiac examination is discussed in the text. (A) An object is contracting in a cyclical manner (4 seconds per cycle). The shape of the object is presented at four points during the cycle. Assume that the contraction rate is too high to scan the whole object in conventional real-time 3D; (B) The object is scanned in three consecutive slices adjacent to each other (1). At least one complete cycle is recorded in real-time 2D ultrasound, thus acquiring many frames per slice. In this example, four frames are recorded in each slice (2). By simultaneous analysis of the tissue movements, the software identifies the beginning of each cycle and sets the time that each frame was acquired in respect of the beginning of the cycle. Knowing the time and position of each frame, the software reconstructs the 3D shape of the complete object in each phase of the cycle (3). The shape is constructed from frames arranged side by side according to their position in the object (hence spatiotemporal). Though each frame composing the object was acquired in a different cycle, their phase in respect of the beginning of the cycle is identical (hence spatiotemporal); (C) The system completes its task by creating an endless loop animation composed of the consecutive reconstructed volumes of the cycle, resulting in a moving volume resembling real-time 3D. The procedure takes only a few seconds; the stored reconstructed volumes are now available for analysis with postprocessing techniques as described in the text; (D) Demonstration of the multiple slices through the heart acquired during a single STIC scan. The dedicated transducer automatically changes its scanning angle, either by means of a small motor in some systems, or electronically by using a phased matrix of elements. (2D: two-dimensional; 3D: three-dimensional; STIC: spatiotemporal image correlation)

Source: Reproduced with permission from Yagel et al.[82] © International Society of Ultrasound in Obstetrics and Gynecology. Permission is granted by John Wiley and Sons Ltd on behalf of ISUOG.

B-flow

B-flow is an old–new technology that images blood flow without relying on Doppler shift; rather, B-flow is an outgrowth of B-mode imaging. With the advent of faster frame rates and computer processing, B-flow directly depicts blood cell reflectors. It avoids some of the pitfalls of Doppler, such as aliasing and signal dropout at orthogonal scanning angles. The resulting image is a live grayscale depiction of blood flow and part of the surrounding lumen, creating sensitive "digital casts" of blood vessels and cardiac chambers **(Figs. 25.3 and 25.4)**. B-flow is also a sensitive acquisition tool for volume measurement. B-flow modality is a direct-volume nongated scanning method able to show blood flow in the heart and great vessels in real time, without color Doppler flow information.[6] B-flow combined with STIC can provide real-time dynamic angiographic features of extracardiac vessels.[7] These capabilities make it an invaluable tool in fetal echocardiography.

Three- and Four-dimensional with Color Doppler, Three-dimensional Power Doppler, and Three-dimensional High-definition Power Flow Doppler

Color and power Doppler have been extensively applied to fetal echocardiography; scanning is incomplete today without color Doppler. Color or power Doppler, and the most recent development, high-definition flow Doppler,

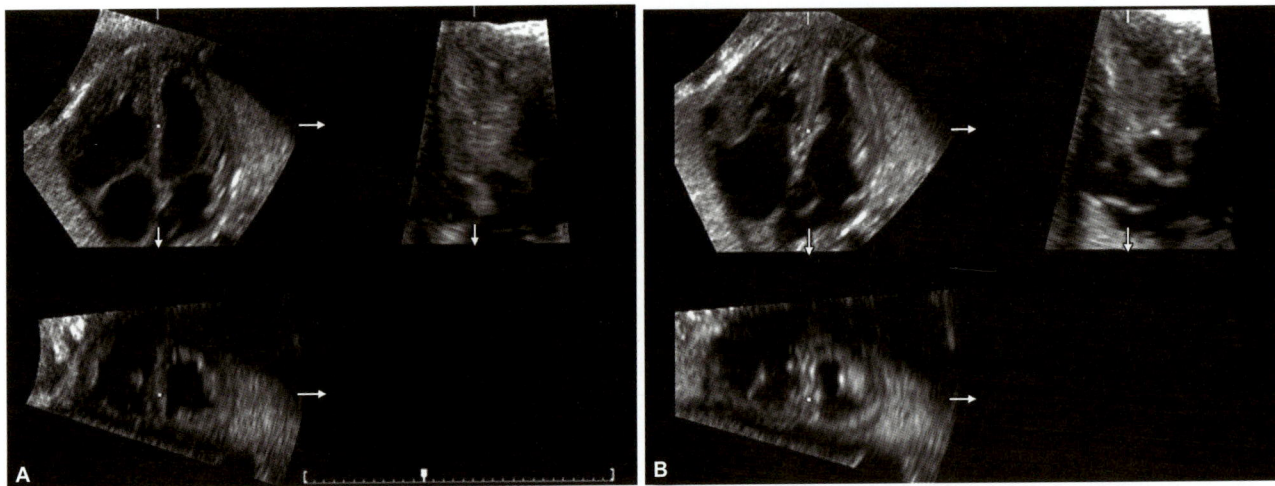

Figs. 25.2A and B: The four-chamber view from a STIC acquisition in a third-trimester fetus in systole (A) and diastole (B). By applying MPR, the operator optimizes the FCV plane, adjusting the image both spatially along the x-, y-, and z-axes, and to the desired stage of the cardiac cycle. The navigation point is placed on the interventricular septum in the A-plane; the B-plane shows the septum en face, and the C-plane shows a coronal plane through the ventricles. (FCV: four-chamber view; MPR: multiplanar reconstruction)
Source: Reproduced with permission from Yagel et al.[82] © International Society of Ultrasound in Obstetrics and Gynecology. Permission is granted by John Wiley and Sons Ltd on behalf of ISUOG.

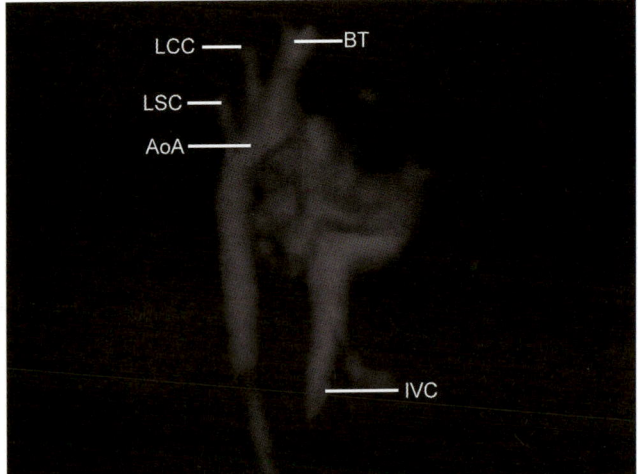

Fig. 25.3: B-flow image of normal heart and aortic arch. BT, LCC, and LSA are seen projecting from the AoA. IVC is indicated. (AoA: aortic arch; BT: brachiocephalic trunk; IVC: inferior vena cava; LCC: left common carotid; LSA: left subclavian artery)
Source: Reproduced with permission from Yagel et al.[82] © International Society of Ultrasound in Obstetrics and Gynecology. Permission is granted by John Wiley and Sons Ltd on behalf of ISUOG.

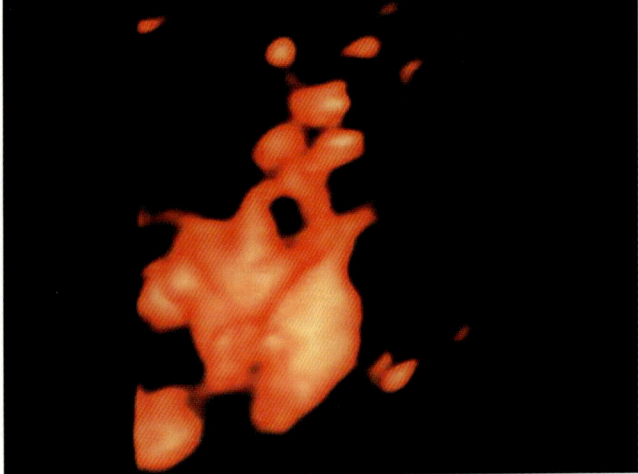

Fig. 25.4: B-flow: A case of aortic ring imaged in B-flow.

can be combined with static 3D direct-volume nongated scanning to obtain 3D volume files with two-color Doppler information or one-color 3D power Doppler (3D PD).

Color Doppler can be used more effectively in 3D/4D when combined with STIC acquisition[8] in fetal echocardiography, resulting in a volume file that reconstructs the cardiac cycle, as above, with color flow information. (Extreme care must be taken when working with Doppler applications in postprocessing, however, to avoid misinterpretation of flow direction as the volume is rotated.) This joins the Doppler flow to cardiac events[1] and provides all the advantages of analysis [multiplanar reconstruction (MPR) rendering, TUI] with color. This combination of modalities is very sensitive for detecting intracardiac Doppler flow signals throughout the cardiac cycle, e.g. mild tricuspid regurgitation occurring very early in systole or very briefly.[9]

Three-dimensional power Doppler is directionless, one-color Doppler that is most effectively joined with static 3D scanning.[1] 3D PD uses Doppler shift technology to reconstruct the blood vessels in the VOI, isolated from the rest of the volume. Using the "glass body" mode in postprocessing, surrounding tissue is not shown, while the vascular portion of the scan is isolated for evaluation. The operator can scroll spatially to any plane in the volume (but not temporally: in this case, color Doppler with STIC is more effective, see above). In 3D PD the vascular tree of the fetal abdomen and thorax is reconstructed,[10,11] obviating the necessity of reconstructing a mental picture of the idiosyncratic course of an anomalous vessel from a series of 2D planes. This has been shown to aid our understanding of the normal and anomalous anatomy and pathophysiology of vascular lesions[12] (**Fig. 25.5**).

High-definition power flow Doppler, the newest development in color Doppler applications, uses high resolution and a small sample volume to produce images with two-color directional information, with less "blooming" of color for more realistic representation of vessel size. It depicts flow at a lower velocity than color or power Doppler, while retaining the advantage of flow directional information, thereby combining high-resolution bidirectional flow Doppler with the anatomic acuity associated with power Doppler. It can be used with static 3D- or 4D-gated acquisition (STIC) and the glass-body mode, to produce high-resolution images of the vascular tree with bidirectional color coding (**Fig. 25.6**). It is particularly sensitive for imaging small vessels. Systolic and diastolic flows are observed at the same time owing to the sensitivity of the modality. For example, when used with STIC acquisition, the ductus venosus is shown to remain filled in both systole and diastole. Doppler applications in 3D/4D US reconstructions have improved steadily over the years and are now providing sharper, more defined appearance of blood flowing in its vessels with two-color information.[13] (**Figs. 25.7A to C**) show a normal heart and vessels imaged with this modality.

Real-time Three-dimensional Ultrasound

Real-time 3D US (RT 3D) with a matrix–array probe and the live xPlane modality provide a moving 3D display of two orthogonal images simultaneously: the primary image scanned by the operator, and the secondary image, which is extracted from the volume along the line placed by the operator on the primary image. This approach has been shown to be a feasible method to image the five

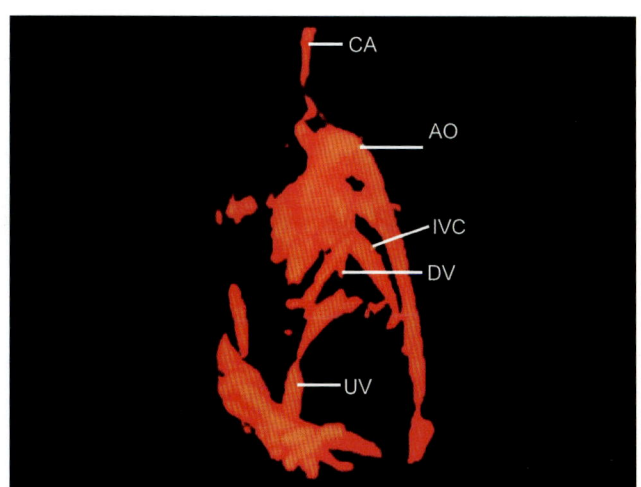

Fig. 25.5: 3D power Doppler of the heart and major vessels. Noted are the CA, AO, IVC, DV, and UV. (3D: three-dimensional; AO: aorta; CA: carotid artery; DV: ductus venosus; IVC: inferior vena cava; UV: umbilical vein)
Source: Reproduced with permission from Yagel et al.[82] © International Society of Ultrasound in Obstetrics and Gynecology. Permission is granted by John Wiley and Sons Ltd on behalf of ISUOG.

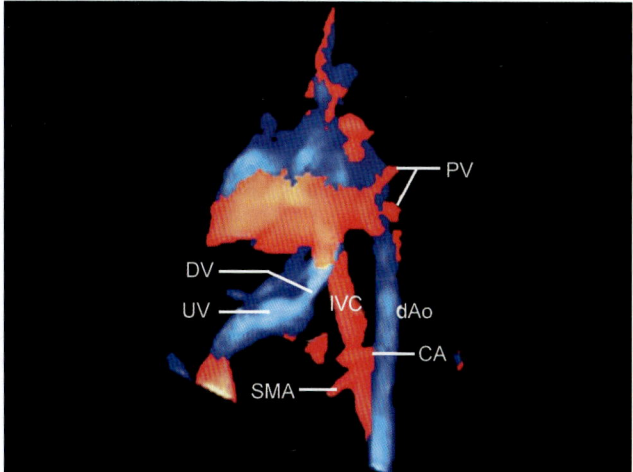

Fig. 25.6: Normal heart and great vessels: STIC acquisition with high definition power flow Doppler. (CA: celiac artery; dAo: descending aorta; DV: ductus venosus; IVC: inferior vena cava; PV: pulmonary veins; SMA: superior mesenteric artery; STIC: spatiotemporal image correlation; UV: umbilical vein.
Source: Reproduced with permission from Yagel et al.[82] © International Society of Ultrasound in Obstetrics and Gynecology. Permission is granted by John Wiley and Sons Ltd on behalf of ISUOG.

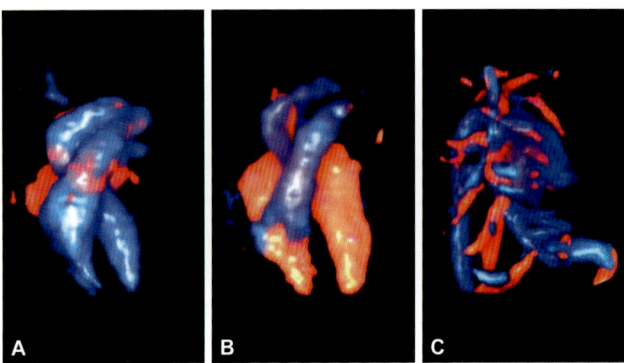

Figs. 25.7A to C: STIC combined with high-definition power Doppler: Normal heart and great vessels from a STIC acquisition with high-definition power Doppler of the heart in: (A) Systole; (B) Diastole; (C) The normal heart and vessels in longitudinal view. (STIC: spatiotemporal image correlation)

planes of fetal echocardiography as well as the ductal arch view, giving it added value in diagnosing conotruncal anomalies, and the interventricular septum.[14-16]

However, this approach may require manual adjustment to accommodate fetal position or an abnormal left ventricular outflow tract (LVOT).[17]

Herberg et al.[18] found that RT3D with a matrix transducer is a valid and reliable method for ventricle volume measurement and showed a strong inter- and intraobserver variability with a mean intraclass correlation coefficient (ICC) of 0.997. In a further study, they compared the visualization rates of specific structures with RT3D, reconstructed 3DUS (3DR), and 2DUS. The investigators found that RT3D had a better visualization rate than 2DUS, and that 2DUS and RT3D had higher sensitivity for identification of anomalies than 3DR.[19]

Zhu et al.[20] applied real-time 3D echocardiography in vivo and in vitro in an animal study to determine the feasibility of this modality to measure fetal stroke volume (SV), left ventricular mass, and myocardial strain, finding excellent correlation with reference values based on a balloon pump model.

Postprocessing Modalities

In postprocessing, various methodologies have been proposed to optimize the acquired volumes to demonstrate the classic planes of fetal echocardiography[21,22] **(Fig. 25.8)**, as well as "virtual planes" that are generally inaccessible in 2D cardiac scanning.[23-27] These views, once obtained, are stored to the patient file, in addition to the original volume, either as static images or 4D motion files. Any of the stored information can be shared for expert review, interdisciplinary consultation, parental counseling, or teaching.

Multiplanar Reconstruction, Three-dimensional Rendering, and Tomographic Ultrasound Imaging

Three- and four-dimensional volume sets contain a "block" of information; this is generally a wedge-shaped chunk of the targeted area. In order to analyze this effectively, the operator displays 2D planes in either MPR mode **(Figs. 25.2A and B)** or 3D volume rendering.

In MPR the screen is divided into four frames, referred to as A (upper left), B, C, and the fourth frame (lower right) showing either the volume model for reference or the rendered image. Each of the three frames shows one of the three orthogonal planes of the volume. The reference dot guides the operator in navigating within the volume, as it is anchored at the point of intersection of all three planes. By moving the point the operator manipulates the volume to display any plane within the volume; if temporal information was acquired, the same plane can be displayed at any stage of the scanned cycle.

From a good STIC acquisition[5] the operator can scroll through the acquired volume to obtain sequentially each of the classic five planes[21] of fetal echocardiography, and any plane may be viewed at any timepoint throughout the reconstructed cardiac cycle loop. The cycle can be run or stopped "frame by frame" to allow examination of all phases of the cardiac cycle, e.g. opening and closing of the atrioventricular (AV) valves.

By comparing the A- and B-frames of the MPR display the operator can view complex cardiac anatomy in corresponding transverse and longitudinal planes simultaneously. So, an anomalous vessel that might be disregarded in cross section is confirmed in the longitudinal plane.

Three-dimensional rendering is another analysis capability of an acquired volume. It is familiar from static 3D applications, such as imaging the fetal face in surface rendering mode. In fetal echocardiography, it is readily applied to 4D scanning. The operator places a bounding box around the region of interest within the volume (after arriving at the desired plane and time) to show a slice of the volume whose depth reflects the thickness of

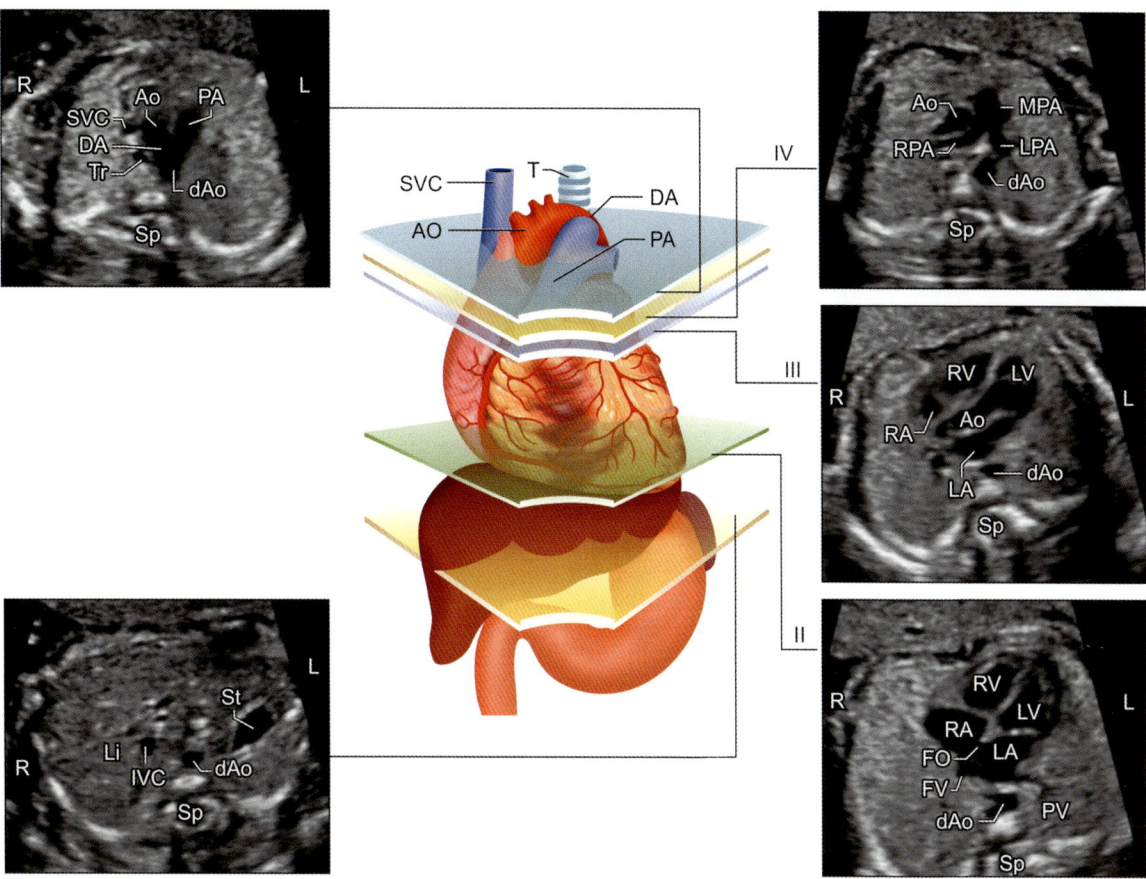

Fig. 25.8: The five short-axis views for optimal fetal heart screening. The color image shows the trachea, heart and great vessels, liver, and stomach with the five planes of insonation superimposed. Polygons show the angle of the transducer and are assigned to the relevant grayscale images (L, left; R, right). (I) The most caudal plane, showing the fetal stomach (ST), cross section of the abdominal aorta (AO), spine (SP), and liver (LI). (II) The four-chamber view of the fetal heart, showing the right and left ventricles (RV, LV) and atria (RA, LA), foramen ovale (FO), and pulmonary veins (PV) to the right and left of the aorta (AO). (III) The five-chamber view, showing the aortic root (AO), left and right ventricles (LV, RV), and atria (LA, RA) and a cross section of the descending aorta (AO with arrow). (IV) The slightly more cephalad view showing the main pulmonary artery (MPA) and the bifurcation of left and right pulmonary arteries (LPA, RPA) and cross sections of the ascending and descending aortae (AO and AO with arrow, respectively). (V) The 3VT plane of insonation, showing the pulmonary trunk (P), proximal aorta ([P]Ao), ductus arteriosus (DA), distal aorta ([D]Ao), superior vena cava (SVC), and the trachea (T).
Source: Reprinted with permission from International Society of Ultrasound in Obstetrics and Gynecology, Carvalho JS, et al. Ultrasound Obstet Gynecol. 2013;41:348-59.56.

the slice. For example, with the A-frame showing a good four-chamber view, the operator places the bounding box tightly around the interventricular septum. The rendered image in the D-frame will show an en face view of the septum. The operator can determine whether the plane will be displayed from the left or right (i.e. the septum from within the left or the right ventricle); the thickness of the slice will determine the depth of the final image, e.g. to show the texture of the trabeculations within the right ventricle **(Figs. 25.9A and B)**.

Figures 25.10 and 25.11 present rendered images of aberrant right subclavian artery and of aortic atresia

that were acquired in STIC with high-definition power Doppler and rendered to display the relevant anatomy.

Tomographic ultrasound imaging application extends the capabilities of MPR and rendering modes. This multi-slice analysis mode resembles a magnetic resonance imaging or computer-assisted tomography display. A matrix displays parallel slices simultaneously, centered around the plane of interest (the "zero" plane). The matrix comprises an adjustable number of sequential views (from 5 to +5, e.g.), dependent on the thickness of the slices, i.e. the distance of one plane to the next, which is regulated by the operator. The upper left frame of the

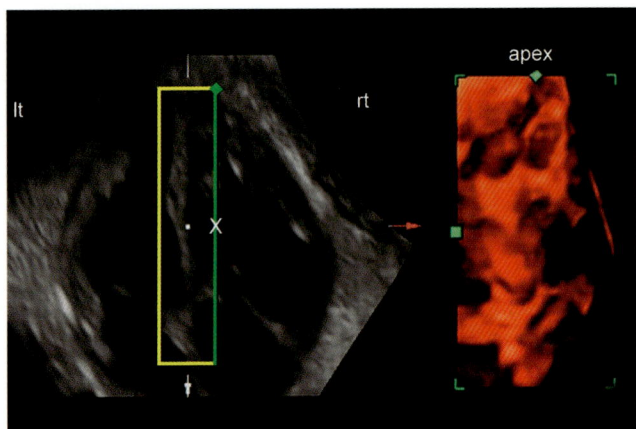

Figs. 25.9A and B: Normal interventricular septum in 3D rendering mode. In frame A (A) the bounding box is placed tightly around the septum with the active side (green line) on the right. The D-frame (B) shows the septum en face: note the rough appearance of the septum from within the trabeculated right ventricle. (3D: three-dimensional) *Source:* Reproduced with permission from Yagel et al.[82] © International Society of Ultrasound in Obstetrics and Gynecology. Permission is granted by John Wiley and Sons Ltd on behalf of ISUOG.

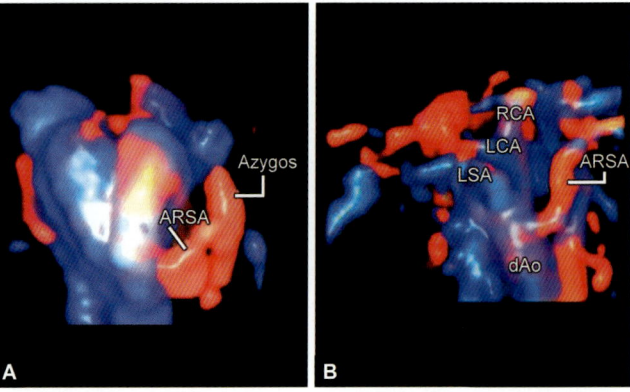

Figs. 25.10A and B: Rendered image of the case of ARSA. Left image (A) shows the 3VT plane with ARSA. The azygos vein (azygos) is marked. Right image (B) shows the ARSA and the relative positions of the aortic branches, the LSA, LCA, RCA, and the dAo. Rendered image derived from a STIC acquisition with high-definition power Doppler of a case of aortic atresia. Arrow indicates reverse flow in the narrow aorta. (ARSA: aberrant right subclavian artery; dAo: descending aorta; LCA: left carotid artery; LSA: Left subclavian artery; RCA: Right carotid artery; STIC: Spatiotemporal image correlation; VT: vessels and trachea)

display shows the position of each plane within the region of interest, relative to the reference plane. This display of sequential parallel planes gives a more complete picture of the fetal heart **(Figs. 25.12 to 25.15)**.

Virtual organ computer-aided analysis mode is a semiautomated 3D measurement mode that performs rotational measurement of volume. The saved volume file is rotated 180° about a fixed central axis through a preset number of rotation steps based on the operator-chosen angle of rotation, 6, 9, 15, or 30%. Setting the rotation angle at 15°, e.g. results in 12 planes available for measurement. The computer mouse is used to manually define the contours of the measured object (for example a heart ventricle) at each plane serially. Alternatively, the operator can opt for the system to draw the contours automatically, according to varying degrees of sensitivity. Once an outline is drawn around each plane of the target, the system reconstructs a contour model of the target. This postprocessing modality has been applied to volume calculation of numerous fetal organs, including heart, lungs, and others.[28-30]

Inversion Mode

Inversion mode is another postprocessing visualization modality that can be combined with static 3D or STIC acquisition.[28,31,32] IM analyzes the echogenicity of tissue (white) and fluid-filled (black) pixels in a volume and

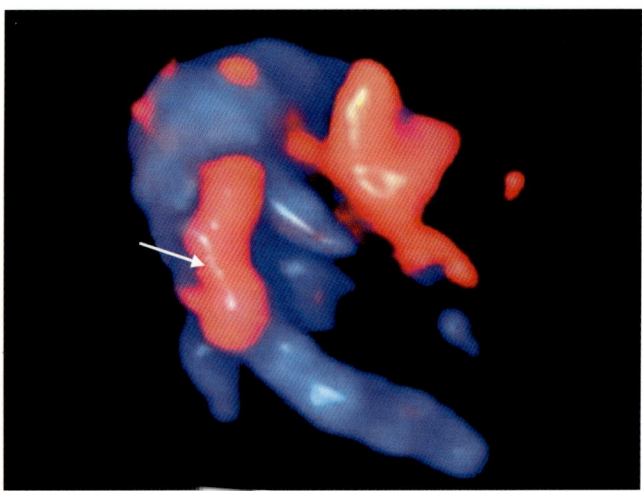

Fig. 25.11: Rendered image derived from a STIC acquisition with high-definition power Doppler of a case of aortic atresia. Arrow indicates reverse flow in the narrow aorta. (STIC: spatiotemporal image correlation)

inverts their presentation, i.e. fluid-filled spaces, such as the cardiac chambers, now appear white, while the myocardium has disappeared. In fetal echocardiography, it can be applied to create "digital casts"[33] of the cardiac chambers, outflow tracts, and great vessels in normal and anomalous cases.[34] It can also produce a reconstruction of the extracardiac vascular tree, similar to 3D PD. IM has the additional advantage of showing the stomach and

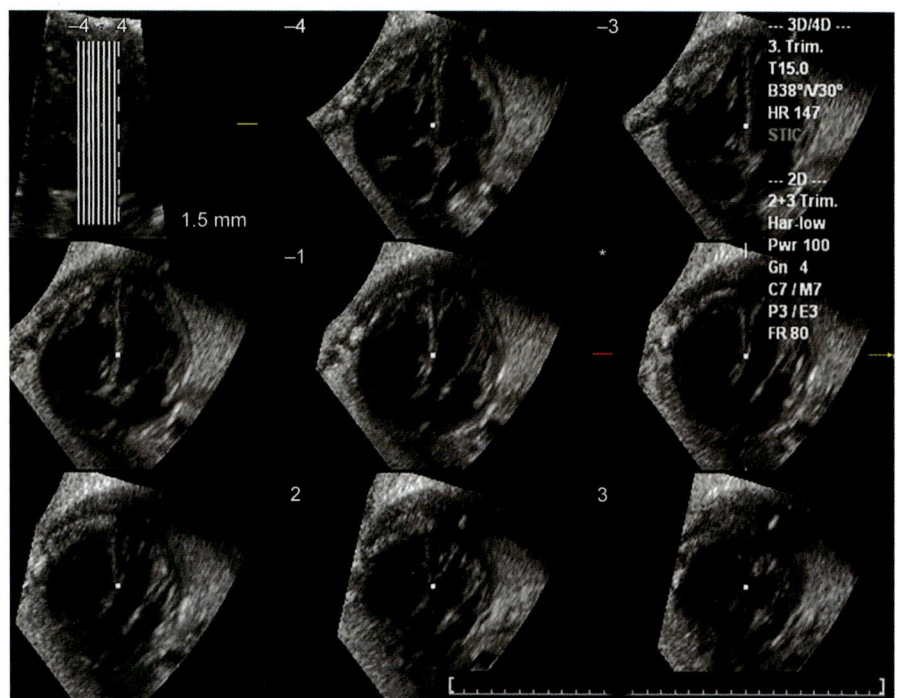

Fig. 25.12: TUI: The −4 plane (top row, center) shows the FCV, while the zero plane (asterisk, middle row, right) shows the outflow tract view, and the +3 plane shows the great vessels (bottom, right). (FCV: four-chamber view; TUI: tomographic ultrasound imaging)
Source: Reproduced with permission from Yagel et al.[82] © International Society of Ultrasound in Obstetrics and Gynecology. Permission is granted by John Wiley and Sons Ltd on behalf of ISUOG.

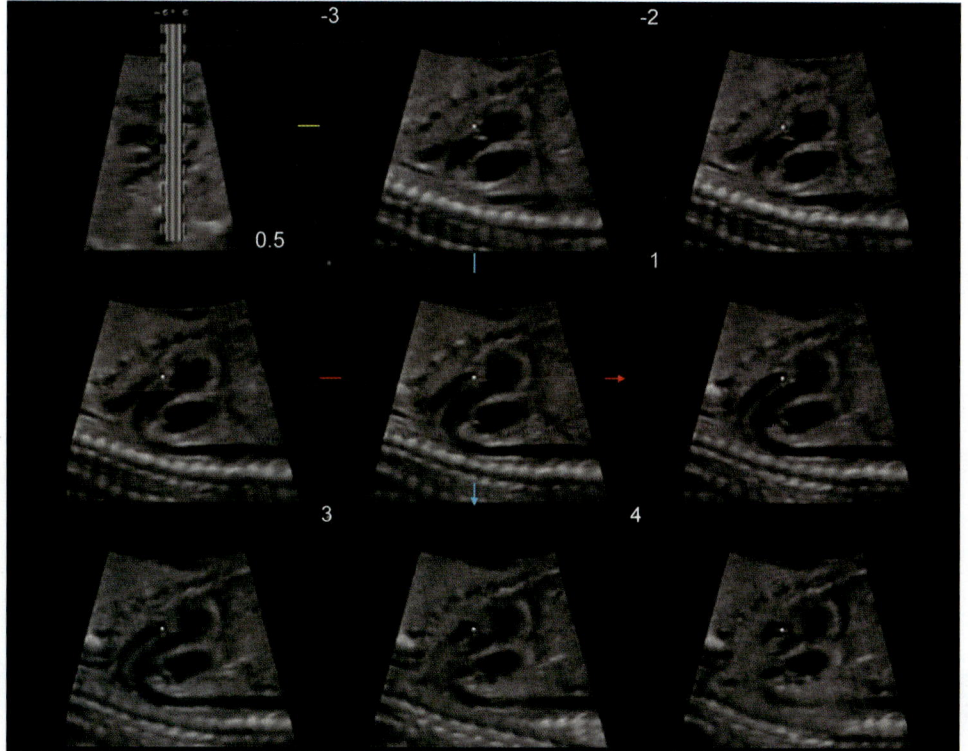

Fig. 25.13: TUI: A TUI image from a Grayscale STIC acquisition showing a case of transposition of the great arteries with parallel vessels. The serial images clearly display the aorta anterior to the pulmonary artery. (STIC: spatiotemporal image correlation; TUI: tomographic ultrasound imaging)

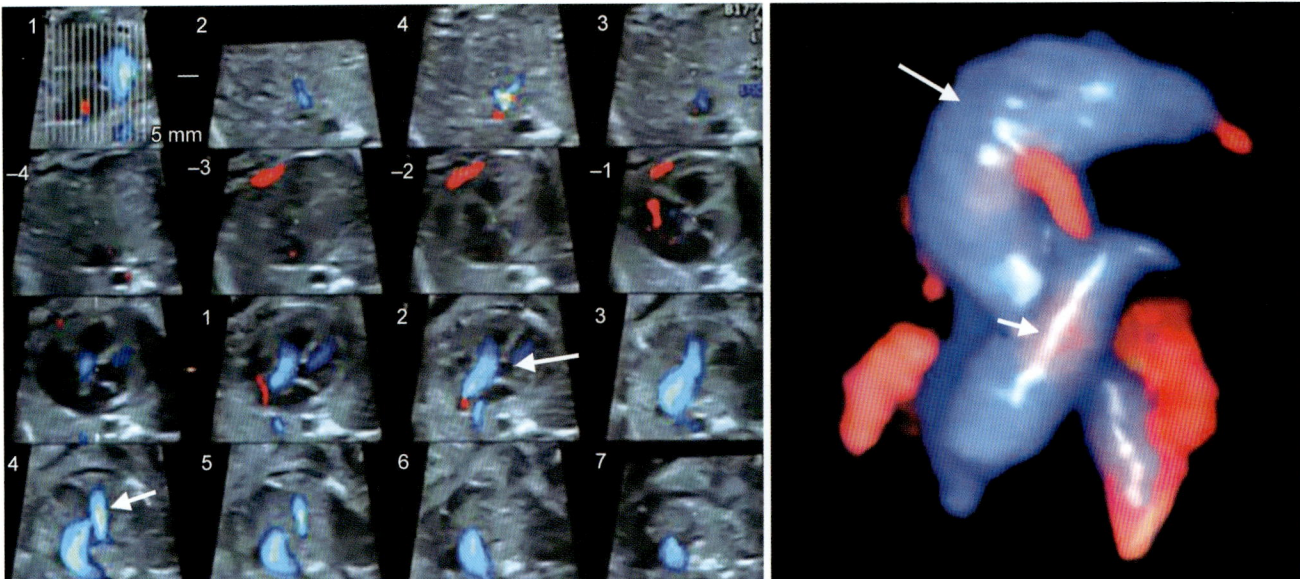

Fig. 25.14: Tetralogy of Fallot shown in TUI (left) and in a rendered image from STIC acquired with high-definition power Doppler (right). TUI image shows the pulmonary stenosis (small arrow) and dilated overriding aorta (long arrow). Rendered image shows the narrow pulmonary artery (small arrow) and dilated aortic arch (long arrow). (STIC: Spatiotemporal image correlation; TUI: Tomographic ultrasound imaging)

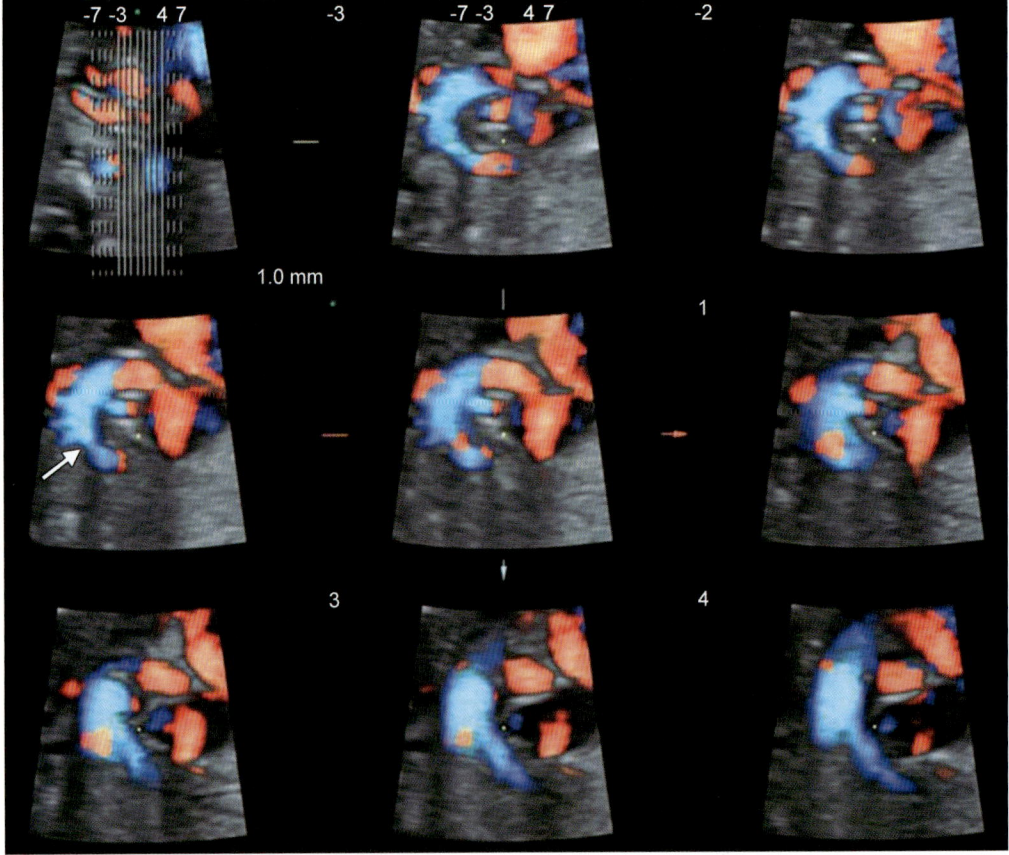

Fig. 25.15: Tomographic ultrasound imaging with color Doppler shows postductal coarctation of the aorta. Arrow indicates the lesion.

gallbladder as white structures, which can aid the operator in navigating within a complex anomaly scan. IM can be joined with STIC and VOCAL to quantify fetal cardiac ventricular volumes or mass and can also be applied to the evaluation of fetal heart function.[28,35,36]

SCREENING EXAMINATION OF THE FETAL HEART WITH THREE- AND FOUR-DIMENSIONAL ULTRASOUND

Guidelines

Guidelines for the performance of fetal heart examination have been published by the International Society of Ultrasound in Obstetrics and Gynecology.[37] These guidelines for fetal cardiac scanning can incorporate 3D/4D applications, and 3D/4D US can enhance fetal cardiac scans, as well as the evaluation of congenital anomalies. Many research teams have applied 3D US and STIC acquisition to fetal echocardiography, and various techniques have been put forward to optimize the use of this modality.

A well-executed STIC acquisition contains all the necessary planes for evaluation of the five classic transverse planes of fetal echocardiography.[21,22] The operator can examine the fetal upper abdomen and stomach, then scroll cephalad to obtain the familiar four-chamber view, the five-chamber view, the bifurcation of the pulmonary arteries, and finally the three-vessel and trachea view. Slight adjustment along the x- or y-axes may be necessary to optimize the images. Performed properly, this methodology will provide the examiner with all the necessary planes to conform to the guidelines, above. However, it must be remembered that STIC acquisition that was degraded by maternal or fetal movements, including fetal breathing movements, will contain artifacts within the scan volume.

Applications

Among the most attractive facets of 3D/4D scanning are the potential for digital archiving and sharing of examination data over a network.[38-43] These capabilities were applied by Vinals et al.[39-41] to increase delivery of prenatal cardiac scanning to poorly served areas. Local practitioners in distant areas acquired and stored 3D volume sets at their centers; they were subsequently sent over an Internet link and analyzed by expert examiners in central locations.[39,40] Rizzo et al. showed that cardiac volumes

acquired by 4D sonography in peripheral centers showed high enough quality to allow satisfactory diagnostic cardiac views.[42] This can have important implications in increasing the penetration of prenatal US services in poorly served or outlying areas of many countries.

Spatiotemporal image correlation also has a role in education and training of examiners.[40,42,44,45] We devised a study to apply STIC specifically to train nonexpert examiners to perform fetal echocardiography.[44] Two sonographers without formal training in fetal echocardiography received theoretical instruction on the five classic planes of fetal echocardiography, as well as STIC technology. They acquired and stored STIC volumes, which were evaluated offline according to a standardized protocol that required the trainee to mark 30 specified structures on the five required axial planes. Volumes were then reviewed by an expert examiner for quality of acquisition and correct identification of specified structures. Trainees succeeded in identifying 97–98% of structures, with a highly significant degree of agreement with the expert's analysis (P <0.001).[44]

DeVore et al. presented the "spin" technique,[25] combining MPR and STIC acquisition to analyze acquired volumes and simplify demonstration of the ventricular outflow tracts. Using this technique, the operator acquires a VOI from a transverse sweep of the fetal mediastinum that includes the sequential planes of fetal echocardiography. In postprocessing the outflow tract view is imaged in the A-plane, and outflow tract and adjacent vessels are then examined by placing the reference point over each vessel and rotating the image along the x- and y-axes until the full length of each vessel is identified.[25]

Abuhamad proposed an automated approach to extract the required planes from an acquired volume, coining the term *automated multiplanar imaging*.[24] Based on the idea that the scanned 3D volume contains all possible planes of the scanned organ, it should be possible to define the geometric planes within that volume that would be required to display each of the diagnostic planes of a given organ, for example the sequential scanning planes of fetal echocardiography. Beginning from the four-chamber view, all the other planes are in constant anatomic relationship to this plane, and a computer-automated program could present those planes once the appropriate volume block is acquired.[24]

Espinoza et al. introduced a novel algorithm combining STIC and TUI[26] to image the diagnostic planes of the fetal heart simultaneously and facilitate visualization of the long-axis view of the aortic arch. Turan et al. proposed a similar approach to employ STIC and TUI to standardize fetal echocardiography; the investigators achieved successful imaging of target views in one panel in 91% of cases.[46]

Yeo and Romero [47] investigated the application of fetal intelligent navigation echocardiography to acquired STIC volumes, to visualize nine diagnostic planes and virtual intelligent sonographer assistance to navigate the anatomy surrounding each plane. The system automatically generates the abdomen/stomach plane, four-chamber, five-chamber (aortic root), LVOT, right ventricular outflow tract (RVOT), and three vessels and trachea views as well as the ductal and aortic arches and the superior vena cava (SVC) and inferior vena cava (IVC) views. Veronese et al.[83] subsequently applied these modalities to STIC volumes of fetuses in the second and third trimesters and found that both modalities, singly or in combination, were effective in identifying the nine diagnostic planes required for fetal echocardiography.[47]

However, in any postprocessing technique, if the original volume was suboptimal, subsequent analysis will be prone to lower image quality and the introduction of artifacts.

Nuchal translucency screening programs will refer approximately 3–5% of patients for fetal echocardiography as high risk,[48,49] increasing demand for fetal cardiac screening programs. The integration of noninvasive prenatal diagnosis to first-trimester screening programs may move targeted anatomy scanning to earlier gestational ages (GAs).[50] STIC acquisition is amenable to younger GAs, as the smaller fetal heart can be scanned in a shorter acquisition time, thus reducing the chance of acquisition degradation from fetal movements. It has been shown to be suitable for use in a screening setting.[51]

Functional Evaluation of the Fetal Heart: Ventricular Volume, Mass, and Functional Measurements

Evaluation of fetal heart functional parameters has long challenged fetal echocardiographers.[52] While duplex and color Doppler flow nomograms have been quantified and are long established in 2D fetal echocardiography, many of the pediatric and adult measures are based on end-systolic and end-diastolic ventricular volumes: SV, ejection fraction (EF), and cardiac output (CO). Without electrical trace or clinically applicable segmentation

methods to determine the ventricular volume, these parameters have eluded practical prenatal quantification. 3DUS opens new avenues for exploration into ventricular volumetry[28,36,53-55] and mass[35,56,57] measurement.

Bhat et al. used nongated static 3D acquisition and STIC to obtain middiastolic scans of fetal hearts, and applied VOCAL analysis to determine cavity volume. The result was multiplied by myocardial density (1.050 g/cm³) to obtain the mass.[56,57] A recent animal study showed the validity of 4DUS-acquired volume analysis to determine ventricular mass in a model of ventricular hypertrophy.[58]

We published[28] a methodology combining STIC acquisition to determine the end-systolic and end-diastolic stages in the cardiac cycle, then IM to isolate the fluid-filled ventricular volume, which was measured using VOCAL analysis **(Fig. 25.16)**. The resulting volumes allowed quantification of SV and EF.[28] It was found that both the IM and VOCAL analysis were highly dependent on operator-determined threshold parameters, which affect the intensity of the signal to be colored and included in the volumetry.

Subsequent studies refined the technique and validated the repeatability and reproducibility of the STIC with VOCAL approach for ventricular volume measurement.[55,59,60] Reference ranges for the ventricular walls

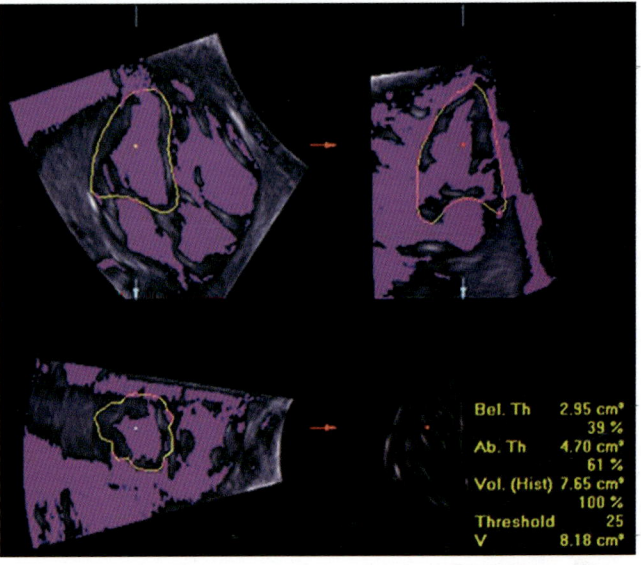

Fig. 25.16: STIC acquisition combined with IM and VOCAL for fetal cardiac ventricle volumetry. The resulting measurements appear in the box, bottom right. (IM: inversion mode; STIC: spatiotemporal image correlation; VOCAL: virtual organ computer-aided analysis)
Source: Reproduced with permission from Yagel et al.[82] © International Society of Ultrasound in Obstetrics and Gynecology. Permission is granted by John Wiley and Sons Ltd on behalf of ISUOG.

and interventricular septum were calculated with this approach,[61,62] which was also shown to be applicable in the cases of congenital heart disease (CHD).[61] 3D/4D US methodologies have also been applied to obtain fetal cardiac functional parameters based on ventricular volumes, including SV, CO, and EF.[18,20,36,54,63-65] The measurements have been validated in mechanical[57,60] and animal models.[20]

Spatiotemporal image correlation combined with IM and VOCAL approach can be extended to mass measurement. We measured fetal ventricular mass[35] based on STIC volumes analyzed with IM and VOCAL. The VOCAL trace included the entire ventricle and walls; IM colors the fluid-filled chamber, which was subtracted from the total volume. The remainder was multiplied by the estimated fetal myocardial density (1.050 g/cm^3). We created scatterplots for fetal right and left ventricular mass in the second half of gestation. Several anomalous cases that were diagnosed during the study period showed deviation from normal values of ventricle mass.[35]

We applied STIC to acquire and analyze fetal tricuspid annular plane systolic excursion (f-TAPSE).[66] f-TAPSE is a modified method to measure the vertical movement of the tricuspid valve annulus. This is traditionally done by M-mode US; it is a recognized measure to assess the fetal right heart. We evaluated the usefulness of STIC M-mode in obtaining it, and compared conventional M-mode and STIC M-mode-based measures of f-TAPSE. First, conventional M-mode was applied to the tricuspid annulus, parallel to the ventricular septum, and the amplitude of the resulting wave was measured. A STIC volume was then acquired and saved; the volume was rotated in postprocessing to show an apical four-chamber view, and f-TAPSE was measured. Scatterplots of f-TAPSE measures obtained with conventional M-mode and with STIC M-mode were created for GA and estimated fetal weight (EFW). f-TAPSE increased linearly with GA and with EFW, and good correlation was found between the two methods (Pearson $R^2 = 0.904$). Inter- and intra-observer variations (ICC) in conventional M-mode and STIC M-mode f-TAPSE measures were 0.94 and 0.97, respectively.[66]

Spatiotemporal image correlation M-mode has also been applied[67] to produce reference ranges of fetal cardiac biometric parameters, including thicknesses of the right and left ventricular walls and intraventricular septum. A subgroup of fetuses with CHD were studied; these cardiac biometric measurements were found to deviate from the reference ranges (>95th centile or <5th centile) in these fetuses.[68]

THREE- AND FOUR-DIMENSIONAL ULTRASOUND IN THE DIAGNOSIS OF CONGENITAL HEART DISEASE

One of the great advantages of a 3D/4D system is its digital archiving capabilities. Examination volumes are stored for later analysis, away from the patient and the time constraints of a busy clinic. In the cases of CHD, other professionals can be invited to view the examination. They can do this anywhere that an Internet link is available.[39] The first examiner can consult with the attending physician, cardiologist, surgical,[69] or other management teams, genetic counselors, and parents. Complex malformations can be elucidated through interdisciplinary discussion and made clear to laymen. In addition, stored data from cases of CHD are invaluable teaching materials for professional education.[44]

Many teams have applied 3D/4D US capabilities to the diagnosis of congenital cardiovascular malformations.

Each of the modalities and applications described above lends itself to different facets of this complex endeavor.

Virtual Planes

As described above, a properly executed STIC acquisition results in a "volume block," which is a reconstructed complete cardiac cycle. This block of spatial and temporal image data contains and makes available many scanning planes that are not readily accessible in 2D US. The term, *virtual planes,* was coined to refer to these rendered scanning planes. The interventricular and interatrial septa planes, and the coronal AV (CAV) plane of the cardiac valves' annuli, have been investigated and applied to the evaluation of CHD.[27] They were shown to have added value in the diagnosis of ventricular septal defect (VSD), restrictive foramen ovale, alignment of the ventricles and great vessels, and evaluation of the AV valves.[67]

Segmental Approach

The segmental approach to CHD has helped to standardize the description of cardiac lesions. In addition, it has contributed to understanding the pathophysiology of the malformed developing fetal heart, and subsequently to our conceptualization and diagnostic imaging. The sequential segmental approach essentially divides the heart into three basic segments: the atria, the ventricles, and the great arteries. These are divided and joined at the level of the AV valves, and at the ventriculoarterial junctions. The segmental approach to diagnosis of CHD is comprehensively and concisely described elsewhere;[70] we follow this sequence in describing the application and added value of 3D/4D in the diagnosis of CHD, through index cases of anomalies diagnosed in our center.

Veins and Atria: Total Anomalous Pulmonary Venous Connection and Interrupted Inferior Vena Cava with Azygos Continuation

Total anomalous pulmonary venous connection (TAPVC) is a many-faceted group of malformations affecting the pulmonary veins.[71] Essentially, in these anomalies the pulmonary veins do not drain into the left atrium, but rather to various other locations: the right atrium, great veins, or abdominal veins. The present case was an intra-diaphragmatic variation with drainage of the pulmonary veins to the portal vein.

Three- and four-dimensional US can have a significant contribution to the understanding of the fetal venous system. **Figure 25.17A** show the use of MPR with the reference point to navigate this complex lesion. Placement of the reference point in the suspected anomalous blood vessel in cross section (A-frame) showed the vessel in longitudinal plane in the B-frame. This confirmed that the finding was not an artifact, but rather the characteristic vertical vein. 3D power flow Doppler displayed the idiosyncratic vascular tree and absence of the pulmonary veins **(Fig. 25.17B)**; rotation of the image in postprocessing allowed overall examination of the lesion in 360°.

Interrupted IVC with azygos continuation is shown in **Figure 25.18**. This cardinal vein anomaly results from primary failure of the right subcardinal vein to connect to the hepatic segment of the IVC.[72] Blood is shunted directly into the right supracardinal vein (which will become the SVC); and blood from the lower body flows through the azygos vein to the SVC. In this instance, B-flow acquisition provided real-time representation of the anomalous course of the IVC and connection to the fetal heart. It showed the azygos vein draining into the SVC, as well as the aorta in one 3D image that would be impossible to obtain with 2D color Doppler scanning. B-flow scanning provided superior imaging of the slower

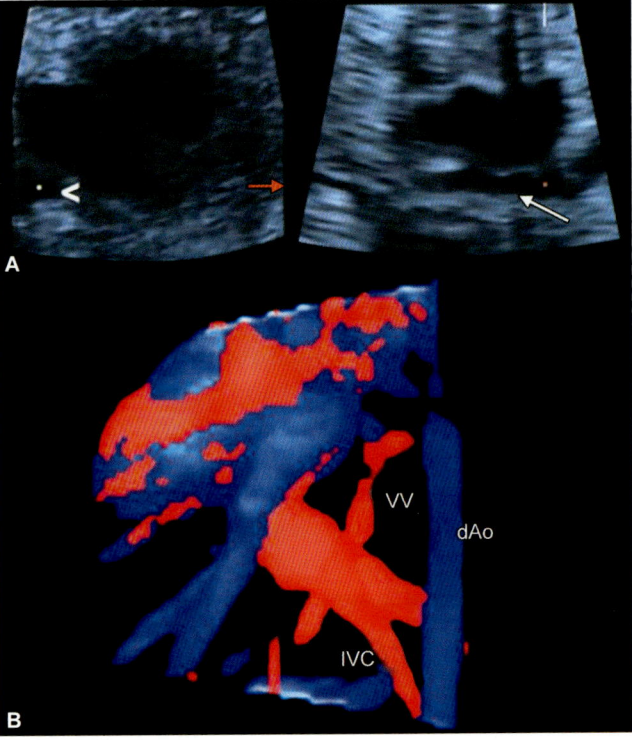

Figs. 25.17A and B: (A) STIC acquisition in a case of TAPVC. The A-plane shown raised suspicion of an anomalous vessel (caret), which is confirmed in the B-plane (arrow); (B) The heart and great vessels of this fetus: STIC acquisition and high-definition power flow Doppler confirmed the characteristic VV. Note also the absence of pulmonary veins (compare Fig. 25.6). (STIC: spatiotemporal image correlation; TAPVC: total anomalous pulmonary venous connection; VV: vertical vein)
Source: Reproduced with permission from Yagel et al.[82] © International Society of Ultrasound in Obstetrics and Gynecology. Permission is granted by John Wiley and Sons Ltd on behalf of ISUOG.

blood flow in the azygos vein than was demonstrated with 3D PD.

Atrioventricular Junction: Atrioventricular Septal Defect and Tricuspid Valve Stenosis

Atrioventricular septal defect (AVSD) is characterized by incomplete atrial and ventricular septation, forming a common AV junction. AVSD has many forms; all involve an abnormality of the AV valves. **Figure 25.19** shows the use of 3D rendering of a STIC volume acquired with color Doppler to demonstrate the anomalous intracardiac flow, resulting from the AVSD.

Another group of AV valve lesions is mitral or tricuspid valve atresia, dysplasia, or stenosis. **Figures 25.20A and B** show the CAV plane in a case of tricuspid stenosis. This

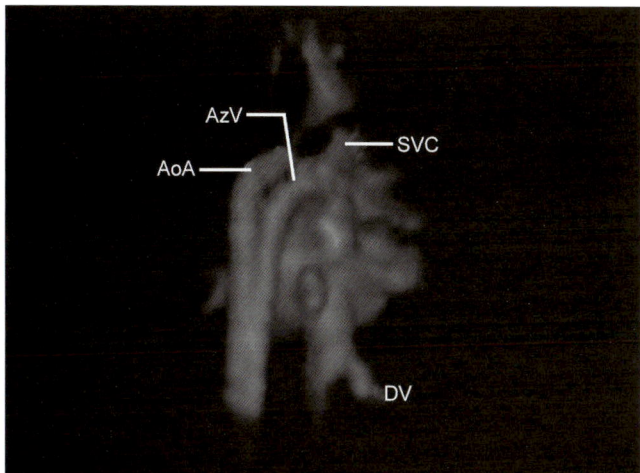

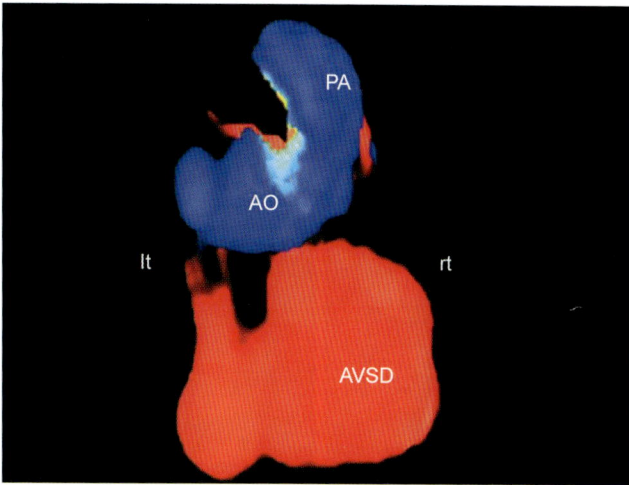

Fig. 25.18: B-flow image of the heart and great vessels in a fetus with interrupted inferior vena cava with azygos continuation. (AoA: ascending aorta; AzV: azygos vein; DV: ductus venosus; SVC: superior vena cava.)
Source: Reproduced with permission from Yagel et al.[82] © International Society of Ultrasound in Obstetrics and Gynecology. Permission is granted by John Wiley and Sons Ltd on behalf of ISUOG.

Fig. 25.19: The coronal atrioventricular plane from STIC acquisition with color Doppler mapping in a case of atrioventricular septal defect. (AO: aorta; AVSD: atrioventricular septal defect; PA: pulmonary artery; STIC: spatiotemporal image correlation)
Source: Reproduced with permission from Yagel et al.[82] © International Society of Ultrasound in Obstetrics and Gynecology. Permission is granted by John Wiley and Sons Ltd on behalf of ISUOG.

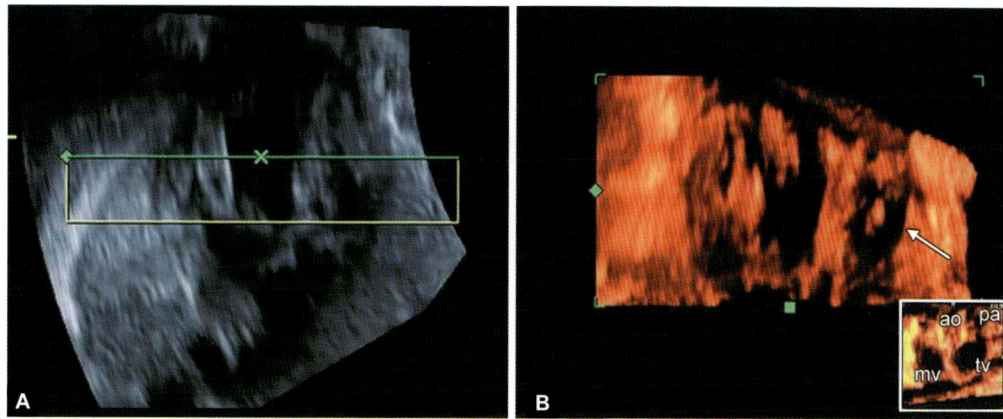

Figs. 25.20A and B: Tricuspid stenosis evaluated with 3D rendering and the CAV plane. The bounding box is placed tightly around the level of the AV valves in the A-frame (A); the D-frame (B) clearly shows the stenotic valve (arrow). Compare normal CAV plane in diastole. (Inset—3D: third-dimensional, ao: aortic valve; CAV: coronal atrioventricular; mv: mitral valve annulus; pa: pulmonary valve; tv: tricuspid valve annulus)
Source: Reproduced with permission from Yagel et al.[82] © International Society of Ultrasound in Obstetrics and Gynecology. Permission is granted by John Wiley and Sons Ltd on behalf of ISUOG.

"virtual plane 2" is obtained from a STIC volume with color Doppler, by placing the bounding box tightly around the level of the AV connection in the four-chamber view, with the superior side active (frame A); the plane is slightly adjusted along the *x*- and *y*-axes; the rendered image (frame D) shows the AV valves with anomalous anatomy (compare normal CAV plane, inset). This virtual plane provides a 3D look at the AV and semilunar valves' annuli,

resembling the surgical plane seen when the heart is opened in surgery.

Ventricles: Ventricular Septal Defects

Ventricular septal defects are perhaps the most common—and most commonly missed—congenital heart defect. Several groups have proposed methods for evaluation of the interventricular septum.[16,27,73,74] By using MPR, with

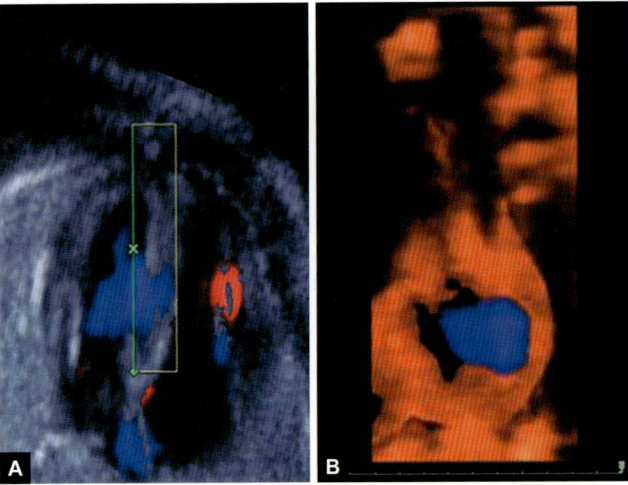

Figs. 25.21A and B: The IVS "virtual plane" with color Doppler in evaluation of VSD. The navigation point is placed on the septum in the A-plane (A); the D-frame (B) shows the rendered IVS with flow across the defect from right to left. (IVC: interventricular septum; IVS: interventricular septa; VSD: ventricular septal defect)
Source: Reproduced with permission from Yagel et al.[82] © International Society of Ultrasound in Obstetrics and Gynecology. Permission is granted by John Wiley and Sons Ltd on behalf of ISUOG.

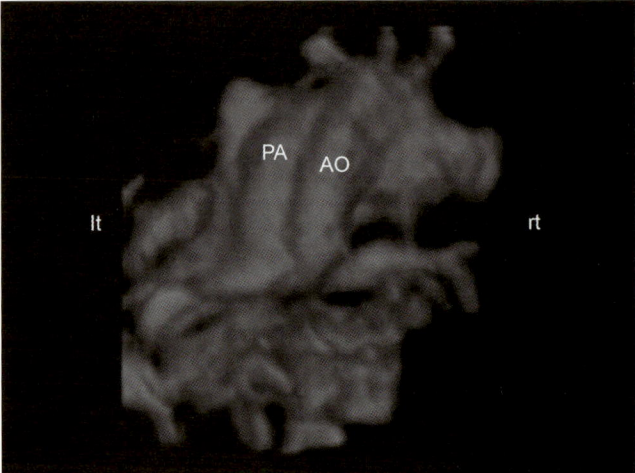

Fig. 25.22: B-flow modality showed the parallel great vessels in a case of transposition. Application of this modality clearly shows the blood flow in the malaligned vessels. (AO: aorta; PA: pulmonary artery.)
Source: Reproduced with permission from Yagel et al.[82] © International Society of Ultrasound in obstetrics and Gynecology. Permission is granted by John Wiley and Sons Ltd on behalf of ISUOG.

the reference point placed on the septum with the four-chamber view in the A-frame, the B-frame will show the septum and defect en face **(Figs. 25.21A and B)**. We recommend, however, the use of the bounding box in 3D rendering from STIC acquisition with color Doppler. The operator places the "active" side of the box to the right or left (i.e. from within the left or right ventricle) and obtains an image (in the D-frame) having more depth, for a more detailed examination of the size and nature (and number) of the VSD(s). The addition of color Doppler demonstrates blood flow across the lesion and shows at what stage in the cardiac cycle and to what degree shunting occurs.

Ventriculoarterial Junctions (Conotruncal Anomalies): Transposition of the Great Arteries, Tetralogy of Fallot

Transposition (or malposition or malalignment) of the great arteries (TGA) is the general name for a complex group of anomalies with widely varying anatomic and clinical presentations. When the sequential segmental approach is applied to systematic diagnosis of CHD,[70] the morphology of each successive anatomic segment is assessed in turn. The morphologic right and left atria and ventricles are established; now the examiner addresses the ventriculoarterial junction and the accordance or discordance of the great arteries and ventricles.

Three-dimensional rendering with color Doppler was applied to the evaluation of suspected malalignment of the great vessels, by examining the CAV ("surgical plane") at the level of the AV and semilunar valves' annuli.

We applied B-flow scanning to the evaluation of TGA and found that it was more effective than 3D PD or IM in visualizing the great vessels' structure and relationships.

Figure 25.22 shows a case of complete dextrotransposition of the great arteries. The B-flow scan clearly showed blood flow into the ventricles and out through the malaligned vessels. This demonstration of the anatomic variant of the anomaly aided our consultations with the parents and their attending physician.

Tetralogy of Fallot is a conotruncal defect characterized by VSD, aortic valve overriding the ventricular septum, narrowing of the RVOT, and right ventricular hypertrophy. **Figure 25.23** shows a case of tetralogy of Fallot imaged in TUI, clearly showing the dilated overriding aorta.

Arterial Trunks: Pulmonary Stenosis and Right Aortic Arch

The use of 3D rendering of a STIC acquisition with or without color Doppler to obtain virtual planes was discussed previously. The CAV plane is an excellent tool for evaluation of the semilunar valves. Once the CAV plane is obtained, the 4D-cinema option is initiated

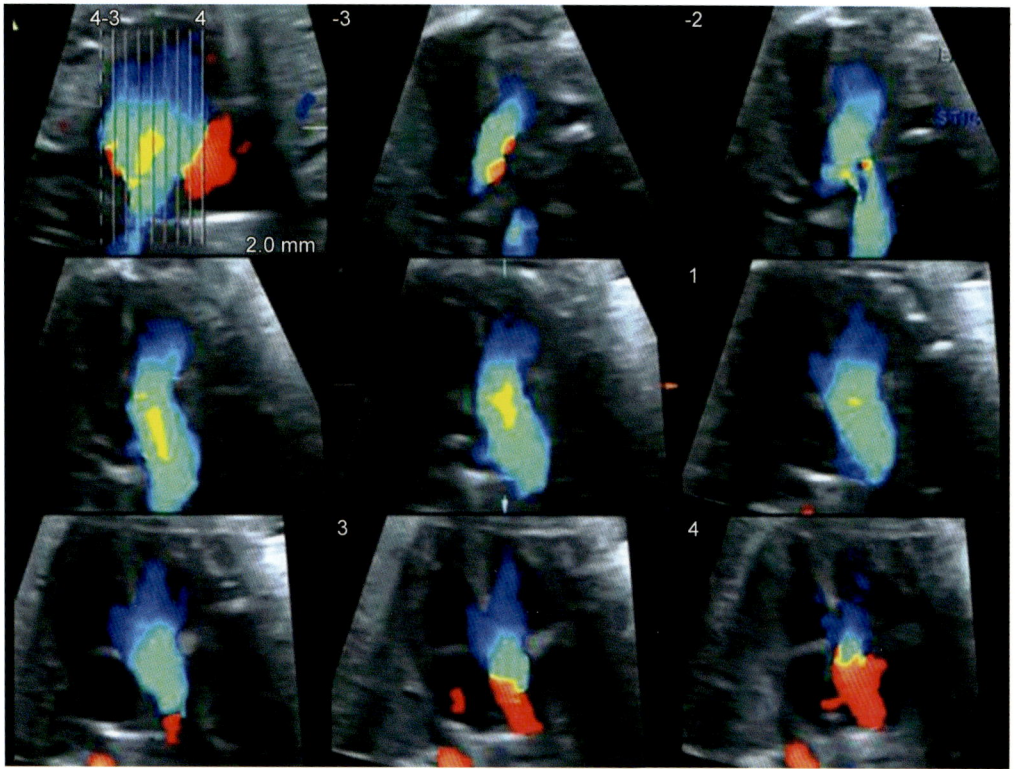

Fig. 25.23: TUI image of the LVOT in a case of tetralogy of Fallot, showing the dilated overriding aorta. (LVOT: left ventricular outflow tract; TUI: tomographic ultrasound imaging)

and blood flow across the valves evaluated through the cardiac cycle. **Figure 25.24** shows a case of critical pulmonary stenosis with retrograde flow in the main pulmonary artery. **Figure 25.25** shows another case of severe pulmonary stenosis with poststenotic dilatation of the pulmonary artery rendered with TUI.

Right aortic arch defect results from persistence of the right dorsal aorta and involution of the distal part of the left dorsal aorta. There are two main types, with or without a retroesophageal component.[72] **Figure 25.26** shows a case of right aortic arch diagnosed with B-flow; this modality showed the characteristic course of the aortic arch to the right of the trachea.

Functional Evaluation

Ventricular Volumes

Messing et al.[28] published a novel methodology combining STIC acquisition with postprocessing application of IM and VOCAL to quantify end-systolic and end-diastolic ventricular volumes. Nomograms were created from right

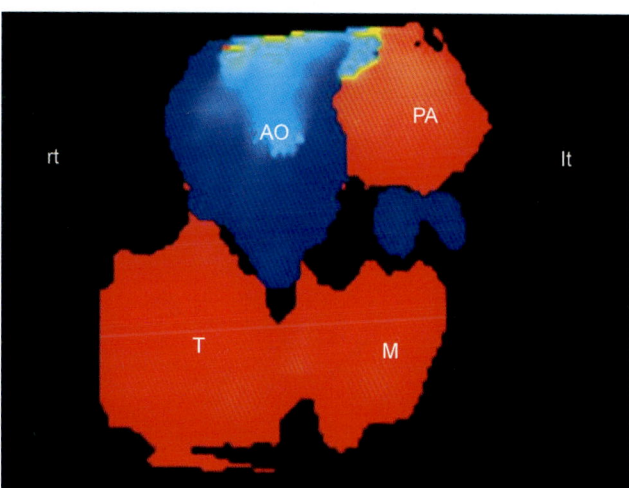

Fig. 25.24: The CAV plane from STIC acquisition with color Doppler mapping in a case of transposition of the great arteries and pulmonary stenosis with retrograde flow in the main pulmonary artery. (AO: aorta; CAV: coronal atrioventricular; M: mitral annulus; PA: pulmonary artery; STIC: spatiotemporal image correlation; T: tricuspid annulus)
Source: Reproduced with permission from Yagel et al.[82] © International Society of Ultrasound in Obstetrics and Gynecology. Permission is granted by John Wiley and Sons Ltd on behalf of ISUOG.

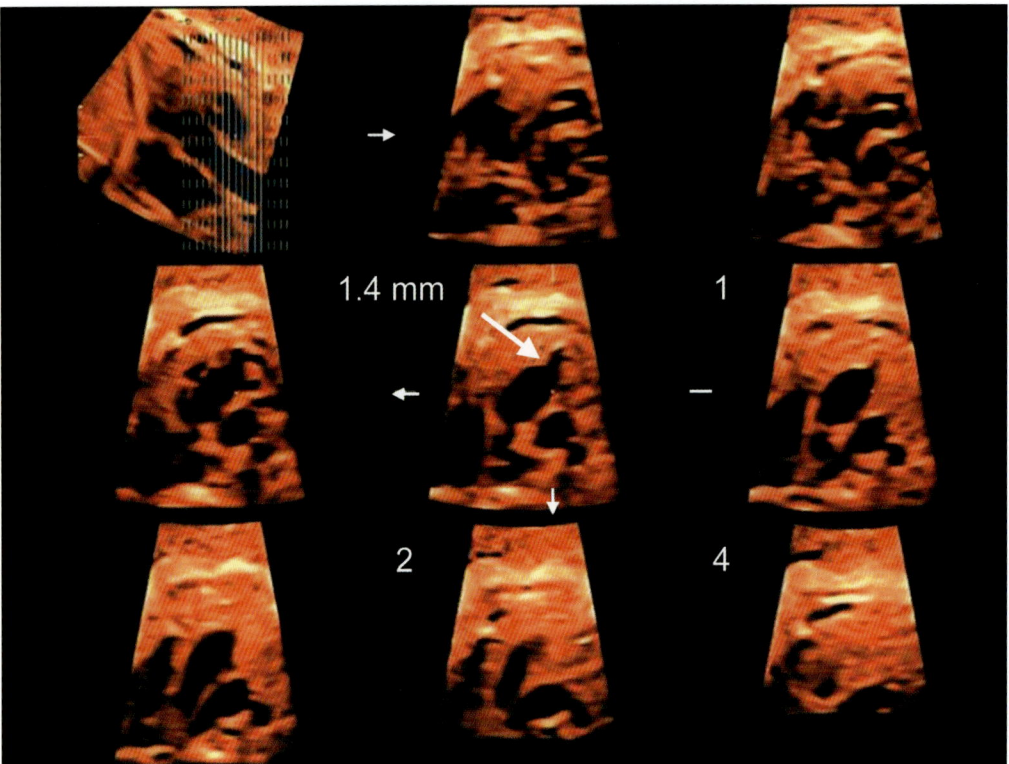

Fig. 25.25: Severe pulmonary stenosis rendered with TUI. Arrow indicates the marked narrowing at the valve and poststenotic dilatation of the pulmonary artery. (TUI: tomographic ultrasound imaging)

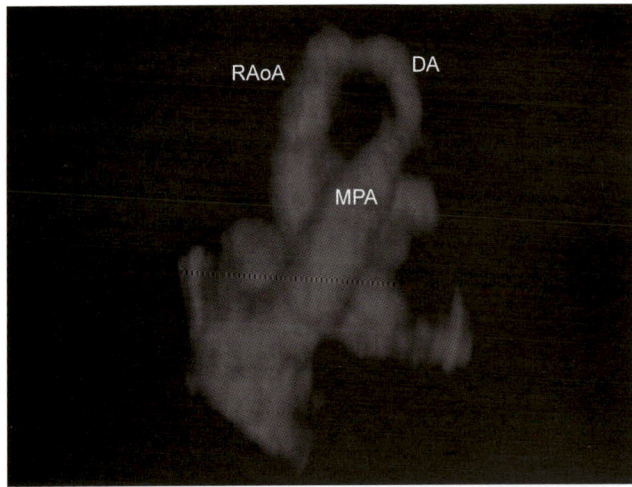

Fig. 25.26: B-flow modality in a case of RAoA. (DA: ductus arteriosus; MPA: main pulmonary artery; RAoA: right aortic arch)
Source: Reproduced with permission from Yagel et al.[82] © International Society of Ultrasound in Obstetrics and Gynecology. Permission is granted by John Wiley and Sons Ltd on behalf of ISUOG.

and left ventricle end-systolic and end-diastolic volumes from 100 fetuses examined between 20 gestational weeks and 40 gestational weeks. The resulting measurements correlated strongly with GA and EFW. The measured volumes were used to create nomograms for fetal SV and cardiac EF.

The methodology was applied to save STIC volumes of cases with cardiac anomaly or dysfunction that involved changes in ventricular volume, SV, or EF. These included critical pulmonary stenosis, twin-to-twin transfusion syndrome with secondary pulmonary stenosis, aortic valve stenosis with hypoplastic aortic arch, Ebstein anomaly, supraventricular tachycardia (SVT), and vein of Galen aneurysm.[28]

Our normal cases showed the effectiveness of fetal heart ventricle volumetry in cardiac evaluation and quantification; such volumetry is not readily available in 2D echocardiography. The pathological cases showed the potential added value of this methodology. In the case of critical pulmonary stenosis, for example, the diagnosis was more serious than suspected by 2D echocardiography. Ventricle volumetry also provided insight into the pathophysiology of lesions, such as SVT and vein of Galen aneurysm, among others.[28]

Subsequently, other teams[36,55] paired STIC with VOCAL to investigate fetal ventricular volume. Hamill et al. found that STIC and VOCAL allowed repeatable and reproducible calculation of ventricular volumes[55] and can be used to quantify normal fetal right and left SV, CO, adjusted CO, and right and left EF. They found that the larger right volume and greater left EF resulted in similar right and left SV and CO.[36] Hamill et al.[65] applied STIC combined with VOCAL in a cross-sectional study of 34 fetuses with umbilical artery pulsatility index (PI) >95th percentile. Ventricular volume at end-systole and end-diastole, SV, CO, adjusted CO, and EF were compared to those of 184 normal fetuses. The investigators found that mean ventricular volumes were lower in fetuses with PI >95th centile, as were mean left and right SV, CO, and adjusted CO. Right ventricular volume, SV, CO, and adjusted CO exceeded the left in these fetuses, while mean EF was greater than that observed in controls. The authors concluded that increased placental vascular impedance to flow is associated with changes in fetal cardiac function.[65]

POTENTIAL PITFALLS OF THREE- AND FOUR-DIMENSIONAL ECHOCARDIOGRAPHY

Three- and four-dimensional fetal echocardiography scanning is prone to artifacts similar to those encountered in 2D US, and some that are specific to 3D/4D acquisition and postprocessing.

Spatiotemporal Image Correlation Acquisition Quality

The quality of a STIC acquisition may be adversely affected by fetal body or "breathing" movements. To improve scan quality the fetus should be in a quiet state and the shortest scan time possible employed. When reviewing a STIC acquisition, the B-frame reveals artifacts introduced by fetal breathing movements **(Fig. 25.27)**. If the B-frame appears sound, the volume is usually acceptable and can be used for further investigation. The quality of the original acquisition impacts on all further stages of postprocessing and evaluation.

Original Angle of Insonation

The original angle at which a scan was performed will impact on the quality of all the planes acquired. It is important to achieve an optimal beginning 2D plane, before starting 3D or 4D acquisition.

Acoustic Shadows

Shadowing artifacts pose a particular problem to 3D/4DUS. When commencing scanning from the 2D plane, acoustic shadows may not be apparent. However, they may be present within the acquired volume block. It is imperative to review suspected defects with repeated 2D and 3D scanning to confirm their presence in additional scanning planes.

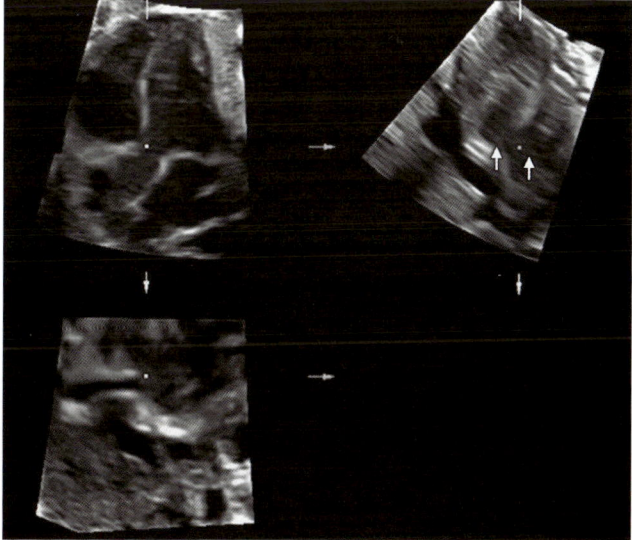

Fig. 25.27: Artifacts and pitfalls. STIC acquisition in a 26-week fetus: the A-frame shows left ventricular outflow tract plane. Note that the B-frame, however, is degraded by fetal breathing artifacts (arrows). (STIC: spatiotemporal image correlation)
Source: Reproduced with permission from Yagel et al.[82] © International Society of Ultrasound in Obstetrics and Gynecology. Permission is granted by John Wiley and Sons Ltd on behalf of ISUOG.

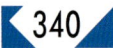

Three-dimensional Rendering

Three-dimensional rendering creates virtual images. Application of some algorithms designed to smooth the image can lead to loss of data from the original scan. 3D rendering should always be used in conjunction with the A-frame 2D image for comparison.

Flow Direction

An acquired volume containing Doppler flow information is available for manipulation and may be sliced and rotated around the x-, y-, and z-axes for analysis. However, rotation of the volume with Doppler directional flow information can mislead the operator: if the directions are reversed, flow data can be misinterpreted. The operator must confirm any suspected pathological flow patterns by confirming the original direction of scanning, whether flow was toward or away from the transducer during the acquisition scan.

ACCURACY

Multiple studies have compared imaging yield between 2D and 3D/4D fetal echocardiography, and others have examined the feasibility of 3D/4D and STIC in screening programs, and still others have described the application of various 3D/4D modalities to diagnosis or evaluation of fetal cardiovascular anomalies. We investigated[23] the contribution of 3D/4D to diagnostic accuracy and precision in our fetal echocardiography screening program. Patients (N = 13,101) underwent complete fetal echocardiography according to our five-planes protocol, as well as examination of the ductus venosus and longitudinal aortic arch planes, performed with 2D US combined with 2D color Doppler, STIC, STIC with color Doppler, and STIC with B-flow. Stored 2D US cinema-loops and 4D US volumes were reviewed separately according to a standardized table of 23 specified structures on five required planes of visualization. During the study, there were 181 diagnosed cases of CHD, and 12 false-negative and 0 false-positive results. In 12 cases, 3D/4D US added to the accuracy of our diagnosis: one right aortic arch with anomalous branching; one transposition of the great arteries with pulmonary atresia diagnosed with TUI; one segmental interrupted aortic arch diagnosed with TUI; one right ventricle aneurysm diagnosed with B-flow; two agenesis of ductus venosus to the coronary sinus diagnosed by MPR and B-flow; two TAPVC diagnosed with MPR; and four VSDs diagnosed with the aid of virtual planes. We found that overall 3D/4D US modalities had impact on diagnostic precision and accuracy in about 6% of cases of fetal anatomical cardiovascular anomalies.[23]

In order to test the reliability and interobserver agreement of 3D/4D US, Espinoza et al.[75] designed a study including seven centers with expertise in 4D fetal echocardiography; each center submitted volume datasets of normal and anomalous cases, which were uploaded onto a centralized server, and blinded analysis by all centers was performed. Intercenter agreement was determined. Ninety volume datasets were randomly selected for analysis. Overall, the median (range) sensitivity, specificity, positive and negative predictive values, and false-positive and false-negative rates for the identification of fetuses with CHDs were 93% (77–100%), 96% (84–100%), 96% (83–100%), 93% (79–100%), 4.8% (2.7–25%), and 6.8% (5–22%), respectively. The most frequent CHDs were conotruncal anomalies (36%). There was excellent intercenter agreement (κ = 0.97). The authors concluded that 4D US volume datasets can be remotely acquired and accurately interpreted by different centers, and that in experienced hands, 4D US is an accurate and reliable method for fetal echocardiography.[75]

Bennasar et al.[76] investigated the accuracy of STIC in the diagnosis of CHD in a referral population. STIC volumes were obtained during the (2D US) referral examinations and stored. The volumes were analyzed at least 1 year later by an examiner blinded to the original results and fetal outcomes. The new diagnoses were compared to 2D US and postnatal or postmortem examinations of the fetuses. The accuracy, sensitivity, specificity, and positive and negative predictive values of STIC to diagnose the presence or absence of CHD were 91.6, 94.9, 88.1, 89.7, and 94.0, respectively. STIC-based diagnoses concurred with the specific postnatal diagnosis of CHD in 74.3% of cases, as compared with 81.7% for 2D US.[76]

Levental et al. compared 2D and nongated 3D US to obtain standard cardiac views.[77] Meyer-Wittkopf et al.[78] evaluated 2D and Doppler-gated 3D in obtaining standard echocardiography scanning planes in normal hearts. They found that 3D provided additional structural depth and allowed a dynamic 3D perspective of valvar morphology and ventricular wall motion.[78]

In evaluating CHD, Meyer–Wittkopf et al.[79] evaluated gated 3D volume sets of 2D-diagnosed cardiac lesions and compared key views of the heart in both modalities. They determined that 3D had added value in a small proportion of lesions.[79] Wang et al.[80] compared 3D and

2D scanning of fetuses in the spine-anterior position. This group found that only in the pulmonary outflow tract was 3D US superior to 2D.

Espinoza et al.[31] examined the added value of IM in the evaluation of anomalous venous connections. The investigators found that IM improved visualization of cases of dilated azygos or hemiazygos veins and their spatial relationships with the surrounding vascular structures.

Benacerraf et al.[81] compared acquisition and analysis times for 2D and 3D fetal anatomy scanning at 17–21 gestational weeks. 3D US compared favorably with 2D in mean scanning time and accuracy of fetal biometry.

The data archiving and networking capabilities of 3D/4D fetal echocardiography with STIC acquisition open new avenues for disseminating fetal echocardiography programs to outlying or poorly served areas. This can have important public health implications in these populations. Michailidis et al.[43] and Vinals et al.[39,40] have shown the feasibility and success of programs based on 3D/4D examination volumes acquired in one center and reviewed by experts in a center connected by telemedicine Internet link.[38]

ACKNOWLEDGMENT

An earlier version of this chapter originally appeared as Yagel S, Cohen SM, Shapiro I, Valsky DV. 3D and 4D ultrasound in fetal cardiac scanning: A new look at the fetal heart. *Ultrasound Obstet Gynecol.* 2007;29:81-95. It is reproduced with permission.[82]

REFERENCES

1. Deng J. Terminology of three-dimensional and four-dimensional ultrasound imaging of the fetal heart and other moving body parts. Ultrasound Obstet Gynecol. 2003;22:336-44.
2. DeVore GR, Falkensammer P, Sklansky MS, et al. Spatio-temporal image correlation (STIC): new technology for evaluation of the fetal heart. Ultrasound Obstet Gynecol. 2003;22:380-7.
3. Falkensammer P. Spatio-temporal image correlation for volume ultrasound. Studies of the fetal heart. Zipf, Austria: GE Healthcare; 2005.
4. Goncalves LFF, Lee W, Chaiworapongsa T, et al. Four-dimensional ultrasonography of the fetal heart with spatiotemporal image correlation. Am J Obstet Gynecol. 2003;189:1792-802.
5. Goncalves LF, Lee W, Espinoza J, et al. Examination of the fetal heart by four-dimensional (4D) ultrasound with spatio-temporal image correlation (STIC). Ultrasound Obstet Gynecol. 2006;27(3):336-48.
6. Volpe P, Campobasso G, Stanziano A, et al. Novel application of 4D sonography with B-flow imaging and spatio-temporal image correlation (STIC) in the assessment of the anatomy of pulmonary arteries in fetuses with pulmonary atresia and ventricular septal defect. Ultrasound Obstet Gynecol. 2006;28:40-6.
7. Hongmei W, Ying Z, Ailu C, et al. Novel application of four-dimensional sonography with B-flow imaging and spatiotemporal image correlation in the assessment of fetal congenital heart defects. Echocardiography. 2012;29:614-9.
8. Goncalves LF, Romero R, Espinoza J, et al. Four-dimensional ultrasonography of the fetal heart using color Doppler spatiotemporal image correlation. J Ultrasound Med. 2004;23:473-81.
9. Messing B, Porat S, Imbar T, et al. Mild tricuspid regurgitation: a benign fetal finding at various stages of pregnancy. Ultrasound Obstet Gynecol. 2005;26:606-9. Discussion 610.
10. Chaoui R, Hoffmann J, Heling KS. Three-dimensional (3D) and 4D color Doppler fetal echocardiography using spatio-temporal image correlation (STIC). Ultrasound Obstet Gynecol. 2004;23:535-45.
11. Chaoui R, Kalache KD, Hartung J, et al. Application of three-dimensional power Doppler ultrasound in prenatal diagnosis. Ultrasound Obstet Gynecol. 2001;17:22-9.
12. Sciaky-Tamir Y, Cohen SM, Hochner-Celnikier D, et al. Three-dimensional power Doppler (3DPD) ultrasound in the diagnosis and follow-up of fetal vascular anomalies. Am J Obstet Gynecol. 2006;194:274-81.
13. Yagel S, Cohen SM, Lipschuetz M, Valsky DV, Messing B. Ep05.08: The Added Value of 3D/4DUS High Definition Power Doppler, Tui and B-Flow to the Evaluation of the Fetal Precordial Venous System. Ultrasound in Obstetrics & Gynecology. 2017;50:283-3.
14. Xiong Y, Chen M, Chan LW, et al. A novel way of visualizing the ductal and aortic arches by real-time three-dimensional ultrasound with live xPlane imaging. Ultrasound Obstet Gynecol. 2012;39:316-21.
15. Xiong Y, Liu T, Gan HJ, et al. Detection of the fetal conotruncal anomalies using real-time three-dimensional echocardiography with live xPlane imaging of the fetal ductal arch view. Prenat Diagn. 2013;33:462 6.
16. Xiong Y, Wah YM, Chen M, et al. Assessment of the fetal interventricular septum using real-time three-dimensional echocardiography with Live 3D imaging. Ultrasound Obstet Gynecol. 2010;35:754-5.
17. Yuan Y, Leung KY, Ouyang YS, et al. Simultaneous real-time imaging of four-chamber and left ventricular outflow tract views using xPlane imaging capability of a matrix array probe. Ultrasound Obstet Gynecol. 2011;37:302-9.
18. Herberg U, Lück S, Steinweg B, et al. Volumetry of fetal hearts using 3D real-time matrix echocardiography—in vitro validation experiments and 3D echocardiographic studies in fetuses. Ultraschall Med. 2011;32:46-53.
19. Herberg U, Steinweg B, Berg C, et al. Echocardiography in the fetus—a systematic comparative analysis of standard

cardiac views with 2D, 3D reconstructive and 3D real-time echocardiography. Ultraschall Med. 2011;32:293-301.

20. Zhu M, Ashraf M, Zhang Z, et al. Real time three-dimensional echocardiographic evaluations of fetal left ventricular stroke volume, mass, and myocardial strain: In vitro and in vivo experimental study. Echocardiography. 2015;32:1697-706.

21. Yagel S, Cohen SM, Achiron R. Examination of the fetal heart by five short-axis views: a proposed screening method for comprehensive cardiac evaluation. Ultrasound Obstet Gynecol. 2001;17:367-9.

22. Yagel S, Arbel R, Anteby EY, et al. The three vessels and trachea view (3VT) in fetal cardiac scanning. Ultrasound Obstet Gynecol. 2002;20:340-5.

23. Yagel S, Cohen SM, Rosenak D, et al. Added value of three-/four-dimensional ultrasound in offline analysis and diagnosis of congenital heart disease. Ultrasound Obstet Gynecol. 2011;37:432-7.

24. Abuhamad A. Automated multiplanar imaging: a novel approach to ultrasonography. J Ultrasound Med. 2004;23:573-6.

25. DeVore GR, Polanco B, Sklansky MS, et al. The 'spin' technique: a new method for examination of the fetal outflow tracts using three-dimensional ultrasound. Ultrasound Obstet Gynecol. 2004;24:72-82.

26. Espinoza J, Kusanovic JP, Gonçalves LF, et al. A novel algorithm for comprehensive fetal echocardiography using 4-dimensional ultrasonography and tomographic imaging. J Ultrasound Med. 2006;25:947-56.

27. Yagel S, Benachi A, Bonnet D, et al. Rendering in fetal cardiac scanning: the intracardiac septa and the coronal atrioventricular valve planes. Ultrasound Obstet Gynecol. 2006;28:266-74.

28. Messing B, Cohen SM, Valsky DV, et al. Fetal cardiac ventricle volumetry in the second half of gestation assessed by 4D ultrasound using STIC combined with inversion mode. Ultrasound Obstet Gynecol. 2007;30:142-51.

29. Peralta CF, Cavoretto P, Csapo B, et al. Lung and heart volumes by three-dimensional ultrasound in normal fetuses at 12-32 weeks' gestation. Ultrasound Obstet Gynecol. 2006;27:128-33.

30. Ruano R, Joubin L, Aubry MC, et al. A nomogram of fetal lung volumes estimated by 3-dimensional ultra-sonography using the rotational technique (virtual organ computer-aided analysis). J Ultrasound Med. 2006;25:701-9.

31. Espinoza J, Gonçalves LF, Lee W, et al. A novel method to improve prenatal diagnosis of abnormal systemic venous connections using three- and four-dimensional ultrasonography and 'inversion mode'. Ultrasound Obstet Gynecol. 2005;25:428-34.

32. Goncalves LF, Espinoza J, Lee W, et al. Three- and four-dimensional reconstruction of the aortic and ductal arches using inversion mode: a new rendering algorithm for visualization of fluid-filled anatomical structures. Ultrasound Obstet Gynecol. 2004;24:696-8.

33. Goncalves LF, Espinoza J, Lee W, et al. A new approach to fetal echocardiography: digital casts of the fetal cardiac chambers and great vessels for detection of congenital heart disease. J Ultrasound Med. 2005;24:415-24.

34. Hata T, Tanaka H, Noguchi J, et al. Four-dimensional volume-rendered imaging of the fetal ventricular outflow tracts and great arteries using inversion mode for detection of congenital heart disease. J Obstet Gynaecol Res. 2010;36:513-8.

35. Messing B, Cohen SM, Valsky DV, et al. Fetal heart ventricular mass obtained by STIC acquisition combined with inversion mode and VOCAL. Ultrasound Obstet Gynecol. 2011;38:191-7.

36. Hamill N, Yeo L, Romero R, et al. Fetal cardiac ventricular volume, cardiac output, and ejection fraction determined with 4-dimensional ultrasound using spatiotemporal image correlation and virtual organ computer-aided analysis. Am J Obstet Gynecol. 2011;205:76.e1-10.

37. Carvalho JS, Allan LD, Chaoui R, et al. ISUOG Practice Guidelines (updated): sonographic screening examination of the fetal heart. Ultrasound Obstet Gynecol. 2013;41:348-59.

38. Adriaanse BM, Tromp CH, Simpson JM, et al. Interobserver agreement in detailed prenatal diagnosis of congenital heart disease by telemedicine using four-dimensional ultrasound with spatiotemporal image correlation. Ultrasound Obstet Gynecol. 2012;39:203-9.

39. Vinals F, Ascenzo R, Naveas R, et al. Fetal echocardiography at 11 + 0 to 13 + 6 weeks using four-dimensional spatio-temporal image correlation telemedicine via an Internet link: a pilot study. Ultrasound Obstet Gynecol. 2008;31:633-8.

40. Vinals F, Mandujano L, Vargas G, et al. Prenatal diagnosis of congenital heart disease using four-dimensional spatio-temporal image correlation (STIC) telemedicine via an Internet link: a pilot study. Ultrasound Obstet Gynecol. 2005;25:25-31.

41. Vinals F, Poblete P, Giuliano A. Spatio-temporal image correlation (STIC): a new tool for the prenatal screening of congenital heart defects. Ultrasound Obstet Gynecol. 2003;22:388-94.

42. Rizzo G, Capponi A, Pietrolucci ME, et al. Satisfactory rate of postprocessing visualization of standard fetal cardiac views from 4-dimensional cardiac volumes acquired during routine ultrasound practice by experienced sonographers in peripheral centers. J Ultrasound Med. 2011;30:93-9.

43. Michailidis GD, Simpson JM, Karidas C, et al. Detailed three-dimensional fetal echocardiography facilitated by an Internet link. Ultrasound Obstet Gynecol. 2001;18:325-8.

44. Avnet H, Mazaaki E, Shen O, et al. Evaluating spatiotemporal image correlation technology as a tool for training non-expert sonographers to perform examinations of the fetal heart. J Ultrasound Med. 2016;35:111-9.

45. Tutschek B, Sahn DJ. Semi-automatic segmentation of fetal cardiac cavities: progress towards an automated fetal

echocardiogram. Ultrasound Obstet Gynecol. 2008;32: 176-80.

46. Turan S, Turan OM, Ty-Torredes K, et al. Standardization of the first-trimester fetal cardiac examination using spatiotemporal image correlation with tomographic ultrasound and color Doppler imaging. Ultrasound Obstet Gynecol. 2009;33:652-6.

47. Yeo L, Romero R. Fetal intelligent navigation echo-cardiography (FINE): a novel method for rapid, simple, and automatic examination of the fetal heart. Ultrasound Obstet Gynecol. 2013;42:268-84.

48. Hyett J, Perdu M, Sharland G, et al. Using fetal nuchal translucency to screen for major congenital cardiac defects at 10-14 weeks of gestation: population based cohort study. BMJ. 1999;318:81-5.

49. Hyett JA, Perdu M, Sharland GK, et al. Increased nuchal translucency at 10-14 weeks of gestation as a marker for major cardiac defects. Ultrasound Obstet Gynecol. 1997;10:242-6.

50. Yagel S, Cohen SM, Benacerraf BR, et al. Noninvasive prenatal testing and fetal sonographic screening: roundtable discussion. J Ultrasound Med. 2015;34:363-9.

51. Uittenbogaard LB, Haak MC, Spreeuwenberg MD, et al. A systematic analysis of the feasibility of four-dimensional ultrasound imaging using spatiotemporal image correla-tion in routine fetal echocardiography. Ultrasound Obstet Gynecol. 2008;31:625-32.

52. Godfrey ME, Messing B, Cohen SM, et al. Functional assessment of the fetal heart: a review. Ultrasound Obstet Gynecol. 2012;39:131-44.

53. Meyer-Wittkopf M, Cole A, Cooper SG, et al. Three-dimensional quantitative echocardiographic assessment of ventricular volume in healthy human fetuses and in fetuses with congenital heart disease. J Ultrasound Med. 2001;20:317-27.

54. Esh-Broder E, Ushakov FB, Imbar T, et al. Application of free-hand three-dimensional echocardiography in the evaluation of fetal cardiac ejection fraction: a preliminary study. Ultrasound Obstet Gynecol. 2004;23:546-51.

55. Hamill N, Romero R, Hassan SS, et al. Repeatability and reproducibility of fetal cardiac ventricular volume calculations using spatiotemporal image correlation and virtual organ computer-aided analysis. J Ultrasound Med. 2009;28:1301-11.

56. Bhat AH, Corbett V, Carpenter N, et al. Fetal ventricular mass determination on three-dimensional echocardio-graphy: studies in normal fetuses and validation experiments. Circulation. 2004;110:1054-60.

57. Bhat AH, Corbett VN, Liu R, et al. Validation of volume and mass assessments for human fetal heart imaging by 4-dimensional spatiotemporal image correlation echocardiography: in vitro balloon model experiments. J Ultrasound Med. 2004;23:1151-9.

58. Liu X, Zhu M, Streiff C, et al. Image-derived assessment of left ventricular mass in fetal myocardial hypertrophy by 4-dimensional echocardiography: an in vitro study. J Ultrasound Med. 2016;35:943-9.

59. Rizzo G, Capponi A, Pietrolucci ME, et al. Role of sonographic automatic volume calculation in measuring fetal cardiac ventricular volumes using 4-dimensional sonography: comparison with virtual organ computer-aided analysis. J Ultrasound Med. 2010;29:261-70.

60. Uittenbogaard LB, Haak MC, Peters RJ, et al. Validation of volume measurements for fetal echocardiography using four-dimensional ultrasound imaging and spatiotemporal image correlation. Ultrasound Obstet Gynecol. 2010;35: 324-31.

61. Barros FS, Rolo LC, Rocha LA, et al. Reference ranges for the volumes of fetal cardiac ventricular walls by three-dimensional ultrasound using spatiotemporal image correlation and virtual organ computer-aided analysis and its validation in fetuses with congenital heart diseases. Prenat Diagn. 2015;35:65-73.

62. Rolo LC, Santana EF, da Silva PH, et al. Fetal cardiac interventricular septum: volume assessment by 3D/4D ultrasound using spatio-temporal image correlation (STIC) and virtual organ computer-aided analysis (VOCAL). J Matern Fetal Neonatal Med. 2015;28:1388-93.

63. DeKoninck P, Steenhaut P, Van Mieghem T, et al. Comparison of Doppler-based and three-dimensional methods for fetal cardiac output measurement. Fetal Diagn Ther. 2012;32:72-8.

64. Uittenbogaard LB, Haak MC, Tromp CH, et al. Reliability of fetal cardiac volumetry using spatiotemporal image correlation: assessment of in-vivo and in-vitro measure-ments. Ultrasound Obstet Gynecol. 2010;36:308-14.

65. Hamill N, Romero R, Hassan S, et al. The fetal cardiovascular response to increased placental vascular impedance to flow determined with 4-dimensional ultrasound using spatio-temporal image correlation and virtual organ computer-aided analysis. Am J Obstet Gynecol. 2013;208:153.e1-13.

66. Messing B, Gilboa Y, Lipschuetz M, et al. Fetal tricuspid annular plane systolic excursion (f-TAPSE): evaluation of fetal right heart systolic function with conventional M-mode ultrasound and spatiotemporal image correlation (STIC) M-mode. Ultrasound Obstet Gynecol. 2013;42: 182-8.

67. Rolo LC, Nardozza LM, Araujo Júnior E, et al. Reference ranges of atrioventricular valve areas by means of four-dimensional ultrasonography using spatiotemporal image correlation in the rendering mode. Prenat Diagn. 2013;33:50-5.

68. Tedesco GD, de Souza Bezerra M, Barros FS, et al. Reference Ranges of Fetal Cardiac Biometric Parameters Using Three-Dimensional Ultrasound with Spatiotemporal Image Correlation M Mode and Their Applicability in Congenital Heart Diseases. Pediatric Cardiology. 2017;38: 271-9.

69. Zidere V, Pushparajah K, Allan LD, et al. Three-dimensional fetal echocardiography for prediction of postnatal surgical approach in double outlet right ventricle: a pilot study. Ultrasound Obstet Gynecol. 2013;42:421-5.

70. Carvalho JS, Ho SY, Shinebourne EA. Sequential segmental analysis in complex fetal cardiac abnormalities: a logical

approach to diagnosis. Ultrasound Obstet Gynecol. 2005;26:105-11.

71. Yagel S, Kivilevitch Z, Cohen SM, et al. The fetal venous system, Part II: Ultrasound evaluation of the fetus with congenital venous system malformation or developing circulatory compromise. Ultrasound Obstet Gynecol. 2010;36:93-111.

72. Moore KL, Persaud TVN. The cardiovascular system. The Developing Human: Clinically Oriented Embryology. Philadelphia, PA: WB Saunders. pp. 349-404.

73. Paladini D, Russo MG, Vassallo M, et al. The 'in-plane' view of the inter-ventricular septum. A new approach to the characterization of ventricular septal defects in the fetus. Prenat Diagn. 2003;23:1052-55.

74. Yagel S, Valsky DV, Messing B. Detailed assessment of fetal ventricular septal defect with 4D color Doppler ultrasound using spatio-temporal image correlation technology. Ultrasound Obstet Gynecol. 2005;25:97-8.

75. Espinoza J, Lee W, Comstock C, et al. Collaborative study on 4-dimensional echocardiography for the diagnosis of fetal heart defects: the COFEHD study. J Ultrasound Med. 2010;29:1573-80.

76. Bennasar M, Martínez JM, Gómez O, et al. Accuracy of four-dimensional spatiotemporal image correlation echocardiography in the prenatal diagnosis of congenital heart defects. Ultrasound Obstet Gynecol. 2010;36:458-64.

77. Levental M, Pretorius DH, Sklansky MS, et al. Three-dimensional ultrasonography of normal fetal heart: comparison with two-dimensional imaging. J Ultrasound Med. 1998;17:341-8.

78. Meyer-Wittkopf M, Rappe N, Sierra F, et al. Three-dimensional (3-D) ultrasonography for obtaining the four and five-chamber view: comparison with cross-sectional (2-D) fetal sonographic screening. Ultrasound Obstet Gynecol. 2000;15:397-402.

79. Meyer-Wittkopf M, Cooper S, Vaughan J, et al. Three-dimensional (3D) echocardiographic analysis of congenital heart disease in the fetus: comparison with cross-sectional (2D) fetal echocardiography. Ultrasound Obstet Gynecol. 2001;17:485-92.

80. Wang PH, Chen GD, Lin LY. Imaging comparison of basic cardiac views between two- and three-dimensional ultrasound in normal fetuses in anterior spine positions. Int J Cardiovasc Imaging. 2002;18:17-23.

81. Benacerraf BR, Shipp TD, Bromley B. Three-dimensional US of the fetus: volume imaging. Radiology. 2006;238: 988-96.

82. Yagel S, Cohen SM, Shapiro I, et al. 3D and 4D ultrasound in fetal cardiac scanning: a new look at the fetal heart. Ultrasound Obstet Gynecol. 2007;29:81-95.

83. Veronese P, Bogana G, Cerutti A, Yeo L, Romero R, Gervasi MT. A Prospective Study of the Use of Fetal Intelligent Navigation Echocardiography (Fine) to Obtain Standard Fetal Echocardiography Views. Fetal diagnosis and therapy. 2017;41:89-99.

Index

Page numbers followed by *b* refer to box, *f* refer to figure, and *t* refer to table.